PLANNING HEALTH PROMOTION PROGRAMS

PLANNING HEALTH PROMOTION PROGRAMS

An Intervention Mapping Approach

L. Kay Bartholomew
Guy S. Parcel
Gerjo Kok
Nell H. Gottlieb

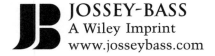

JOSSEY-BASS
A Wiley Imprint
www.josseybass.com

Published by Jossey-Bass
A Wiley Imprint
989 Market Street, San Francisco, CA 94103–1741   www.josseybass.com

Jossey-Bass books and products are available through most bookstores. To contact Jossey-Bass directly call our Customer Care Department within the U.S. at 800–956–7739, outside the U.S. at 317-572-3986, or fax 317-572-4002.

Jossey-Bass also publishes its books in a variety of electronic formats. Some content that appears in print may not be available in electronic books.

Library of Congress Cataloging-in-Publication Data

Planning health promotion programs: an intervention mapping approach/L. Kay Bartholomew . . . [et al.].—1st ed.
     p.; cm.
  Includes bibliographical references and index.
   ISBN-13 978-07879-7899-0
   ISBN-10 0-7879-7899-X (cloth)
 1. Health promotion. 2. Health promotion—Planning—Methodology. 3. Health education.
   [DNLM: 1. Health Education. 2. Health Promotion. 3. Evidence-Based Medicine. 4. Planning techniques. 5. Program Development—methods. WA 590 P712 2006] I. Bartholomew, L. Kay.
   RA427.8.P553 2006
   362.1—dc22

                                                            2005036844

Printed in the United States of America
FIRST EDITION
HB Printing   10 9 8 7 6 5 4 3 2 1

CONTENTS

LIST OF FIGURES AND TABLES

Figures

Tables

PREFACE

The practice of health promotion (used synonymously here with health education) involves four major program-planning activities: conducting a needs assessment, developing the program, implementing the program, and evaluating the program's effectiveness. Since the 1980s, significant enhancements have been made to the conceptual base and practice of health education and promotion, especially in needs assessment (Green & Kreuter, 2005), program evaluation (Windsor, Clark, Boyd, & Goodman, 2003), adoption and implementation (Rogers, 2003), and the use of theory (Glanz, Lewis, & Rimer, 2002; DiClemente, Crosby, & Kegler, 2002). However, the health education community has been slow to specify the processes involved in program design and development. Applications of behavioral and social science theories to intervention design are given important consideration, but even in this regard, the processes involved are not typically made explicit in the research or practice literature. Researchers often discuss intervention development and design in only a few sentences.

This book and the Intervention Mapping process are the products of our frustration in teaching health education students the processes involved in planning an intervention. Although the literature provides helpful models for conducting a needs assessment and program evaluation, as well as ecological models for conceptualizing the multiple levels of health education intervention (Simons-Morton, Green, & Gottlieb, 1995; McLeroy, Bibeau, Steckler, & Glanz, 1988), it lacks comprehensive frameworks for program development. In our experience, students have been able to understand theories of behavior and social change but have not been able to use them to design a coherent, practical health education intervention. Students frequently ask the following questions:

- When in the planning process do I use theory to guide my decisions?
- How do I know which theory to use?
- How do I make use of the experience of others and the results of other program evaluations?
- How do I decide which intervention methods to use?
- How can I get from program goals and objectives to the specific intervention strategies for the program participants?
- How do I link program design with planning for program implementation?
- How do I address changing the behavior of other people in the environment when they are not at risk for the health problem but are important to changing conditions that affect those at risk?

Motivated by these questions, we began to examine programs we had developed through our work as researchers and practitioners and to identify general principles and procedures in intervention design that were common to most of our work. One of our early case examples was the Cystic Fibrosis Family Education Program, an intervention designed to improve self-management skills, the interaction between patient and health care provider, and the health and quality of life of children with cystic fibrosis and their families (Bartholomew et al., 1997; Bartholomew et al., 2000; Bartholomew et al., 1991; Bartholomew, Parcel, Swank, & Czyzewski, 1993; Bartholomew, Seilheimer, Parcel, Spinelli, & Pumariega, 1989; Bartholomew et al., 1993).

To substantiate the steps of Intervention Mapping and to further delineate the tasks required for each, we then conducted a retrospective review of several large demonstration projects in the United States (Mullen & Bartholomew, 1991; Mullen & Diclemente, 1992; Parcel, Eriksen, et al., 1989; Parcel, Taylor, et al., 1989; Perry et al., 1992; Perry et al., 1990) and the Netherlands (De Vries & Dijkstra 1989; Mesters, Meertens, Crebolder, & Parcels, 1993; Schaalma, Kok, Poelman, & Reinders, 1994; Siero, S., Boon, Kok, & Siero, F., 1989). This review led to a working framework for health education program development, the process of Intervention Mapping. Analogous to geographic mapping, Intervention Mapping enables the planner to discover relations, locate desired destinations, plan a route for getting from one place to another, and execute a plan for covering distance. Intervention Mapping also has a visual component, including numerous diagrams and matrices that are used as landmarks to logical program development.

To further develop the steps of the process, we applied Intervention Mapping prospectively to ongoing projects that involved health education and promotion

program development. The following projects are among those that we used to
test, revise, and refine our proposed Intervention Mapping steps and tasks:

- *Long Live Love*, an HIV prevention program for Dutch adolescents that is described in Chapter Eleven (Schaalma & Kok, 1995; Schaalma, Kok, Bosker, et
  al., 1996; Schaalma, Kok, & Paulussen, 1996)
- The *Partners in Asthma Management Program*, a self-management program for children with asthma that is described in Chapter Twelve (Bartholomew, Gold, et
  al., 2000; Bartholomew, Shegog, et al., 2000; Shegog et al., 2001)
- *Five a Day*, a nutrition education program for nine- to twelve-year-old girls (Cullen,
  Bartholomew, & Parcel, 1997; Cullen, Bartholomew, Parcel, & Kok, 1998)

Additional experience with and refinement of the Intervention Mapping
process has occurred throughout the course of ten years of graduate instruction
in health promotion planning and implementation at the School of Public
Health, University of Texas Health Science Center at Houston; at the Schools
of Health Sciences and Psychology, University of Maastricht, the Netherlands;
and elsewhere.

After the first edition of *Intervention Mapping* appeared in 2001, a number of
new projects have applied the Intervention Mapping process to patient adherence
(Heinen, Bartholomew, Wensing, Van de Kerkhof, & Van Achterberg, in press),
diet (Hoelscher, Evans, Parcel, & Kelder, 2002), screening (Hou, Fernandez, &
Parcel, 2004), stroke treatment (Morgenstern et al., 2002; Morgenstern
et al., 2003), HIV prevention (Van Empelen, Kok, Schaalma, & Bartholomew,
2003), and the new application in Chapter Fourteen of this 2006 edition. Other
recent publications have described the usefulness of applying Intervention Mapping to various topics (Brug, Oenema, & Ferreira, 2005; Kok, Schaalma, Ruiter,
Brug, & Van Empelen, 2004; Van Bokhoven, Kok, & Van der Weijden, 2003).

We present Intervention Mapping as an additional tool for the planning and
development of health education and promotion programs. It serves as a way to
map the path of intervention development from recognizing a need or problem
to identifying and testing potential solutions. The steps and tasks included in Intervention Mapping provide a framework for making and documenting decisions
about how to influence change in behavior and conditions to promote health and
to prevent or improve a health problem. This documentation provides a means
to communicate to everyone involved in the process a logical and conceptual basis
for how the intervention is intended to work to make change possible. The level
of specificity included in each of the products of Intervention Mapping enhances
the possibility that a planned program will be effective in accomplishing its goals
and objectives. In addition, by making explicit the pathways and means by which
change is expected to occur and by examining the assumptions and decisions

made in each step and task of the Intervention Mapping process, program planners, users, and participants can better explain why a program succeeds or fails. It is our hope that this new tool will contribute to more effective health promotion programs and better explication of these programs and will result in an enhanced knowledge base for research and practice.

Chapter One presents the perspective from which Intervention Mapping was conceived, as well as its purpose. Before using Intervention Mapping, a planner should have at least an elementary grasp of the use of behavioral science theory in planning. Chapters Two through Four offer an overview of methods for accessing appropriate behavioral science theories and empirical evidence in the planning process and a review of applicable social and behavioral science theories. Chapters Five through Ten present a step-by-step guide to Intervention Mapping, and Chapters Eleven through Fourteen provide detailed case examples of the application of Intervention Mapping to public health programs.

January 2006

L. Kay Bartholomew
Houston, Texas

Guy S. Parcel
Houston, Texas

Gerjo Kok
Maastricht, The Netherlands

Nell H. Gottlieb
Austin, Texas

ACKNOWLEDGMENTS

Many people have been kind enough to offer suggestions and encouragement during the development of this text. Others have contributed through their contributions to health education and promotion, from which we have greatly benefited. Still others have allowed us to steer project teams down loosely defined pathways in order to test new ideas. We offer thanks to our friends and colleagues Charles Abraham, Stuart Abramson, Robin Atwood, Tom Baranowski, Karen Basen-Engquist, Judy Bettencourt, Cor Blom, Martine Bouman, Lex Bouter, Johannes Brug, Theresa Byrd, Noreen Clark, Matt Commers, Jennifer Conroy, Karin Coyle, Karen Cullen, Sharon Cummings, Danita Czyzewski, Marijn de Bruin, Evelyne de Leeuw, Hein de Vries, Nanne de Vries, Dirk-Jan den Boer, Elia Diez, Anton Dijker, Arie Dijkstra, Margot Dijkstra, Polly Edmundson, Cees Egmond, Michael Eriksen, Alexandra Evans, María Fernández-Esquer, Amy Fetterhoff, Brian Flay, Barbara Giloth, Phyllis Gingiss, Karen Glanz, Gaston Godin, Robert Gold, Bob Goodman, Patricia Goodson, Larry Green, Merwyn Greenlick, Jan Groff, Jong Long Guo, Arada Halder, Karol Kay Harris, Paul Harterink, Amy Jo Harzke, Maud Heinen, Helen Hill, Jeffrey Hill, Deanna Hoelscher, Carole Holahan, Harm Hospers, Dorothy Husky, Aimee James, Ruud Jonkers, Jolanda Keijsers, Steve Kelder, Gerda Kraag, Doug Kirby, Connie Kohler, Marieke Kools, Marshall Kreuter, Randi Bernstein Lachter, Cheryl Lackey, Sue Laver, Alexandra Loukas, Barbara Low, Alfred McAlister, Amy McQueen, Ree Meertens, Ilse Mesters, Barbara Meyer, Anna Meyer-Weitz, Jochen Mikolajczak,

Aart Mudde, Nancy Murray, Marita Murrman, Brian Oldenburg, Theo Paulussen, Cheryl Perry, Bobbie Person, Gjalt-Jorn Peters, Fred Peterson, Gopika Rama- murthy, Priscilla Reddy, Lori Roalson, Barbara Rimer, Michael Ross, Rob Ruiter, Ann Saunders, Dale Schunk, Dan Seilheimer, Bruce Simons-Morton, Michele Murphy Smith, Gail Sneden, Marianna Sockrider, Teshia Solomon, Alan Steckler, Mary Steinhardt, Victor Strecher, Paul Swank, Peggy Tate, Wendell Taylor, Jasmine Tiro, Mary Tripp, Theo van Achterberg, Patricia van Assema, Bart van den Borne, Pepijn van Empelen, Katy van den Hoek, Angelique van der Kar, Nicole van Kesteren, Olga van Rijn, Sarah Veblen-Mortenson, Peter Veen, Sally Vernon, Rachel Vojvodic, Pjer Vriens, Marsha Weil, Henk Wilke, and Barry Zimmerman.

We are indebted to our students who allowed us to class-test the first edition of the text. We attempted to make it better each time we taught it. We also benefited from the review and class-testing by our colleagues Omowale Amuleru-Marshall, Morehouse School of Medicine; Julie Baldwin, Northern Arizona University; Michael Barnes, Brigham Young University; Dan Bibeau, University of North Carolina at Greensboro; Brian Colwell, Texas A&M University; Carolyn Crump, University of North Carolina at Chapel Hill; Debra Krummel, West Virginia Uni- versity; Michael Pejsach, Central Michigan University; Rick Petosa, Ohio State University; Janet Reis, University of Illinois, Urbana-Champaign; and Ruth Saun- ders, University of South Carolina.

Our thanks to our colleagues who contributed case studies to the second edi- tion: Carlo DiClemente, María Fernández, Alicia Gonzales, Chris Markham, Pa- tricia Dolan Mullen, Sylvia Partida, Herman Schaalma, Ross Shegog, Guillermo Tortolero-Luna, and Shellie Tyrrell.

Some of our friends and colleagues provided extraordinary support. Com- prehensive reviews of the first edition by John Allegrante and Kenneth McLeroy enabled us to fine-tune the manuscript. Patricia Dolan Mullen not only con- tributed her ideas to the book but unflaggingly believed in the usefulness of In- tervention Mapping.

The following individuals have our deep gratitude for contributions to the second edition:

- *Patricia Dolan Mullen,* professor of Health Promotion and Behavioral Sciences at the School of Public Health, University of Texas Health Science Center at Houston, teaches classes on program evaluation and on systematic review and meta-analysis. She has served on many review groups, expert panels, and most re- cently on the U.S. Community Preventive Services Task Force to produce the new *Guide to Community Preventive Services.* She contributed to sections in Chapter Two on evidence reviews.

- *Herman Schaalma* is associate professor and holds the Dutch AIDS Fund Chair in AIDS Prevention and Health Promotion at the School of Psychology, Maastricht

University, The Netherlands. In 1995 he completed his doctoral thesis on the theory- and evidence-based development of school-based AIDS education. He is principal investigator of projects using Intervention Mapping for the development of HIV- prevention programs targeting youth in Sub-Saharan Africa and migrant women in the Netherlands. Dr. Schaalma contributed greatly to the plan for the second edition.

•   *María Fernández* is assistant professor of Health Promotion and Behavioral Sci- ences at the University of Texas Health Science Center at Houston, School of Public Health Center for Health Promotion and Prevention Research. Her re- search focus is the development and evaluation of interactive multimedia health promotion programs, particularly in the area of cancer control for Hispanic pop- ulations. Since the mid-1990s Dr. Fernández has contributed to the refinement of Intervention Mapping through her teaching and use of the framework in program development. She also contributed to conceptualizing how to incorporate issues related to cultural competence and relevance within the Intervention Mapping planning process for the current edition of the text.

•   *Christine Markham* is assistant professor in Health Promotion and Behavioral Sciences at the University of Texas Health Science Center at Houston. Her re- search area is child and adolescent health with emphasis on sexual and repro- ductive health and substance use prevention. She has been instrumental in demonstrating the use of Intervention Mapping as an effective approach for adapting existing programs to meet the needs of a new target population and has taught Intervention Mapping in the United States and the Netherlands.

•   *Helen Clark* is a doctoral student at the School of Public Health, University of Texas Health Science Center at Houston. She managed the references for the sec- ond edition and provided unflagging support and goodwill to the authors.

•   *Karyn Popham* is a biomedical editor and reference manager at the Center for Health Promotion and Prevention Research, School of Public Health, University of Texas Health Science Center at Houston.

Finally, the four coauthors thank each other. It seems that we discussed, wrote, argued over, and rewrote every part of *Intervention Mapping* again in the second edi- tion, testing and deepening our friendships.

L.K.B.
G.S.P.
G.K.
N.H.G.

THE AUTHORS

L. Kay Bartholomew is associate professor of Health Promotion and Behavioral Sciences and associate director of the Center for Health Promotion and Prevention Research at the School of Public Health, University of Texas Health Science Center at Houston. Dr. Bartholomew has worked in the field of health education and health promotion since her graduation from Austin College in the mid-1970s, first at a city-county health department and later at Texas Children's Hospital. Currently, in her research center and faculty roles, she teaches courses in health promotion intervention development and conducts research in chronic disease self-management. Dr. Bartholomew received her M.P.H. degree from the School of Public Health, University of Texas Health Science Center at Houston and her Ed.D. degree in educational psychology from the University of Houston College of Education. Dr. Bartholomew has won the Society for Public Health Education Program Excellence Award for the Cystic Fibrosis Family Education Program as well as numerous other professional association and media awards.

Guy S. Parcel is dean of the School of Public Health, the John P. McGovern Professor in Health Promotion, and the M. David Low Chair in Public Health at the University of Texas Health Science Center at Houston. He also serves as a professor in the Division of Health Promotion and Behavioral Sciences at the School of Public Health. Dr. Parcel has directed research projects to develop and evaluate programs to address sexual risk behavior for adolescents, diet and physical activity in children, self-management of childhood chronic diseases, smoking prevention, sun protection for preschool children, and the diffusion of health promotion programs. Dr. Parcel received his B.S. and M.S. degrees in health education at Indiana University and his Ph.D. degree at Pennsylvania State University with a major in health education and a minor in child development and family relations. Dr. Parcel has authored or coauthored more than two hundred scientific papers and received the American School Health Association 1990 William A. Howe Award for outstanding contributions and distinguished service in school health.

Gerjo Kok is dean of the Faculty of Psychology at Maastricht University, the Netherlands. He also holds the Dutch AIDS Fund–endowed chair for AIDS prevention and health promotion. Currently a professor of applied psychology, from 1984 to 1998 he was professor in health education at Maastricht University. A social psychologist, he received his doctorate in social sciences from the University of Groningen, the Netherlands. His main interest is in the social psychology of health education.

Nell H. Gottlieb is professor and coordinator of health education programs in the Department of Kinesiology and Health Education at the University of Texas at Austin and professor of behavioral science at the University of Texas Health Science Center at Houston School of Public Health. Dr. Gottlieb is the author of numerous articles and two textbooks. She received her Ph.D. degree in sociology from Boston University. Her interests are in multilevel health promotion intervention development and evaluation, particularly in the area of chronic disease prevention and control. Dr. Gottlieb has served as chair of the executive board of the Health Education and Promotion Section of the American Public Health Association and as president of the Society for Public Health Education.

PLANNING HEALTH PROMOTION PROGRAMS

PART ONE

FOUNDATIONS

CHAPTER ONE

OVERVIEW OF INTERVENTION MAPPING

Reader Objectives

- Explain the rationale for a systematic approach to intervention development
- Describe an ecological approach to intervention development
- Explain the types of logic models that can be used to conceptualize various phases of program development
- List the steps, processes, and products of Intervention Mapping

In this chapter we present the perspective from which Intervention Mapping was conceived as well as its purpose. We also present a preview of the program-planning framework, which is detailed in the remaining chapters.

The purpose of Intervention Mapping is to provide health promotion program planners with a framework for effective decision making at each step in intervention planning, implementation, and evaluation. Health promotion has been defined as "Any combination of education, political, regulatory and organizational supports for actions and conditions of living conducive to the health of individuals, groups or communities" (Green & Kreuter, 2005, p. G-4), and health education is a subset of health promotion strategies that are primarily based on education. We recognize this distinction but also the fact that many people in the health field practice health promotion; some of them specialize in health education. Often the boundaries are quite blurred. This book uses the terms *health educator, health promoter,* and *program planner* interchangeably when a subject is needed to mean someone who is planning an intervention meant to produce health outcomes. An intervention can be designed to change environmental or behavioral factors related to health, but the most immediate impact of an intervention is usually on a set of well-defined determinants of behavior and environmental conditions.

A difficulty that planners may encounter is that of delineating tasks for the development of health promotion or education programs that are based on theory, empirical findings from the literature, and data collected from the at-risk population. Existing literature, appropriate theories, and additional research data are basic tools for any health educator; but often it is unclear how and where these tools should be used in program planning. In Intervention Mapping, these tools are systematically applied in the steps of program development.

Box 1.1. Mayor's Project

Imagine a health educator in a city health department. The city's mayor, who has recently received strong criticism for inattention to a number of critical health issues, has now announced that a local foundation has agreed to work with the city to provide funding to address health issues. Youth violence, adolescent smoking, and other substance abuse as well as the high incidence of HIV/AIDS are among the issues competing for the mayor's attention. Not only does the allocated sum of money represent a gross underestimation of what is needed to address these issues, but also the city council is strongly divided on which health issue should receive priority. Council members do agree, however, that to dilute effort among the different issues would be a questionable decision, likely resulting in little or no impact on any single issue. As a response to increasing pressures, the mayor makes a bold political move and presents a challenge to the interest groups lobbying for public assistance. The mayor agrees to help secure funds on a yearly basis, contingent on the designated planning group's demonstrating significant, measurable improvements in the issues at hand by the end of each fiscal year.

The head of the health promotion division of the city health department is a social psychologist. She intends to use the mayor's challenge as a testing ground for her favorite behavioral science theory, but she has appointed the health educator to lead the project. Although apprehensive about the professional challenge as well as the complications inherent in facilitating a highly visible political project, the health educator is encouraged by the prospect of working with community and public health leaders.

The first step the health educator takes is to put together the planning group for the project. She considers the stakeholders concerned with youth health in the city. These are individuals, groups, or other entities that can affect or be affected by a proposed project. She develops a list of community and public health leaders and invites these individuals to an initial meeting whose purpose is to expand this core group. She uses a "snowball" approach whereby each attendee suggests other community members who may be interested in this project. The superintendent of schools begins the process by suggesting interested parents, teachers, and administrators. Later these individuals may have additional suggestions. After the first meeting, the health educator has a list of 25 people to invite to join the planning group.

Twenty-five people is a lot of people for one group, and the health educator knows that this multifaceted group will have to develop a common vocabulary and understanding, work toward consensus to make decisions, maintain respect during conflicts, and involve additional people throughout the community in the process. Members must be engaged, create working groups, believe that the effort is a partnership and not an involuntary mandate, and work toward sustainability of the project (Cavanaugh & Cheney, 2002). The health educator knows that she has taken on a complex task, but she is energized by the possibilities.

The composition of the city's planning group is diverse, and group members are spurred by the mayor's challenge and enthusiastic to contribute their expertise. With this early momentum, the group devotes several weeks to a needs assessment, guided by the PRECEDE model (Green & Kreuter, 1999, 2005). The members consider the various quality-of-life issues relevant to each of the health problems, the segments of the population affected by each issue, associated environmental and behavioral risk factors for each health problem, and determinants of the risk factors.

Members recognize the relative importance of all three issues, but they select youth violence because violence is a particular problem in their community, which disproportionately affects underserved minorities. Also, they are challenged by the lack of effective or evaluated violence prevention programs in the field (Tolan & Guerra, 1994, 1996; World Health Organization, 2002; Centers for Disease Control & Oak Ridge Institute for Science and Education, 2003), and the interests and expertise of the individual group members are well suited to working on this problem. The results of the needs assessment indicate that violence is the leading cause of death among young people aged fifteen to twenty-four in the United States and the primary cause of death among Hispanics and African Americans in this age group (Singh & Yu, 1996). Moreover, for every violent death, conservative estimates suggest that 100 nonfatal injuries result from violence (Rennison, Rand, & U.S. Department of Justice, 2003). The group reviews the literature to identify the behavioral and environmental causes of violence and finds that the factors related to violence are diverse.

For example, socioeconomic status, education, and job mobility are all factors that may be related to personal involvement in violence. The lack of conflict resolution and communication skills are enabling factors related to personal violence. At the same time, the sudden occurrence of situational antagonism, such as verbal or physical assault, is a contextual factor that is also likely to incite violent behavior (Reiss, Miczek, & Roth, 1993). The planning group reviews a long list of factors related to violence. They recognize that their one-year program can address certain of these. However, they also realize that broad social problems such as poverty and lack of opportunities for success in school and employment must be taken into account even though they are not easy to address. Further investigation reveals that little empirical evidence is available on the effectiveness of existing programs that address a broad array of determinants of violent behavior (Tolan & Guerra, 1994).

Even though the planning group comprises many segments of the city's leadership, health sector, and neighborhoods, the members realize that they do not have a deep enough perspective on youth violence in their community. A subgroup takes on the role of community liaison to meet with members of various communities within the city that have been disproportionately affected by violence. The community liaison group wants to understand community members' perceptions of their needs, but it is equally concerned with understanding the strengths of the communities and their unique potential contributions to a partnership to prevent violence. The subgroup invites members of each interested neighborhood to join the planning group. Jointly, the planning group, the communities, and the funders agree to select this problem as the focus of a health education and promotion intervention.

The group's work on the needs assessment facilitated group cohesion and cultivated even greater enthusiasm about generating a solution for the health problem. Several members of the group even began to imagine the victory that would be had if the group were to produce a change in half the allotted time because so much of the needed background information had already been gathered. The health educator remains apprehensive about the time frame yet comfortable with the group's pace and productivity. Now that the group has decided which issue to address, it faces the challenge of moving to the program-planning phase. In her previous work the health educator had implemented and evaluated programs designed by others, but she had not created new programs. However, bolstered by its good work, the group schedules the first program-planning meeting.

What the health educator hadn't anticipated was that in the course of conducting the needs assessment, each group member had independently begun to conceive of the next step in the planning process as well as to visualize the kind of intervention that would be most suitable to address the problem. The day of the meeting arrived, and on the agenda was a discussion of how the group should begin program planning. What follows is a snapshot of dialogue from the planning group that illustrates several differing perspectives.

Participant A: As we see from the needs assessment, violence is a community problem. According to community development techniques, we have to start where the people are. I think we should begin by conducting a series of focus groups and have the kids tell us what to do.

Participant B: But why do you use the kids to develop a program for the community? I say we address violence at the family level, using a series of conflict resolution training workshops for kids and their parents.

Participant C: Community and family are only two dimensions of the problem. The literature says you have to address multiple levels in a comprehensive approach. Plus, onetime workshops have no long-term impact. I say we find a nonprofit group to serve as a community coordinating center from which various interventions and services can be implemented. That way, programs are sustainable, and a variety of activities can be offered.

Participant D: One of the national violence prevention centers has great brochures and videos—in three languages. We have numerous testimonials from kids, teachers, and parents about how motivated they were by these interventions. This approach is quick and easy; it's low cost; and I've already made sure we can get the materials. Plus, if the materials come from a national center, they must be effective.

Participant B: But are those materials really powerful enough? How would you address the different levels of the community? Moreover, violence is a human problem. The root of the problem is that kids don't have anyone or anything they can relate to. In school we always started with learning objectives that reflect the needs of the specific patient population.

Participant E: Yes, but we know it takes more than learning information to change behavior. We have to address factors such as attitudes and self-efficacy. But how do we measure a change in attitudes? I think we should measure behavior directly.

Participant F: Well, clearly we have to begin by designing a curriculum. What are our learning objectives?

The health educator in our example must first consider what steps to follow to construct the intervention and then must consider how to design each step to incorporate the needs, ideas, training, and experience of the various members of the planning group. The planning group began well by completing a comprehensive needs assessment using an effective model that has been applied to many health issues (Green & Kreuter, 2005). The members began the program-planning phase armed with an ecological perspective, that is, the belief that one must intervene at individual, organizational, community, and societal levels to resolve a problem (McLeroy, Bibeau, Steckler, & Glanz, 1988; Simons-Morton, Greene, & Gottlieb, 1995; Kreuter, De Rosa, Howze, & Baldwin, 2004). But, as the group dialogue indicates, each group member brought a different set of experiences and training to the meeting. This is a common experience in group activities. Although group members may become critical of other perspectives, each member makes an important and relevant contribution worthy of consideration in the creation of the intervention.

Perspectives

Intervention Mapping is based on the importance of planning programs that are based on theory and evidence. We also take into consideration the social and physical environmental causes of health problems and risk behavior.

Theory and Evidence

We agree with Kurt Lewin's adage that nothing is as useful as a good theory (Hochbaum, Sorenson, & Lorig, 1992). We believe this is especially important in health promotion planning. The use of theory is necessary in evidence-informed health promotion to ensure that we can describe the aspects of programs that are generalizable and robust interventions that actually address all of the determinants necessary to achieve change. In general, the use of theory can help us protect against type III error, that is, failing to find intervention effectiveness because the program is poorly designed or implemented (Green, 2000). Still, given this assertion, more guidance is needed regarding the application of theory in health promotion and health education practice. Few teachers of health promotion would debate the importance of teaching behavioral and social science theories, but many observers would question whether teachers use effective methods to teach students to *use* theory (McLeroy et al., 1993). Some authors argue that many practitioners find theory nearly irrelevant to their practices (Hochbaum et al., 1992; Jones & Donovan, 2004).

Furthermore, program planners, even those who are scientists, often approach theory in a way that is fundamentally different from either the theory generation or the single theory–testing process. Health promotion planners are likely to bring multiple theoretical and experiential perspectives to a problem rather than to define a practice or research agenda around a specific theoretical approach. Teachers of health promotion and education suggest that the field will be well served with better guidance in how to use theory to understand health and social problems (Burdine & McLeroy, 1992; DiClemente, Crosby, & Kelger, 2002; Earp & Ennett, 1991; Glanz, Lewis, & Rimer, 1997; Glanz, Lewis, & Rimer, 2002; Hochbaum et al., 1992; Kok, Schaalma, de Vries, Parcel, & Paulussen, 1996; Jones & Donovan, 2004).

To understand a problem, the planner begins with a question about a specific health or social issue (Veen, 1985; Kok et al., 1996). The planner then accesses social and behavioral science theories and research evidence of causation at multiple levels. These or other theories may also suggest intervention points and methods, and the planner proceeds to accumulate evidence for the effectiveness of these methods. By the term *evidence*, we mean not only data from research studies as represented in the scientific literature but also opinion and experience of community members and planners. In this way theoretical and empirical evidence are brought to bear on meeting a health or social need. Intervention Mapping provides a detailed framework for this process.

An Ecological Approach to Health Promotion Program Planning

The World Health Organization (WHO) defines health as an instrumental value in service of a full, gratifying life (WHO, 1978, 1986). We recognize the interaction of health and quality of life, and Robertson and Minkler (1994) point out the existence of both a micro level or individual dimension to health and a macro level structural dimension. Our primary focus, consonant with health education and health promotion, is that of health as it is mediated by both behavior and environment (Parcel et al., 1987). In Intervention Mapping we argue for a social ecological approach in which health is viewed as a function of individuals and of the environments in which individuals live, including family, social networks, organizations, communities, and societies (Stokols, 1996; Berkman & Kawachi, 2000; Marmot, 2000). Individual behavior is influenced by determinants at these various environmental levels. The social ecological paradigm focuses on the interrelationships among individuals with their biological, psychological, and behavioral characteristics and their environments. These environments include physical, social, and cultural aspects that exist across the individual's life domains and social settings. A nested structure of environments allows for multiple influences both vertically across levels and horizontally within levels. The picture that emerges is a complex web of causation as well as a rich context for intervention. Looking for the most effective leverage points within this web, across levels, reduces the complexity and is necessary for developing effective multilevel interventions.

Planners can look at the relationship between individuals and their environments in two ways. First, mechanistically, the individual and the environment can be viewed as mechanisms in a general system in which small changes in the social environment, for example, can lead to large changes in individual behavior (Green, L. W., personal communication, February 26, 1997). This view tends toward an emphasis on higher-order intervention leverage points such as policy or social norms as external determinants of the individual's behavior, health, and quality of life. Second, the various levels are viewed as embedded systems. In Figure 1.1, higher-order systems set constraints and provide inputs to lower-order systems, and the lower-order systems provide inputs to systems at a higher level. New properties emerge at each system level, but each level incorporates the lower levels of embedded systems. For example, social norms exist independently of the individual even though the individual perceives them. An intervention may influence both levels (that is, the actual norms and the individual perception), and these may in turn influence both health behavior and health.

Multiple levels may be influenced by an intervention at one level. For example, a program aimed at convincing organizations to conduct health-related lobbying may influence a legislature to pass laws that may influence individual health behavior. For example, one of our colleagues worked with a coalition in a large metropolitan area to use media and social advocacy to influence the police department and the U.S. Department of Labor to crack down on the use of young Hispanic children as dancers in bars and nightclubs (an activity that can lead to health risk behaviors of substance abuse and prostitution). In this example, intervention at the individual or interpersonal levels would have been difficult. Families felt helpless to control the girls' activities, and the monetary incentives to dance were strong in impoverished neighborhoods. However, once social change began to occur, parents expressed more empowerment to manage their children.

A program may be aimed at any ecological level and have effects on that level and all the levels nested within it. For example, individuals may not engage in physical activity due to determinants at each level: personal lack of self-efficacy for exercise, lack of social support from family and friends at the interpersonal level, lack of fitness norms and facilities at the work site or organizational level, and barriers to physical activity in the built environment at the societal level. Figure 1.1 denotes embedded reciprocal systems with individual, group, organization, community,

FIGURE 1.1. SCHEMATIC OF THE ECOLOGICAL APPROACH IN HEALTH PROMOTION PROGRAMS.

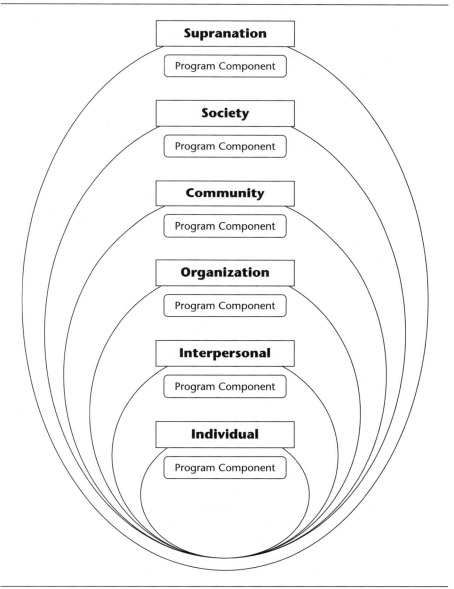

Source: Adapted from Potvin, Kishchuk, Prlic, & Green, 1996.

society, and supranational levels. This figure indicates that the individual exists within groups, which in turn are embedded within organizations and higher-order systems. The individual is influenced by these systems and can in turn influence them directly or through groups and organizations. We acknowledge the hazards of trying to plan from such a complex formulation, but we judge the hazards of oversimplicity to be greater. Nevertheless, we agree with Green that complexity can breed despair, and we encourage the reader to bear with the process (Green, Richard, & Potvin, 1996). Intervention Mapping helps the planner take on this complexity in a structured systematic way, thereby making it more manageable without oversimplifying.

Agency in the Environment

We draw the approach to change at the various ecological levels from three traditions. The first is that of Kurt Lewin, who focused on the gatekeepers within channels (McGrath, 1995). The second is social exchange theory, which focuses on the positions or roles of persons within the social system (Coleman, 1990). And the third is the MATCH model, which has been used to plan multilevel interventions for health education (Simons-Morton, Greene, & Gottlieb, 1995; Simons-Morton, Simons-Morton, Parcel, & Bunker, 1988).

In each of these views, the key to understanding social reality at each of the ecological levels and ways to change conditions at each level is tied to understanding the positions that compose the level and exert influence on its conditions. For example, Lewin described two channels by which food gets to a family's table: the grocery channel and the garden channel (McGrath, 1995). In the grocery channel, various gatekeepers act to influence what foods are selected to move along the channel, from the food manufacturer's product-line managers to the buyers at the wholesale grocer's, to the grocery chain buyers, to the individual store managers, to the shopper for the family. At each point an array of forces helps or hinders passage through the gates along the channel. The product-line manager, for example, acts on findings from consumer marketing surveys, cost and availability of ingredients, and fit to the company's manufacturing facilities. Consumer demand for low-fat products could influence the food manufacturer to produce these foods. Moving down the channel to the end of the line, the family shopper may be influenced by forces that include motivations to provide healthy food for the family, to please the family, to save money, and to purchase food that is easily prepared. By understanding the determinants of these gatekeeper behaviors at several levels, the health educator is better able to plan where to intervene to create the most effective and efficient interventions for change.

Throughout the book we have adopted the approach of Simons-Morton and colleagues (1988, 1989) of looking at agents (decision makers or role actors) at each systems level: interpersonal (for example, parents), organizational (for example, managers of school food services), community (for example, newspaper editors), or societal (for example, legislators). The focus of interventions at the various levels are agents (individuals or groups, such as boards or committees) in positions to exercise control over aspects of the environment.

The Need for a Framework for Intervention Development

When the authors of the often-used PRECEDE model (Green, Kreuter, Deeds, & Partridge, 1980) began development more than thirty years ago, they were concerned with the focus of the field of health education on intervention. Health education programs often did not have firm epidemiological foundations, and outcomes sometimes were not documented in terms of change in behavior, environment, health, or quality of life. Green, Kreuter, and colleagues (Green et al., 1980) intentionally steered away from a focus on intervention (Green, L. W., personal communication, February 26, 1997) and acknowledge the impact of other pioneers in the field such as Mayhew Derryberry, who cautioned against a focus on activities rather than outcomes. After thirty years of developments in the field, we believe that we can cautiously steer back toward an intervention focus.

We believe that everyone with a health education or health promotion role must have the knowledge and skills to develop effective interventions. Anyone with the responsibility to help individuals or communities change health risk behavior, initiate health-promoting behavior, change environmental factors, or manage illnesses must design or adapt existing effective interventions and develop plans to implement them. With the movement toward best practices and evidence-based public health (Green & Kreuter, 2002; Centers for Disease Control and Prevention & Oak Ridge Institute for Science and Education; 2003; Truman, Smith-Akin, Hinman, Gebbie, Brownson, Novick, et al., 2000; International Union for Health Promotion and Education & European Commission, 1999; Cameron, Joslin, Walker, McDermott, & Gough, 2001) and evidence-based public health following in the footsteps of evidence-based medicine (Zaza, Briss, & Harris, 2005; Task Force on Community Preventive Services, 2000, p. 5; Briss, Rodewald, et al., 2000; Briss, Zara, et al., 2000), some planners may think that they are superfluous, that their jobs are over. Nothing could be further from the truth.

First, there are certainly not enough well-evaluated and effective interventions to meet every, or even most, needs. The United States Task Force on Community

Preventive Services (Zaza, Lawrence, Mahan, Fullilove, Fleming, Isham, et al., 2000; Zaza et al., 2005; Guide to Community Preventive Services, 2004) systematically reviewed many interventions. In 50 percent of the interventions reviewed for the first edition of the Guide, however, there was insufficient evidence to make any recommendation; and planners may face a problem for which there is little intervention guidance.

Furthermore, although collections of interventions reviewed by the task force were grouped to be as similar as possible, in view of the diverse interventions tested in the original studies, program planners will still be faced with some need for planning exactly what to adapt and implement for their communities (Zaza et al., 2000; Zaza et al., 2005; Guide to Community Services, 2004) Some groupings in the Guide are helpful, as for example, the recommendation that client reminder (vaccination is due) or recall (vaccination is late) systems increase vaccination coverage among children and adults. The recommendation is the same regardless of the delivery method (telephone, postcard, or letter) or message (specific or general) (Briss, Rodewald, et al., 2000). In other cases, however, the grouping of interventions is less helpful. Another example from those aimed at increasing vaccination coverage is the recommendation for multi-component interventions that include education. To be sure, a note describes the frequency of component interventions in the multi-component interventions on which the recommendation was based, but these include client reminders, provider education, expansion of the hours of access, and so forth—a grouping with diverse components. Thus, the advent of such resources of evidence-based interventions will greatly facilitate the job of intervention development some of the time and merely assist more of the time.

Some best practices are actually planning processes as described by Freudenberg and colleagues (1995, pp. 297–299), who suggested that programs should do the following:

- Be tailored to specific populations and settings
- Involve participants in planning, implementation, and evaluation
- Integrate efforts aimed at changing individuals, social and physical environments, communities, and policies
- Link participants' concerns about health to broader life concerns and to a vision of a better society
- Use resources within the environment
- Build on the strengths of participants and communities
- Advocate for resources and policy changes needed to achieve the desired health objectives
- Prepare participants to become leaders

- Support the diffusion of innovation
- Seek to institutionalize successful intervention components and replicate them in other settings

Best practices for intervention are often labeled as such based on reviews that emphasize the importance of their internal validity rather than generalizability. Any program, even one that has been labeled as a good program, must undergo a process for selection for a new use (Kahan & Goodstadt, 1998, 2001). Programs shown to be effective in one setting must be adapted for each new community and implementation (Glasgow, Marcus, Bull, & Wilson, 2004; Glasgow, Lichtenstein, & Marcus, 2003; Green, 2001).

There remains some confusion about how planners can integrate the wealth of information, theories, ideas, and models to develop interventions that are logical and appropriate in their foundations and are practical and acceptable in their administration. The complexity of intervention development is sometimes overlooked in health education training. When we began the development of Intervention Mapping, researchers and practitioners seldom wrote in depth about the process of intervention development, and complicated interventions were often reduced to several sentences in evaluation articles. This situation is slowly changing, and health promotion and other journals have become more hospitable to articles about intervention development. The introduction of a practice-oriented journal in the field has been particularly useful for the description of interventions and their development (Briss et al., 2000; Dodge, Janz, & Clark, 2002; Levy, Anderson, Issel, Willis, Dancy, & Jacobson, 2004; van Empelen, Kok, Schaalma, & Bartholomew, 2003; Lytle & Perry, 2001).

We describe planning processes out of a desire to enable health educators to create programs that are feasible and that have a high likelihood of being effective. Good program planning provides the basis for creative health education practice and provides the vehicles for communicating program specifications to production specialists such as writers and artists. Thorough planning at the beginning of a project can lead to creative developmental and production processes, enhance the intervention's deliverability, and result in the desired outcomes.

Intervention Mapping Steps

Each step of Intervention Mapping comprises several tasks (Figure 1.2). The completion of the tasks in a step creates a product that is the guide for the subsequent step. The completion of all of the steps serves as a blueprint for designing, implementing, and evaluating an intervention based on a foundation of theoretical,

FIGURE 1.2. INTERVENTION MAPPING.

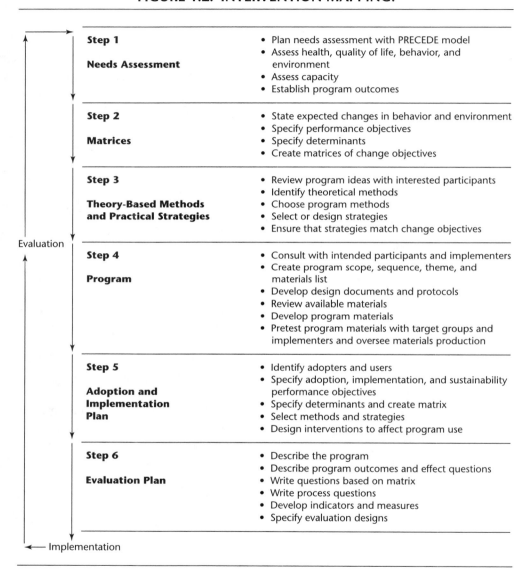

Step 1 **Needs Assessment**	• Plan needs assessment with PRECEDE model • Assess health, quality of life, behavior, and environment • Assess capacity • Establish program outcomes
Step 2 **Matrices**	• State expected changes in behavior and environment • Specify performance objectives • Specify determinants • Create matrices of change objectives
Step 3 **Theory-Based Methods and Practical Strategies**	• Review program ideas with interested participants • Identify theoretical methods • Choose program methods • Select or design strategies • Ensure that strategies match change objectives
Step 4 **Program**	• Consult with intended participants and implementers • Create program scope, sequence, theme, and materials list • Develop design documents and protocols • Review available materials • Develop program materials • Pretest program materials with target groups and implementers and oversee materials production
Step 5 **Adoption and Implementation Plan**	• Identify adopters and users • Specify adoption, implementation, and sustainability performance objectives • Specify determinants and create matrix • Select methods and strategies • Design interventions to affect program use
Step 6 **Evaluation Plan**	• Describe the program • Describe program outcomes and effect questions • Write questions based on matrix • Write process questions • Develop indicators and measures • Specify evaluation designs

Evaluation

Implementation

empirical, and practical information. Even though we present Intervention Mapping as a series of steps, the process is iterative rather than completely linear. Program developers move back and forth between tasks and steps as they gain information and perspective from various activities. However, the process is also cumulative. Developers base each step on the previous steps, and inattention to a step can jeopardize the potential effectiveness of the intervention by narrowing the scope and compromising the validity with which later steps are conducted. Sometimes planners can get carried away by momentum in the process of the planning group and forget a step, or they may perform a step with less than optimal rigor. Fortunately, most of the time planners can backtrack and include, repeat, or elaborate on a neglected step.

The six fundamental steps of the Intervention Mapping process are the following:

1. Conduct a needs assessment or problem analysis
2. Create matrices of change objectives based on the determinants of behavior and environmental conditions
3. Select theory-based intervention methods and practical strategies
4. Translate methods and strategies into an organized program
5. Plan for adoption, implementation, and sustainability of the program
6. Generate an evaluation plan

These steps are completed using core processes including the following:

- Posing planning problems as questions that facilitate finding answers from theory, the existing literature, and new research
- Brainstorming answers to planning questions
- Searching the literature for empirical evidence
- Evaluating the strength of the evidence
- Using the issue, concept, and general theories approaches to access theory and empirical evidence to answer the questions
- Addressing the importance of new research for unanswered questions in the planning process

Chapter Two presents these core processes.

Step 1: Needs Assessment

In Step 1 (Chapter Five) before beginning to actually plan an intervention, the planner assesses the health problem, its related behavior and environmental conditions, and their associated determinants for the at-risk populations. This assessment encompasses two components: (1) a scientific, epidemiologic, behavioral, and social analysis of an at-risk group or community and its problems and (2) an effort to get to know and begin to understand, the character of the community, its members, and its strengths. The product of this first step is a description of a health problem, its impact on quality of life, behavioral and environmental causes, and determinants of behavior and environmental causes.

In Step 1 the planner must complete the following tasks:

1. Establish a planning group that includes potential program participants and plan the needs assessment (Note: This group will evolve over the course of the planning process.)
2. Conduct the needs assessment using the PRECEDE model (Green & Kreuter, 2005) to analyze health and quality of life problems and their causes and to decide on priorities
3. Balance the needs assessment with an assessment of community capacity.
4. Link the needs assessment to evaluation planning by establishing desired program outcomes

Step 2: Matrices of Change Objectives

Step 2 (Chapter Six) provides the foundation for the intervention by specifying who and what will change as a result of the intervention. The product of Step 2 is a set of matrices of selected ecological levels (that is, individual through societal) that combines performance objectives for each level with selected personal and external determinants to produce change objectives, the most immediate target of an intervention. In order to develop performance objectives beyond the individual, the planners identify roles of environmental agents at each selected ecological level. For example, superintendents, principals, and teachers may have roles for school environmental change. Statements of what must be changed at each ecological level and who must make the change are more specific intervention foci than are traditional program goals and objectives. For example, the mayor's planning committee constructed matrices that focused on the school environments in the city, on neighborhood environments including supervised youth activities, and on community cohesion—not only on the behavior of the youths themselves. For another example, in a program to increase fruit and vegetable consumption by children in elementary school, matrices would be created for both the child and the food service. The food service matrix might contain more than one role: for example, the manager's purchasing practices, the dietitian's menu development, and the cooks' recipe choices.

In Step 2 the planner must complete the following tasks:

1. State the expected change or program outcomes for health-related behavior and environmental conditions
2. Subdivide behavior and environmental conditions into performance objectives

3. Select important and changeable personal and external determinants of at-risk group behavior and environmental conditions
4. Create a matrix of change objectives for each level of intervention planning (individual, interpersonal, organizational, community, and societal) by crossing performance objectives with determinants and writing change objectives

Step 3: Theory-Based Methods and Practical Strategies

In Step 3 (Chapter Seven), the planner seeks theory-informed methods and practical strategies to change the health behavior of individuals and related small groups and to change organizational and societal factors to affect the environment. An intervention method is a defined process by which theories postulate and empirical research provides evidence for how change may occur in the behavior of individuals, groups, or social structures. One example of a theory-informed method is modeling, which is frequently used to facilitate behavior change. In Step 3 the planner lists intervention methods that correspond to the change objectives developed in Step 2. These are then used to begin to formulate program activities that will result in achieving the change objectives (Chapter Eight). Whereas a method is a theory-based technique to influence behavior or environmental conditions, a strategy is a way of organizing, operationalizing, and delivering the intervention methods. The translation of selected methods into action is completed through the development of strategies. Examples of strategies include a meeting with community members to form community development task forces for empowerment, a diary for self-monitoring, role-model stories for modeling, a pledge for commitment, and self-talk for cognitive-behavioral rehearsal. A planner working from the food service matrix mentioned in Step 2 might use the methods of persuasion and modeling to influence the food services manager's purchasing practices. Strategies might include testimonials by food service personnel who had incorporated healthier buying practices. If the planner discovered that school district policy was a barrier to changing purchasing practices, he or she would return to Step 2, identify roles at the district level that could influence the policy, write performance objectives for these roles, specify determinants, and construct matrices. These district-level policy changes would then functionally be methods for change at the next lower ecological level, the food service managers and cooks.

In Step 3 the planner must complete the following tasks:

1. Review program ideas with the intended participants and use their perspectives when choosing methods and strategies
2. Use core processes to identify theoretical methods that can influence changes in determinants and identify the conditions under which a given method is most likely to be effective

3. Choose program theoretical methods (Note: The planner must be sure to distinguish between theoretical methods and practical strategies, ensure that all program components contain appropriate methods, and consider preliminary ideas on the program in light of information from theory and evidence.)
4. Select or design practical strategies for delivering the methods to intervention groups
5. Assure that the final strategies (still) match the change objectives from the matrices

Step 4: Program

The products in Step 4 (Chapter Eight) include a description of the scope and sequence of the components of the intervention, completed program materials, and program protocols. This step demands the careful reconsideration of the intended program participants and the program context. It also requires pretesting and pilot testing of program strategies and materials with intended implementers and recipients (Chapter Nine). This step gives specific guidance for communicating program intent to producers (for example, graphic designers, videographers, and writers). The planners of the food service change might organize all their change methods and strategies into creating a program called the *Creative Cooks for Healthy Kids Cooking School*. The "school," however, might include on-the-job training, policy change, newsletters featuring role models, and social reinforcement—or whatever was planned in Step 3 to produce the changes specified in Step 2.

In Step 4 the planner must complete the following tasks:

1. Consult again with the intended participants for a health education and promotion program and bring their preferences to program design
2. Describe program scope and sequence, themes, and needed program materials
3. Prepare design documents that will aid various professions in producing materials that meet the program objectives and adhere to specific guidelines or parameters for particular methods and strategies
4. Review available program materials for possible match with change objectives, methods, and strategies
5. Develop program materials
6. Pretest program materials and oversee the final production

Step 5: Adoption and Implementation

The focus of Step 5 (Chapter Nine) is program adoption and implementation (including consideration of program sustainability). Of course, considerations for program implementation actually begin as early as the needs assessment and are revisited in this step. The step requires the process of matrix development exactly like that in Step 2, except that these matrices have adoption and implementation performance objectives juxtaposed to personal and external determinants. The linking of each performance objective with a determinant produces a change objective to promote program adoption and use. Methods and strategies are then matched to these objectives to form theory-informed plans for adoption and implementation. For example, the promoters of the food service change would ask the following questions:

- Who is in charge of food service at the school district and at individual schools?
- Who would perceive a need, develop awareness of a program, and choose to adopt the program to make changes in the food service?
- Who would be in charge of implementing the program?
- What, specifically, would these people have to do?

For example, a principal might have to order the program for review, ask the food service manager for his or her opinion of the program, and form a task force for food service change. The planner then uses theory and evidence to hypothesize determinants of the principal's adoption and implementation performance objectives. The product for Step 5 is a detailed plan for accomplishing program adoption and implementation by influencing behavior of individuals or groups who will make decisions about adopting and using the program.

In Step 5 the planner must complete the following tasks:

1. Identify potential users of the health promotion program (revisit the planning group and linkage system to assure representation)
2. Specify performance objectives for program adoption, implementation, and sustainability
3. Specify determinants of adoption, implementation, and sustainability and create change-objective matrices for program use
4. Select methods and strategies to address the change
5. Design interventions and organize programs to affect change objectives related to program use

Step 6: Evaluation Planning

In Step 6 (Chapter Ten), the planner completes an evaluation plan that is actually begun in the needs assessment and is developed along with the intervention map. In the process of Intervention Mapping, planners make decisions about change objectives, methods, strategies, and implementation. The decisions, although informed by theory and evidence from research, still may not be optimal or may even be completely wrong. Through effect and process evaluation, planners can determine whether decisions were correct at each mapping step (Rossi, Lipsey, & Freeman, 2004; Windsor, Clark, Boyd, & Goodman, 2003; Steckler & Linnan, 2002). To evaluate the effect of an intervention, researchers analyze the change in health and quality-of-life problems, behavior and environment, and determinants of performance objectives. All these variables have been defined in a measurable way during the preceding steps. Effect evaluation may show positive, negative, or mixed effects or show no effect at all. Planners want to understand the reasons behind the effects that were achieved, regardless of what those effects were. They need to know more about the process and the changes in intermediate variables. They ask such questions as the following:

- Were determinants well specified?
- Were strategies well matched to methods?
- What proportion of the priority population did the program reach?
- Was the implementation complete and appropriate?

The product of Step 6 is a plan for answering these questions.

In Step 6 the planner must complete the following tasks:

1. Describe the program and complete the logic model
2. Write evaluation questions based on the program outcome objectives for quality of life, health, behavior, and environment
3. Write evaluation questions based on the matrix, that is, concerning performance objectives and determinants as expressed in the change objectives
4. Write process evaluation questions based on the descriptions of methods, conditions, strategies, program, and implementation
5. Develop indicators and measures
6. Specify evaluation design

Navigating the Book

The process of Intervention Mapping is unchanged from the first edition text. However, we have rearranged the presentation of some aspects of the process. We also have made more explicit use of logic models in the Intervention Mapping steps, and we have introduced the concept of logic models in this section.

Changes from the First Edition

Users familiar with the first edition of *Intervention Mapping* will find several changes that may have an impact on their practice and teaching. The first is the inclusion of needs assessment as a step in Intervention Mapping rather than a preliminary process. Further, we have clarified and sometimes slightly changed the tasks within each step. In Step 2, the development of matrices, we have tried to decrease confusion about terminology concerning objectives: We now call all objectives within matrix cells change objectives, and we do not refer to the components of the matrices as proximal program objectives.

Other changes will primarily affect navigation of the book: Needs assessment has been moved into the steps sequence (from Chapter Two to Chapter Five). Theories are now presented in two chapters: Chapter Three for theories pertaining to individuals and Chapter Four for theories pertaining to groups and communities. The theoretical material on methods has been moved from Step 3 (Chapter Seven) into the theories chapters.

Foundations

Chapter Two presents the core processes for making empirical literature, formative qualitative and quantitative research and theory accessible and useable in intervention development. It covers core process applications for understanding determinants of behavior, defining health behavior, and generating intervention methods. Chapter Three provides an overview of behavior-oriented theories, which focus on understanding or changing behavior. Chapter Four provides an overview of environment-oriented theories, which focus on understanding or changing environmental conditions.

The Formulation of Matrices as the Program Foundation

In Intervention Mapping, matrices that combine performance objectives with their determinants are the basis for intervention development. They are used in both planning a program (Step 2) and in planning its adoption and implementation (Step 5). If an intervention method or strategy is not intended to change the objectives in the matrices, then either it does not belong in the program or the matrix is not adequate and should be revisited.

We use matrices as a foundation for promoting adoption and implementation because of the importance of promoting a program's use. A program with modest effectiveness could have a great impact if it reached the entire population, while a highly efficacious program would have little or no impact if it was not adopted or implemented fully. Health education programs may be difficult to implement and sustain because they are innovations that cause change in organizational systems. Program planning must include strategies to ensure that those people who will use it with the intended populations adopt the program (Orlandi, 1986, 1987; Smith, Steckler, McCormick, & McLeroy, 1995). In addition, there is a difference between the potential program efficacy and actual program effectiveness when interventions are transported from their developers to extended use in practice. Program implementation may tend to decline in amount and quality over time. Practitioners must know what is an acceptable level of implementation (Ottoson & Green, 1987) and must plan strategies for program maintenance. As a result of increasing awareness of problems with program diffusion, implementation, and maintenance, health educators have recently been giving more attention to the factors affecting program use (Basen-Engquist, O'Hara-Tompkins, Lovato, Lewis, Parcel, & Gingiss, 1994; Gingiss, Gottlieb, & Brink, 1994; Goodman & Steckler, 1989; Mullen & Mullen, 1983; Oldenburg, Hardcastle, & Kok, 1997; Orlandi, Landers, Weston, & Haley, 1990; Ottoson & Green, 1987; Paulussen, Kok, & Schaalma, 1994; Paulussen, Kok, Schaalma, & Parcel, 1995; Scheirer, 1990; Scheirer & Rezmovic, 1983).

An Iterative Process

In order to describe the intervention and program development process, we have laid out a series of steps. This orderly presentation sometimes wrongly suggests to the reader that every step is completed only once and in a rigid order. This is not the case. Even though each step should provide the basis for the next, only rarely does a step need no revision as the next steps are completed. New information is acquired with each step. And with increasing ideas about the program, knowledge about the intended groups to benefit from the program, community participation, and research and theory, a planner often needs to revisit and fine-tune a previous step. For example, a planning group in the Netherlands included in Step 3 strategies for delivery of role modeling to teens in an HIV-prevention program in schools. When working with teachers on the program in Step 4, planning group members discovered that the teachers were uncomfortable leading role playing, and they had to revisit Step 3 to rethink some of the strategies before completing the program design.

In addition to the process of revisiting prior steps, some "steps" actually weave in and out of the process. For example, evaluation planning begins in the needs assessment and continues in each step until the final plan is completed in Step 6, evaluation. In another example, community participation, including potential program implementers, is begun at the very beginning of a project, continued in each step, and revisited in Step 5, adoption, implementation, and sustainability.

Themes and Conventions Throughout the Book

Several concepts arise repeatedly in the descriptions of Intervention Mapping throughout the book. The first is the set of core processes of accessing, evaluating, and using empirical literature, theory, and formative research, which is introduced in Chapter Two and used throughout the steps.

Another important concept is that of a logic model to present the relations among concepts, which is introduced in this chapter and used throughout the book. Like the logic model, the concepts of community participation and cultural competence are woven into most chapters. Finally, each chapter on a step in the Intervention Mapping process includes a section on implications for evaluation, which link closely to Step 6, in Chapter Ten.

Core Processes. Core processes are common techniques for thinking with theory and evidence. These techniques include asking questions related to aspects of the health problem and its solutions, brainstorming provisional answers, and then using evidence from the literature (both empirical and theoretical), theory, and new data to add to and tighten the logic in the provisional list. These techniques are core intellectual processes for use in program planning, and the Intervention Mapping framework provides the structure for when and how to use them.

Logic Models. Logic models are graphic representations of the demonstrated or hypothesized causal relationships between concepts such as program activities, program output, and outcomes or benefits (Julian, Jones, & Deyo, 1995; Sartourious, 1991; Chen, 1990; Julian, 1997). Logic models can help program developers take into account the complexity of health problems and possible solutions; make explicit the implicit pathways of program effects; and make clear the rationale for program activities (Kirby, 2004). Logic models are commonly being used in program development and evaluation and are a requirement for many funding agencies. (W. K. Kellogg Foundation, 1998; ActKnowledge and Aspen Institute Roundtable, 2004; United Way of America, 1996).

In the process of Intervention Mapping, the planner will build three types of logic models. The first is an *etiologic model* or theory of the problem. Figure 1.3 is based on PRECEDE, a model often used in health education and promotion, and presents the first type of logic model: the description of the causes of health and quality of life problems. In the needs-assessment step (Chapter Five), the planner analyzes and depicts the health, quality of life, behavioral and environmental problems. The planned changes in these will become the program outcomes (Centers for Disease Control & Oak Ridge Institute for Science and Education, 2003; Green and Kreuter, 2005, pp. 103–112).

A second type of logic model is a *change model* created in the matrix step (Chapter Six) and depicting what the program intends to change in the behavior of the risk group and in the environment, as well as the expected determinants of the change. Some authors refer to this as developing a theory of change, theory

FIGURE 1.3. LOGIC MODEL OF RISK.

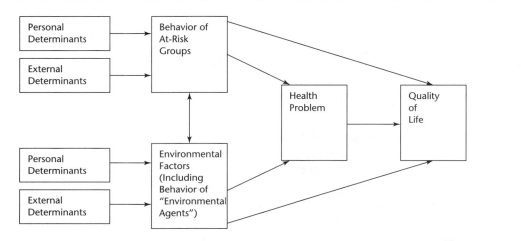

Source: Adapted from Green & Kreuter, 2005.

of the program, or a tacit theory (Connell & Kubisch, 1996; Rossi, Lipsey, & Freeman, 2004; Weiss, 1997). We refer to it as the logic of change. These models explain how the program components or activities are thought to influence the social or health problem. Kirby describes these models as behavior, determinants, intervention (BDI) logic models (Kirby, 2004). All of these logic models are intended to carefully describe the variables that must change in order for the program to be effective. Figure 1.4 presents this type of logic within the third type of logic model, the *intervention logic model,* which depicts program components, resources, and activities (program inputs and outputs) along with the outcomes they are meant to effect. In the program development and implementation steps (Chapters Eight and Nine), the planner describes program inputs and outputs. Rossi, Lipsey, and Freeman (2004) call these the service utilization and organizational schematic. This model has the implementation resources as inputs, program activities as outputs, and program effects as outcomes. Kirby (2004) describes a model in which intervention methods, strategies, and program activities are main inputs; while the proposed changes in behavior, environment, and their determinants are the intermediate outputs and changes in health and quality of life, the terminal outputs. The main purpose of logic-model building in this book is to depict the effects of the proposed intervention on health behavior, environmental causes of health problems, health problems themselves, and quality of life.

FIGURE 1.4. INTERVENTION LOGIC MODEL.

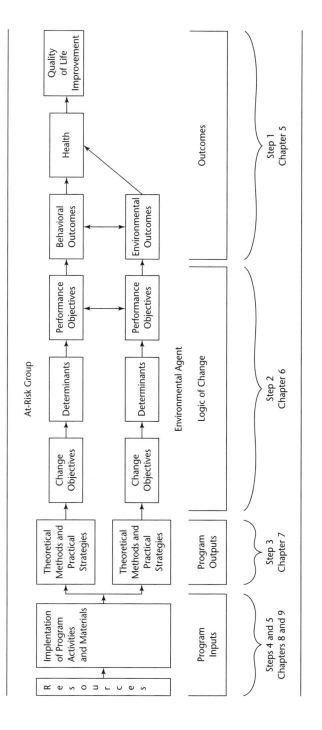

In addition to the logic model that is pieced together as intervention development progresses, we present a number of more detailed logic models to help clarify relations among concepts, such as theoretical constructs (Chapters Three and Four). We also use other graphic devices that do not imply causal relations, such as Figure 1.2, a depiction of the steps involved in Intervention Mapping. When a figure is a logic model, that is, implies causal relations, we clearly label it as such. This intervention logic model is developed throughout the Intervention Mapping steps and is used as the basis of evaluation planning (Chapter Ten).

Participation in Planning. In Intervention Mapping our commitment is to bring both a community and a multidisciplinary professional perspective to the process of planning health promotion. Despite the hazards that the health educator in our mayor's project scenario faced, work groups are a critically important fact of life for health educators. Programs cannot be developed in a vacuum, nor should they be developed without stakeholders' participation (Wallerstein, 1992; Israel, Schulz, Parker, Becker, Allen, & Guzman, 2003; Sullivan, Chao, Allen, Kone, Pierre-Louise, & Krieger, 2003; Yoo, Wood, Lampa, Mbondo, Shado, & Goodman, 2004; Hunt, Lederman, Potter, Stoddard, & Sorensen, 2000; Krieger, Allen, Cheadle, Ciske, Schier, Senturia, et al., 2002; Minkler, Thompson, Bell, Rose, & Redman, 2002). Whether health educators develop programs as group participants, or as formal group leaders, they should have a goal of encouraging full participation to bring multiple perspectives to bear on a problem and to create the most intelligent, productive, and sustainable consensus possible. No matter how many so-called experts are involved in program development, the individuals for whom the intervention is intended can best convey the subjective meaning of the health problem and its antecedents. The people who will deliver the program can best convey the realities of the program setting. Ongoing interaction between program planners and potential program users and participants is necessary for the planner to fully understand and convey the real-world program context.

Beginning in Step 1, needs assessment, a very early task for the planner is to establish a planning group that includes stakeholders for the program. Stakeholder groups are all of those who have an interest in a program and its outcomes. The planning group should include representatives of those who are intended to benefit from the program as well as those who will be important to the adoption of the program and its implementation. Orlandi and colleagues (1990) refer to this as a "linkage system" that helps ensure successful program adoption (Chapter Nine).

Cultural Competence. Another theme that appears in each step of Intervention Mapping is the need to create culturally relevant programs for diverse groups. Often health educators work with groups of people who are members of a cultural group different from themselves; often these are underserved groups. The literature documents the critical issue of health disparities (Institute of Medicine, Committee on Understanding and Eliminating Racial and Ethnic Disparities in Health Care, 2003; Pamuk, Makuc, Heck, Rueben, & Lochner, 1998; Fiscella, Franks, Gold, & Clancy, 2000; Thomas, 2001; Vinicor, Burton, Foster, & Eastman, 2000; Williams & Jackson, 2000). The Healthy People 2010 objectives highlight the health disparities between racial and ethnic groups, with particular emphasis on eliminating those disparities in infant mortality, cancer screening and management, cardiovascular disease, diabetes, HIV/AIDS, and childhood and adult immunizations (U.S. Department of Health and Human Services, 2005). For example, in comparison to whites in the United States, infant mortality rates are 2.5 times higher for African Americans and 1.5 times higher for Native Americans. The prevalence of diabetes in Hispanics is nearly twice that of whites (Pamuk, Makuc, Heck, & Lochner, 1998). In order to address these and many other priority health issues effectively, health educators must be able to develop culturally appropriate programs.

In addition to this explicit association of cultural diversity with race and ethnicity, there are many ways to be a culturally diverse group, and health educators will use the same skills in cultural competence in all program development. For example, in the Netherlands van Kesteren and colleagues are developing an HIV prevention and sexual health program for HIV-positive men who have sex with men (van Kesteren, Hospers, Kok, & van Empelen, 2005). Van Kesteren and colleagues described a specific subgroup structure with definable cultural characteristics, social support mechanisms, and organizations that required the sensitive interaction and reflection in program development (N.M.C. van Kesteren, personal communication, May 2003).

Each planning step requires a specific aspect of a culturally competent approach. In Step 1, needs assessment (Chapter Five), we cover aspects of becoming a more culturally competent practitioner as a prerequisite for beginning a needs assessment and encouraging community participation. In this step we also present the idea of cultural assessment as a part of defining the priority population for the program. In Step 2, matrices (Chapter Six), we discuss the importance of working with the priority population to adequately define the performance objectives and determinants. Without the culturally correct matrix components, no program materials will be salient to the intended cultural group. In Steps 3 and 4, methods, strategies, and programs (Chapters Seven and Eight), we reiterate the importance of maintaining the participation of the intended audience in materials development, and we discuss approaches to creating culturally relevant materials.

Evaluation. Program evaluation always begins with a thorough description of the program to be evaluated and its proposed causal pathways and activities. This description is accomplished step-by-step in Intervention Mapping. First, in the needs assessment, the planner begins to formulate goals for program outcomes in health and quality of life. These become part of the plan for evaluating effects (Chapter Ten). In Step 2 the planner specifies desired changes in behavior and environment as well as their determinants, which again become further outcomes for evaluating effects. Steps 3, 4, and 5 guide the specification of program components and implementation plans that link closely to process evaluation. Step 3 also contains discussion of pretesting and pilot-testing or formative evaluation of the program.

Summary

Intervention Mapping is presented as a series of steps and processes to help health promotion and health education planners develop theory- and evidence-informed programs. Well-designed and effective interventions should be guided by theory and informed by empirical evidence regarding the target behavior. For example, meta-analyses of cancer-screening interventions have found that larger effect sizes are achieved when interventions are based on theory (Stone, Morton, Hulscher, Maglione, Roth, Grimshaw, et al., 2002; Yabroff, O'Malley, Mangan, & Mandelblatt, 2001; Yabroff & Mandelblatt, 1999). However, no one theoretical model completely predicts or explains health behaviors (Rakowski & Breslau, 2004; Institute of Medicine, 2004; Rimer, 2002). Therefore, a system is needed to help intervention developers choose useful theories and integrate relevant constructs from multiple theories to describe health problems and develop health promotion and health education solutions (van Bokhoven, Kok, & van der Weijden, 2003; Kok, Schaalma, Ruiter, van Empelen, & Brug, 2004).

Specifically, Intervention Mapping ensures that theoretical models and empirical evidence guide planners in two areas:

- The identification of behavioral and environmental determinants related to a target health problem
- The selection of the most appropriate methods and strategies to address the identified determinants

Intervention Mapping has been used to develop intervention programs for asthma management (Bartholomew, Gold, Parcel, Czyzewski, Sockrider, & Fernandez, 2000; Fernandez, Bartholomew, Lopez, Tyrrell, Czyzewski, & Sockrider, 2000; Shegog, Bartholomew, Parcel, Sockrider, Masse, & Abramson, 2001; Bartholomew, Shegog, Parcel, Gold, Fernandez, Czyzewski, et al., 2000), nutrition (Cullen, Bartholomew, Parcel, & Kok, 1998; Cullen, Bartholomew, & Parcel, 1997; Hoelscher, Evans, Parcel, & Kelder, 2002), sun protection (Tripp, Herrmann, Parcel, Chamberlain, & Gritz, 2000), adolescent risk taking (Tortolero, Bartholomew, Abramson, Sockrider, Jones, Tyrrell, et al., 2005), violence (Murray, Kelder, Parcel, & Orpinas, 1998), HIV prevention (van Empelen, Kok, Schaalma, & Bartholomew, 2003), cervical cancer screening (Hou, Fernandez, & Parcel, 2004; Hou, Fernandez, Baumler, & Parcel, 2002; Hou, Fernandez, & Parcel, 2004), mammography (Fernandez et al., 2005), colorectal cancer screening (Vernon, 2004), leg ulcers (Heinen, Bartholomew, Wensing, van de Kerkhof, & van Achterberg, 2005) and acute stroke therapy (Morgenstern, Bartholomew, Grotta, Staub, King, & Chan, 2003; Morgenstern, Staub, Chan, Wein, Bartholomew, King, et al., 2002). Even though Intervention Mapping has not been directly compared to other processes for developing interventions, planners working on these projects think that the systematic process has been useful and will strengthen future program development (Hoelscher, Evans, Parcel, & Kelder, 2002).

CHAPTER TWO

CORE PROCESSES: USING EVIDENCE, THEORY, AND NEW RESEARCH

Reader Objectives

- Pose planning problems as questions that facilitate finding answers from theory, the existing literature, and new research
- Brainstorm answers to planning questions
- Search the literature on the topic at hand (evidence that can be either empirically or theoretically based, or both) to answer planning questions
- Use multiple approaches to access and use theory to answer the planning questions
- Evaluate the strength of the evidence
- Work from the evidence to revise the brainstormed list of planning question answers
- Decide when to conduct new research to address unanswered questions in the planning process
- Formulate a working list of answers to the planning question

Health promoters deal with questions regarding specifying desired behavior change, identifying determinants of that change, differentiating the intended program recipients, selecting methods, creating strategies, and developing implementation plans. To answer these questions, they survey the wealth of information available in the existing empirical and theoretical literature related to health and health behavior, and they conduct new research. In this chapter we focus on finding and using evidence and theoretical constructs in the planning of health education programs. We encourage the reader to consult other sources for guidance on literature synthesis (Cooper & Hedges, 1994; Lipsey & Wilson, 2001; Briss, Mullen, & Hopkins, 2005), qualitative research methods (Huberman & Miles, 1994; Kreuger & Casey, 2000; Merriam, 1988, 1991; Yin, 2002; Strauss & Corbin, 1990; Dey, 1999; Patton, 1990, 2001; Petticrew & Gilbody, 2004; Payne, 2004; Stake, 1995), and quantitative research and evaluation (Shadish, Cook, & Campbell, 2002; Rossi, Lipsey, & Freeman, 2004; Stake, 1995; Windsor, Clark, Boyd, & Goodman, 2004; Petticrew & Gilbody, 2004; Payne, 2004).

Box 2.1. Mayor's Project

The health educator knows that as the violence prevention planning group moves toward intervention development, it will need effective processes for defining problems. Group members must ask questions about what causes violence, using an ecological perspective that includes environmental, social, and psychological determinants. They must ask questions about who is at risk for perpetrating violence and who is likely to be a victim. They must formulate ideas of how to intervene with the determinants of violence in their community.

They know that a simple answer that suggests the need to intervene on a single behavioral or environmental risk factor (for example, more parental supervision) probably would be inadequate. They also wonder whether theory might help them understand determinants, and they think about planning new research. The health educator knows that once the planning group understands determinants of the behavior and environmental conditions and decides on program objectives, it must ask equally important questions about effective intervention methods. The way group members structure the questions related to these issues and the processes they use to formulate the answers will underlie the success of their program-planning efforts.

Perspectives

Here we present two perspectives on theory use in health promotion. We propose that program planners have the job of piecing together theories of problems and solutions rather than the job of theory testing, and we suggest the need for a multi-theory approach.

Theory: Problem Focus Versus Theory Testing

A person who wants to find a solution to a public health problem has a different task than one who wants to test a theory. To state this more forcefully: A scientist devising a test of a theory will be more likely to contribute to knowledge about the theory than to solving a practical problem in a real world situation. Problem-driven applied behavioral or social science may use one or multiple theories, empirical evidence, and new research both to describe a problem and to solve a problem. In this approach the main focus is on problem solving, and the criteria for success are formulated in terms of the problem rather than the theory. Resulting contributions to theory development may be quite useful, but they are peripheral to the problem-solving process. In Intervention Mapping we work from a problem-driven perspective. Choices have to be made in the process of developing an intervention, and theories are one tool to enable us to make better choices.

Box 2.2. Mayor's Project

When the mayor's planning group met to discuss the causes of violence and to decide how to intervene in their community, they focused their discussion on the questions: "What are the factors related to violence in youth?" One member wanted to focus on the impact on children of violence in the media (Centerwall, 1993; Eron, Huesman, Lefkowitz, & Walder, 1996). The group members discussed the importance of this idea and the social cognitive theory construct of modeling as it helps explain the effects of media violence, but they did not stop their discussion of determinants of violence with this one construct or theory.

The group did not find in its literature search a unified theoretical model describing the risk factors for perpetrating violence or describing the determinants of those factors in children and adolescents (American Psychological Association, Commission on Youth and Violence, 1993). However, group members did come up with theoretical and empirical evidence that helps explain or describe the causes of violence. They wanted to understand what all the information meant and to try to develop a comprehensive perspective on the predictors of violence. They analyzed many possible determinants of aggressive behavior in children and adolescents and sorted them into personal, behavioral, and social-environmental factors (Perry & Jessor, 1985).

Some of the theory-related personal factors were beliefs that support aggression and aggressive attributional bias (Dodge & Cole, 1987; Slaby & Guerra, 1988). They discussed theory-related behavioral risk factors such as inadequate problem-solving skills and the viewing of media with violent role models (Cen-

---

terwall, 1993; Eron et al., 1996; Slaby & Guerra, 1988). Social-environmental factors related to theories of parenting included coercive family interactions, hostile or rejecting parenting, inconsistency, permissiveness, disintegrated family unit, and little parental monitoring (Patterson, 1986; Patterson & Stouthamer-Loeber, 1984; Perry, Perry, & Boldizar, 1990; Yoshikawa, 1994).

The health educator realized that the group's understanding of violence included other determinants that were not clearly related to theory, for example, the effects of brain injury, lead exposure, low academic achievement, poverty, easy access to weapons, family violence, and parental criminality (Baker, O'Neill, Ginsburg, & Li, 1992; Farrington, 1995; Loeber & Dishion, 1983; Loeber, Stouthamer-Loeber, van Kammen, & Farrington, 1991; Needleman, Riess, Tobin, Biesecker, & Greenhouse, 1996; Webster, Wilson, Duggan, & Pakula, 1992; Yoshikawa, 1994).

With the beginnings of a comprehensive picture of what causes violence in youth, the planning group could begin to figure out important and changeable determinants and proceed with planning an intervention. The group has quite a bit more work to do, and the health educator realizes that a slightly more systematic approach might have been helpful. She is pleased, however, with the problem-focused approach and realizes how different it is from the approach group members would have taken had they been theory centered—applying one set of theoretical constructs to violence and measuring how well the theory predicted the outcomes. Or as sometimes seems to happen, they might have failed to search for causation of violence and launched directly into an intervention.

Need for a Multitheory Approach

In a problem-driven context, then, all theories, theoretical models, and constructs are potentially useful within the parameters that the theory describes (Kok, Schaalma, Ruiter, van Empelen, & Brug, 2004). The challenge is to find the best theory or combination of theoretical constructs first to understand and then to solve the problem at hand. Limiting the pool of candidate theories too soon may lead to an inadequate solution of a practical problem or, worse, to conclusions that are counterproductive. When planners were originally confronted with the challenge of developing HIV-prevention programs, they looked first, with some success, at theories that had been useful for other preventive activities, such as the Theory of Planned Behavior (TPB) (Ajzen, 1988; Montaño & Kasprzyk, 2002), Social Cognitive Theory (SCT)(Bandura, 1986; Baranowski, Perry, & Parcel, 2002), and the Transtheoretical Model (TTM) (Prochaska, Redding, & Evers, 2002). However, when new questions came up, such as how to prevent HIV transmission by HIV-positive persons or how to prevent stigmatization of people with HIV or AIDS, other theoretical perspectives were needed. For those who are HIV-positive, preventing partners from becoming infected with HIV is protecting someone else instead of protecting oneself. Of course, the earlier mentioned theories would be relevant to these issues, but some other theoretical constructs are more specifically relevant to protecting others: altruism (Batson, 1991), taking responsibility (Schwartz & Howard, 1982), and empathy (Batson et al., 1997). And when developing interventions to prevent or reduce the negative effects of stigma, the program planner might profit from such theoretical constructs as emotional reactions to stigma (Dijker, Kok, & Koomen, 1996), functions of stigmatization (Herek & Capitanio, 1998), attributions and stigmatization (Weiner, Perry, & Magnusson, 1988), and the two-factor model—in this case, the stigma of AIDS related to the stigma of homosexuality (Pryor, Reeder, & Landau, 1999).

Core Processes for Intervention Mapping

Sometimes the processes involved in understanding a problem or answering a question with empirical data and theory are complex and time-consuming. Many planners do not persevere through the difficulties. Consequently, understanding often is incomplete, and the intervention is faulty. Therefore, we provide considerable detail about how to undertake these core processes (Figure 2.1). The core processes begin with asking a question, continue through figuring out what the planning team already knows about potential answers to the question, reviewing the literature for both theory- and evidence-based "answers" to the question, assessing and addressing needs for new data, developing a working list of answers, and then moving on to the next question.

Posing Questions

The first task for the core processes is to pose a question. The first questions asked are often to facilitate the analysis of the health problem. Veen (1985) and Kok, Schaalma, De Vries, Parcel, and Paulussen (1996) suggest asking questions to clarify all aspects of the problem. The most basic questions include the following:

- What is the problem?
- What is the evidence that this is a problem?
- For whom is it a problem?
- Who has labeled a certain phenomenon a problem?
- What might be the causes of the problem?
- Is the problem likely to be resolved?
- What are the costs and benefits of solving the problem?

FIGURE 2.1. CORE PROCESSES:
HOW TO USE THEORY, LITERATURE, AND NEW DATA.

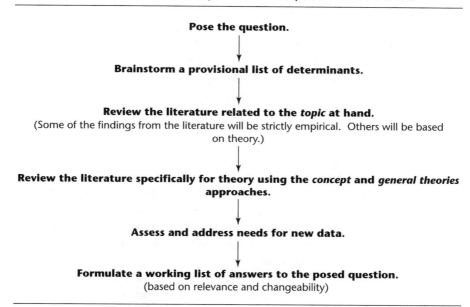

Pose the question.

Brainstorm a provisional list of determinants.

Review the literature related to the *topic* at hand.
(Some of the findings from the literature will be strictly empirical. Others will be based on theory.)

Review the literature specifically for theory using the *concept* and *general theories* approaches.

Assess and address needs for new data.

Formulate a working list of answers to the posed question.
(based on relevance and changeability)

Careful consideration of multiple dimensions of a problem may prevent spending time on irrelevant problems or on problems that require approaches from outside the realm of health promotion. The planner should state the problem as a question using the terms *what, why,* or *how;* and state a new question or questions for each step of the program-planning process: health problems, behavior and environmental conditions, determinants, methods, strategies, adoption, and implementation.

Although these questions are concerned with, among other things, explanations and solutions, they are not meant to offer adequate answers at an early stage but simply to clarify the problem. For example, if a solution to a problem appears quite obvious, it may be useful to examine why no one has tried this solution in the past. It is possible that the organization responsible for solving the problem was resistant to the most obvious solution or that an earlier solution led to more unanticipated consequences than expected. The resistance or the unanticipated consequences may put the problem in another light and call for redefining the problem in terms of both questions about its causes and questions about proposed solutions.

Common mistakes that planners make in attempting to understand a problem are to accept another person's or organization's definition of a problem without further considering the problem or asking questions about the problem that make assumptions about its causes. In 1980 one of us was involved in a campaign concerned with road safety in a small Dutch town. The town council undertook a campaign when it noticed that its rate of crashes at intersections was higher than in similar towns. The health educators working on the problem allowed it to remain defined in terms of the excess morbidity and mortality resulting from traffic accidents. The consultants accepted the question as this: What can be done regarding public education to solve the health problem? This question focused on the solution. The consultants failed to first ask a question about the causes of the problem. They assumed that the accidents were due to a failure to adhere to traffic laws, and the health educators began a local campaign about right-of-way rules. In the middle of the education campaign, the health educators discovered that the majority of all right-of-way accidents happened at only one point: the exit of the parking lot near the supermarket. They discovered the environmental problem at this location and realized it could be solved with an environmental intervention such as pruning the shrubs that obscured the view or introducing a traffic light at that intersection. In this case the planning group should have asked questions to determine the nature of the problem, and group members should have made sure that the questions asked did not entail assumptions about the solutions to the problem.

To further illustrate the process of posing questions, a work group in one of our health education methods classes began work on a project to prevent HIV and other sexually transmitted infections (STI) transmission and pregnancy among urban adolescents. Over the course of the project, they asked a number of questions related to the following areas:

• Health problem. They first asked a question related to the health problem: What is the health problem related to HIV and STIs in adolescents (age 13–18) in the United States?

• Behaviors. They then asked: What are important risk behaviors for the transmission of HIV and STIs and for pregnancy among adolescents? How do these risk behaviors vary for different groups such as boys and girls? (They were thinking of sexual intercourse as the predominant transmission route for the infections, but they also had to consider intravenous [IV] drug use.)

• Determinants. After defining the health problem and the behavioral risks, the group asked a question concerning determinants of the risk behavior of not using condoms: Why do adolescents have sexual intercourse without using condoms? Because they had discussed several possible group differences in behavior in the previous question, they posed several additional questions to elicit more detailed explanations: Why don't adolescent males use condoms when having vaginal sex with steady girlfriends? Why do girls have sex with boys who do not use condoms? And so forth.

- Change methods. Then the focus of the questions shifted to potential solutions or methods: How can we help specific subgroups of adolescents use condoms? Which theoretical methods can be translated into appropriate practical strategies?
- Program implementation. Finally, much later in the process, when the group was working on a school-based program, the problem shifted to the implementation process. The work group asked about determinants of adoption and implementation behaviors: What influences health professionals to adopt and implement programs that help adolescents learn to use condoms? Shifting to the implementation intervention, the group asked: How can we motivate and train health professionals to implement programs that help adolescents use condoms?

Project Parents and Newborns Developing and Adjusting (PANDA) (Chapter Thirteen) provides a very good example of careful wording of the questions about the risk behavior. Mullen and colleagues (Chapter Thirteen) were concerned about smoking after pregnancy in women who had stopped smoking before the birth of the baby. It might have been natural given their familiarity with the work of Marlatt and Gordon (1985) to frame the question in terms of relapse. After all, these were women who had stopped smoking cigarettes and then started again. The question might easily have contained a perspective on the intervention had it been: Why do women *relapse* after pregnancy? Thus, the question would have brought the relapse literature into the picture and implied a solution: Focus on training for coping with risky situations to prevent relapse. Fortunately, Mullen and colleagues framed the question more openly and asked: Why do women who have stopped smoking during pregnancy return to smoking at high rates during the first six months after the birth? They looked at theory, but they also interviewed women and realized that the women had different reasons for their actions: Some women relapsed; others never fully changed their behavior; and some had only stopped for the pregnancy and fully intended to resume smoking. Framing the problem with this broader question had a huge impact on intervention development. (See Chapter Thirteen.)

Brainstorming Provisional Answers

The second core process task for the planning group is to brainstorm a provisional list of answers to the question. The brainstorming process is in response to a specific question, but it can lead to clarification of other questions as well. Before searching the literature for empirical evidence and theory, brainstorming clarifies what members of the planning group already know, or think they know. Of course, this presumes some familiarity with the problem from practice or from the literature.

Making a provisional list of answers to a question is a creative process that primarily involves free association with the aim of generating as many explanations as possible in response to a question (Veen, 1985; Kok et al., 1996). The planners can later drop explanations that are poorly supported from the literature. Planners should avoid getting stuck on a single explanation too soon. In formulating these provisional explanations, health educators, as applied behavioral scientists, typically use theoretical and empirical knowledge, whether consciously or not. Doing so is unavoidable at this stage, but the brainstorming should be as open as possible and should not be limited to data- or theory-informed items.

The group of students working on determinants for condom use generated the provisional list in Table 2.1 in response to the question: Why do adolescents have sexual intercourse without using condoms? The work group brainstormed determinants based on what they knew from many sources about condom use. They stimulated creativity by asking related questions, by taking the sexually active adolescent's perspective, and by narrowing the question to particular populations and situations. When they became stuck, they reversed perspectives and asked themselves the radical question: How can the problem be increased—how would we reduce the use of condoms? Reversing perspective helped them recognize the barriers to condom use.

At this stage of the brainstorming, there is no reason to favor one explanation over another. However, in the subsequent steps, health educators should begin to take into account two criteria for good answers: An explanation should describe a process, and it should be plausible. By the term *process*, we mean an explanation that suggests a mechanism of cause. For example, socioeconomic status on Table 2.1 is not a very helpful explanation. What about socioeconomic status contributes to not using condoms? A useful aid is to represent the explanation in a logic model schematic that shows causation (Earp & Ennett, 1991). A plausible explanation is one that can survive when it is depicted visually and examined critically, using logic to evaluate the relationships between the various elements in the model.

Reviewing the Literature Systematically for Findings from Research

The next steps are to support or refute provisional explanations from the brainstorming with empirical evidence, theoretical constructs, and new research. A focused literature review should yield new explanations, cause deletion of some explanations from the provisional list, and raise new questions to answer by means of additional research (Kok et al., 1996). Although team members likely did their brainstorming with a sense of previous research about the problem, after brainstorming the provisional list of determinants, they should systematically examine the literature to help them decide which factors should remain on the list and how

TABLE 2.1. PROVISIONAL LIST: DETERMINANTS OF LACK OF CONDOM USE AMONG SEXUALLY ACTIVE ADOLESCENTS.

Original Provisional List	Additions from Empirical Literature	Additions from Theory
Personal Determinants		
Lack of knowledge of HIV or STI transmission	Alcohol and drug use	Intention to use condoms (Theory of Planned Behavior)
Perceived group norm	Use of hormonal contraceptives	Subjective norms (Theory of Planned Behavior)
Perceived benefits of condoms	Type of relationship (steady versus casual)	Perceived barriers to condom use (Health Belief Model)
Attitude toward condom use		Self-efficacy and skills for putting on condoms (Social Cognitive Theory)
Experience with condom use		
Gender		
Salience (knowing someone with AIDS)		Self-efficacy and skills regarding negotiation of condom use (Social Cognitive Theory)
Lack of confidence to use condoms		
Cultural beliefs		Outcome expectations (Social Cognitive Theory)
External Determinants		
Partner's insistence on not using condoms	Community characteristics (poverty, low education, unemployment, access to family planning services)	
Mass media portrayal of sexual activity		
Availability of condoms	Coercive parenting	
Socioeconomic status	Lack of parental supervision	

these factors are related to the behavior. This topic is introduced here as a core process and covered in more depth under skills for core processes.

Systematic reviews have recently received much attention in public health, with the appearance of reports from the United States Task Force on Community Preventive Services (Zaza, Briss, & Harris, 2005). Procedures and new norms for what is now known as a systematic review are well established in medicine. The Cochrane Collaboration (Alderson, Green, & Higgins, 2004) is one example and treatment guidelines for problems such as tobacco use from the Agency for Healthcare Research and Quality are another (U.S. Department of Health and

Human Services, Agency for Healthcare Research and Quality, 2000). Basically, the systematic review process is like that used for research studies:

1. Specify study aims: What questions do you want to answer?
2. Set inclusion criteria: What evidence will address the questions?
3. Design the recruitment strategy: How will you find the evidence you want?
4. Screen potential participants: Which evidence from the search process meets your criteria?
5. Decide on measures and design the data collection protocol: Which characteristics will you code?
6. Select an appropriate metric to represent the strength of the findings: How will you represent findings from individual studies?
7. Collect the data: What are your coding procedures?
8. Analyze and display the data using appropriate methods.
9. Draw conclusions based on the data and the limitations.

Not only are the steps between a systematic review and a primary study similar, but both are expected to report the methods that were used so that the process is replicable.

Not All Evidence Is Equal

The approach to selecting the primary sources for a literature review that many planners learned is the equivalent of saying, "Look up everything you can find on the subject." And yet literature reviews should all be systematic reviews as we discussed earlier and should be as well planned as any other research study. As planners search for and find evidence to guide intervention development, they weigh many aspects of the literature. They should address two overarching questions:

- Which evidence is relevant to my questions?
- What conclusions can safely be drawn regarding the nature of the relationships between variables of interest?

Figure 2.2 is a checklist for determining the quality of a literature review. It will also be helpful in determining the quality of one's own systematic review.

Despite the reassuring term, the literature is not always a nice neat package with easily defined boundaries, nor are the findings necessarily self-evident. In reality, the literature is often an admixture of diverse study aims, research designs, constructs, and indicators, let alone times, settings, contexts, and populations. Looking critically at the individual pieces of evidence, it is a wonder that readers can make any strong conclusions. We return to these considerations later in this chapter.

FIGURE 2.2. CONSIDERATIONS IN EVALUATING REVIEWS: A CHECKLIST.

☐ What was the *purpose* of the review? What were the questions to be answered? What was the hypothesis? Is the question, hypothesis, or objective clearly and specifically stated?

☐ Are the *criteria* for including or excluding studies clearly stated? What is the rationale for these criteria? Is this an appropriate rationale in my context? Looking at the criteria plus search strategies should ensure a fair representation of the available evidence.

☐ How was the *search* done that located the studies? Was the search systematic? Is it fully described so that it can be replicated? Did it go beyond computerized databases to include expert writings, bibliographies of articles already retrieved, or bibliographies of other relevant written materials such as government reports, books, monographs? (Note: Some reviewers restrict the studies they will include to those that have been peer reviewed. Peer review is a higher standard in some journals than in others. Published articles can vary markedly in quality on statistical and many other aspects of study design.)

☐ Are *study characteristics* clearly noted? Study characteristics include study design, sample, variables, and measures. Are tables and charts or a structured narrative used to display important study characteristics for all the included studies? To interpret the review's conclusions, the same information must be obtained about every study.

☐ Is the *intervention* well specified? Interventions include intended methods and strategies; vehicles and communication channels; and participant contact points, frequency, and duration.

☐ Is a common *metric,* such as standard deviation units used? Does the reviewer avoid relying on tests of significance to tell the outcome of studies? Are such indicators as the percent achieving some behavior in the control and experimental groups or the mean difference and confidence interval included? A review must show a measure of effect size so that (1) meaningful, consistent differences can be separated from problems of low study power, and (2) small, unimportant differences can be separated from large numbers (excessive power).

☐ Are *dependent variables* examined separately? Some reviews, particularly quantitative reviews or meta-analyses, have combined knowledge and belief measures with behavior and physiologic effects as if these were all measuring the same construct.

☐ Are *findings* interpreted in depth? Are non-average findings, positive and negative, examined closely? Are the lessons that can be derived from such outliers clearly articulated? Does the reviewer pursue the reasons for these?

Source: Adapted from Mullen, 1993.

Here, we focus on the study design and on how this important characteristic of studies should influence the reviewer's conclusions about the relationship between potential determinants and a behavior of interest. Thus, the main question is how certain we can be that a relationship described by a study is causal and important. The degree to which the results could be sorted into the categories of evidence—such as barriers and facilitators, correlates, predictors, risk factors and determinants—is in large part dependent on the study design and methods of data analysis (Rakowski & Breslau, 2004). For example, consider the variety of possibilities in retrospective study designs: Respondents may have been asked directly why they performed a behavior or not; they may have been asked to provide sociodemographic characteristics; they could have been asked about specific beliefs and perceived norms; or they could have been interviewed with open-ended questions and skillful probes to build rich descriptions. Samples could have been created in many different ways, for example to be representative of a population, to be impressionistically representative, or simply to be convenient.

Despite the use in Intervention Mapping of the term *determinants* to indicate a factor that may be the target of intervention, we understand that most cross-sectional surveys yield correlates but rarely determinants, despite the claims of enthusiastic authors. Not only should the modest term *correlates* be applied to most findings from cross-sectional studies, but the reader should take a further step in recognizing the ambiguity of the direction of the relationship by first stating one variable as a cause of the other and then the reverse. For example, cross-sectional studies were a basis for premature conclusions that youth were influenced to smoke by friends who smoked. This directional interpretation gave rise to a social-influence explanation (youth had been influenced by their friends to smoke) for the observation that youth smokers were more likely to have friends who were smokers than were youth who did not smoke. Reversing the order of influence would have made it clearer that a social-affiliation explanation (youth who smoke affiliate with other youth who smoke) was also plausible from cross-sectional studies.

Sometimes the importance of the relationship is difficult to determine. For example, in studies of the same variables, one study may test the variables one at a time; another may use multivariate techniques that control for sociodemographic variables; and a third may use multivariate techniques to control for psychosocial variables. What does one make of the varying conclusions? Laying out the study findings in evidence tables can help clarify the relative contributions of findings from different types of studies.

Prospective, longitudinal studies are generally more reliable in producing findings that provide evidence for a variable's causal relationship to a behavior when the variable is from an earlier time than the behavior. Prospective experimental and quasi-experimental studies testing interventions are theoretically the highest quality of evidence for many of the questions embedded in health promotion planning steps. In practice, however, precise descriptions of the intervention often are not reported, and key indicators of objectives are not measured, so it may not be possible to identify the proximal factors that were affected by the intervention or their effect on the study outcomes. Planners must take care in interpreting and presenting study results used in planning.

The student group in our example looked for what others had found regarding adolescents' condom use. In this topical approach to the literature, broadening the topic to include other behaviors related to sexual activity would be relevant to the question at hand. Mindful of this, the group also looked for information on other risk-taking behaviors in adolescents (Jaccard, Blanton, & Dodge, 2005; Turbin, Jessor, & Costa, 2000) and for other behaviors related to sexual activity, such as contraception use (Manlove, Ryan, & Franzetta, 2004; Commendador, 2003; Fortenberry, Costa, Jessor, & Donovan, 1997).

From the topical review, the planners refine the provisional list of answers to the posed question. From their search the student work group added to Table 2.2 the relationship between lack of condom use with other risky behaviors, such as alcohol and drug use (Tapert, Aarons, Sedlar, & Brown, 2001), with partner type (steady or casual) (Manlove et al., 2004; Gebhardt, Kuyper, & Greunsven, 2003), and with hormonal contraceptive use (Manlove et al., 2004).

Accessing and Using Theory

A significant focus of the core processes is how to find and use aspects of theory. For all the various questions and decisions that are part of the steps of Intervention Mapping, we need appropriate theories. In Table 2.2 we provide examples of theories that might be applied for the various decisions in the Intervention Mapping process. Notice that these theories do not apply equally to all steps and that adequate use of the core processes enables the professional to apply multiple theories or models throughout the planning process. A theory that is helpful in making one decision might not be very helpful for making another. Of course, some theories cover a broad area of phenomena: Social Cognitive Theory, for example, could be applied to determinants, methods, and implementation. Even when applying such a theory, it may still be necessary to find and use other helpful theories.

TABLE 2.2. EXAMPLES OF THEORIES FOR INTERVENTION MAPPING STEPS.

Types of Planning Decisions	Possible Theories
Needs assessment	Quality-of-life theories
Behaviors	Self-regulatory theories
Environmental conditions and external determinants	Power theories
Personal determinants	Value expectancy theories
Methods, strategies, intervention	Persuasive communication theories
Implementation	Diffusion theories

The next core process task is to continue to refine, add to, and discard provisional answers based on theoretical concepts. We suggest three approaches to search the literature for applicable theories. These are the topic, concept, and general theories approaches (Veen, 1985).

Topic Approach. Planners have usually begun their review of the literature by using a topic or issue approach and have discovered both theory-informed and atheoretical approaches to the question(s) they have asked. Probably, however, they will want to revisit the literature on their health, behavior, or environmental topic with a particular focus on theory. For example, the student group working on HIV as a health problem had posed a question about the predictors of condom use and had searched for provisional explanations in the literature specifically related to HIV and condom use. Group members then used the topic of condom use to approach the literature and found studies that used the Health Belief Model (HBM) (Lux & Petosa, 1994; Laraque, McLean, Brown-Peterside, Ashton, & Diamond, 1997) and the Theory of Planned Behavior (TPB) (Basen-Engquist & Parcel, 1992; Gage, 1998; Gebhardt et al., 2003). From these theories they considered adding to their list any of the constructs that were not already present, such as barriers from the HBM and intention to perform the behavior from the TPB. Also from the TPB (Ajzen, 1988), the group redefined perceived norms as subjective norms to include both the perception of whether significant others support performance of a behavior and the motivation to comply with the wishes of those others. If the work group had had a low yield through this narrow search, group members might have looked for theories in a literature on a related behavior such as contraception (Chambers & Rew, 2003) or at a more general set of risk-taking behavior by adolescents (Turbin et al., 2000).

As a matter of fact, the group did expand its search to the issues of adolescent pregnancy and STI prevention in general because group members wanted to think about the problem slightly more broadly before they were satisfied with focusing on condom use. They chose to expand because they noticed, as they worked with their provisional list, that a focus on condom use narrowed their list of determinants to predominantly those determinants within the individual or quite close to the individual. The group was also interested in the wider social context of why adolescents might not protect against pregnancy and STIs. They found that researchers had demonstrated that community characteristics, such as proportion of families living below the poverty line, low levels of education, and high unemployment, were highly related to birthrates among young teenagers (Kirby, Coyle, & Gould, 2001). They also found that other neighborhood characteristics, such as access to family planning services, had been linked to adolescent contraceptive use (Averett, Rees, & Argys, 2002). This broader search also located evidence that lack of parental supervision, association with deviant peers (that is, those participating in other risk behaviors), and coercive parenting were associated with engaging in sexual risk taking (Metzler, Noell, Biglan, Ary, & Smolkowski, 1994). (See Table 2.1, column 2.)

Concept Approach. The concept approach enables planners to track the concepts on the provisional list to theoretical constructs and then to their parent theories. Going to the construct enables full understanding of the meaning of a concept on the list and orientation to other constructs from the theory. For example, "confidence" on the student work group's provisional list (Table 2.1) is similar to the construct of self-efficacy in the SCT (Bandura, 1986; Mulvihill, 1996). When group members explored the construct of self-efficacy, expressed in their provisional list as confidence, they found considerable useful information. This new information guided them to look at two kinds of self-efficacy: self-efficacy for negotiating condom use as separate from self-efficacy for applying a condom. The work group also found that self-efficacy is closely related to skills, so group members added skills for negotiating condom use and applying a condom to the list. Further, they encountered methods for influencing self-efficacy and began to think ahead about the intervention. None of this useful information would have been available if the group had not looked beyond the concept of confidence.

Working with the construct-related approach also means that planners may apply the theory fully. Most of the time, a theory will have constructs in addition to the constructs on the provisional list that led to the theory. For instance, the work group found the construct of self-efficacy by exploring the concept of confidence. Group members also found that social cognitive theory contained other constructs, such as outcome expectation, skills, reciprocal determinism, and modeling. They then added some of these constructs to their provisional list.

General Theories Approach. In the general theories approach, planners look at their question through the lens of a determinants theory or a change theory, depending on the question. They also think about how the specific constructs in that theory apply to their question. Applying the general theories approach, for instance, by using the index of a textbook to locate theories, may lead planners to theories with which they are not yet familiar. If the question concerns determinants of behavior, as in the case of condom use, they may go to the TPB, for example, and consider subjective norms, attitudes, self-efficacy expectations, and behavioral intentions, in the unlikely event that they haven't encountered this theory through the earlier processes (Ajzen & Madden, 1986). Clearly, the construct and general theories approaches are limited by the number of theories with which a planner is familiar, and we devote the next two chapters to a brief review of multiple theories commonly used in health education. We also suggest that the reader review theories from more complete sources (Glanz, Lewis, & Rimer, 2002; DiClemente, Crosby, & Kegler, 2002).

Identifying and Addressing Needs for New Data

At this point the planner will have assembled a set of answers from both the theoretical and empirical literature that fit with, change, or add to the provisional explanations. In some cases this information provides insight into the exact processes of the provisional answers. The information may at the same time give cause for further examination of some variables and raise questions that the planning team had not thought of before. For example, the planners would want to know whether certain theoretical constructs that look promising were actually explanatory in their population. They would also want to know the particular way a factor is expressed in their group.

In general, a combination of qualitative and quantitative techniques is used to explore the question of interest in the population (De Vries, Weijts, Dijkstra, & Kok, 1992; Steckler, McLeroy, Goodman, Bird, & McCormick, 1992). During this process the theories that have been applied to this point can serve as a guide for the qualitative and quantitative study questions. For a question regarding determinants, for example, planners first search the available theoretical and empirical literature on the cause of the behavior or environmental condition of interest to find theories and data. They might then use a qualitative method to find out the population's own ideas about determinants of their behavior and then conduct a quantitative study using a structured questionnaire with questions that are based on the results of the qualitative phase. Some factors cannot be measured by just asking the population because perceptions may be different from reality, so planners need information from key persons and observations. Of course, in some situations qualitative and quantitative methods are used independently rather than sequentially to shed light on a question, or qualitative methods are used later in the research process to better understand the findings from a quantitative approach (Steckler, McLeroy, et al., 1992).

Formulating the Working List of Answers

At this point the planning team is ready to summarize and complete its provisional list of answers into a working list for which the evidence is sufficient. The planners already have considered the criteria of plausibility and process. Now, they use two further general criteria: relevance and changeability. *Relevance* is the strength of the evidence for the causal relationship between the determinant and the behavior or environmental factor we want to change. *Changeability* is the strength of the evidence that the proposed change can be realized by an intervention. The latter criterion requires health educators to consider that some determinants may be changed by interventions directed at the individual and others by interventions directed at the environment. For determinants questions, answers that remain on the list will be factors that are both important and changeable. For a solutions or methods question, answers that remain on the list will be processes that have been shown to produce significant change in similar situations. Later in this chapter, we present two case studies, one on determinants and one on methods, and provide more detail about this selection process.

Skills for Core Processes: Literature Review

In order to conduct a basic systematic literature review, the health promoter must first describe a clear research question and match a search strategy to the question. Once articles are found, tasks revolve around judging the validity of the evidence and selecting articles to be summarized in the review.

The Research Question for a Literature Review

The first part of planning a literature review is posing the question that the review is intended to answer (Alderson, Green, & Higgins, 2004). Richardson, Wilson, Nishikawa, & Hayward (1995) and Counsell (1997) suggest several components of good questions. These include the following:

1. Description of what types of people are of interest, including what people have the problem and what specific population and settings are the focus
2. Types of interventions or other study questions that will be the focus, including the types of comparisons (control or comparison groups) that will be acceptable
3. Types of outcomes that will be considered
4. Types of study designs that can answer the question

For example, the group interested in condom use first asked the question: What factors are related to not using a condom in adolescence? Group members then had to include in their question the characteristics of the population(s) and sample(s) of interest including demographic and risk characteristics. The planning group would want to specify the age range encompassing adolescence as well as any combination of sociodemographic, institutional, or behavioral markers of risk, such as social class, ethnicity, residence in a public housing project, or sexual contact with multiple partners. They also included the range of study dates in which they were interested. They were interested in both intervention studies of theory-informed interventions targeted at condom use and in determinants studies that did not test an intervention. Further, they specified that they were interested in three outcomes: condom use at last intercourse, condom use on first intercourse, and reported routine condom use. They were interested in both longitudinal and cross-sectional studies and in both randomized clinical trials and quasi-experimental studies. They were not interested in simple pre- and posttest designs with no comparison group.

The boundaries of a question and related search can be narrow or broad, as long as they are clear. An example of a broad criterion for a search for interventions of interest is this: any educational intervention conducted that has the objective of increasing use of protection during sex. Because of the diverse interventions that could meet this criterion, it would be essential to categorize the various intervention characteristics that could affect the outcome, such as contact time, type of contact, content, determinants targeted, and intervention objective (for example, protection against pregnancy or against HIV and other STIs). These variables could even be used in a meta-analysis multivariate procedure (Cooper & Hedges, 1994) to help sort out the relative effectiveness of intervention features. Another approach might emphasize population characteristics, modifying the broad criterion to this: any educational intervention (regardless of techniques, number of sessions, or aim) with low-income Mexican American boys in middle school or junior high. Alternatively, the health educator could set narrow boundaries based on other considerations, such as any educational intervention conducted with a subpopulation identified by their stage of change, for example, precontemplators, that is, individuals who are not thinking about beginning to use condoms.

Specific criteria are not sufficient, however. They must also be appropriate for the questions that are guiding a particular search. A group of planners, for example, is interested in developing a sun protection intervention. The planners already know that sales of sunscreens with a sun protection factor (SPF) of 15 are a significant part of total product sales and that the low SPF is not optimal for protection. The planners want to answer the question: What methods and strategies have been used to influence substitution of higher SPF sunscreen for lower SPF sunscreen at the marketplace? When the group set criteria that the search had to cover sunscreen product substitution, group members could find no references. They had to find other criteria that would ensure the inclusion of studies related to their question. They brainstormed other health protection substitutions, such as interventions to discourage use of full-fat dairy products in favor of low-fat or nonfat products, and they broadened their criteria. After reading about such interventions, the group came up with the strategy of point-of-purchase labeling (for example, shelf labels) of both desirable and undesirable products, with the insight that such strategies and the implied method, mild fear-arousal with simultaneous presentation of a means of reducing risk, might be usefully applied to one segment of the intended group, individuals who already purchase sunscreen (Palmer, Mayer, Eckhardt, & Sallis, 1998).

Another example of relevance, one in which a conceptual bridge had to be built to a different population, comes from the PANDA case study (Chapter Thirteen). The problem was to develop an intervention to reduce the number of women who stop smoking successfully during pregnancy but who return to smoking after giving birth. One issue was that no such programs had been reported in the published literature. In this case, the task of identifying populations that would be relevant meant that those populations would have to be conceptually relevant and not necessarily the same type of population (pregnant women who had quit smoking). The development team asked for suggestions from colleagues who knew the smoking literature, which led to a search of the literature on preventing return to smoking by victims of heart attacks who, largely because of hospital policy, were not able to smoke while they were hospitalized. The idea of stopping smoking because of a temporary, acute event and external constraints had some parallels; on the other hand, the population was older and primarily male. Nevertheless, some of these studies revealed the importance of attributions for stopping smoking and other hypotheses regarding moderating variables that would be important in developing the PANDA intervention (Mullen et al., 1999). Thus, fortunately, relevance may be achieved without a perfect match to the topic, population, or question at hand.

Finally, planners should set criteria with conservation of resources in mind: They should be efficient. For example, health educators who are researching what's been tried to reduce HIV and STI risk among adolescents who attend school unfortunately could encounter studies of motivational speeches at school assemblies or of pamphlets mailed to every student's home. Scanning abstracts from a vaguely defined computer search sounds easy, but such searches frequently turn up hundreds of abstracts. Efficient criteria will help the planner conserve resources that will be better spent comparing the relative effectiveness of a limited set of interventions with the highest promise of success, lowest cost, or widespread use.

A Validity Framework for Judging Evidence

We have presented the development of search criteria in terms of their relation to the study question. A second method for establishing criteria is a validity framework suggested in the synthesis literature by Bryant and Wortman (1984), advocated by Mullen and Ramirez (1987), and used by others (Mullen et al., 1997). This framework is based on the four major types of validity described by Cook and Campbell (1979) and updated by Shadish et al. (2002):

- Construct validity
- External validity
- Statistical conclusion validity
- Internal validity

These validity types form two pairs.

Construct and external validity refer to the validity of generalizations about a study's intervention and measurement operations from a study's samples, settings, and times to the populations, setting, and times of interest. The concept of generalization captures the question: Is this study really relevant to the study question? To use a common, problematic example, a search of the intervention literature for studies evaluating the use of peer educators will net a wide range of definitions of the term *peer educator*, from individuals that students select from their own group to honors students that school personnel select as exemplary in their eyes. If the results of this broad range of operations are to be interpreted in designing an intervention, it is essential to be clear about what constitutes the construct of *peer*. Inevitably, some of the studies should be discarded from the group, lest their negative results be misunderstood as indicating that peer educators are ineffective.

The second pair of validity types, statistical conclusion and internal validity, pertain to the study design and refer to the validity of conclusions about the strength and direction of relationships. We discussed some aspects of this issue earlier in this chapter. In the particular case of a review of evaluation studies of intervention effectiveness, criteria set by important review groups may be informative. They have set different criteria for rigor of design, depending on the level at which the intervention took place, so that the searchers recognize that communitywide interventions will be evaluated with different designs than are individual-level interventions. For example, the hierarchy of study designs used by the Community Preventive Services Task Force puts other controlled trials together with randomized trials in the best evidence category and recognizes the value of repeated measures and time series designs in the next highest category of evidence—with both categories included in the evidence base (Briss, Zaza, et al., 2000; Briss et al., 2005). The same strategy was adopted earlier by the Centers for Disease Control and Prevention HIV-AIDS Prevention Research Synthesis project (Sogolow, Peersman, Semaan, Strouse, & Lyles, 2002).

Creating Evidence Tables

A systematic review calls for a systematic presentation of the data from each of the studies consulted. Evidence tables are an essential method for describing the findings of a review and for drawing conclusions about a particular body of evidence. They do not have to be complex, but they do require some thought about how to organize the information in ways that are consistent with the questions that users want to answer. In a typical table, the individual studies form the rows, and the columns organize study characteristics and findings. The variable that creates the most important subgroups of studies is usually the row subheading. For example, in the systematic review of trials of youth sexual–risk behavior interventions, about half of the studies took place in regular school classes, while the others were in such places as juvenile detention centers, boys' and girls' clubs, and on school grounds in all-day workshops led by nonschool personnel on Saturday (Table 2.3) (Mullen, Ramirez, Strouse, Hedges, & Sogolow, 2002). Because these two groups of studies differed widely in the selection of participants and in the constraints on the content of the intervention and in other factors that could potentially affect the study outcome, in-classroom and out-of-classroom studies formed subgroups of the rows (studies) of the evidence table. One more variable, the broad category of intervention (behavioral versus social) as defined in the project (Sogolow et al., 2002), was combined with the setting to create row subgroups that shared two characteristics, as behavioral interventions in classroom.

Column headings display the study citation, important characteristics of the intervention (for example, content, theoretical method, strategies, timing, duration), study participants (for example, age, gender, ethnicity), and study design (for example, individual or group assignment, number of participants or groups, random or other method of assignment), the presence or lack of a treatment in the control or comparison group, measures (for example, timing of follow-up), and outcomes (effect sizes or another descriptor). In the evidence table for sex risk behavior, a structured description of the intervention content formed an important narrative cell, followed by the number of sessions—a widely varying study characteristic and the most readily available indicator of intervention intensity. Sample characteristics at baseline included an important contextual variable, the percentage of study participants who had ever had sex. Because the majority of the studies had a design in which clusters, such as schools, classes, residential centers, and the like, were the unit of intervention and assignment, the number of units, unit of assignment, and method of assignment (random, not random) were stacked in a single column. Findings based on several types of measures, condom use, number of partners, and a behavioral index made up of the two variables were all converted to odds ratios with 95 percent confidence intervals (see the following section on effect size), and findings from studies with insufficient information to calculate an odds ratio were summarized qualitatively with text (Mullen et al., 2002).

Another example of an evidence table is from a review of predictors. Table 2.4 shows the inevitable variation in studies that are purportedly answering similar questions. In this case the review question was: What are the predictors of returning to smoking postpartum by women who stopped smoking during

TABLE 2.3. PROFILE OF PRIMARY STUDIES AND STUDY OUTCOMES BY INTERVENTION TYPE AND SETTING.

	Intervention Characteristics			Baseline Characteristics				Design Characteristics			Findings ORs (95 Percent CI)[a]		
Author (Year)	Content	Sessions (Number)	Percent Female	Age (Years)	Race and Ethnicity (Percent)[b]	Sex Ever (Percent)	Number of Units No Study Groups Assignment	Follow-Up (Months)	Comparison Group Treatment	Sex Without Condoms	Partners (Number)	Mixed Behavioral Risk Index
Behavioral Interventions in Classroom (k = 6)												
Boyer, Shafer, & Tschaan (1997)	Risk enhancement; interpersonal, personal, and technical skills with practice	< 6	59	< 16	45 Asian 16 Black 20 Hispanic 10 White	22	4 schools 2 groups Not random	≤ 1	Some	1.53 (.70–3.33)	1.11 (.60–2.03)	—[c]
Fisher, Fisher, Bryan, & Misovich (1998)	Risk enhancement; interpersonal and technical skills with practice; social support; other content	≥ 6	58	< 16	0 Asian 57 Black 28 Hispanic 5 White	50	4 schools 4 groups Not random	≤ 1	None	.24 (.04–1.50)	—	—
Kirby, Korpi, Barth, & Cagampang (1997)	Risk enhancement; interpersonal skills with practice; technical skills without practice	≥ 6	54	< 16	13 Asian 9 Black 64 Hispanic 5 White	8	102 classes 2 groups Random	≥ 4	Some	1.28 (.68–2.39)	—	—
Levy, Perhats, Weeks, Handler, Zhu, & Flay (1995)	Interpersonal and personal skills with practice; other content	≥ 6	50	< 16	0 Asian 60 Black 12 Hispanic 24 White	35	15 school districts 3 groups Random	≤ 1	None	.46 (.10–2.04)	.94 (.65–1.35)	—

Siegel, DiClemente, Durbin, Krasnovsky, & Saliba (1995)	Interpersonal and personal skills without practice	≥ 6	≈ 50	< 16	41 Asian 38 Black 9 Hispanic 6 White	23	3 schools 2 groups Not random	2–3	None	—	—	.59 (.23–1.47)
Walter & Vaughn (1993)	Risk enhancement; interpersonal and technical skills with practice; referrals	≥ 6	58	< 16	0 Asian 37 Black 35 Hispanic 0 White	33	4 schools 2 groups Not random	2–3	None	—	—	.67 (.50–.90)

Behavioral Interventions Outside Classroom (k = 9)

Jemmott, Jemmott, & Fong (1992)	Interpersonal skills with practice; technical skills without practice	< 6	0	< 16	100 Black	83	n = 79 Individuals 2 groups Random	≤ 1	Some	.30 (.12–.75)	.59 (.30–1.15)	—
Jemmott, Jemmott, & Fong (1998)	Risk enhancement; interpersonal and technical skills without practice; responsibility enhancement; self-esteem	< 6	53	< 16	100 Black	25	n = 66 Individuals 3 groups Random	2–3	Some	.53 (.38–.76)	—	—

[a] Odds ratio (OR) <1 = less risk

[b] Percentages might not total 100 because of rounding or "other" category.

[c] No data reported for this outcome.

Source: Adapted from Mullen, Ramirez, Strouse, Hedges, & Sogolow, 2002, pp. 96–97.

pregnancy? The studies were first divided based on study design, with one subgroup of the cross-sectional surveys with retrospective reports of smoking during pregnancy and the other subgroup of prospective studies that recruited quitters during pregnancy and followed them postpartum. The prospective study group is shown in Table 2.4 (Mullen, 2004). Further, important features in interpreting these studies were the researchers' definitions of "quitting during pregnancy," ranging from self-report of one week or longer to a biologically confirmed quit by the twentieth week with no disconfirming biologic samples before the birth. Because of this variation, the small number of studies in the prospective subgroup (four) and the large number of independent variables that were tested in these studies, in this table the studies formed the columns, and the predictor constructs were grouped for the rows. The definitions of pregnancy and postpartum smoking and study population could be highlighted with the study citation in the column heading. The number of rows could have been much larger if all the specific variables had been listed in separate rows; in service of analytic lumping, the reviewer grouped the specific variables in more general constructs—marital status or weight, for example, with the particular operations for a study described in the cell formed by the construct row and study column.

Creating and Interpreting Effect Sizes

The reviewer of the literature needs to know how strong the relationship is between a barrier or predictor and the health behavior of interest, not only whether it is statistically significant. The latter tells us that the relationship is unlikely to be the result of chance alone. Traditionally, researchers have used a .05 alpha level, which means the chance of finding a relationship when there is none is 1 in 20. Two erroneous conclusions are often made: (1) that $p > .05$ indicates no effect and (2) that $p < .05$ indicates an effect of significant magnitude (Rosnow & Rosenthal, 1996; Rosnow, 2003; Rosenthal, Rosnow, & Rubin, 2000). But statistical significance is influenced by both the magnitude or strength of the relationship and the sample size. Therefore an effect size is needed to interpret whether the results from significance tests are practically meaningful (Cohen, 1992). Additionally, because effect-size measures are based on standard metrics, they are useful for making comparisons across studies. For example, the three right-hand columns in Table 2.3 show the findings for all of the studies as odds ratios and 95 percent confidence intervals.

Meta-analytic methods have grown in popularity and are used to combine primary studies to estimate an overall effect size across studies, with individual studies weighted according to the precision of their point estimate, usually a function of sample size. (Compare the width of the confidence intervals (CI) for the studies by Boyer, Shafer, Tschann, 1997, CI = .70–3.33, and Jemmott, Jemmott, & Fong, 1998, CI = .38–76.) Meta-analysis methods can be used to test whether different study factors, such as design or gender of the sample, influenced the effects observed. Meta-analyses are useful both for synthesizing potentially conflicting results in the literature but also for correcting for errors in the primary studies such as small sample size, measurement error, range restriction, and artificial dichotomization (Hunter & Schmidt, 1996).

Although previous manuals had encouraged researchers to report effect sizes along with each test of statistical significance, the 5th edition of the *Publication Manual of the American Psychological Association* has made the reporting of effect sizes a requirement (American Psychological Association, 2001). Many individual journals have made similar changes to their publication policies, and guidance for achieving this aim is available (Vacha-Hasse & Thompson, 2004; Trusty, Thompson, & Petrocelli, 2004; Cortina & Nouri, 2000; Grissom & Kim, 2005; Rosenthal, Rosnow, & Rubin, 2000; Capraro & Capraro, 2002).

Each statistical test has its own effect-size index, which can generally be classified into three major types: standard mean differences, strength of association (correlation), and ratios (relative risk, odds ratio) (Rosnow, 2003). When primary studies do not report measures of effect size for each of their outcomes, various formulas can be used to estimate the effect size from other information provided (for example, means, standard deviations, cell sizes) (Cooper & Hedges, 1994; Hunter & Schmidt, 1996; Lipsey & Wilson, 2001), and web-based or Excel-based calculators are now available on the Internet.

Effect sizes can only be interpreted within the context of the literature to date in the particular field of study, because no single effect size is appropriate or meaningful for all situations. Health promoters interpreting effect-size estimates should not simply follow Cohen's rules of thumb (1988, 1992) for small, medium, and large effect sizes. An effect size that is not sufficiently large may suggest that more research is needed to examine additional factors, because differences between groups have not been fully accounted for (Rosnow & Rosenthal, 1996).

Planning and Executing a Search

We provide the bare essentials of thinking about search strategies. Most searches will benefit from consultation from the start with a good reference librarian.

Using the Research Question to Plan a Search.

To plan a search of the literature, the health promoter will use the key components of the research question to locate and select studies. Determining how many search components are needed to turn up the desired literature may take some trial and error. Too many parameters such as "condom use," "adolescents," "behavioral intervention," and "HIV" and "randomized clinical trial" together may cause the searcher to miss studies, while "condom use" alone will turn up hundreds of irrelevant reports.

TABLE 2.4. PREDICTORS OF POSTPARTUM SMOKING FROM MULTIVARIATE ANALYSES.

	McBride, Pirie, & Curry, 1992	O'Campo, Faden, Brown, & Gielen, 1992	Mullen, Richardson, Quinn, & Ershoff, 1997	Kahn, Certain, & Whitaker, 2002
Citation				
N, Source	106, age ≥ 18, Minnesota clinics, 95 percent white	100 white, 148 black, private and public clinics, Baltimore	127, California HMO, age ≥ 18; entered care ≤ 17 weeks	1249, 1988 National Maternal and Infant Health Survey
Pregnancy[a] Measures	Validated quit ≥ 28 weeks; average quit = 32 weeks	Quit when planning pregnancy or first trimester	Validated quit ≤ 20 weeks + no positive urine before birth	Quit ≥ 1 week
Postpartum[a] Measures (Timing; Percent Smoking)	Validated, < vs. ≥ 7 cigarettes past week (6 weeks, 24 percent)	Resumed smoking by postpartum interview (6–12 weeks, 28 percent white, 46 percent black)	No puffs vs. any (6 months, 37.1 percent)	Not smoking vs. smoking now (17 ± 5 months, 72.0 percent)
Sociodemographic Characteristics				
Age	+[b] younger[c] relative risk (RR)[d] = .9 (.9, 1.0)	0[e] < 25 years vs. ≥ 25 OR = 1.1 (.5, 2.7)	0 < 20 vs. 20–29 vs. ≥ 30	0 < 20 vs. ≥ 30 OR = .5 (.2, 1.1)
Race/Ethnicity	n/a	0 black vs. white OR = 1.5 (.6, 3.7)	0 black vs. white vs. other	0 Hispanic vs. white OR = .6 (.3, 1.1) 0 black OR = 1.6 (1.0, 2.7)
Marital Status	0 married or living as RR = .4 (1.0, 2.4)	0 unmarried OR = 1.2 (.4, 3.4)	0 married	0 formerly married OR = 1.9 (1.0, 3.7)
Current Pregnancy				
Live Births	0 previous pregnancies OR = 1.4 (.6, 3.2)	0 1 vs. ≥ 2	0 first child 0 first pregnancy	0 ≥ 1, OR = .7 (.5, 1.0)

Mother's Health	n/a	0 "excellent" 0 nausea often	n/a
Alcohol	n/a	n/a	0 ≥ 1 per week OR = 1.0 (.4, 2.1)
Weight	+ likely return to desired weight ≤ 6 months postpartum RR = 1.2 (.9, 1.8) 0 satisfied with weight postpartum 0 importance of return to prepregnancy weight	0 "too much" weight gain in pregnancy 0 "overweight" postpartum 0 exercise ≤ once a week postpartum	0 > 40-pound gain OR = .8 (.6, 2.1)
Smoking	0 weeks abstinent	0 quit before first visit + puffs third trimester rate ratio = 2.4 (1.2, 4.6)	n/a
Smoking Context	+ partner smokes RR = 2.7 (0.7, 4.0) 0 most close family smoke vs. few vs. 0 RR = 1.9 (1.0, 3.5)	+ partner smokes rate ratio = 2.6 (1.6, 4.2) + > 2 friends smoke rate ratio = 1.9 (1.2, 3.1) 0 smokers in household 0 ETS exposure > 1 hour per day	+ ≥ 1 household smoker OR = 3.9 (2.6, 6.0)

[a] Unless otherwise noted, all measures are self-reported.

[b] Statistically significant positive (+) or negative (−) independent effect for the variable as described in the cell, based on a multivariate analysis.

[c] If the variable was dichotomized, there is no reference value ("vs").

[d] Relative risk, odds ratio, and rate ratios (confidence interval) adjusted for all other variables reported for the study that also have an effect measure.

[e] 0 = Non-significant independent effect in bivariate analysis, if no measure of effect is provided. If a measure of effect is shown in the cell, then the variable had a nonsignificant independent effect in a multivariate analysis.

Source: Mullen, 2004, pp. S217–S238.

Electronic Databases. Index Medicus (MEDLINE, published by the U.S. National Library of Medicine) and Excerpta Medica (EMBASE, published by Elsevier) index health care journals. PubMed (http://www.ncbi.nlm.nih.gov) is an online MEDLINE database that also includes citations that are not yet indexed. EMBASE is often considered to be the European counterpart to MEDLINE, and even though the journals indexed overlap considerably, most searches are not complete without using both databases.

Search Terms. With an eye to the research question, the planner should determine which search terms to use. Both MEDLINE and EMBASE have standardized subject terms (not the same in the two indexes) that indexers assign to articles. These terms are a good way to find articles because researchers may use different terms to describe the same concepts. That being said, however, the terms are only as good as the indexer and may not be a foolproof way of finding articles. A simple strategy can be to identify a small set of articles pertinent to the question using the standardized terms and then note both common text words and the words that indexers have used for the articles. The Cochrane Collaboration suggests that an electronic search strategy should usually have terms related to (1) the health problem, (2) the intervention, and (3) the types of studies able to answer the question (Alderson, Green, & Higgins, 2004). A note of advice: Seek a librarian with expertise in electronic searching to design the search strategy. You can save yourself a world of time and effort.

Nonelectronic Search Strategies. Other search mechanisms, especially ones that would discover unpublished sources, are available and should be used when comprehensiveness is a major concern. For example, this would be a major issue when trying to determine whether certain types of interventions are effective because of the bias toward the publication of significant findings (Dickersin, 1997). Other ways of searching include hand searching, which involves looking through a journal's contents. Conference proceedings are particularly important to hand search because they contain studies that are not yet (and perhaps never will be) more widely published. Abstracts have been shown to be the source of about 10 percent of the studies reviewed in Cochrane Reviews (Mallet, Hopewell, & Clarke, 2002). A particularly effective method is checking reference lists of relevant articles (especially review articles) and then checking the *Science Citation Index* for references to identified articles. Talking to colleagues is also very helpful.

Documenting the Strategy. Like any other study, a literature search should be something that others can replicate. For electronic searches the planner will want to keep the following information about the search (Alderson et al., 2005):

- Databases searched
- Name of the host and version
- Date of the search
- Years covered by the search
- Complete search strategy used, including all search terms
- Language restrictions of the search

The planner will also want to document nonelectronic strategies, including hand searching, conference proceedings, and efforts to identify unpublished sources. The planner should document a brief summary of procedures for each source.

Skills for Core Processes: Qualitative and Quantitative Methods

The program planner who practices Intervention Mapping often uses a process referred to as triangulation. Triangulation brings findings from multiple data sources, methods, and investigators together, allowing planners to increase the validity of their findings (Thurmond, 2001; Manfredi, Lacey, Warnecke, & Balch, 1997; Koelen, Vaandrager, & Colomer, 2001; Levy et al., 2004; Nakkash et al., 2003; Goldberg, Rudd, & Dietz, 1999).

Quantitative methods such as surveys and disease registries enable the planner to estimate the incidence and prevalence of health problems and related behaviors in the at-risk population. Quantitative methods also enable estimates of the strength of the correlation of determinants with risk behaviors. On the other hand, qualitative methods such as ethnographic interviews (McDonald, Thomas, & Eng, 2001; Braithwaite, Bianchi, & Taylor, 1994), focus groups (Basch, 1987; Kreuger & Casey, 2000; Gilmore & Campbell, 1996), the problem-posing methods from Freire's education for critical consciousness (1973a) (Wang, Cash, & Powers 2000), critical incident technique (Witkin & Altschuld, 1995; McNabb, Wilson-Pessano, & Jacobs, 1986), and nominal group process (Delbecq, 1983; Delbecq, Van de Ven, & Gustafson, 1975; Dewar, White, Posade, & Dillon, 2003), and photovoice (Wang, 2003) help health educators to understand communities, health problems, behavioral and environmental causes, and determinants from the perspectives of the people involved. For example, Nakkash and colleagues (2003) describe their formative work on a community-specific cardiovascular disease (CVD) prevention program as using triangulation of sources and methods. First, they surveyed 2,486 community residents to describe the "what": the problem of CVD and its risk factors of sedentary lifestyle, obesity, and smoking. Following the survey, planners conducted eight focus groups to identify the "why":

barriers and facilitators to a CVD-preventive lifestyle. Finally, members of the community coalition served as natural discussion groups to garner information on the "how": issues of interventions and their feasibility and sustainability.

Qualitative and quantitative approaches to problem analysis are not simply two different techniques to arrive at the same answer. They are essentially different, in their philosophical origins and approaches to knowledge. They are so different that some researchers would argue that they cannot be used together. The health education field, although historically dominated by quantitative work, is adopting a paradigm integrating the two approaches. We think that using the two approaches or methods together produces a more usable, comprehensive, and accurate assessment product based on better information about and from members of the intended community throughout Intervention Mapping. However, each approach must be used under its own assumptions, and the reader should look to other texts for instruction in quantitative (Shadish et al., 2002) and qualitative (Berg, 2003; Miles & Huberman, 1994; Patton, 2001; Wolcott, 1994) methods.

The methods in each tradition differ in the research object and in design, data collection, and analysis (De Vries et al., 1992). In general, qualitative approaches are the following (Patton, 1990, 2001):

- Inductive
- Discovery oriented
- Iterative
- Question and theory generating
- Subjective and valid with the self as the instrument
- Not usually amenable to counting
- Case-oriented
- Not generalizable

Quantitative methods are the following:

- Deductive
- Theory verification–oriented
- Question answering
- Objective and reliable, subject to reliable counting
- Population-oriented
- Generalizable

Steckler, McLeroy, and colleagues (1992) present a useful diagram of four ways that qualitative and quantitative methods can be used in program evaluation (Figure 2.3). Those research models are equally appropriate in other steps of

FIGURE 2.3. INTEGRATING QUALITATIVE
AND QUANTITATIVE METHODS.

Model 1
Qualitative methods are used to help develop quantitative measures and instruments.

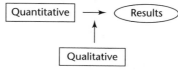

Model 2
Qualitative methods are used to help explain quantitative findings.

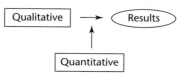

Model 3
Quantitative methods are used to embellish a primarily qualitative study.

Model 4
Qualitative and quantitative methods are used in an equal and parallel way.

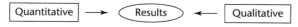

Source: Adapted from Steckler, McLeroy, et al., 1992.

Intervention Mapping. In Model 1 the planner uses qualitative data-gathering methods, such as focus groups, nominal group technique, observation, ethnographic interviews, or semistructured interviews, in order to begin to hear perceptions of health problems, related behavioral and environmental causes, determinants, and quality of life in the community.

After the qualitative phase, surveys are developed to document the prevalence of the issues that emerged from a qualitative study (Thompson, Gifford, & Thorpe, 2000; Desvousges & Frey, 1989; O'Brien, 1993). Beginning with qualitative methods gives the planner a better chance of asking pertinent and intelligible questions during a survey phase. This sequence of using qualitative methods to inform survey design may also enable the researcher to develop new hypotheses or to refine hypotheses before the quantitative phase of the research. For example, O'Brien (1993) used focus groups in a study of the social relationships of gay and bisexual men to inform questionnaire development. He learned the language that the men in the groups used to discuss relationships and sexual experiences. His discussions led to a survey that contained careful definitions of the terms *primary relationship* and *safer sex*, two very important and potentially ambiguous concepts. The focus groups also led to the addition of several questions that the larger study would address.

In another example, Thompson and colleagues (2000) studied an Aboriginal community in Melbourne to better understand the role of food among those at high risk for diabetes. They found that food was clearly segregated by its social meaning into three types: family food, fast food, and diet food. Understanding more about the meaning and context of food, and especially that diet food was isolated from the normal meaning of food, contributed to the development of a culturally grounded epidemiologic risk-factor survey for the next phase of the study.

In Model 2 planners use qualitative techniques to better understand the meaning of their quantitative findings. In a needs assessment, health educators might use census or epidemiologic data to describe the health problem, behavioral or environmental risk, or determinants and then conduct qualitative research to better understand the perceptions of the at-risk group (Wingood, Hunter-Gamble, & DiClemente, 1993). For example, Wingood and colleagues used the focus group technique to better understand the determinants of HIV-associated risk behaviors in African American women. They found that the women they spoke with could bring up with their partners the conversational topic of safer sex, but they could not effectively negotiate condom use. Demanding that a partner use condoms could imply lack of trust in a relationship, violate a woman's conflict-avoiding stance, and prove difficult or even dangerous to a woman.

In Model 3 the health educator conducts a qualitative study in order to document the problems or needs in a community and then uses quantitative data to verify and establish the magnitude of the primarily qualitative needs assessment. Bartholomew and colleagues (2005) recently completed interviews of 180 older adults to assess barriers to immunization in older adults of three racial or ethnic groups. Once the barriers were described, they then conducted a prevalence survey to document the distribution of the various barriers in the different groups (Bartholomew, Selwyn, Livoti-Debellis, Chronister, Sablotne, Hodgson, et al., 2005).

In Model 4 both qualitative and quantitative methods are used in parallel to shed light on an issue or a problem (Saint-Germain, Bassford, & Montaño, 1993). For example, Levy and colleagues (2004) used data sources at the individual, family, community, and public policy ecologic levels to describe the influences on CVD and diabetes in two Chicago communities. They conducted focus groups, administered the Behavioral Risk Factor Surveillance Survey (BFRSS), and used a community mapping tool (Curtis & Jones, 1999). These three methods used together increased their understanding and helped them guard against misinterpretations in any one source. For example, members of the community mapping team interpreted the absence of gang tags (graffiti) as positive, whereas community members explained that without gang tags, residents cannot discern safe areas from those that are unsafe.

De Vries and colleagues (1992) suggest an iterative or spiral approach for use in intervention development. In their description a planner alternates qualitative and quantitative approaches both in the development of interventions and in their evaluation. Figure 2.4 presents the approach to alternating qualitative and quantitative methods used in the various stages of the development of the Cystic Fibrosis Family Education Program (CF FEP). Qualitative and quantitative processes were alternated and used to inform each phase of the program development, evaluation,

FIGURE 2.4. INTEGRATING METHODS: CF FEP.

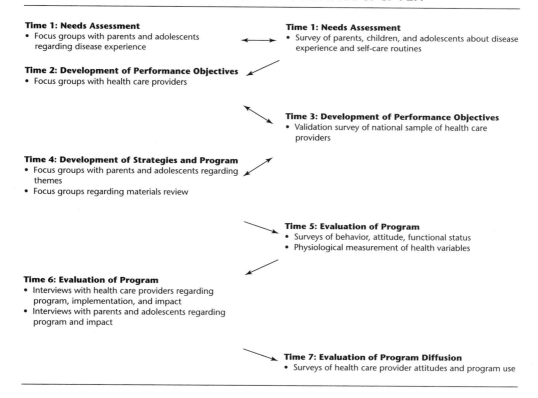

Time 1: Needs Assessment
• Focus groups with parents and adolescents regarding disease experience

Time 1: Needs Assessment
• Survey of parents, children, and adolescents about disease experience and self-care routines

Time 2: Development of Performance Objectives
• Focus groups with health care providers

Time 3: Development of Performance Objectives
• Validation survey of national sample of health care providers

Time 4: Development of Strategies and Program
• Focus groups with parents and adolescents regarding themes
• Focus groups regarding materials review

Time 5: Evaluation of Program
• Surveys of behavior, attitude, functional status
• Physiological measurement of health variables

Time 6: Evaluation of Program
• Interviews with health care providers regarding program, implementation, and impact
• Interviews with parents and adolescents regarding program and impact

Time 7: Evaluation of Program Diffusion
• Surveys of health care provider attitudes and program use

and diffusion process (Bartholomew et al., 1997; Bartholomew, Czyzewski, Swank, McCormick, & Parcel, 2000; Bartholomew, Seilheimer, Parcel, Spinelli, & Pumariega, 1989; Bartholomew, Sockrider, et al., 1993). Dodge, Janz, and Clark (2002) provide another excellent example of the iterative use of qualitative and quantitative methods.

Core Processes Applied to Determinants: The Case of Child Restraint Devices

The first case concerns the determinants of child restraint devices before the use of car seats for children was both legislated and normative.

Posing the Question

When this project took place, the Dutch Foundation for Traffic and Safety had had a long history of educating parents on the consistent use of child restraint devices (CRDs) to protect young children against the consequences of an automobile accident. However, children were still injured in a high number of car accidents. The Foundation board engaged a consulting team to find out why their educational programs did not work and how to improve them. When the team began thinking about the problem as conceptualized by the Foundation board as a program failure, the members realized that no question regarding causes of the problem had ever been asked. The team asked a first question: What are the reasons parents do not always use CRDs?

Brainstorming Provisional Answers

The consulting team brainstormed a provisional list of answers to the question of why parents don't use CRDs (Table 2.5). They discussed the many possibilities shown in the table, including parents' perceptions that the child is not at risk and practical problems, for example, that parents actually own a CRD but do not use it consistently because they have two cars or because more than one child has to be transported at the same time. This discussion highlighted the difference between acquisition of a CRD and its use.

Searching the Literature

After the brainstorming, the consultants searched the literature on CRD use. Because they found very little CRD research, they also looked for information on seat-belt use. They found information on prevalence of injury related to use and

TABLE 2.5. PROVISIONAL LIST: DETERMINANTS OF LACK OF CRD USE.

Original Provisional List	Additions from Empirical Literature and Theory	Additions from New Data
Parents' educational level	Outcome expectations—prevention of harm (replaces "lack of knowledge of CRDs")	Delete "Lack of exposure to information that CRDs prevent serious injury to children"
Practical problems, such as two cars or children riding in the cars of others		
CRD expense	Risk perception—unrealistic optimism based on perception of control, stereotypical perception of the type of parents who run risks, overestimation of comparable efforts to take precautions (replaces "underestimation of child's risk in an accident" and "underestimation of being in an accident")	Self-efficacy specifically for handling the child's disruptive behavior
Lack of exposure to information that CRDs prevent serious injury to children		Outcome expectations regarding handling the child's disruptive behavior
Lack of knowledge of CRDs—understanding that CRDs are especially meant to avoid serious injury from accidents		Skills to handle the child's disruptive behavior
Underestimation of child's risk in an accident		
Underestimation of being in an accident	Perception of control	
Overestimation of benefits of other ways of protecting child, such as holding or using seat belts	Delete "parents' educational level"—not a process, no evidence	
	Self-efficacy and behavioral effectiveness	
	Subjective norms	
	Parents have tried and stopped using CRDs	

nonuse of CRDs and seat belts (Johnston, Hendricks, & Fike, 1994; Kaplan & Cowley, 1991; Russell, Kresnow, & Brackbill, 1994), risk factors (Thompson & Russell, 1994), and the effects of regulation (Escobedo et al., 1991; Walter & Kuo, 1993). However, they learned little about their actual question and almost nothing that brought theory to bear on the problem.

Accessing and Using Theory

The consultants had already entered the literature through their topic and had found little that was theory-related. Using the concept approach and working from their provisional list, the team pursued the concepts of risk and found that theories such as the Protection Motivation Theory (PMT) (R. Rogers, 1983), HBM (Janz & Becker, 1984), SCT (Mullen, Gottlieb, Biddle, McCuan, & McAlister, 1988; Allen & Bergman, 1976; Goebel, Copps, & Sulayman, 1984), and risk perception theories (Weinstein, 1988) have explained other risk-taking phenomena (see Chapter Three). Based on Weinstein's Precaution Adoption Process Model (PAPM), the group thought that parent drivers might believe they control children's risks, as parents who plan to hold children in case of an accident might. The parents' beliefs might partly be due to stereotypical perceptions of parents who run risks. They also might overestimate their efforts to take precautions compared to other parents (Van der Pligt, Otten, Richard, & Van der Velde, 1993). From this review the consultants clarified the concept of risk on their provisional list (see Table 2.5).

Other risk perception models, such as the HBM (Becker, 1974a, 1974b; Janz & Becker, 1984; Rosenstock, Strecher, & Becker, 1988) and the PMT (R. Rogers, 1983), cover more than just risk perception. They helped the consultants describe under what circumstances parents' risk perceptions might lead to adequate action. The threat of risk may motivate parents to acquire and use a CRD, provided that they are convinced that such a seat constitutes an effective means of protection (behavioral effectiveness) and that they believe they are able to acquire such a seat and use it consistently (self-efficacy).

The consultants then approached theory using the general theories approach and reviewed Ajzen's Theory of Planned Behavior (TPB) (1991). The consultants explored social influence effects and found the possible importance of subjective norms (the partner's expectation that a CRD should be used and the motivation to comply with the reference person), as well as the overt behavior of other parents (modeling). In addition, the team assumed that a number of people would be motivated (favorable attitude) but probably would not be able to adopt the behavior (low self-efficacy).

The consultants then applied McGuire's Persuasion Communication Matrix (PCM) (1985) to address their question of why parents don't use CRDs. The team used the communication matrix to list a series of possible reasons for lack of use, from a first exposure to CRDs to the maintenance of use:

1. Attention: They have never heard of CRDs.
2. Comprehension: They do not understand the purpose of the CRD.
3. Attitude: They are not convinced of the advantages of the CRD.
4. Social support: The partner does not consider it necessary.
5. Self-efficacy: It is too much trouble when they have two cars.
6. Behavioral change: They do not think of it at the moment.
7. Behavior maintenance: They tried but do not sustain the behavior.

Some of these reasons had been included in the provisional explanations, but some were new. From this list the team added behavior maintenance to the provisional list.

Addressing Needs for New CRD Data

The consultants needed to collect new data after reviewing the literature for three reasons: (1) They might not know enough about the possible reasons for parents not using CRDs. (2) They do not know which are the most important determinants or how determinants are expressed in their particular population. (3) They had uncovered little empirical evidence supporting the theoretical constructs they had discussed as possible determinants of CRD.

The consultants were fortunate to have the time and resources to conduct a study (Pieterse, Kok, & Verbeek, 1992). They questioned parents at the exit from a parking lot about their reasons for acquiring and using CRDs (or not). The consultants were guided by the constructs on their provisional list, particularly the components of attitudes derived from Ajzen (1988). They paid particular attention to practical barriers. In short, the researchers discovered that safety of the children (risk perception, attitude) is the main reason that parents acquired CRDs and that more than 90 percent of parents were positively disposed to use CRDs.

However, the most important reason for not using the CRD for these parents was the child's response. When a child became restless and disruptive while riding in a seat, parents often did not know how to cope with the behavior and consequently removed the child from the seat. In theoretical terms the child's behavior is punishing to the parents for using the CRDs. These negative consequences may result in low perceived self-efficacy to continue the behavior. The consultants realized that the impact of emphasizing the risks of not using CRDs without raising the parents' skills and self-efficacy for dealing with unruly children might have a contrary effect. Research has demonstrated that increasing negative outcome expectations, or risk perception, under conditions of low self-efficacy results in a condition, similar to learned helplessness, in which individuals are unlikely to acquire and perform the behavior (Hale & Dillard, 1995). In this case, high self-efficacy for using CRDs and managing children would be an important requisite for effectively coping with risk information. Again the consultants began to think about solutions. With this additional information, they realized that the intervention emphasis should be on increasing self-efficacy for managing children in CRDs rather than only on risk perception. From new research the group substantially improved its provisional explanations.

Formulating the Working List of Answers

In general, it seems that the determinants of CRD use center around motivational issues related to risk perception and around self-efficacy for dealing with the behavior of a child restrained in a car seat. The group first deleted some items based on the criteria of process and plausibility. For example, the explanation that more highly educated parents use CRDs more often than do less educated parents does not reflect a process. A process explanation might be that the more highly educated parents are relatively more convinced of the usefulness of CRDs. Another might be that they are relatively less concerned about the high price of these seats. But the group had no data on which to base either explanation. In terms of plausibility, the group knew that in health centers parents consistently receive health education about CRDs. Therefore, most parents being unaware of the existence of CRDs would not be a very plausible explanation.

The consultants completed the provisional list of answers and discussed which were the most important predictors of CRD use and which the most changeable. They evaluated all determinants on the list in terms of relevance and changeability (see Table 2.6). The last three determinants are the most relevant: outcome expectations, skills, and self-efficacy for handling the child's disruptive behavior. Skills and self-efficacy needed to be improved. Outcome expectations for using CRDs were also relevant, and this determinant needed to be reinforced. All the relevant determinants seemed to be changeable, so the consultants selected these four determinants for a future intervention.

The resultant causal diagram (Figure 2.5) depicts their decisions. As the figure indicates, it seemed to the consultants at the end of their analysis that parents obtain and try to use car seats because they perceive their children to be at risk from car accidents. However, parents discontinue use because they are unable to manage their children's behavior. Therefore, intervention solutions might increase

TABLE 2.6. SELECTING DETERMINANTS: RELEVANCE AND CHANGEABILITY.

Determinants from List *(Selected Determinants in Italics)*	Relevance	Changeability
Practical problems	+	+
High cost of CRDs	0	+
Overestimation of the benefits of other ways to prevent harm	+	+
Outcome expectations (prevention of harm)	++	++
Risk perception–unrealistic optimism	+	++
Perception of control	+	+
Subjective norms	++	+
Self-efficacy for handling child's disruptive behavior	+++	++
Outcome expectations for handling child	+++	++
Skills for handling child's disruptive behavior	+++	++

FIGURE 2.5. CAUSAL MODEL FOR CRD USE.

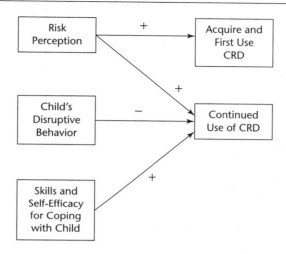

the intensity of the risk perception while providing skills and self-efficacy for managing children who are riding in car seats.

Core Processes Applied to Methods: HIV Infection in Drug Users

The second case addresses methods for changing safe-sex behavior in drug users.

Staff in the local health services in Maastricht and Heerlen in the Netherlands were worried about the increase of HIV infection in drug users. AIDS is still an incurable disease, and moreover, HIV-positive drug users appeared to be the source of the majority of heterosexual HIV transmissions in the Netherlands (van Empelen, Kok, Schaalma, & Bartholomew, 2003; van Empelen, Kok, van Kesteren, et al., 2003). The major behavioral risk factors for HIV infection among drug users are needle sharing and unprotected sexual intercourse (especially for noninjecting drug users). Most HIV-preventive activities for this group have been directed at safe needle use, with some success. Unprotected sexual intercourse was becoming a more important HIV transmission route within the drug-using community but had not received much attention from prevention workers (van Empelen, Kok, van Kesteren, et al., 2003).

The local health services in Maastricht and Heerlen partnered with a national Dutch organization, Mainline, which supports drug users with information on health and quality of life, and researchers from Maastricht University to form a project team.

The project team performed a needs assessment and set a priority to promote condom use (van Empelen, Kok, Schaalma, et al., 2003). They came up with a list of program objectives that can be summarized as follows:

1. Drug users are aware of their personal risk of HIV (risk perception) when not using condoms.
2. Drug users see the benefits and accept the disadvantages of condom use (attitude).
3. Drug users perceive and receive positive social influence for condom use (norms, environment).
4. Drug users are confident that they are able to use condoms consistently and correctly (self-efficacy and skills).

Posing the Question: Risk Perception

The next task for the team was to find appropriate methods and strategies to address each objective. They knew that methods would be different for the various objectives, and they ordered the objectives based on determinants. The first question for the team was this: How can we influence personal risk perception of HIV infection with drug users? The remainder of this example presents the process the team used for finding answers to this question. Where the team members in the CRD example looked for answers to the question of explaining behavior, the team working on HIV infection was looking for answers to questions concerning how to change determinants of behavior. Team members started with a question about risk but then turned to other questions about attitude, norms, and self-efficacy. Here we address only the question about changing risk perception because the process is the same for all determinants.

Brainstorming Provisional Answers for Methods

Team members shared their experiences and knowledge about various aspects of the question. Safe sex was not an issue in the literature on drug users and HIV prior to this work, so most of the brainstorming was based on knowledge from working with drug users. The brainstorming led to a provisional list of answers (Table 2.7). The group identified the possibilities of giving drug users information about risks, confronting drug users with their own risk, trying to scare them with

TABLE 2.7. PROVISIONAL LIST: METHODS FOR CHANGING RISK PERCEPTION AMONG DRUG USERS.

Original Provisional List	Additions from Empirical Literature	Additions from Theory
Information	Community-based program	Consciousness raising (replaces "information")
Confrontation with own risk	Peer education	
Feedback on what might go wrong without planning	Role-model stories	Dramatic relief, anticipated regret
	Free condoms	
Fear tactics		Reevaluation
Hand out condoms		Personalizing risk of own behaviors (replaces "confrontation with own risk")
		Self-efficacy
		Skills training
		Modeling
		Scenario information (replaces "feedback on what might go wrong without planning")
		Delete "fear tactics"

the horrible consequences of getting HIV, and giving drug users feedback on what might happen if they did not anticipate and plan for safe sex. Finally, some team members were in favor of handing out condoms in order to ensure that drug users would have condoms available when needed.

Reviewing the Literature: Risk Perception

Once the project team generated a provisional list of methods, team members searched the literature using the topic approach for information on methods for changing HIV risk perception among drug users. The team found only limited literature on sexual risk taking among drug users (van Empelen, Kok, van Kesteren, et al., 2003). Therefore, they also looked at studies on safe needle use among drug users and studies about safe-sex promotion among groups other than drug users. Articles about promoting safe sex in drug users presented only general descriptions and categorized interventions as small-group, community-level, and individual interventions (van Empelen, Kok, Schaalma, et al., 2003; van Empelen, Kok, van Kesteren, et al., 2003). From the descriptions, it seemed that interventions were seldom tailored to psychosocial determinants. The few interventions that had been shown to be effective did not rely on a single theory but made use of multiple theories and aimed at changing relevant determinants. For changing risk perception, effective community-level interventions with drug users often used peer education, role-model stories, and free condoms (van Empelen, Kok, Schaalma, & Bartholomew, 2003; van Empelen, Kok, van Kesteren, et al., 2003). The team added these methods to the list of provisional methods.

Accessing and Using Theory: Risk Perception

In reviewing the literature through the topic approach, the team had found some studies that were theory-related. The theories that were applied to the CRDs could be characterized as theories of the problem, explaining behavior; here the team was looking for theories of action, changing behavior (Glanz et al., 2002) (see also Chapters Three and Four). The HBM describes more about the determinants related to the health behavior than about methods for change. However, the planners interpreted the model to indicate that messages in their program should include four types of information: personal risk, severity of outcomes, effectiveness of preventive behavior, and self-efficacy about preventive behavior. The team learned from the HBM that risk information needs to be accompanied by behavior information, especially self-efficacy improvement and skills training.

The Transtheoretical Model (TTM) describes the stages that people go through when changing their behavior. The model starts with raising awareness to move people from precontemplation to contemplation and suggests various methods that may change risk perception. Consciousness raising stimulates finding and learning new facts, ideas, and tips to support a behavior change. Dramatic relief involves experiencing the negative emotions that go along with the behavioral risk. Environmental reevaluation helps people to realize the negative impact of the unhealthy behavior and the positive impact of the healthy behavior.

The AIDS risk reduction model suggests that people go through stages to recognize and label their own risk, make a commitment to reduce risk, and take preventive action. Possible influences to bring people to recognize their risk include knowledge of risk behaviors, personal risk perception, positive attitude toward HIV preventive actions, and social norms. However, the model does not say much about methods to reach those objectives.

SCT provides many suggestions for methods to change behavior, with one very effective method being modeling, for example, observing models becoming aware of their personal risk for HIV infection. While adding this method to the provisional list, the team discussed the importance of taking the theoretical parameters into account (Kok et al., 2004). For example, modeling can be a very effective method for change when interventions use a coping rather than a mastery model, reinforce the model for the desired behavior, teach skills for performing the behavior, and choose a model with whom the priority population can identify (see Chapter Seven).

Working from the provisional list, the team pursued the concept approach to finding theory. First, team members clarified what they meant by the terms *information* and *confrontation*. They decided that the TTM methods of consciousness raising, dramatic relief (including anticipated regret), and reevaluation were closer to what the group thought would work than were information and confrontation. Elaborating on dramatic relief, the team realized that this method relates to the method of anticipated regret: asking people to imagine how they would feel after a risk behavior, for instance, after having had unsafe sex with someone they later discover is HIV-positive (Richard, Van der Pligt, & de Vries, 1995). The team added anticipated regret to the list of methods (see Table 2.7).

Team members moved to the concepts of risk and feedback to drug users about what can go wrong without planning. They found risk perception and risk communication theories such as PMT (R. Rogers, 1983), PAPM (Weinstein & Sandman, 2002), and theoretical ideas such as unrealistic optimism (Weinstein, 1988) and scenario-based risk information (Hendrickx, Vlek, & Oppewal, 1989). PMT, like the HBM, suggests giving information on personal risk and effective behavior alternatives, and providing skills for action. The PAPM proposes stages of change with a focus first on people (see Chapter Three) who are unaware of a problem. The group discussed raising awareness by mass media and using interpersonal influence to promote decision-making. The team members noted that theories that define stages of change all suggest that interventions that are matched to the stage will be more effective. At this point, though, they did not know how they might tailor the messages or methods to the stage.

The team also considered the concept of unrealistic optimism, in which people think that they run less risk than others because they perceive that they protect themselves better than others do and they have a stereotypical image of high-risk people (for example, prostitutes). To improve risk perception, the team thought it might give information about the ways other drug users protect themselves and about the risks of certain behaviors, such as judging a partner's HIV status on the basis of external characteristics even though one actually cannot see from these whether a partner is HIV-positive or -negative.

A further consideration for methods discovered by the team is that theories on risk perception and decision making suggest that people base their risk judgments on the frequency of the outcome plus images of the ways in which a particular outcome may occur (Hendrickx et al., 1989). Therefore, team members proposed scenarios that include both a cause and an outcome rather than ones presenting the outcome by itself. They thought, for example, that they could present credible scenarios in which drug users have good intentions (without planning), but the good intentions alone do not prevent them from being in situations that lead to unprotected sexual intercourse.

The team then returned to the discussion of scare tactics or fear-arousing communication. Some team members argued that the only way to attract people's attention is to confront them with very threatening information about the severity of AIDS. Others argued that, although popular, these methods have not been shown to be effective and could even be countereffective if not designed using theoretical principles. A number of theories explain that making people afraid will lead to preventive behavior only when the individuals have an effective alternative behavior in combination with the necessary skills and confidence to perform the alternative behavior (Witte & Allen, 2000). If these conditions are not present, the person who is confronted with a fear-arousing message may take up defensive reactions and ignore the risk altogether. The team summarized the literature as suggesting a focus on personal risk and training in effective alternative behavior and skills, while avoiding messages that dramatize the severity of the risk outcome by itself (Ruiter, Abraham, & Kok, 2001). The team decided to follow this advice.

Peer education and community-based interventions refer to the process of interpersonal communication and social influence: how people are influenced by communicating with their peers and members of their community. Most of the theories that the team looked at were at the individual level, focusing on changing perceptions of drug users. But the social environment is often crucial for individual changes, as the team learned from SCT. Perceptions of risk are influenced by social norms. The team now linked methods for promoting risk awareness with methods for promoting social norms for avoiding risk and using condoms.

Posing the Question and Brainstorming: Social Norms

The team decided to proceed with brainstorming the question: How can we influence social norms for condom use among drug users? One of the first issues that came up in the brainstorming was the question: Is it at all possible to change social norms among drug users? The answer from the field workers was positive; they recalled how quickly social norms within the drug-using community had changed with respect to using clean needles.

The brainstorming led to a provisional list of methods (Table 2.8). Based on the earlier analysis of the literature, team members remembered that peer education and community-based interventions were potentially successful. The field workers suggested outreach interventions, combining peer education with professional counseling.

TABLE 2.8. PROVISIONAL LIST: METHODS FOR CHANGING SOCIAL NORMS AMONG DRUG USERS.

Original Provisional List	Additions from Empirical Literature	Additions from Theory
Peer education	Modeling	Vicarious learning, modeling
Community-based interventions	Ownership	Behavioral journalism approach
Outreach interventions	Mobilizing supportive social norms	Mobilizing social networks
Professional counseling	Resistance to non-supportive social norms	Interpersonal skills training
Communication with peers		Persuasive communication

Reviewing the Literature: Changing Social Norms

Again, the team turned to the limited number of studies on this topic (van Empelen, Kok, van Kesteren, et al., 2003) and learned that interventions directed at social norms may either mobilize social norms when these are supportive of the desired behavior or train the target group to resist social norms when these are not supportive. A second outcome of the review was the insight that social norms are often more positive, and social support more available, than people think, and the intervention has only to stimulate people to talk about the behavior with their peers to find this out. The group expanded the list of provisional answers.

Indeed, the shift in social norms within the drug-using community with respect to safe needle use was documented, as was the potential positive effect of peer education and community-based interventions (Coyle, 1998). Some of the community-based interventions included outreach activities that attempted to create ownership of the program by the drug-using community. Modeling was the most frequently used method in interventions. The field workers in the project group warned the team that, in their experience, interventions that used only persuasive communication by peers were not effective; drug users became distrustful of the motives of these so-called peers. However, peer models in a supportive environment, with outreach activities involving professionals and the target group, were promising.

Accessing and Using Theory

The team looked again at the literature on promoting safe sex among drug users (topic approach) and found that interventions that use modeling to change social norms refer to SCT and highlight the importance of reinforcement of role models

(Baranowski et al., 2002). In fact, through modeling, people learn what behaviors are being reinforced in their social environments.

The team was particularly interested in the SCT method of behavioral journalism. Interventions based on behavioral journalism use role-model stories based on authentic interviews with the priority group to illustrate and reinforce the behavior of interest. These are distributed through networks within the community.

From the provisional list, the team pursued the concepts (concept approach) of communication with peers, mobilization of social networks, and community-based interventions to promote adoption of new behavior. The key word here is *adoption*, because that concept brings the team to the Diffusion of Innovations Theory (DIT) (E. M. Rogers, 2003). According to DIT, new behaviors are more likely to be adopted when they are relatively advantageous, compatible with prevailing social norms, and simple to use and when they yield observable, tangible outcomes. Methods to change prevailing norms are mobilizing social networks, modeling, and increasing interpersonal skills. The team added these methods to the list. The theory also suggests that early adopters may function as role models for later adopters, confirming their selection of behavioral journalism (van Empelen, Kok, Schaalma, et al., 2003).

At this point, the group accessed theories using the last approach: general theories and looked for theories that might provide some further insight into change for either risk perceptions or social norms. What seemed to the group to be missing at this point was any reference to the persuasive communication process. Team members explored both the Persuasive Communication Matrix (W. J. McGuire, 1985) and the Elaboration Likelihood Model (ELM) (Petty & Cacioppo, 1986a, 1986b; Petty, Barden, & Wheeler, 2002). What the team learned from McGuire's matrix was the importance of deciding very carefully how the content of the message, the source of the message, and the communication channel would have an optimal fit with the target group of drug users, in order to promote exposure, attention, comprehension, and yielding. However, the team realized that the idea of behavioral journalism that came up in an earlier stage could be an answer to exactly this challenge.

The ELM was also helpful because it warns against optimism with respect to persuasion effects. Sometimes people process information through the central route, carefully looking at the arguments, but other times they use the peripheral route, meaning that they are influenced by relatively irrelevant aspects of the message, such as the attractiveness of the source or the print quality of the materials. This model suggests two ways to promote central processing: making the message more personally relevant and unexpected and repeating the message.

Identifying and Addressing Needs for New Data

The team members considered how certain they were about the validity of their answers so far. They decided that they were quite sure they had identified the most relevant and potentially most effective methods methods.

However, they decided that it was necessary to pilot-test all materials in the intervention to make sure that they had indeed taken into account the theoretical conditions for all methods (see Table 2.9). For example, after being exposed to role models, drug users should recognize that the model was a coping model, that the model was reinforced, that the modeled behavior is feasible, and that they could identify with the model. Also, after being exposed to role-model stories with scenario information, they should appreciate that the scenario is credible and realistic, that it has a cause and an outcome, and that they themselves could have ended up in a comparable situation, against their initial intentions.

Formulating Working Answers for Risk and Shifting Norms

The team summarized members' ideas on effective methods for influencing drug users' risk perceptions and social norms. For risk perception, relevant methods were scenario information and anticipated regret, and for changing norms, role modeling on condom use and anticipating risky situations, interpersonal communication, and outreach. All methods could be part of a behavioral journalism approach, working with authentic role-model stories in combination with outreach activities in the community. The team decided to select methods for the program by evaluating all the listed ideas on relevance and changeability (see Table 2.10). The determinants selected earlier were risk perception (relevance: +) and social norms (relevance: ++). The most effective methods seemed to be behavioral journalism, including role-model stories; anticipated regret; personalizing

TABLE 2.9. THEORETICAL CONDITIONS FOR METHODS.

Theoretical Methods	Conditions for Methods
Scenario information	Cause and effect, easy to imagine
Anticipated regret	Easy to imagine
Modeling	Identification, reinforcement, coping, skills
Behavioral journalism	Adequate role models from the community

TABLE 2.10. SELECTING METHODS: RELEVANCE AND CHANGEABILITY.

Methods from List (Selected Methods in Italics)	Relevance	Changeability
Hand out condoms	+	+++
Community-based program, ownership	++	+
Peer education	+	+
Role model stories	++	+++
Consciousness raising	+	+
Dramatic relief, anticipated regret	+	+++
Reevaluation	+	+
Personalizing risk of own behaviors	+	+++
Scenario information	+	+++
Skills training	++	+
Modeling	++	+++
Outreach interventions	++	++
Mobilizing social norms, social networks	++	++
Resistance to social pressure	++	++
Communication with peers	++	++
Behavioral journalism	++	+++
Interpersonal skills training	++	+
Persuasive communication	++	++

risk; scenario information; modeling; social norms; resistance to social pressure; and persuasive communication. The team decided to distribute the behavioral journalism materials using an outreach intervention by field workers, who also promote communication with peers, mobilize social networks, and hand out condoms.

Translating these methods into practical strategies and an integrated program is a creative process that will lead to a specific intervention with well-produced materials. However, it is important to make sure that the original methods with the conditions that are necessary for the methods to be effective are still in place (Kok et al., 2004). Remember that we limited our discussion to risk perception and changing norms. In reality, we also would have applied the core processes to find methods for changing attitudes and for promoting self-efficacy and skills.

CHAPTER THREE

BEHAVIOR-ORIENTED THEORIES USED IN HEALTH PROMOTION

Reader Objectives

- Describe a social ecological approach to health-related behavior and environments
- Identify and use behavior-oriented theories and theoretical constructs to explain behavior of at-risk individuals and agents at each ecological level
- Select behavior-oriented theoretical constructs to inform methods to change determinants of behaviors

The purpose of this and the next chapter is to identify theories that are applicable to health education and promotion problems. The primary focus is health-related behavior, the supporting social and physical environments for this behavior, and the environments related directly to health. We review theories that help to explain or to change the health-related behavior of the at-risk group or the behavior of individuals who are responsible for health-related aspects of environments. In this chapter we review behavior-oriented theories: theories in which understanding and changing human behavior are the major processes of interest. In Chapter Four we focus on environment-oriented theories: theories in which understanding and changing environmental conditions for health are the major processes of interest.

In Chapter One we explained that health promoters start with an assessment of health and quality-of-life problems, describe who has the problem and who is at risk for it, and explore behavioral and environmental conditions that contribute to the problem. Planners then must search for causes of the behaviors or conditions and choose methods to influence those determinants. In this process the health educator can look to theory for help with the following:

- Describing the at-risk and intervention groups
- Understanding the health-promoting behavior and environmental conditions
- Describing possible determinants of both risk and healthful behavior and environments
- Finding methods to promote change in the determinants, behavior, and environmental conditions

Table 3.1 presents some uses of theory in health promotion planning and examples of theories for each use. An understanding of theoretical constructs applicable to health promotion can broaden the planner's ability to complete all the planning tasks.

TABLE 3.1. WHEN TO USE THEORY IN INTERVENTION PLANNING.

Task	Examples
To describe and select intervention groups	Stages of Change Models Diffusion of Innovations Theory Agenda-Building Theory
To define behaviors	Theories of Self-Regulation Organizational Development Theory Diffusion of Innovations Theory
To define environmental conditions	Social Cognitive Theory Theories of Social Support Organizational Development Theory
To understand possible determinants of behavior and select intervention targets	Theory of Planned Behavior Social Cognitive Theory Health Belief Model
To choose methods to promote change and to translate theoretical methods into practical strategies	Persuasion Communication Matrix Organizational Development Theory Conscientization

Perspectives

In this chapter we focus on the importance of an ecological understanding of health problems and their solutions. We also encourage planners to break away from their habitual approaches to developing programs and to use a variety of theories to enhance their practice.

Ecological Interventions

Once a health educator understands a health problem, including the behavior, the environmental conditions, and their determinants, the next use of theory is to identify intervention levels and methods. The choice of environmental levels can depend on identifying the level of the problem and its determinants as individual or interpersonal, organizational, community, societal or supranational environment (Steuart, 1993; L. Richard, Potvin, Kishchuk, Prlic, & Green, 1996). (See Figure 1.1.) The model by L. Richard and colleagues also assumes that the ultimate focus of health promotion interventions is the health of at-risk individuals, even though the intervention may not directly address these persons. We discussed various paths by which interventions might work in Chapter One.

As shown in Figure 3.1, we look at the determinants of the behavior of both the at-risk population and of agents who influence the environmental conditions that influence the at-risk individuals' behavior and health. Questions regarding what influences the behavior of individuals and environmental decision-makers increase our understanding of the determinants of these behaviors as in the following nutrition example. At the individual level, we might ask: What influences the individual to eat more fruits and vegetables? At the higher levels, we might ask: What influences the decision-making agent to make the healthful decision? Why, for example, do the decision-making agents buy fruits and vegetables for the home, purchase or modify healthful foods for the school cafeteria, develop feature articles on how families are changing the way they eat for health and well-being, or pass legislation subsidizing healthful school meals for low-income children? As with individual health behavior, agent decision making is influenced by personal and external determinants. At the higher-order system levels, however, the complexity increases, and different variables come into play. First, the decisions related to environmental changes are often made by larger bodies, such as school boards or legislatures, composed of environmental agents. Emergent processes unique to each level constrain the behavior of individual agents, and the action by the larger body changes the environmental condition. Second, individuals at the higher levels act within roles. We discuss this more fully in Chapter Four.

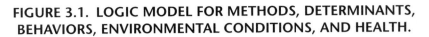

FIGURE 3.1. LOGIC MODEL FOR METHODS, DETERMINANTS, BEHAVIORS, ENVIRONMENTAL CONDITIONS, AND HEALTH.

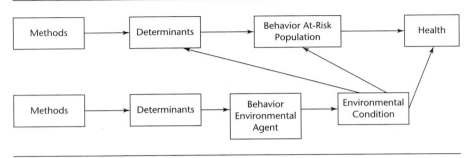

Figure 3.1 presents a logic model for the relationships among theoretical intervention methods, determinants, behaviors, environmental conditions, and health. Among the contributors to health are the behavior of the at-risk group and environmental conditions. We search for determinants of the at-risk group behavior. We also search for agents that could act on the environmental condition and for the determinants of these agents' behavior. Finally, we identify theoretical methods and practical strategies that might influence both sets of determinants. As we ask the questions pertinent to each step in the logic model, theories will be one source of answers.

Political, Practical, and Habitual Influences on Intervention Planners

Health educators often work within settings, such as public health departments, schools, work sites, hospitals, or community agencies with particular missions and funded projects. Also, health educators may have specialized training or particular skills and talents that influence them to focus on a particular level or type of intervention, for example, community organization, media advocacy, small-group facilitation, or counseling. In addition, health educators often have their own favorite theories or ways of understanding health problems, risk factors, and determinants. Health educators and those who direct their work may intervene habitually with methods and strategies based on the one or two theories with which they are most comfortable. However, using a favorite explanation for every problem and intervening in every situation with the same method may be like knowing Grandmother's recipe for only one type of soup. The recipe is familiar, and sometimes it works, depending on what ingredients the cooks have at hand

and on their skill in the kitchen. But sometimes it doesn't work, and the cook needs both new ingredients and new recipes (Kok, Schaalma, Ruiter, van Empelen, & Brug, 2004).

In this chapter and the next, we present brief reviews of selected theories to give the reader an overview of the use of theories in health promotion. A description of each theory is followed by a summary of the theory's contribution to our understanding. More than anything, this chapter should alert the reader to the need to delve further into theories (Conner & Norman, 1996; R. J. DiClemente, Crosby, & Kegler, 2002; Gilbert, Fiske, & Lindzey, 1998; Glanz, Lewis, & Rimer, 2002; Minkler, 1997a).

In our summaries of the theories, we indicate the contribution of each theory to the following:

- Intervention groups: How and why do we differentiate members of a group of program participants into subgroups?
- Behaviors: How can we describe relevant behaviors for intervention?
- Environments: What are relevant environmental conditions for interventions?
- Determinants: What are the determinants of behavior and environments?
- Methods: What are appropriate methods to create change in determinants of behavior and environment?

Box 3.1. Mayor's Project

The mayor's planning committee found itself in a predicament. Everyone in the planning group had his or her favorite recipe for intervention. They had brainstormed some determinants of violent behavior and used the core processes (Chapter Two), but the health educator seemed hard-pressed to get the group members to see beyond their own pet theories. Some group members, including the health educator's supervisor, thought that theoretical eclecticism was forbidden to academically well-trained individuals. What to do? The health educator was determined to help the group construct a useful model of the problem. She had successfully used this approach in her previous job. She wanted to help the group develop a hypothetical causal model of the problem and then to think about intervention levels and methods. But how would she get the group to come along?

The health educator approached the group management problem as she would any other planning process question. What were the determinants of the group members' behavior? What was holding them back from really working with theory? The health educator brainstormed a list: Some group members knew only one theory; some wanted a venue for theory testing; others just wanted to get the intervention done and weren't sure that theory was helpful at all. Looking at this short list, the health educator decided that if the group members had better knowledge of multiple theories and of ways to apply them to the problem of violence, they might be more willing to continue with the planning process.

The health educator took all the literature that the group had gathered and sorted the articles first by the underlying theories and then by whether the articles discussed causes of violence or interventions. To each set of violence-related articles, the health educator attached an article that reviewed the relevant theory. Small groups from the task force (which contained twenty-five members) then were assigned to summarize a set of articles and present them to the larger group. The small groups answered the following questions: What do these articles say about the causes of violent behavior? Which of these causes are psychosocial determinants of individual behavior, and which are environmental conditions? If the causes are environmental, does the article contain data or theories that suggest the determinants of the environmental cause? With crossed fingers and held breath, the health educator awaited the results.

Overview of Theories

We have organized this and the next chapter by arranging theories by ecological levels and describing representative theories. In this chapter we present individual- and interpersonal-level theories, and in Chapter Four we review environmental theories as presented in Table 3.2 (R. J. DiClemente et al., 2002; Glanz et al., 2002; McLeroy, Bibeau, Steckler, & Glanz, 1988). This presentation is a simplification because theories often link systems levels. For example, Social Cognitive Theory (SCT) includes determinants from the social and physical environments, and the Theory of Planned Behavior (TPB) has as a key predictor of behavior the normative expectations of others (in the environment) as perceived by the individual. The health educator can look outside the more obvious boundaries of a particular theory and work with the causal determinants from higher-order levels. For example, a planner working with concepts from the TPB could think about the sources of the normative beliefs and, moving to a more sociological frame of reference or to communications theory, look at how social norms are created and transmitted. Thus, even though individual theory may not

TABLE 3.2. THEORIES ARRAYED BY LEVEL.

Problem and Intervention Levels	Theories
Chapter 3 Individual	Learning theories Information-processing theories Health Belief Model Protection Motivation Theory Theory of Planned Behavior Goal-related theories Habitual behavior Transtheoretical Model Precaution Adoption Process Model Attribution Theory Relapse Prevention Theory Persuasion Communication Model Elaboration Likelihood Model Theories of Self-regulation
Interpersonal environment	Social Cognitive Theory Diffusion of Innovations Theory
Chapter 4 Interpersonal environment Organization	Theories of social networks and social support Stage Theory of Organization Change Organizational Development Theory Interorganizational Relationship Theory
Community	Models of community organization Conscientization
Society and government	Agenda-Building Theory Policy Windows Theory

explicitly link levels of analysis, a planner can use an eclectic approach to theory to develop hypothetical causal maps of how systems work to determine specific behavior or environmental changes.

In addition, many theories are potentially applicable to all ecological levels and also to the understanding and promotion of program adoption and implementation. When available, we give examples of applications outside each theory's more common application. The TPB, for example, is often applied to individual health behavior (Godin & Kok, 1996) but can be applied to explain the behavior of environmental agents such as politicians (Flynn et al., 1998; N. H. Gottlieb et al., 2003) and program implementers as well (Paulussen, Kok, Schaalma, & Parcel, 1995).

From Theories of the Problem to Theories of Action

Some theories are primarily explanatory (that is, theory of the problem); some are primarily focused on change (that is, theory of action); and others have elements of both types. The link between theories of the problem and theories of action is often not very clear. Some theories provide both explanations of behavior and ways to change it; some theories give only one or the other. Theories of the problem suggest *what* to change; theories of action ideally tell *how* to change it. In practice, the jump from objectives about what to change to methods for creating change may sometimes be difficult.

Witte (1995) suggests an interesting approach to this challenge. She organizes the results of the determinants analysis in a list of relevant categories (for example, beliefs, social influences, self-efficacy, values) and then decides which determinants need to be changed, which need to be reinforced, and which need to be introduced. For example, in a program for HIV prevention for Hispanic men, the men's belief that condoms were unclean needed to be changed; the importance of family values needed to be reinforced; and the belief that condoms could prevent HIV infection needed to be introduced.

Intervention Mapping suggests a link between theories of the problem and theories of action through the link between the two steps: matrices of change objectives and theoretical methods. Theories of the problem help planners formulate appropriate objectives ordered by *determinant;* theories of action point to *methods* that can change the determinants. For example, using the TPB, the educator may have formulated a program objective in terms of perceived social expectations. Using SCT, the educator may select modeling and guided practice to improve resistance to social pressure (Hardeman et al., 2002). In discussing the theories, we pay attention to methods for change—such as cues, feedback, implementation intentions, persuasion, tailoring, and modeling—that may be linked to only one theory. In Chapter Seven we provide lists of methods, ordered by the determinant that these methods are able to influence. In the discussion of each theory in the current chapter, we first present its contribution to understanding behavior and then its contribution to methods.

Cultural Sensitivity of Theories

Resnicow, Braithwaite, Dilorio, and Glanz (2002) summarize the current state of the art with respect to cultural sensitivity. Cultural sensitivity is defined by two dimensions: surface and deep structures. Surface structure involves matching intervention materials and messages to observable, superficial (but important) characteristics of a priority population. This may involve using people, places, language, music, food, and clothing familiar to, and preferred by, the target audience. Surface structure refers to how well interventions fit within a specific culture. Deep structure involves incorporating the cultural, social, historical, environmental, and psychological forces that influence the target health behavior in the proposed population. Whereas surface structure generally increases the population's receptivity to or acceptance of messages, deep structure imparts salience.

Our position is, with Resnicow and colleagues (2002), that theories are descriptions of processes that can be generalized over groups and over cultures. The weight of each different variable in a theory, for instance, the TPB, may vary over cultures as it varies over subpopulations. In fact, the theory predicts this. The variables in the Health Belief Model (HBM), for instance, have been useful in understanding health behavior in various cultures, even though the relative importance of the variables varies (Janz, Champion, & Strecher, 2002). The specific content of the variables within theories—surface as well as deep structure variables—may be very different. For instance, the meaning of health, environmental factors, life styles, determinants of behaviors, media characteristics, or settings may differ across cultural groups. In other words, beliefs may be different, but beliefs will influence behavior. Self-efficacy expectations may vary, but they will still predict behavior changes. The role models used in interventions will reflect the cultural background of the intended audience, but modeling should be a useful method for change in any culture. Self-management of diseases will take different forms, but the process of monitoring, evaluating, and moving to action is the same (Kaaya et al., 2002; Manders et al., 2001; Meyer-Weitz, Reddy, van den Borne, Kok, & Pietersen, 2003; Laver, van den Borne, Kok, & Woelk, 1997; Reddy, Meyer-Weitz, van den Borne, & Kok, 2000). So the challenge of cultural sensitivity is in determining the content and the application, not in deciding whether the use of theory in general is advantageous.

Theories and Common Constructs

Because theories reflect reality, many of the ones we discuss have similar elements but use different names for the constructs. Some agreement is emerging in the health promotion and behavioral health fields regarding important theoretical constructs across theories. For example, five major behavioral science theorists agreed on a set of eight variables as key determinants of behavior (Institute of Medicine, 2002b; Fishbein et al., 2001; Fishbein, 1995):

1. The person has formed a strong positive intention (or made a commitment) to perform the behavior.
2. No environmental constraints make it impossible for the behavior to occur.

3. The person has the skills necessary to perform the behavior.
4. The person believes that the advantages of performing the behavior outweigh the disadvantages (attitude).
5. The person perceives more social (normative) pressure to perform the behavior than not to do so.
6. The person perceives that performing the behavior is more consistent than inconsistent with his or her own self-image (personal norms, personal standards).
7. The person's emotional reaction to performing the behavior is more positive than negative.
8. The person perceives that he or she has the capability to perform the behavior under a number of different circumstances (perceived self-efficacy, perceived behavioral control).

The five theorists saw the first three variables as necessary and sufficient and the remaining five as influencing the strength and direction or intention.

Many of these eight key variables have different names in different theories. For example, attitudes are termed outcome expectations and expectancies in social cognitive theory, benefits and barriers in the HBM, behavioral beliefs and values in the TPB, and pros and cons in the Transtheoretical Model (TTM). Self-efficacy in SCT is very similar to perceived behavioral control in the TPB. Self-standards, perceived norms, and emotional reactions are seen by some theorists as self-representation (Abraham, Sheeran, & Johnston, 1998) and by others as included in outcome expectations and expectancies. Emotional reactions also come back as, for instance, dissatisfaction with self in self-regulatory theories or as anticipated regret in the TPB. When we discuss theories, we attempt to point out similar or related constructs from other theories.

Learning Theories

Learning theory is the foundation of most behavioral science theories. The term *learning* refers to any enduring change in the way an organism responds based on its experience (R. Schwartz, Wasserman, & Robbins, 2001; Westen, 1997). Learning theories assume that experiences shape behavior and that learning is adaptive. Two major learning theory perspectives are classical conditioning and operant conditioning.

Classical Conditioning

Classical conditioning is the learning of an association between an unconditioned stimulus (UCS) and a conditioned stimulus (CS). A UCS produces a response that does not have to be learned (for example, nausea as a result of chemotherapy). A conditioned response is a response that people learn as a result of the learned association of the CS with the UCS (for example, certain food aversions in cancer patients who have eaten the food while they experienced nausea during chemotherapy). The association is most effective when the time interval is short and the CS precedes the UCS. People generalize from one CS to another, in case of similar CSs (for example, one food to another food in the case of chemotherapy nausea; fear of one dog to fear of another dog), but they also discriminate between CSs (for example, fear of dogs but not of cats). Extinction (forgetting or unlearning) will occur when the stimuli are unpaired, when the CS is repeatedly presented without the UCS.

Operant Conditioning

Operant conditioning refers to the reinforcement of a behavior, resulting in more or less frequent occurrence of the behavior. Whether the behavior increases or decreases in frequency depends on the kind of reinforcer. Presentation of a stimulus that is rewarding (for example, a present) is positive reinforcement and makes a behavior more likely to occur, whereas the removal of a stimulus that is punishing (for example, silencing a loud noise) is termed negative reinforcement but has the same positive effect of making the behavior more likely to occur. Punishment, on the other hand, is the application of an unpleasant stimulus and decreases the probability that a behavior will recur.

There are several important characteristics of reinforcement:

- Reinforcement can be internal to the individual. For example, one may have positive feelings in response to performing a behavior.
- The more continuous the reinforcement schedule is, the faster the learning process. However, the more intermittent (less continuous) the reinforcement schedule is, the stronger the resistance to extinction of the learned behavior.
- A shorter time interval between the behavior and the reinforcer leads to a faster learning process.
- Reinforcers may vary among individuals and among cultures.

People learn to discriminate between situations that lead to reinforcement and situations that do not. People also learn to discriminate between behaviors that are reinforced immediately and those for which reinforcement is delayed (R. Schwartz et al., 2001). Most people will prefer a smaller immediate reward (tasty food) over the large delayed reward (good health). Interestingly, when forced to choose at an earlier stage when neither reinforcer will be immediate (both reinforcements are now delayed), most people will choose the larger delayed reward. It may thus be helpful to let people make an early commitment to healthier choices and help them develop self-control and skills to follow through.

The reinforcing effects of positive feelings form the basis for social cognitive theories. The basic assumption of social cognitive theories is that what is crucial to learning is not the environmental stimulus itself but the perception of the environmental stimulus. Perceptions of environmental stimuli include, for instance, outcome expectations and self-efficacy expectations (Bandura, 1986; Baranowski, Perry, & Parcel, 2002).

Zajonc (1980) showed that people become more positive about stimuli the more times they are exposed to them, even if they are not consciously aware of the process. This effect is probably limited to stimuli that are associated with a relatively neutral attitude at the start. One way to change people's attitudes in a more positive direction would be to expose them repeatedly to the new behavior or object. For instance, adolescents may be shown condoms repeatedly in classroom HIV-prevention education.

Methods from Learning Theory

Feedback and reinforcement have been shown to be effective methods to create changes in various determinants and behavior (Bandura, 1986; Mullen, Green, & Persinger, 1985; Mullen, Mains, & Velez, 1992). *Feedback* is information given to the learner regarding the extent to which the learner is accomplishing learning or performance (for example, reduction in fat intake, increase in aerobic exercise) or the extent to which change is having an impact (for example, reduction in blood pressure and weight, increase in physical conditioning). Feedback functions as a method for the learner to become aware of learning and performance, but it can also function to raise the learner's awareness regarding risk (Prochaska, DiClemente, & Norcross, 1997). *Reinforcement* is any component of the intervention that is designed to reward or punish the learner for the behavior after the learner has enacted the behavior. Bandura (1986) distinguishes among three types of directly applied reinforcement:

- Social reinforcement: praise from other people
- Vicarious reinforcement: observation of reinforcement of another who is functioning as a model for a behavior
- Self-reinforcement: giving oneself a reward

Another relevant prediction of learning theory is that one learns behaviors through positive reinforcements but very slowly unlearns them by lack of reinforcement (R. Schwartz et al., 2001). Letting people experience a lack of reinforcement or even negative outcomes will not immediately lead to their unlearning the behavior. People accept, for instance, losing a number of sports games (punishment) if they sometimes win (positive reinforcement). Experiencing that an unhealthy behavior sometimes has negative consequences may not have much influence as long as these behaviors sometimes lead to positive reinforcement. To stimulate unlearning of a behavior, it may be necessary to create a continuous lack of positive reinforcement.

Maibach and Cotton (1995) cite direct experience (enactment) as a method for changing outcome expectations. Modeling, as a form of indirect experience, is also powerful, especially if it is clear that the model's behavior resulted in a lower risk and positive health or other attributes. One caution is advisable when using direct experience as a method: Although this may enhance outcome expectations, direct experience may also lower them in the presence of unpleasant results from the behavior, such as discomfort during a mammogram or decreased sensation during condom use.

Summary: Learning Theory in Problem Analysis and Intervention Methods

- Intervention groups: groups of people with the same learning history
- Behaviors: all human behavior
- Environment: origin of many stimuli in physical and social environments
- Determinants: association of conditioned stimuli with unconditioned stimuli, responses to short-term positive reinforcement, negative reinforcement, punishment, attitude
- Methods: short-term dissociation or association of CS with UCS, feedback and reinforcement, short-term positive reinforcement for healthy behaviors, removal of punishing stimuli for healthy behaviors, punishment of unhealthy behaviors, direct experience, modeling, and repeated exposure

Theories of Information Processing

Conventional wisdom long held that giving people information could help them change their behavior and thereby solve health and social problems. However, knowledge does not generally lead directly to behavior change. Furthermore, ensuring that the members of the population attain knowledge is not necessarily an easy task. Theories of information-processing provide several concepts that suggest methods for successfully conveying information. Kools, Ruiter, van de Wiel, and Kok (2004) show that the health education field could make much better use of most of the evidence-based principles related to the coherence of textual material.

Chunking

Theories of information processing are concerned with how information is perceived, stored, and retrieved. Drawing from the Gestalt school of psychology (Koffka, 1935), These theories suggest that the senses perceive information in the context of what people already know. People perceive information actively to make sense of incomplete stimuli. For instance, someone who sees only eyes and a forehead will tend to perceive a face in order to complete the expected pattern in the act of perception. Theorists suggest that people then use their short-term memory, also called working memory, to complete the pattern. Working memory is a small "space," and its effectiveness can be increased by a method called chunking. A *chunk* is a stimulus pattern that may be made up of parts but that one perceives as a whole, for example, the term *FBI* (Federal Bureau of Investigation) or *ER* (emergency room). One might use chunking by assigning an acronym or a summary slogan to a process so that the entire process can be encoded into memory. For example, children in the asthma self-management program learned a rap song with the words "Watch, discover, think, and act" for the stages of self-management (see Chapter Twelve) (Bartholomew, Gold, et al., 2000; Bartholomew, Shegog, et al., 2000). Other slogans are "Stop, drop, and roll" for burn prevention; "Slip, slap, and slop" for use of hats and sunscreen, and "Stop, look, and listen" for traffic safety.

Advance Organizers and Images

Theories of information processing also present some ideas about how knowledge is stored in long-term memory. Long-term memory comprises information about events, concepts, and procedures (how to do something). The storage is described as a network of nodes (cognitive units of concepts and propositions) with links between the nodes that enable activation of a single node to spread to linked nodes (J. R. Anderson, 1983). Other theorists describe schemas that have both passive and active qualities. In other words, schemas contain related information that people can activate passively by perceiving an object or actively by consciously thinking of a group of concepts in order to compare a new perception with an existing category (Rumelhart, 1980). The idea of schemas suggests that a health message will be better understood if it activates existing schemas, if the receiver has a handy place to store the information and some conscious ideas regarding where the information is stored. An important method related to schemas is the advance organizer, a presentation of an overview of the material with familiar and concrete examples, that enables a learner to activate relevant schemas so that new material can be associated (Derry, 1984; Mayer, 1984). Kools, Van de Wiel, Ruiter, Crûts, and Kok (2005) show that graphic organizers, a form of advance organizers using images, could improve the understandability of health education materials substantially.

Others have shown that the use of imagery, the encoding of pictures with concepts to be stored in long-term memory, improves storage (Glover, Ronning, & Bruning, 1990). Hamilton and Ghatala (1994) relate the ancient Greek method of loci, in which orators mentally attached parts of long speeches to landmarks on well-known travel routes. One might imagine a patient educator helping a learner memorize a long self-care process by attaching the steps in the procedure to landmarks on a familiar daily route. Verbal images or analogies are also helpful for encoding information to long-term memory. If material is too foreign or discrepant, it will not be learned. Therefore, analogies to more common events, concepts, or processes may be a helpful method, especially if learners can be guided to create their own analogies.

Preexisting schema that contradict an informational message certainly may interfere with the encoding of the message for long-term memory. For example, a child who knows ivy as a plant may activate an entirely wrong schema when told in the hospital about an IV (intravenous administration of medication). In cultures in which the etiology of certain diseases is thought to be an imbalance in temperatures, an explanation of immunizations may not readily activate an appropriate schema, making it difficult for the individual to process the information.

Elaboration and Cues

Getting information into long-term memory is only the first part of learning. Usually, the learner must also get the information back out (retrieval). Retrieving information from memory is easier when the memory is a strong one. Strong memories are made when encoding requires effort. Promoting skills for information processing is a relevant issue in the Elaboration Likelihood Model (ELM), which provides methods for increasing these skills and also for increasing motivation to process information more carefully (Petty, Barden, & Wheeler, 2002). Effort requires the learner to add to the meaning of the material, to elaborate on it. Elaboration is particularly effective if it helps tie the information together. Rehearsal of information is more effective in promoting remembering when the rehearsal is elaborative, when the learner adds something to the information being learned. For example, a leader who is working on more effective group management and who wants to remember three new skills for the next meeting could simply rehearse the concepts of summarizing, gatekeeping, and connecting. However, once he or she is in the meeting, these abstract concepts may be hard to retrieve. Elaborating the concepts with images may help. The leader might use the visual image of a gate for gatekeeping, letting people and their ideas into the conversation. Adding to the image of the gate, the leader puts all the sheep (ideas) into the corral, summarizing and then pairing (or connecting) them up two by two. Elaboration could also be done with concepts. The group leader could take each concept and think of specific ways to implement it in the next meeting. Although it seems counterintuitive to have to learn more in order to remember, the method of elaboration does create stronger memories.

Providing cues is another method for getting information out of memory. For a cue to be effective, it should be present at the time of encoding and at the time of retrieval. Providing cues has many implications for health educators. For example, for teens who are learning to negotiate condom use, the cues present during learning and practice, such as what the partner says and the situation or setting, should be as similar as possible to what teens will actually encounter when they try to retrieve and apply the steps of negotiation (R. I. Evans, Getz, & Raines, 1991; Godden & Baddeley, 1975; Tulving & Thomson, 1973). Cues work best when people are allowed to select and provide their own cues.

Summary: Theories of Information Processing in Problem Analysis and Intervention Methods

- Intervention groups: preexistence of schema as facilitators or barriers to information processing
- Methods: chunking, advance organizers, imagery, rehearsal, and cues

Health Belief Model (HBM)

Historically, a number of theories have focused directly on health and risk-related behavior (Weinstein & Sandman, 2002). A model that has been used in a wide range of health-related contexts is the HBM (M. H. Becker, 1974a, 1974b; Janz et al., 2002; Janz & Becker, 1984; Rosenstock, Strecher, & Becker, 1988). The basic components of the HBM are based on psychological expectancy-value models (Janz et al., 2002). These models hypothesize that human behavior depends mainly on the value that an individual places on a particular goal and on the individual's estimate of the likelihood that a given action will achieve that goal. With respect to health, the components are the desire to avoid illness or to get well and the belief that specific behavior will prevent or reduce illness.

The original HBM comprises the following four psychological variables (Janz & Becker, 1984):

- Perceived susceptibility: a person's subjective perception of the risk of contracting a particular condition or illness (perceived personal risk)
- Perceived severity: a person's feelings concerning the seriousness of contracting an illness
- Perceived benefits: a person's beliefs regarding the effectiveness of various actions available to reduce the threat of a disease
- Perceived barriers: potential negative aspects of a particular health action

In other words, an individual's decision to engage in a health action is determined by his or her perceptions of personal susceptibility to, and the severity of, a particular condition or illness balanced against perceived benefits and barriers. According to the HBM, this decision-making process is triggered by a cue to action, which may be internal (for example, symptoms of a disease) or external (for example, a health education message or a friend with the disease).

Although an impressive body of research findings has linked HBM dimensions to health actions (Harrison, Mullen, & Green, 1992; Janz & Becker, 1984), recent research has demonstrated the importance of factors that were not originally examined in the context of the model (Janz et al., 2002). For example, many health-related behaviors are undertaken for ostensibly nonhealth reasons, suggesting that people's barrier-benefit analysis should include costs and benefits other than health beliefs (Ajzen, 1988). Current general social psychological models suggest that an individual's behavior, including health-related behavior, is also determined by perceptions of social influences and self-efficacy (Ajzen; Bandura, 1986). In later descriptions of the HBM, researchers incorporated these variables, self-efficacy specifically and the role of social influences more generally (Rosenstock et al., 1988; Strecher, DeVellis, Becker, & Rosenstock, 1986). The HBM may be most helpful in understanding relatively simple health behaviors, such as mammography screening or immunization (Janz et al., 2002). However, HBM has been shown to have some predictive validity for other problems, such as diabetes self-care.

Health Belief Model and Behavior Change

The HBM is a descriptive model of determinants of behavior and can sometimes provide clear direction for what factors should be changed (Janz et al., 2002). It does not suggest specific methods for behavioral change, except for the cue to action, which, among the constructs in the theory, has demonstrated the weakest relation to health behaviors thus far (Janz et al., 2002). In its use in intervention studies, other methods, such as counseling, have been used to shift HBM determinants. For example, Champion, Ray, Heilman, and Springston (2000) increased uptake of mammography screening among low-income women by providing for counseling regarding susceptibility, benefits, and barriers.

Summary: HBM in Problem Analysis and Intervention Methods

- Intervention groups: groups differentiated according to their perceptions of susceptibility and seriousness
- Behaviors: originally for health-protective behaviors, currently for health-promoting behaviors as well

- Environment: perceived environmental barriers in relation to perceived benefits
- Determinants: perceived susceptibility, perceived severity, perceived benefits, and perceived barriers
- Methods: cues to action

Protection-Motivation Theory (PMT)

An alternative to the HBM is a model that has the same basic ingredients: the PMT (Boer & Seydel, 1996; Floyd, Prentice-Dunn, & Rogers, 2000; Milne, Orbell, & Sheeran, 2002; R. Rogers, 1975; 1983; Salovey, Rothman, & Rodin, 1998). PMT suggests that people will try to control both the danger and the fear associated with it. Low response efficacy (the effectiveness of a certain response to decrease the danger) and low self-efficacy (self-confidence in the ability to perform the protective behavior) may lead to maladaptive behavior. The person at risk may avoid the health education message but not the behavior. Research studies show that a high threat may result in health-promoting behavior but only in combination with high self-efficacy (Eagly & Chaiken, 1993; Floyd et al., 2000; Milne et al., 2002; Ruiter, Abraham, & Kok, 2001).

Fear

Fear arousal has been suggested as a method to raise awareness of risk behavior and to change the risk behavior into health-promoting behavior. Using fear may be intuitively appealing to the health educator, and research on fear-arousing communication has a long tradition in social psychology and public health education (Hale & Dillard, 1995; Maibach & Parrott, 1995; McGuire, 1985). In their extensive review, Eagly and Chaiken (1993) summarize the inconclusive state of the art with respect to fear arousal. Most relevant theories and the available empirical data suggest that fear, as a result of subjective appraisals of personal susceptibility and severity, motivates an individual to action. However, the type of action is dependent on both outcome expectations and self-efficacy expectations. For instance, smokers may become afraid of cancer when they recognize their own susceptibility to cancer and the severity of the disease. Their fear may motivate them to stop smoking but only when they are convinced that quitting is really effective in preventing cancer (response efficacy or outcome expectation) and when they feel confident that they are able to quit (self-efficacy). In this particular example, low self-efficacy may be the most important barrier to quitting for most smokers.

What happens when people are afraid but are not convinced of the effectiveness of the alternative behavior or of their own self-efficacy? Most data suggest that under those conditions, the resulting behavior may be defensive, more oriented toward avoidance than action (for example, avoidance of the antismoking message) (Eagly & Chaiken, 1993; Floyd et al., 2000; Milne et al., 2002; Ruiter et al., 2001). Smokers may deny the risks of cancer, and messages that arouse extreme fear may result in more smoking.

What does this response mean for the use of fear-arousing communication as a method? Our understanding of the underlying process of fear arousal is still insufficient to make definitive statements, but there seem to be two important methodological points. First, fear is a motivator to behavior change, that is, no fear, no action. Second, fear motivates health-promoting behavior but probably only if the individual has high outcome expectations and high self-efficacy expectations. In cases in which people are not aware of their risk (as for some people in the precontemplation stage for a behavior), some fear arousal may be effective. In situations in which people are aware of their risk but lack self-efficacy for engaging in a health-promoting alternative behavior, messages should focus on improving self-efficacy. A word of caution: Precontemplation may, for some people, be the result of denial; and in that case, those precontemplators will not react positively to fear-arousing messages.

Negative and Positive Appeals and Message Framing

Monahan (1995) analyzes the effects of negative and positive appeals and concludes that, to be effective, emotional appeals in a message should be congruent with the target's existing feelings. In line with that conclusion, Salovey and colleagues (1998) report that messages with a loss frame (not doing the behavior results in a negative outcome) are more effective with detection behaviors, whereas messages with a gain frame (doing the behavior results in a positive outcome) are more effective with preventive behaviors. For example, missing early detection of cancer by not getting a Pap test every year can cost you your life (loss frame). Doing weight bearing exercise every day will maintain healthy bones (gain frame).

Summary: PMT in Problem Analysis and Intervention Methods

- Intervention groups: groups differentiated according to their risk perceptions
- Behaviors: originally for health-protective behaviors, currently for health-promoting behaviors as well
- Environment: perceived environmental barriers in relation to perceived benefits
- Determinants: perceived susceptibility, perceived severity, perceived benefits (for example, outcome expectations), and perceived barriers (for example, self-efficacy)
- Methods: tailoring to determinants, cues to action, framing, fear arousal (under appropriate conditions)

Theory of Planned Behavior (TPB)

Ajzen's TPB (1988) is an extension of the Theory of Reasoned Action (Conner & Sparks, 1996; Fishbein & Ajzen, 1975; Godin & Kok, 1996; Montaño & Kasprzyk, 2002). Both theories focus primarily on determinants of behavior and can be seen as expectancy value theories. Although they do not give specific methods for behavior change, these theories help health educators understand the specific variables that need to be changed (Hardeman et al., 2002; Witte, 1995). The TPB has successfully been applied to many types of health behavior (Montaño & Kasprzyk, 2002). It can be applied in situations in which people are aware of the negative consequences of their behavior, for instance, when they realize they are eating a high-fat diet (Brug, Hospers, & Kok, 1997; Brug, Van Assema, Kok, Lenderink, & Glanz, 1994) or not getting enough exercise (Ronda, Van Assema, & Brug, 2001). When people are not aware, they first have to become aware of the problem before determinants can be analyzed.

The TPB postulates that intention, the most proximal determinant of behavior, is determined by three conceptually independent constructs: attitude, subjective norms, and perceived behavioral control. Perceived behavioral control is not really different from Bandura's self-efficacy (Bandura, 1986; Salovey et al., 1998).

The TPB describes an attitude as a disposition to respond favorably or unfavorably to an object, behavior, person, institution, or event. Health educators are concerned mostly about the attitude toward a behavior, "the individual's positive or negative evaluation of performing the particular behavior of interest" (Ajzen, 1988, p. 117). To understand attitudes toward a behavior, there must be correspondence, meaning that attitudes may predict behavior when both concepts are assessed at identical levels of action, context, and time. The attitude toward the behavior is determined by salient beliefs about that behavior. Each behavioral belief links the behavior to a certain outcome or to an attribute (for example, "Going on a low-fat diet reduces my blood pressure"). Beliefs are weighted by the evaluations of those outcomes ("A reduced blood pressure is very good for me").

The construct of subjective norms (perceived social expectations) is a function of beliefs that specific, important individuals or groups (social referents) approve or disapprove of performing the behavior. Beliefs about specific social referents, such as "my partner thinks . . ." or "my mother thinks . . ." are termed normative beliefs. Relative to normative beliefs, some authors distinguish between social expectations and social pressure, describing the latter as a much stronger influence (De Vries, Backbier, Kok, & Dijkstra, 1995; Evans et al., 1978).

Perceived behavioral control (Ajzen, 1988) or self-efficacy (Bandura, 1986) refers to the subjective probability that a person is capable of executing a certain course of action (for example, "For me to go on a low-fat diet would be [easy versus difficult]") (Conner & Sparks, 1996). Ajzen sees perceived behavioral control as influencing behavior through intention and as influencing behavior directly (Montaño & Kasprzyk, 2002).

Current Developments in TPB

Some authors have suggested determinants in addition to the three that are currently in the theory. One suggestion is the addition of personal moral norms and anticipated regret. Personal moral norms are measured, for instance, as "I personally think I should always use a condom" (Godin, Fortin, Michaud, Bradet, & Kok, 1997; Godin, Savard, Kok, Fortin, & Boyer, 1996; Manstead & Parker, 1995). Anticipated regret is measured, for example, as "How would you feel afterward if you had unprotected sex?" (R. Richard, Van der Pligt, & de Vries, 1995). Note that anticipated regret can also be applied as a method for attitude change: Having people imagine how they would feel after they behaved in a risky way helps them to refrain from that behavior. Abraham, Sheeran, and Johnston (1998) integrated these various ideas and identified a concept that they called self-representation. Self-representations are concerned with the principles of a person about certain behavior. Such principles may be based on moral values, including personal feelings of responsibility, or they may be closely related to an individual's self-identity, focusing on societal rather than personal values. For example, a person with HIV might see herself as someone who would never expose another individual to infection.

Another current development is attention to the relation between intention and behavior. Studies on implementation intention show that helping people make plans to behave in a certain way (for example, "Exactly when and how do you think you will . . .") can improve the intention-behavior link (Orbell, Hodgkins, & Sheeran, 1997). Later in this chapter, under goal-directed behavior, we discuss implementation intentions in more detail.

Measuring TPB Determinants

The TPB gives very clear guidelines for measuring the determinants of behavior. The theorists suggest starting with open, qualitative methods such as interviews and focus groups to find all the salient factors, the prevalence and strength of which are then summarized through quantitative methods (De Vries et al., 1994). One well-researched topic, for example, is the onset of smoking in youth (De Vries et al., 1994, 1995; Kok, Schaalma, De Vries, Parcel, & Paulussen, 1996). First, young people age ten to fifteen were asked about smoking, nonsmoking, and regular smoking in interviews or open response questionnaires to elicit salient outcome beliefs, normative beliefs, self-efficacy expectations, and intentions. Based on this eliciting procedure, structured questionnaires were developed to measure the following:

- Beliefs and evaluations of the consequences of smoking (for example, "If I smoke or should start to smoke, this is very [sociable versus unsociable]")
- Normative beliefs and corresponding motivations to comply with respect to various social referents (for example, mother, father, brothers, sisters, friends, classmates)
- Perceived behavioral control or self-efficacy expectations (for example, students' perceived ability to refuse offers of cigarettes, to provide arguments against smoking, to resist social pressures to smoke)
- Intentions regarding both initial and regular smoking (for example, smoking with friends, smoking at parties)

The young people's answers to these questions differentiated smoking from nonsmoking youth. For example, nonsmokers are more likely than smokers to endorse that smoking causes bad health consequences (such as cancer, coughing, nausea) and that there are negative social expectations regarding smoking (from parents, other relatives, friends, and classmates). Young smokers are more likely than nonsmokers to endorse the personal advantages of smoking as a good way to increase sociability, be nice, show off, relax, relieve boredom, and be part of a group that does what others do (conformity). Nonsmokers had higher self-efficacy for not smoking when friends smoke, refusing cigarettes, staying nonsmokers, and explaining that they did not want to smoke. As a matter of fact, smokers reported negative self-efficacy about stating reasons to refuse cigarettes, not smoking when friends smoke, and becoming nonsmokers.

Using TPB at Higher Ecological Levels

The TPB is most often applied at the individual level. However, it can be applied to other ecological levels as well. For example, TPB has been used to examine the voting intentions of state legislators in North Carolina, Vermont, and Texas (Flynn et al., 1998; N. H. Gottlieb et al., 2003). Legislators' general attitudes and norms concerning cigarette tax increases were predictive of their intentions to vote for a cigarette tax. Normative influences were perceived interests of the tobacco industry, constituents, the legislature, and the health sector. Legislators who intended to vote for enforcement of the minors' access legislation held strong outcome beliefs and evaluations about the public health impact. The strongest normative be-liefs were for health and medical lobbyists (for example, "Medical lobbyists expect me to . . ."), and motivation to comply was strongest for voters and medical lob-byists (for example, "I care about what voters and lobbyists expect me to do"). The perceived impact of the cigarette tax legislation on retail sales, public health, and loss of political support for the next election—along with perceived behavioral control for getting the bill out of committee, voting for it, and passing it—were each associated with the legislators' voting intention. These types of TPB findings can provide guidance to health educators who plan messages for advocacy efforts.

TPB has also been used to plan the implementation of health education pro-gram innovations (Paulussen, Kok, & Schaalma, 1994; Paulussen, Kok, Schaalma, & Parcel, 1995). Differences in beliefs, perceived social expectations, and self-efficacy were associated with teachers' different rates of diffusion, adoption, and implementation of an HIV-prevention program. Diffusion was associated with the social influence of colleagues through professional networks; adoption with out-come expectations such as expected student satisfaction; implementation with self-efficacy expectations about the proposed teaching strategies and with teachers' moral opinions on sexuality. Surprisingly, the effectiveness of the program had no influence on teachers' implementation decisions.

Shifting Subjective Norms

Thinking about how to shift subjective norms may require more information about the nature of the construct. The subjective social norm is a special case of social influence: the impact of others on people's perceptions and behaviors (Forsyth, 1998). TPB focuses on the perceived expectations of others, whereas so-cial cognitive theory focuses on vicarious learning or modeling, the observation of the behavior of others. Interestingly, the perception of others' expectations may be incorrect; children may, for instance, incorrectly assume that most peers expect them to smoke. De Vries, Backbier, Kok, and Dijkstra (1995) distinguish among subjective social norms, modeling, social support for the health-promoting behavior, and social pressure for the risk behavior, the latter being a much stronger form of social expectations.

More generally, social psychology textbooks will refer to conformity processes and social comparison (Forsyth, 1998). Conformity refers to the social influence of a majority on a minority, an influence that has been shown to be very strong, especially in the situation of a group against a minority of one person. Confor-mity can lead to public compliance but also to internalized change. Social com-parison theory (Suls, Wheeler, & Suls, 2000) explains why social influences are effective:

1. People like to be right, so when direct information or experience is lacking, people turn to others to decide about the right course of action.
2. People like to feel good, and they think they will feel good if they become more accepted by relevant others by agreeing with them or joining in their behavior.

The first process explains why conformity may end in internalized change: People accept others' ideas as correct. Social comparison processes have been described in the area of patient education (Suls et al., 2000), in which both processes lead to upward and downward comparison of patients with other patients. Upward comparison with patients who do better will provide information on how to cope with the disease; downward comparison with patients who do worse will make people feel better about their own situation. Use of a patients' self-help group may serve both purposes and provide social support (see Chapter Four).

There are three ways to influence the social expectations in TPB:

1. Influence normative beliefs by making peer expectations visible
2. Influence motivation to comply by building resistance to social pressure to engage in risk behavior or by increasing motivation to comply with positive social pressure

Finally, if we are unable to shift either the norm or the motivation to comply, we can do the following:

3. Hide the behavior or shift attention from the behavior

For example, assume that young women do not want to ask their partners to use a condom for AIDS prevention because they expect the partners to react negatively to the idea that the women suspect them of having HIV. An approach of the first type would be to mobilize peers to talk about safe sex to make the norms for using condoms more visible. This approach assumes that positive peer experiences are available for discussion in the environment—both that young men are willing to wear condoms and that young women agree to ask the boys to wear them. The second approach might be to build resistance to social pressure, which in this case might mean that women learn effective refusal skills when the partner does not want to use a condom. The third approach, hiding or shifting attention from the behavior, might be translated into methods and strategies in which women learn to shift attention from using a condom to prevent HIV infection by telling the partner that they want to use a condom to prevent pregnancy.

Methods for changing social influences and for improving self-efficacy are sometimes the same, when they both relate to self-efficacy and skills. Resistance to social pressure, for instance, can be seen as a skill. How can we teach people to resist social pressure? A summary of the literature (McGuire, 1985) suggests five methods:

- Training refusal skills
- Modeling resistance
- Committing to earlier intention and behavior
- Relating intended behavior to values
- Performing a psychological inoculation against pressure

Summary: TPB in Problem Analysis and Intervention Methods

- Intervention groups: groups that can be differentiated according to their beliefs and intentions
- Behaviors: useful for understanding health risk behaviors when people are aware of the negative outcomes associated with continuing the behavior
- Environment: environmental barriers in relation to perceived self-efficacy; all constructs used to explain behavior of agents at every ecological level
- Determinants: beliefs, attitudes, perceived social expectations, perceived behavioral control
- Methods: does not directly suggest methods; other theories provide anticipated regret, the process of making social expectations visible, resistance skills building, shift in focus, skills building for self-efficacy and skills improvement

Theories of Goal Setting

Goal setting leads to better performance because people with goals exert themselves to a greater extent, persevere in their tasks, concentrate more, and if necessary, develop strategies for carrying out the behavior (Locke & Latham, 1990, 2002). Theories of goal setting are clearly theories of action and describe a particular method for behavior change. In AIDS prevention, for example, the health educator may attempt to associate safe sex with important goals for students, such as careers that might be threatened by the consequences of unsafe sex. In this way safe sex becomes part of the strategy to attain long-term goals.

Goal setting in health education also may be directly related to the health behavior. In the Cystic Fibrosis Family Education Program, for example, parents and children work with health care providers to set goals regarding self-care, such as increasing calories a certain amount or keeping a record of symptom change to provide the context for the self-care goals. Health care providers also work with the families to clarify goals that may indirectly relate to cystic fibrosis care, (Bartholomew et al., 1991). For example, a child may set a goal to try out for the school tennis team. She may need to gain weight and improve her fitness to do so; therefore, she sets specific eating and exercise goals.

Characteristics of Goals

A goal should be behaviorally specific and measurable or observable. Strecher and colleagues (1995) advise that goals should be stated in terms of behavior (for example, exercise behavior and food intake) instead of health outcomes (for example, weight loss). Locke and Latham (1990, 2002) have demonstrated that setting a challenging goal, a goal that is feasible though somewhat difficult, leads to a better performance than does setting an easy goal or no goal at all. This positive effect of difficult goals occurs only if a person accepts the challenge and has sufficient experience, self-efficacy, and feedback to be able to perform adequately. The rewards for reaching the goal are not only the expected outcomes but also a sense of self-satisfaction. Goal setting probably will not be effective when the task is too complex. In that case the educator can help the client set subgoals and suggest strategies (for example, not to quit smoking permanently but first to abstain for one week and then set a new goal).

Summary: Theories of Goal Setting in Problem Analysis and Intervention Methods

- Intervention groups: different goals for people who are high or low in self-efficacy and skills
- Behaviors: all behaviors in which feedback is feasible
- Determinants: Self-efficacy and skills
- Methods: somewhat difficult goals, acceptance of goal, match of goal complexity and difficulty with skills, and feedback

Theories of Goal Directed Behavior

Gollwitzer (1999) presents a series of studies on goal intentions and implementation intentions. Goal intentions ("I intend to pursue X," as in TPB) result in a commitment to realize a wish or desire. Implementation intentions ("I intend to initiate behavior X when conditions Y are met") connect a certain goal-directed behavior with an anticipated situation. The purpose of an implementation intention is to lay down a specific plan to promote the initiation and efficient execution of goal-directed activity. Gollwitzer shows that by forming implementation intentions, people pass the control of the behavior over to the environment. Situations and means are turned into cues to action that are hard to forget, ignore, or miss. It appears that forming an implementation intention is a conscious cognitive act that has automatic consequences.

Facilitating Formation of Implementation Intentions

An important method to help people realize their intentions is to facilitate their forming implementation intentions: to get people to stipulate when, where, and how they intend to achieve their goals. (See also the discussion of relapse prevention later in this chapter.) Having people form clear implementation intentions has been shown for various behaviors to be an effective method for changing behavior for people who are motivated to change. Health behaviors that have been studied include reducing dietary fat intake (Armitage, 2004), initiating exercise and quitting smoking in patients with coronary heart disease (Johnston, Johnston, Pollard, Kinmonth, & Mant, 2004), initiating exercise (Milne et al., 2002), engaging in workplace health and safety (Sheeran & Silverman, 2003), participating in cervical cancer screening (Sheeran & Orbell, 2000), performing testicular self-examination (Steadman & Quine, 2004), and using condoms (Svenson, Ostergren, Merlo, & Rastam, 2002). Adding implementation intentions to an intervention based on PMT was shown to be more effective than the original intervention (Milne et al., 2002).

Implementation intentions are hypothesized to trigger two types of psychological processes that facilitate initiation of action (Gollwitzer, 1999). Implementation intentions lead to heightened activation of situational cues, and they automatize action initiation. To be effective, implementation intentions should very clearly link the initiation of the intended behavior to specific environmental cues. Gollwitzer presents studies that show how implementation intentions lead to immediate responses to environmental cues without conscious intent, obviously having characteristics of automated behavior or habits. Interestingly, implementation intentions also help in overcoming undesirable habits. For example, a smoker who has regularly smoked with friends while drinking alcohol may find that, although successfully resisting smoking during the day, he or she experiences very strong desires for a cigarette while drinking and, seemingly without thinking, asks friends for a cigarette (Abraham et al., 1998). To disrupt this context-prompted, automatic behavior, a person would need a clear understanding of why the craving happens; self-monitoring of the automatic desires; and conscious initiation of alternative, cognitively rehearsed implementation intentions. The person would need to declare the craving and ask for social support as soon as he or she felt the desire. Implementation intentions are therefore a potentially effective method for influencing habitual behaviors.

Summary: Theories of Goal Directed Behavior in Problem Analysis and Intervention Methods

- Intervention groups: people who are motivated for change
- Behaviors: goal-directed behaviors, habitual behaviors
- Environment: behavior influenced by environmental stimuli
- Determinants: habits, environmental influences
- Methods: implementation intentions, environmental cues

Theories of Automatic Behavior and Habits

Much of health promotion research and theory is based on the assumption that people are consciously and systematically processing information in order to construe and interpret their world and to plan and engage in courses of action. Bargh and Chartrand (1999) argue, however, that most of our moment-to-moment psychological life occurs through nonconscious means. They present evidence that goal-directed behavior may start consciously but may become automatic over time. An example is driving style: During the first lessons, the aspiring driver is fully aware of the actions required to perform the most basic driving activities, for example, starting a car. For the experienced driver, however, driving a car is largely automatic. Also, environmental cues may guide behavior outside of awareness. An example can be found in the effects of priming, in which people are exposed to a stimulus and later their actions are congruent with the stimulus. In one example of this process, elderly participants were exposed either to words related to the stereotype of the elderly or to words unrelated to that stereotype. Participants exposed to stereotyped words behaved more in line with that stereotype; for instance, they walked more slowly. In social interaction, people tend to change their behavior as a function of other people's behavior. For instance, participants in a study liked other participants better (who were in fact confederates of the experimenter) who deliberately mimicked the participants' mannerisms and body postures. In all these cases, the participants were not aware of these behaviors and behavior changes. Bargh and Chartrand point out that automatic behavior is a necessity for living; without it we could not function. If all life's simple decisions and actions involved deliberate and careful thought, people would simply not have enough time and resources for the demands of living. Because a large part of behavior is conducted on automatic pilot, people are, for instance, able to do two things at the same time.

Attitudes can also be activated automatically (Fazio, 2001). Exposure to stimuli with a subjective negative evaluation activates negative attitudes; exposure to stimuli with a positive evaluation activates positive attitudes. The activated attitude determines a first reaction, whether negative or positive, to the next stimulus, without a person being completely aware of that reaction. The negative or positive automatic reaction may make a person more likely to visually notice something, more likely to categorize objects or people in categories that match with the attitude, and more likely to behave in negative or positive ways toward categories of objects or people. The last case may lead to prejudice and discrimination. Automatically activated attitudes impose selectivity in the perception of behavioral choices. For example, people who habitually drive to work will, when asked about a way to travel to a holiday destination, automatically activate a positive car-use attitude and may have difficulty even considering alternative ways of transportation.

Verplanken and Aarts (1999) define habits as a special case of automatic behavior. The most prominent characteristics of habits are that they are efficient and occur without much awareness. Habits are also goal-directed and, to some extent, controllable. Habits are significant predictors of future behaviors in addition to intentions, especially when individuals repeatedly perform the behaviors and when the habit is strong (which it is likely to be after enough repetition). When people have an intention to eat healthy foods but a habit of eating fatty foods, their eating pattern will often be unhealthy.

Changing Habits

Habits are difficult to change, and they are not particularly influenced by information for two reasons (Verplanken & Aarts, 1999). First, information influences attitude and intentions, but these do not change behavior when they have to compete with a strong habit. Second, people with strong habits are usually not very interested in new information. On the one hand, health promoters know this phenomenon and therefore actually try to make new and healthy behavior a habit. On the other hand, it is very hard to change existing strong and unhealthy habits. Interestingly, forming new habits may be the best method to change old habits. Forming implementation intentions (see the discussion of goal-directed behavior earlier in this chapter) may be a useful start to creating new habits that may replace old ones. New cue-response links can be formed and after some time may turn into new habits. However, the new cue-response links may not be as rewarding as the earlier ones; so applying implementation intentions as a method for changing habits needs to be paralleled by applying other methods, such as relapse prevention (see the discussion of attribution theory and relapse prevention later in this chapter).

Summary: Theories of Automatic Behavior and Habits in Problem Analysis and Intervention Methods

- Behaviors: automatic, unconscious behaviors; those behaviors that could become habitual
- Environment: behavior guided by external stimuli
- Determinants: habits, environmental influences, automatic activation of attitudes
- Methods: implementation intentions, environmental cues

Transtheoretical Model (TTM) of Behavior Change

The TTM has two major sets of constructs: stages of change and processes of change (Prochaska & DiClemente, 1984; Prochaska et al., 1997; Prochaska, Redding, & Evers, 2002). This model has been used to describe cessation of addictive behaviors and more recently to predict uptake of health-promoting behaviors (Prochaska et al., 2002). Further, both the stages of change and the processes of change are suggestive of intervention methods to stimulate change. An important contribution of the model is the specific tailoring of educational efforts to include different methods for individuals in different stages of change.

Stages of Change

In the stages of change, people are thought to move from having no motivation to change to internalizing the new behavior. The early stages are defined by the level of intention to change a problem behavior, whereas the later stages are defined by the length of time a person has engaged in the new behavior. The stages are as follows:

- Precontemplation, in which people have no intention of changing their behavior
- Contemplation, in which people are thinking about changing the problem behavior in the next six months
- Preparation, in which people are planning to change this behavior in the short term (one month) and are taking steps to get ready for the change
- Action, in which people have recently changed the behavior
- Maintenance, in which people have performed the new behavior for more than six months

People in the action or maintenance stages may lapse and then recycle to action or relapse to contemplation or even precontemplation. There is still considerable debate on the validation of the stages of change, but most authors agree that the model makes a useful contribution to understanding and promoting change (Adams & White, 2004; Brug, Schols, & Mesters, 2004; Prochaska et al., 2002).

Processes of Change

Prochaska and colleagues (1997, 2002) describe processes of change that may be stimulated by different methods (Table 3.3). Other authors have suggested processes for the various stages as well. Processes sometimes are clearly determinants of moving to the next stage; at other times they are very close to methods for promoting change. Holtgrave, Tinsley, and Kay (1995) suggest methods based on risk-perception theories for the first two steps. Maibach and Cotton (1995) suggest methods based on social cognitive theory. De Vries and Backbier (1994) and Marlatt and Gordon (1985) provide additional methods. Table 3.3 defines the processes suggested by the authors of TTM and by others.

Reevaluation. Prochaska and colleagues (2002) mention methods for bringing precontemplators to contemplation and preparation. In self-reevaluation a person combines cognitive and affective assessments of self-image with and without a particular unhealthy habit. For example, a person can compare his or her image as a sedentary person to a possible image as an active person. Clarifying values, having healthy role models, and using mental imagery are methods that can move people to a more realistic evaluation of their current behavior.

Environmental reevaluation combines both affective and cognitive assessments of how the presence or absence of a personal habit affects one's social environment. For example, a father might assess the effect of his smoking on his children. It can also include the awareness that one can serve as a positive or negative role model for others. Methods such as empathy training and viewing of documentaries may lead to such assessments. In Project Parents and Newborns Developing and Adjusting (PANDA), the intervention designed by Mullen and colleagues (see Chapter Thirteen) included messages to stimulate new fathers to assess their potential impact as role models for their children and to prepare smoke-free environments to help mothers stay off cigarettes.

Self-reevaluation can be compared to constructs in other theories. The second stage in self-regulation theories is evaluation, in which a person compares current performance to a personal standard. In Chapter Seven, where we present methods for changing determinants, we treat variables related to self-presentation as a group of attitudinal variables including self-evaluation ("I am satisfied with my performance"), personal moral norm ("I feel I should do X") and anticipated regret ("How would you feel after you did X?"). Some other authors see those variables as a separate cluster (Abraham et al., 1998). Self-evaluations may be

TABLE 3.3. CHANGE PROCESSES
IN THE TRANSTHEORETICAL MODEL.

Process	Definition
From Precontemplation to Contemplation	
Consciousness raising	Finding and learning new facts, ideas, and tips to support a behavior change
Dramatic relief	Experiencing the negative emotions (fear, anxiety, worry) that go along with unhealthy behavioral risks
Environmental reevaluation	Realizing the negative impact of the unhealthy behavior and the positive impact of the healthful behavior
Risk comparison	Comparing risks with similar dimensional profiles: dread, control, catastrophic potential, and novelty
Cumulative risk	Processing cumulative probabilities instead of single-incident probabilities
Qualitative and quantitative risks	Processing both qualitative and quantitative expressions of risks
Positive framing	Focusing on success framing instead of failure framing
Self-examination related to risk	Risk perception: likelihood information, personalization, impact on others
Reevaluation of outcomes	Emphasizing positive outcomes of alternative behaviors and reevaluating outcome expectancies
Perception of benefits	Perceiving advantages of the healthy behavior and disadvantages of the risk behavior
From Contemplation to Preparation and Action	
Self reevaluation	Realizing that the behavioral change is an important part of a person's identity
Self-efficacy and social support	Mobilizing social support; skills training on coping with emotional disadvantages of change
Decision-making perspective	Focusing on decision-making perspective
Tailoring on time horizons	Incorporating personal time horizons
Focus on important factors	Incorporating factors with the highest importance
Trying out new behavior	Changing something about oneself and gaining experience with that behavior
Persuasion of positive outcomes	Promoting new positive outcome expectations and reinforcing existing ones
Modeling	Showing models to overcome barriers effectively

TABLE 3.3. CHANGE PROCESSES
IN THE TRANSTHEORETICAL MODEL, Cont'd.

Process	Definition
From Preparation to Action	
Self-liberation	Making a firm commitment to change
Skill improvement	Restructuring environments to contain important, obvious, socially supported cues for the new behavior
Coping with barriers	Identifying barriers and planning solutions to the behavior-change obstacles
Goal setting	Setting specific and incremental goals
Modeling	Perceiving models who receive social reinforcement of health behaviors
From Action to Maintenance	
Helping relationships	Seeking and using social support for the healthy behavior change
Counter conditioning	Substituting healthier alternative behaviors and cognitions for the unhealthy ones
Contingency management	Increasing the rewards for the positive behavioral change
Stimulus control	Removing reminders or cues to engage in the unhealthy behavior and adding cues or reminders to engage in the healthy behavior
Skills enhancement	Restructuring cues and social support; anticipating and circumventing obstacles; modifying goals
Dealing with barriers	Understanding that setbacks are common and can be overcome
Self-rewards for success	Feeling good about progress; reiterating positive consequences
Maintenance	
Coping skills	Identifying high-risk situations; selecting solutions; practicing solutions; coping with lapses

Sources: Prochaska, DiClemente, and Norcross, 1997; Holtgrave, Tinsley, and Kay, 1995; Maibach and Cotton, 1995; De Vries and Backbier, 1994; Marlatt and Gordon, 1985.

activated by setting goals and giving feedback (Bandura, 1986). Personal moral norms may be enhanced by counseling or small group discussions on values and moral norms (Godin et al., 1996). Anticipated regret may be enhanced literally by asking people to imagine how they would feel after having had, for instance, unsafe sex (R. Richard et al., 1995).

The strategy of gaps analysis applies reevaluation in the context of organizational development. The organization compares the current situation to organizational values or to a vision of the preferred future. For example, surveys of organization members to determine the existing cultural norms and practices are conducted and the findings discussed in relationship to the culture that the members desire. This provides the motivation and direction for intervention (Allen & Bellingham, 1994; Cummings & Worley, 1993).

Mobilizing Social Support. Prochaska and colleagues (2002) also describe helping relationships as a process of change related to mobilizing social support. These relationships combine caring, trust, openness, and acceptance as well as support for the behavioral change. Rapport building, therapeutic alliances, counselor calls, and buddy systems can be sources of social support. In contrast to this counseling approach to increasing social support, the California Department of Mental Health conducted a media campaign, called *Good Friends Make Good Medicine,* designed to increase awareness of the importance of social support and to suggest specific actions individuals could take to strengthen their support networks (Hersey, Klibanoff, Lam, & Taylor, 1984).

Improving Self-Efficacy and Skills. Prochaska and colleagues (2002) mention various processes of and methods for change that are related to self-efficacy improvement and skills training:

- Self-liberation is both the belief that one can change and the commitment to act on that belief. Public commitment and testimonies and multiple, rather than single, choices may enhance persistence.
- Counterconditioning requires the learning of healthy behaviors that can substitute for problem behaviors. Relaxation, assertion, desensitization, and positive self-statements are strategies for finding safer substitutions.
- Contingency management provides specified consequences (mostly rewards) for taking steps in a particular direction.
- Contingency contracts, overt and covert reinforcements, and group recognition are procedures for reinforcement when the person meets contingencies.
- Stimulus control removes cues (avoidance and environmental reengineering) for unhealthy habits and adds prompts for healthier alternatives.

- Social liberation requires an increase in social opportunities or alternatives. Advocacy, empowerment procedures, and appropriate policies can be used to help people change.

The efficacy construct is also applicable to groups, communities, and societies. *Collective efficacy* refers to the group's shared belief in its capacity to organize and carry out actions required to produce goals. The most effective way to increase collective efficacy is through successful performance.

Relevance, Tailoring, and Individualization.

Relevance, tailoring, and individualization have all been shown to be effective basic methods in health education interventions; and they can be traced to a number of theories, such as social cognitive theory and TTM. We will discuss these methods here because they fit with TTM's stages approach. Adapting the program to the knowledge, beliefs, circumstances, and prior experience of the learner, as assessed by pretesting or other means, can create relevance (Mullen et al., 1985, 1992). Computer programs enable one to tailor interventions to measured characteristics of the individual, such as stage of change, beliefs, attitude, and self-efficacy (Brug et al., 1994; Brug, Glanz, Van Assema, Kok, & van Breukelen, 1998; Brug, Oenema, & Campbell, 2003; Campbell, DeVellis, Strecher, Ammerman, Devellis, & Sandler, 1994; Kreuter, Farrell, Olevitch, & Brennan, 2000; Skinner, Strecher, & Hospers, 1994; Strecher et al., 1994; Strecher, 1999).

Tailoring will be effective only when there is a clear link between characteristics of the person and the messages that are supposed to address those characteristics (Brug et al., 1998). Witte (1995) points out that tailoring the message to salient beliefs of the intervention group would increase people's motivation and ability to process the message carefully, thereby increasing the chance of persistent changes in attitudes and behavior. Salovey and colleagues (1998) stress the importance of tailoring interventions to laypeople's beliefs about illness, such as causes, consequences, duration, and cure. Witte (1995) proposes a protocol for defining types of important beliefs from a health communication perspective.

Individualization is the provision of opportunities for learners to have personal questions answered or instructions paced according to their individual progress (Mullen et al., 1985, 1992). It may also include the ability to offer instruction that is geared to specific needs and disease characteristics. The *Watch, Discover, Think, and Act* asthma computer application (Chapter Twelve) individualizes instruction to each child's asthma triggers and symptoms based on information the child types in (Bartholomew, Gold, et al., 2000; Bartholomew, Shegog, et al., 2000).

Both individualization and tailoring are related to the concept of cultural competence, which we discuss further in Chapter Eight. Both program methods and strategies not only must be acceptable to the intervention groups but must fit the culture in order to foster empowerment and program effectiveness. Development of a culturally competent program requires the community's participation as program planners. The Pathways to Early Cancer Detection in Four Ethnic Groups project, for example, developed specific interventions for early cancer detection for Latinos, Vietnamese women, and a multiethnic indigent population who used emergency rooms for health care. Although the interventions' goals, objectives, and theoretical base were similar, there were some specific differences in the mode of intervention (for example, mass media vs. interpersonal communication); use of role models and lay health workers; staffing patterns; content of messages; and the language, idiom, and designs of the print material for specific populations (Pasick, D'Onofrio, & Hiatt, 1996).

Summary: TTM of Behavior Change in Problem Analysis and Intervention Methods

- Intervention groups: different groups for people in precontemplation, contemplation, preparation, action, and maintenance
- Behaviors: originally helpful for addictive behaviors; currently work in a variety of behaviors
- Environment: suggests environmental barriers for change and also relevant for considering behavior change of agents at the various environmental levels
- Determinants: determinants of various behaviors different for each stage
- Methods: methods tailored to stages; methods guided by processes of change (counterconditioning, reevaluation, self-evaluation, anticipated regret, consciousness raising, and mobilization of social support)

Precaution-Adoption Process Model (PAPM)

Another stage theory, the PAPM integrates almost all theoretical constructs that we have discussed in the PMT and the TTM sections (Weinstein, 1988; Weinstein & Sandman, 2002). PAPM pays more attention to the issue of awareness of the risk compared to TTM and to the difficulty of reaching resistant groups. Compared to the TTM, PAPM incorporates determinants and methods for change that are supported by popular health promotion theories, especially SCT (Bandura, 1997). The model defines the stages this way:

1. Unaware of the problem
2. Aware, but not thinking about changing

3. Thinking about acting
4. Decided not to act
5. Decided to act
6. Action
7. Maintenance

As in other stage theories, Weinstein (1988) suggests that people in different stages need different tactics to help them change and to help them move through the stages. People who have decided not to act are a particularly difficult group because they may be quite well informed but tend to dispute or ignore information that challenges their decision. One relevant factor in deciding not to act may be that people systematically underestimate their own risk (see the following discussion of unrealistic optimism).

Weinstein and Sandman (2002) list a number of factors or issues that are likely to determine progress between the stages (Table 3.4).

TABLE 3.4. THE PRECAUTION-ADOPTION PROCESS MODEL.

Stage Transitions	Factors or Issues
Stage 1: Unaware of the problem to Stage 2: Aware but not thinking about changing	Media messages about the hazards and precautions
Stage 2 to Stage 3: Thinking about changing	Communications from significant others
	Personal experience with the hazard
Stage 3 to Stage 4: Decided not to act or Stage 5: Decided to act	Beliefs about hazard likelihood and severity
	Beliefs about personal susceptibility
	Beliefs about precaution effectiveness and difficulty
	Behaviors and recommendations of others
	Perceived social norms
	Fear and worry
Stage 5 to Stage 6: Action	Time, effort, and resources needed to act
	Detailed "how-to" information
	Reminders and other cues to action
	Assistance in carrying out action

Unrealistic Optimism. People often underestimate their risk, a condition that risk-perception theorists call unrealistic optimism (Brug et al., 1994; Van der Pligt, Otten, Richard, & Van der Velde, 1993). The main reasons for unrealistic optimism are that people underestimate what techniques others undertake to protect themselves and that they have stereotypes of people who run high risks (Salovey et al., 1998). To illustrate, adolescents may refrain from condom use because they think that other adolescents do not use condoms to protect themselves, that other adolescents have multiple partners whereas they have regular partners, and that only adolescents who often change partners are at risk for contracting HIV. Health educators should assist in making clear each person's risks, preferably through undeniable feedback, and should also indicate that risk is a matter of risk behavior rather than of what risk groups the person belongs to. Janz and colleagues (2002) suggest the following methods for changing risk-perception variables:

- Define the risk levels of the population at risk
- Personalize risk based on a person's behavior
- Make perceived susceptibility more consistent with the individual's actual risk
- Specify consequences of the risk

Risk Communication

Holtgrave and colleagues (1995) suggest various methods to effectively communicate risks. Health educators can, for example, compare risks on the same dimensions (dread, control, catastrophic potential, equity, and novelty) or compare risks with similar dimensional profiles. Sometimes people become angry when a risk over which they have no control, such as air pollution, is compared to a risk over which they do have control, such as smoking. Health educators can give cumulative risk information and can emphasize cumulative probabilities instead of single-incident probabilities. Holtgrave and colleagues (1995) suggest that health educators avoid giving the probability of getting infected with HIV in one unprotected sexual encounter; instead, the message should encourage a person to think about how many times he or she is likely to have sex and to realize that unsafe sex presents a cumulative risk of HIV infection. Health educators can provide both qualitative and quantitative expressions of risks; they can say both "90 percent chance" and "extremely likely." Finally, health educators can choose what is known as success framing of the message instead of failure framing when the message relates to the effectiveness of a health behavior. For example, they can state that "condom use is 95 percent effective" rather than "the failure rate is only 5 percent."

Currently, work is being done to apply economic theory to the specification of risk. Allegrante and Roizen (1998) calculate biological age of coronary bypass patients based on unmodified risk factors. They counsel patients to compare biological with chronological age as a way of concretizing risk.

Raising Awareness

Awareness is often described as the first step in the change process. In the theories of self-regulation and coping, the first step in an intervention is some form of need recognition or problem appraisal. However, these theories do not provide clear methods for stimulating need recognition. Often, self-regulatory and coping theories are applied in situations in which people have a disease, such as asthma, cystic fibrosis, or AIDS (Wenzel, Glanz, & Lerman, 2002). Individuals are taught appraisal skills to detect a problem related to disease or self-management as well as other skills with which to solve the problem (Bartholomew, Sockrider et al., 1993). Without these additional problem-solving skills to raise self-efficacy and outcome expectations, avoidance of thinking about the risk may ensue. For people who are not motivated to perform appraisal, methods for awareness may be applied, such as risk information, confrontation, and fear arousal.

People are often not aware of the negative outcomes of their behavior. The TTM suggests that cognitive and affective methods raise awareness of negative outcomes, thereby moving people from precontemplation to contemplation (Prochaska et al., 2002). Consciousness raising involves increased awareness about a risk behavior as a cause of a particular health problem, about the consequences of the risk behavior, and about the consequences of possible health promotion behaviors. Intervention methods that can induce consciousness raising include feedback, confrontation, and interpretation. Dramatic relief initially produces increased emotional experiences followed by reduced affect if appropriate action is taken. Psychodrama, role-playing, grieving, and personal testimonies are examples of strategies for operationalizing dramatic relief.

Hendrickx, Vlek, and Oppewal (1989) state that people may base their risk judgments on information that aids the construction of an image of the ways in which a particular outcome may occur. An essential parameter for this method is that the information includes a plausible scenario with a cause and an outcome, instead of only an outcome.

Maibach and Cotton (1995) stress that messages to promote awareness should focus on self-evaluation related to risk and reevaluation of outcome expectations, rather than on action. Messages could include personalization by reminding someone of recent episodes of the risk behavior and potential consequences of the person's risk behavior on significant others. At a higher ecological level, mass media gatekeepers must also become aware of an issue as a necessary condition for featuring health-promoting issues (McGrath, 1995).

Summary: PAPM in Problem Analysis and Intervention Methods

- Intervention groups: people in different stages of precaution adoption
- Behaviors: all health behaviors, but especially risk behaviors that people are not aware of
- Environment: lack of environmental resources as barriers for change
- Determinants: different determinants in different stages
- Methods: tailoring of methods to stages

Attribution Theory and Relapse Prevention

An important variable in many models that try to explain determinants of behavior is self-efficacy, the self-confidence for performing a particular behavior. But what are the determinants of self-efficacy? Weiner (1986) suggests that self-efficacy, or expectancy of success as he calls it, is determined by the perceived stability of the attributions for success and failure. Attribution theory describes the impact of the way people attribute the outcomes of behavior on their future cognition and behavior across the three dimensions of stability, locus, and controllability (Weiner).

Stability is the relevant dimension for the understanding of success expectations for health behavior change. A person attributing a failure to a stable cause (for example, ability) will have a lower expectancy of success for performing the same task again compared to somebody who attributes a failure on the same task to an unstable cause (for example, bad luck). In the case of success, this effect is reversed. If a person succeeds, attributing the success to a stable cause (for example, talent) will be associated with a higher expectation of success than if the success is attributed to an unstable cause (for example, fortunate circumstance). Furthermore, attribution theory suggests that lower success expectancy leads to less adaptive task behavior; people will invest less energy in the task at hand. Hospers, Kok, and Strecher (1990) report an attribution explanation of health behavior in a study of success of participants in a weight-reduction program. They found that success was positively related to the participants' self-efficacy at the start of the program. Self-efficacy was inversely related to stability of attributions for earlier failures, and both relationships were independent of the number of failures.

Attributional Retraining and Relapse Prevention

One method for changing attributions to improve self-efficacy is called attributional retraining, or reattribution (Kok et al., 1992). The health educator or counselor tries to help people reinterpret previous failures in terms of unstable attributions ("You were in a very difficult situation there") and previous successes in terms of stable attributions ("You are the type of person who has been able to stay off cigarettes during your whole pregnancy").

Attributional retraining is often used in attempts to prevent relapse (Marlatt & Gordon, 1985). Relapses are caused by a lack of coping response when a person lapses in a high-risk situation. Self-efficacy expectations and perceived skills are relevant not only for new behavior but also for the maintenance of behavior changes. Relapse-prevention theory describes the process of lapses, attributions, self-efficacy estimations, and successes and failures in maintaining the behavior change (see Figure 13.2). The major distinction between success and failure is the presence or absence of a coping response for high-risk situations (Dimeff & Marlatt, 1998; Marlatt & Gordon, 1985; Shiffman, 1984). High-risk situations are those situations that invite or pressure people to take up their risk behavior again. For instance, a worker who has quit smoking goes to the coffee shop where colleagues are smoking. If the worker has an adequate coping response, she will be more likely to maintain her health-promoting behavior and may develop an even higher estimation of self-efficacy. However, if she does not have an adequate coping response to the high-risk situation at the coffee shop, she may lapse into her earlier risk behavior and experience a sense of failure. She may attribute this failure to stable and uncontrollable causes and develop lower self-efficacy and a higher chance of complete relapse as a result.

How can health promotion programs help people prevent relapse? The theory suggests a series of primarily face-to-face or group methods that involve helping the person at risk identify high-risk situations, plan coping responses, and practice the responses until they become automatic (Marlatt & Gordon, 1985). It also suggests reattribution training for incidental lapses so that the at-risk person attributes failure to an unstable cause.

Summary: Attribution Theory and Relapse Prevention in Problem Analysis and Intervention Methods

- Intervention groups: people who make stable versus unstable attributions for failure
- Behaviors: all behaviors with success or failure characteristics
- Environment: real barriers that may be too difficult even with high self-efficacy
- Determinants: stable versus unstable attributions for failure
- Methods: attribution retraining, relapse-prevention training, planning coping responses

Persuasion-Communication Matrix (PCM)

One general theory for behavior change is McGuire's PCM (1985). It is used in public health education somewhat differently from the way McGuire originally intended (Kok et al., 1996). In the original model, McGuire distinguishes the following stages (Hamilton & Hunter, 1998):

1. Exposure to the message
2. Attention to the message
3. Comprehension of the arguments and conclusions
4. Acceptance of the arguments
5. Retention of the content resulting from information integration
6. Attitude change

Health educators use this model to describe an individual's progression from an initial response to an educational message, through intermediate processes, to change of behavior in the desired direction.

Table 3.5 presents McGuire's PCM (1985) as it was adapted to health education by including variables from social cognitive theories (attitude, social influences, and self-efficacy) and stage theories (maintenance). The first steps posit that successful communication should result in the receiver's attention and comprehension. The subsequent steps refer to the receiver's changes in attitudes, social influences, self-efficacy, and behavior; and the last step refers to the maintenance of that behavior change. McGuire argues that educational interventions should match each step. Choices of the message content, the program audience, the communication context, and the message source depend on the step that is addressed. For instance, certain mass media messages, such as statements by famous sports heroes, may attract a lot of attention but may have negative effects on self-efficacy. An important contribution of PCM is that every method that uses communication will have to go through the steps for successful communication in order to have any effect at all. Protocols for pretesting of educational materials should apply these steps, and in practice most of them do (U.S. Department of Health and Human Services, 2002). Applying the PCM to all program communications is a basic method for change; see Table 3.5.

PCM can accommodate a host of social psychological variables that have been found to influence attitude and behavior (McGuire, 1985). However, for many of these variables, the relationship to attitude and behavior change is ambiguous. McGuire explains this ambiguity by distinguishing differential effects on reception of the message (that is, successful communication) and yielding to the message (that is, attitude and behavior change). For instance, the use of celebri-

TABLE 3.5. PERSUASION COMMUNICATION MATRIX.

	Message Content	Target Group	Communication Context	Message Source
Attention				
Comprehension				
Attitudes				
Social Influence				
Self-Efficacy				
Behavior				
Maintenance				

ties in persuasive messages can have a positive effect on reception but may have a negative effect on yielding. Almost no variables have a universal, unidirectional effect on attitude and behavior change.

Summary: PCM in Problem Analysis and Intervention Methods

- Intervention groups: intended program recipients at different stages of awareness, comprehension, attitude change, social support, sufficient self-efficacy, behavior change, or maintenance
- Behaviors: applicable to any behavior that can be influenced by communication
- Environment: information processing disturbed by information complexity and external factors
- Determinants: different by stage
- Methods: increasing thoughtful information processing, tailoring intervention methods to stage, use of the matrix to plan all communication decisions

Elaboration Likelihood Model (ELM)

Petty and Cacioppo (1986a, 1986b) and Petty, Barden, and Wheeler (2002) have created a dramatic new perspective on persuasion effects with the ELM. The basic idea of the ELM is that people differ in the ability and motivation for thoughtful information processing. These authors explain two ways of processing information: central and peripheral (also called systematic versus heuristic; see Chaiken, 1987). Central processing occurs when a message is carefully considered and compared against other messages and beliefs. Peripheral processing occurs when a message is processed without thoughtful consideration or comparison. For example, a student learning about self-efficacy for the first time can process the information centrally by comparing his or her own self-efficacy for several different behaviors. The student can continue the central processing by trying to find situations wherein self-efficacy seems to be important in choosing to attempt a behavior or to maintain effort. Pollay and colleagues (1996) suggest that peripheral cues are systematically used in tobacco advertisements for youth because these cues tend to bypass logical analysis. A variable—for instance, the source credibility of a sports hero as a role model—may have a positive effect when receivers process the message through the peripheral route but a negative effect when they follow the central route. In the sports hero example, people realize that their behavioral capabilities are different from those of the sports hero. For example, a well-known cyclist might be used in a mass media campaign to promote physical activity among youth. With peripheral processing, an overweight, sedentary teen might admire the athlete and react favorably to the ad for a brief time. However, with central processing, the same teen might compare the attributes of the athlete to her own fitness and end up with lower self-efficacy for physical activity than before the campaign. The same variable, source credibility, may also influence the motivation and ability to think, thus shifting people from the peripheral route to the central route or vice versa (Petty & Wegener, 1998).

The ELM has been very successful in explaining persuasion effects retrospectively, but is as yet less successful in predicting persuasion effects. Research findings suggest that thoughtful information processing is related to a higher persistence of attitude change, a higher resistance to counterpersuasion, and a stronger consistency between attitude and behavior (Petty & Cacioppo, 1986). Health educators would thus like to promote thoughtful information processing as much as possible. The ELM suggests three ways to stimulate motivation to think about the message: make the message personally relevant, make it unexpected, and repeat it.

Successful Communication

Successful communication is a prerequisite for any other change method (McGuire, 1985). A program cannot have any effect if the population is not exposed, does not pay attention to the program, or does not understand the message. Any program that includes methods for changing determinants and behavior should also include methods to achieve successful communication.

The ELM suggests that people only process the message seriously, through the central route, when they are motivated and able to do so (Petty & Cacioppo, 1986a, 1986b). An illustration is the program *Sex, Games, and Videotapes,* an HIV-prevention program for homeless mentally ill men in a New York shelter, that made messages personally relevant, surprising, and repeated by embedding them in playing competitive games, storytelling, and watching videos, activities that were salient pastimes in the shelter (Susser, Valencia, & Torres, 1994). Petty and colleagues (2002) mention additional motivational methods for stimulating central processing: making the message personally relevant through tailoring, making people feel responsible or accountable, and making people believe that they are part of a minority that practices the behavior. Additional methods that improve skills for information processing are using media that allow self-pacing by the target individuals, environments without distractions, and the use of language that people easily understand. Anticipation of interaction over the message and direct instructions to process the message carefully can help centralize the processing (Petty & Wegener, 1998). When the intervention group has the time and the behavioral capability, active learning can be used to promote central information processing based on the evidence that getting individuals to search for answers to questions they pose as a result of some stimulus leads to better information processing and learning, followed by more change in determinants and behavior.

However, even with high involvement, messages that are too discrepant from the receivers' positions will not have much effect (McGuire, 1985). When people process the health message through the central route, the quality of the argument is essential. An argument's quality can be determined only by pretesting the arguments with the target population.

Persuasion

One of the most widely used intervention methods for attitude change is the presentation of arguments in a persuasive message. The ELM predicts that high-quality arguments are effective only when the receivers process the message through the central route, not when they use the peripheral route. Because attitude change through the central route is more persistent, more resistant to change, and more related to behavior, health promoters should want to promote central information processing. A higher number of arguments does not ensure quality and, in fact, may negatively affect attitude change (Petty & Wegener, 1998). A greater number of arguments may be convincing for people who process the information through the peripheral route, but they will be less convincing for people who process through the central route. Petty and Wegener suggest that the following characteristics determine the quality of arguments, that is, their effectiveness after careful processing:

- Expectancy value: people like outcomes that are likely and desirable and avoid outcomes that are likely and undesirable.
- Causal explanations: a causal explanation will convince receivers of the likelihood of the outcome.
- Functionality: arguments that match the way people look at the world are more convincing.
- Importance: the relevance of outcomes determines the argument's effectiveness.
- Novelty: an unfamiliar or unique argument has more impact than does a familiar argument.

Persuasive arguments may be used at the individual level to encourage people to adopt healthful behaviors and may also be used for agents at higher ecological levels. For example, viewing a television broadcast on the health consequences to children from environmental tobacco smoke and the benefits of protecting children from smoke may influence a mother to declare her home smoke free. Seeing other legislators receive media attention for promoting, healthy policy may lead legislators to vote for health legislation. Both outcome expectations and expectancies must be high. For example, a city council must be persuaded both that fluoridation prevents dental caries and that the prevention of dental caries is something to value because of its effect on children's health. A persuasive argument about the extent of dental disease in children in the community and the outcome to their overall health that uses facts and personalized models might influence the council to accept both beliefs and to change the way it votes.

Summary: The ELM in Problem Analysis and Intervention Methods

- Intervention groups: different stages and different tendencies to process the messages with either high or low elaboration likelihood
- Behaviors: any behavior that can be influenced by communication
- Environment: information processing disturbed by information complexity and external factors
- Determinants: different by stage
- Methods: persuasive communication, increasing thoughtful information processing, active learning, tailoring to the individual's stage, use of the PCM to plan successful communication decisions and new arguments

Theories of Self-Regulation

Self-regulatory conceptualizations have to do with how individuals function to self-correct behavior (Baumeister & Vohs, 2004; Boekaerts, Pintrich, & Zeidner, 2001). Creer (2000) argues that *self-management,* the term that has often been used in the health domain, and *self-regulation*, the term used in psychology (Cleary & Zimmerman, 2000; B. Zimmerman, 2000) and in education (Schunk & Ertmer, 2000) refer to the same phenomena: an active, iterative process of setting a goal, choosing strategies, observing oneself, making judgments based on observation (as opposed to ones based on habit, fear, or tradition), reacting appropriately in the light of one's goal, and revising one's strategy accordingly (N. M. Clark, 2003; N. M. Clark & Zimmerman, 1990). The process is iterative, because feedback loops, through which one sees discrepancies between goals and outcomes and feels dissatisfaction, play an essential part in self-regulation (Scheier & Carver, 2003). Various authors' descriptions of this process are presented in Table 3.6.

Recently, Rothman, Baldwin, and Hertel (2004) have extended self-management stages and argue that the recycling process leads from trying the new behavior, to continuing, to maintenance, and finally to habit formation. They also point out that the determinants for change and the methods to promote change vary over these stages, comparable to the other stage models that we described earlier.

In a review of thirteen successful theory-based interventions for disease management, N. M. Clark (2003) notes that eight of the programs (N. M. Clark et al., 1997; N. Drummond et al., 1994; D. Evans et al., 1987; A. C. Israel, Guile, Baker, & Silverman, 1994; Janz et al., 1999; Lieberman, 2001; Sawicki, 1999; Scorpiglione et al., 1996) used self-regulatory approaches, which encourage the executive cognitive processes of setting goals, observing behavior, and revising goals.

TABLE 3.6. SELF-REGULATORY THEORY.

Authors	Construct Names		
	Monitoring	**Evaluation**	**Action**
Clark & Zimmerman, 1990	Self-observation	Self-judgment	Self-reaction
Kotses, Lewis, & Creer, 1990	Monitoring	Comparing to personal best	Normal activity Control of asthma
Creer, Kotses, & Wigal, 1992	Information collection	Information processing and evaluation	Self-management skills Self-instruction Treatment steps
Lazarus & Folkman, 1991	Appraisal	Problem description	Generation of flexible solutions
Thorensen & Kirmil-Gray, 1983	Self-monitoring	Self-evaluation	Action Self-reinforcement

Self-regulatory theory is useful for designating health-promoting behaviors for the self-management of chronic disease. For example, in a family-oriented pediatric asthma self-management program, Bartholomew, Gold, and colleagues (2000) conceptualized both asthma-specific skills (for example, taking control medications) and self-regulatory skills (for example, monitoring for symptoms of asthma) (Chapter Twelve) (Bartholomew, Gold et al., 2000; Bartholomew, Shegog et al., 2000; Shegog, Bartholomew, Gold, Parcel, et al., 1999; Shegog, Bartholomew, Gold, Pierrel, et al., 1999). The teaching of self-regulatory skills has been demonstrated in the school setting (Schunk, 1998; Schunk & Zimmerman, 1994). In the asthma program, the skills were called watch, discover, think, and act. Children were taught to watch or monitor their asthma symptoms, discover whether there was a problem and what might be causing it, decide on a plan of action to solve the problem or to prevent a future problem, and take action.

In another example of the application of self-regulatory theory to the delineation of self-management behavior, Cox, Gonder-Frederick, Julian, and Clarke (1994) taught diabetics to prevent both hypoglycemia and hyperglycemia by providing self-regulatory skill training and practice. They increased sensitivity to symptoms, promoted identification of external events such as insulin administration or food intake that can change the likelihood of blood sugar peaks and dips, and helped participants create effective responses to internal and external cues.

Summary: Theories of Self-Regulation in Problem Analysis and Intervention Methods

- Intervention groups: people who are trying to incorporate complex behaviors into their lifestyles
- Behaviors: performance objectives for self-regulatory behaviors, that is, monitoring, evaluation, action
- Environment: helps the learner explicitly consider the role of the environment in the performance of certain behaviors, for example, to appraise the environment in the monitoring phase
- Determinants: can be seen as a determinant of behavioral capability
- Methods: skill training for self-regulation

Social Cognitive Theory (SCT)

Bandura's social cognitive theory (1986) is an interpersonal theory that covers both determinants of behavior and the process of behavior change (Bandura, 1997; Baranowski et al., 2002). SCT explains human behavior "in terms of a model of reciprocal determinism in which behavior, cognitive and other personal factors, and environmental events all operate as interacting determinants of each other" (Bandura, 1986, p. 18). Major determinants of behavior described by SCT are outcome expectations, self-efficacy, behavioral capability, perceived behavior of others, and environment.

Outcome Expectations, Self-Efficacy, and Behavioral Capability

An *outcome expectation* is a judgment of the likely consequence that a certain behavior will produce ("When I use a condom consistently, I will prevent sexually transmitted infections" [STIs]). *Outcome expectancies,* on the other hand, are the values that individuals place on a certain outcome (Baranowski et al., 2002). Outcome expectations are comparable to behavioral beliefs in the TPB, and outcome expectancies are comparable to evaluations.

Self-efficacy is a judgment of a person's capability to accomplish a certain level of performance ("I am confident that I can use a condom consistently"). Bandura (1986, p. 392) is very explicit about the interrelation between outcome expectations and self-efficacy: "The types of outcomes people anticipate depend largely on their judgments of how well they will be able to perform in given situations." When people are not confident that they can use a condom consistently, they may also not expect to prevent STIs. Some studies have found an interaction effect between self-efficacy and outcome expectations. When a person is in a situation in which outcome expectations are positive and strong but self-efficacy for that behavior is low, a situation of avoidance or denial may occur; and the person is unlikely to attempt the behavior (Bandura, 1986). In addition to personal self-efficacy, Bandura (1997) describes perceived collective efficacy, belief in the performance capability of a social system as a whole (Chapter Four).

The concept of behavioral capability is that if people are to perform a particular type of behavior, they must know what the behavior is (knowledge of the behavior) and how to perform the behavior (skill). Self-efficacy is a person's perception; capability is the real thing. Health promotion programs should go beyond providing knowledge to providing behavioral capability, which is closer to actual performance. The development of behavioral capability is the result of the individual's training, intellectual capacity, and learning style. The behavioral training technique called mastery learning provides procedural knowledge of the activities to perform, practice in performing those activities, and feedback about successful performance.

Observational Learning and Environment

Most human behavior is learned through observation of models (vicarious learning). By observing others, a person can form rules for behavior; and on future occasions this coded information can serve as a guide for action. Four constituent processes govern modeling:

- Attention to and perception of the relevant aspects of modeled activities (including characteristics of the observer and the model)
- Retention and representation of learned knowledge and remembering
- Production of appropriate action
- Motivation as a result of observed positive incentives and reinforcement.

When providing models to encourage the learning of certain behaviors, the health educator should find a role model from the community or at-risk group that will encourage identification. The model should present a coping model (for example, "I tried to quit smoking several times and was not successful, then I tried . . . Now I have been off cigarettes for . . .") rather than a mastery model (for example, "I just threw my pack away, and that was it"). Learners should be able to observe models being reinforced for their behavior (for example, being congratulated by friends for staying off cigarettes or having a partner say how fresh the ex-smoker smells).

Perceived behavior of others is distinguishable from perceived social expectations: Smoking parents may be contributing to their child's taking up smoking (a model) while they may expect their child not to smoke (perceived social expectation).

The term *environment* refers to an objective notion of all the factors that can affect a person's behavior but that are physically external to that person. The social environment includes, for instance, family members, peers, and neighbors. The physical environment includes availability of certain foods, indoor and outdoor air quality, restrictions for smoking, and so on. Individuals may or may not be aware of the strong influence that the environment has on their behavior. Likewise, health promoters may underuse the role of environment in their program planning; keeping the concept of reciprocal determinism in mind will help planners avoid this pitfall. Planners should always try to create a facilitating environment for health-promoting change.

SCT and Behavior Change

SCT integrates determinants of behavior with methods for behavior change. All SCT interventions are based on active learning that promotes performance during the learning process. Perceived behavior of others is not only a determinant of behavior, it is also a very effective method for behavior change: modeling. A general method of SCT is reinforcement. Modeling, in which a person experiences vicarious reinforcement, is a special case of reinforcement. A person may experience vicarious reinforcement by observing a model receiving reinforcement. Reinforcements may be external (receiving money) or internal (doing something that one perceives as right). Self-efficacy and behavioral capability may be improved through the following (Bandura, 1997):

- Enactive mastery experiences with feedback to serve as indicators of capability
- Vicarious experiences (modeling) that alter efficacy expectations through perception of competencies and comparison with the attainment of others
- Verbal persuasion and allied types of social influences that suggest the person, agent, or group possesses certain capabilities
- Enhancement or reduction of physiological and affective states (for example, anxiety) from which people partly judge their own capability, strength, and vulnerability to dysfunction

Facilitation

All learning has to be complemented by facilitation, the provision of means for the learner to take action or means to reduce barriers to action (Bandura, 1986; Mullen et al., 1985, 1992). Facilitation often means creating a change in the environment. For instance, a program that targets improvement in drug users' self-efficacy for using clean needles must also facilitate clean needles being easily accessible. People with higher self-efficacy will exert more effort, although actual barriers ultimately mediate what the effect will be.

Summary: Social Cognitive Theory in Problem Analysis and Intervention Methods

- Intervention groups: no specification
- Behaviors: any behavior, but usually applied to behaviors that are complex and require considerable behavioral capability
- Environment: actual barriers difficult even with high self-efficacy, strong impact of the social and the physical environment
- Determinants: outcome expectations, self-efficacy expectations, behavioral capability, perceived behavior of others, social and physical environment
- Methods: active learning, reinforcement, modeling and guided practice, persuasion

Diffusion of Innovations Theory (DIT)

An *innovation* is an idea, practice, or product that is new to the adopter, which may be an individual or an organization (Oldenburg & Parcel, 2002). Healthy behavior, for example, physical activity, cessation of smoking, and use of contraceptives may be innovations for individuals. Health promotion programs to encourage these behaviors may be innovations in an organization. For example, patient self-management programs may be an innovation in an organization because they change the power relationship between patients and providers (Mullen & Mullen, 1983). For many years E. M. Rogers (1983, 1995, 2003) has studied the process of diffusion, beginning with a focus on individual adopters of new technology. Rogers's individual model is useful for health education because it describes the decision-making process not only of individuals but also of change agents and program implementers.

E. M. Rogers (1983, 1995, 2003) and others over several decades have laid the groundwork for how to get innovations adopted, implemented, and continued over time (Steckler et al., 2002). Diffusion is thought of as moving from awareness of a need or of an innovation, through decisions to adopt the innovation, to initial use and maintenance. The individual must become aware of the innovation, develop an interest, try it out, adopt it, and maintain it.

From an organizational perspective, there are essentially three stages (Steckler, Goodman, McLeroy, Davis, & Koch, 1992; Goodman, Steckler, & Kegler, 1997; Shediac-Rizkallah & Bone, 1998; Parcel, Perry, & Taylor, 1990; Parcel et al., 1995):

1. Adoption, which depends on knowledge of an innovation, awareness of an unmet need, and the decision that a certain innovation may meet the perceived need and will be given a trial
2. Implementation, the use of the innovation to a fair trial point
3. Sustainability, the maintenance and institutionalization of an innovation or its outcomes

Some authors have written about dissemination taking place prior to adoption (Parcel, 1995; Parcel, Eriksen, et al., 1989; Parcel, Taylor, et al., 1989). Dissemination can be seen as something someone does to make potential adopters aware of and favorably disposed toward the innovation.

Characteristics of Adopters and Innovations

Of course, potential adopters can decide not to adopt an innovation. This decision can be either an active process or simply a passive failure to become familiar with the innovation and to decide. Classic diffusion theory has dealt with characteristics of both adopters and innovations. Adopters adopt at different times following the introduction of the innovation into their social system; and the population can be segmented into innovators, early adopters, early majority, late majority, and laggards, based on the point at which they adopt the innovation. E. M. Rogers (1995, 2003) described the process of adoption as a normal, bell-shaped distribution that places majority adopters within one standard deviation on either side of the mean of the curve, early and late adopters two standard deviations away, and laggards and innovators three standard deviations away. These categories of adopters have been shown to have different characteristics: Innovators are venturesome; early adopters are opinion leaders; early majority are deliberators; late majority are skeptical; and the laggards are traditional. All individual adopters go through a process of awareness, interest, trial, and adoption of the innovation; but the time required to complete these stages increases across the categories, with innovators having the shortest period between awareness and adoption.

Innovations are often communicated through two different channels: media and interpersonal communication. Initially, media increase awareness of the innovation. As people hear about the innovation and begin to adopt it, they talk with others about their interest and experience. The interpersonal channel thus becomes more important as more members of the population adopt the innovation. More potent outreach and incentives are needed for late adopters and laggards, who have not adopted even though the innovation has been communicated through the media and the majority of members of the population have adopted the innovation. Thus, for intervention planning, it is important to know the adopter category (Green, Gottlieb, & Parcel, 1991; E. M. Rogers, 1995).

SCT provides explanations of the psychological mechanisms by which diffusion occurs (Bandura, 1997). For people to adopt, implement, and maintain a new behavior, they must be aware of the innovation, hold positive outcome expectations and expectancies for it, and have sufficient self-efficacy and behavioral capability for both adoption and implementation. Adolescents adopting condom use, for example, must know that condoms are available, expect that condoms help prevent HIV and STIs, and have positive self-efficacy expectations about talking to their partner about condoms and about using condoms adequately. In Chapter Four we discuss adoption, implementation, and sustainability at the organizational and community levels; and in Chapter Nine we focus on diffusion of health promotion programs. Also important in the consideration of interventions to promote diffusion of behavior change are the characteristics of innovations (Oldenburg & Parcel, 2002; E. M. Rogers, 1995). These characteristics are the potential adopters' perceptions of what the innovation is like. They include the following:

- Relative advantage of the innovation compared to what is being used
- Compatibility with the intended users' current behavior
- Complexity
- Observability of the results

- Impact on social relations
- Reversibility or case of discontinuation
- Communicability
- Required time
- Risk and uncertainty
- Required commitment
- Ability to be modified

Each of these characteristics of an innovation must be considered as either a predictor of or a barrier to adoption and implementation both in innovation design and in the creation of an intervention to aid diffusion.

Diffusion of Innovations Theory suggests methods and strategies to influence the determinants and accomplish the performance objectives for adoption, implementation, and sustainability of new behavior (E. M. Rogers, 2003). Many of the determinants of adoption, implementation, and sustainability are comparable to determinants from other theories, such as the TPB, SCT, and the TTM; and they may be influenced by the same type of methods. Communication within the community about the innovation is essential for the diffusion process; the health promoter will want to stimulate communication and mobilize social support for the innovation. One effective method is to speed this process by communicating through mass media the stories of people who have been successful in adopting the new behavior. These early adopters then serve as role models for the early majority in the target community, and the early majority serves as models for the late majority. One way to do this is by using behavioral journalism (McAlister, 1995; van Empelen, Kok, Schaalma, et al., 2003). Combining DIT with SCT, behavioral journalism includes the use of appropriate role-model stories (for example, those of early adopters) based on authentic interviews with the target group and the use of mass media and networks within the community to distribute those role-model stories to the target population (for example, early majority).

Summary: Diffusion of Innovations Theory in Problem Analysis and Intervention Methods

- Intervention groups: adopter categories, such as innovators, early adopters, early majority, late majority, and laggards
- Behaviors: adoption, implementation, and sustainability of the new behavior
- Environments: may be applied to any behavior that is new to the person: at-risk individuals, environmental agents, or program users

- Determinants: adopter characteristics, such as being venturesome individuals, opinion leaders, deliberators, skeptical, and traditional; innovation characteristics, such as relative advantage, compatibility, complexity, observability, impact on social relations, reversibility, communicability, time, risk and uncertainty, commitment, and ability to be modified
- Methods: increase the rate of diffusion by linkage, participation, organized communication about the innovation, mobilizing social support, role-modeling, and behavioral journalism

CHAPTER FOUR

ENVIRONMENT-ORIENTED THEORIES

Reader Objectives

- Identify theories to describe environmental conditions that promote behavior and health
- Identify potential environmental agents whose role behavior influences the environmental conditions
- Describe determinants of the behavior of the environmental agents and theoretical methods to change these behaviors
- Discuss the differences due to role and power in methods used as one goes to higher socioecological levels

The purpose of this chapter is to identify environment-oriented theories and models that are useful for planning health promotion interventions. We first discuss how to describe and select environmental conditions to be changed, and then we suggest how to change these conditions. The theories and models are organized by environmental level: interpersonal, organizational, community, and societal.

As we discussed in the previous chapters, the individual is embedded within social networks, organizations, community, and society; and each lower level is embedded within higher levels. A facilitating environment that makes the health promoting behavior the easiest behavior to perform (Milio, 1981) is key to a change in the behavior of the at-risk population, as well as to a change of environmental conditions. Examples of environmental conditions include social influences (such as norms, social support, and reinforcement) and structural influences (such as access to resources, organizational climate, and policies). Barriers to performing a health behavior are often structural, such as lack of health insurance, inconvenient clinic hours, lack of transportation, high-fat cafeteria foods, high cost of healthy foods, intense advertising of cigarettes and alcohol, and unsafe neighborhoods for jogging or walking.

Perspectives

In this section, we discuss our logic model for the relations among environmental methods, determinants, agents, conditions, and health as they relate to environmental change and the influence that power plays in environmental change.

Model for Change of Environmental Conditions

Figure 4.1, the logic model for the relationships among methods, determinants, behaviors, environmental conditions, and health that we introduced in Chapter Three, has the environmental path through the environmental agent. The environmental condition is a state of a given environment that is more or less promoting of health either directly or through behavior. The accessibility of hiking and bicycling trails, for example, is an environmental condition that facilitates physical activity. The presence of toxic agents in the air acts directly on health.

FIGURE 4.1. LOGIC MODEL FOR RELATIONSHIPS BETWEEN METHODS, DETERMINANTS, BEHAVIORS, ENVIRONMENTAL CONDITIONS, AND HEALTH.

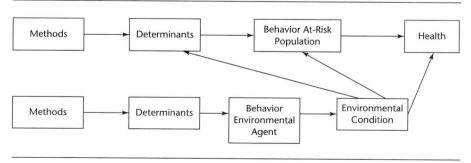

For each environmental condition, human agents act or behave in ways that influence the existence or intensity of the environmental condition. A city council allocates money to build hiking and bicycling trails, and Congress may authorize money for use by cities to build such trails. Members of city councils and federal legislators are environmental agents in this case, and their respective behaviors are proposing and voting to allocate funds. Note that agents and actions at different levels are directed at the same environmental condition in this example. Working to influence change at multiple ecological levels is synergistic in producing and sustaining changes in environmental conditions.

Once the agents and behaviors have been identified, the planner can select behavior-oriented determinants and methods to change them. In Chapter Three theoretical constructs were identified that described determinants for behavior, as were theoretical methods to change specific determinants. These constructs and methods apply to behavior of both the at-risk population and the environmental agent. For example, positive outcome expectations of the behavior would influence a legislator to vote to allocate funds (for example, "If I vote to allocate funds for trails, people in my district will have more opportunities to exercise"), as well as to influence the at-risk population to jog (for example, "If I jog, I will reduce my level of stress"). Similarly, persuasive communication is a method to influence the outcome expectations of both the population at risk and the environmental agents. Thus, theories from both Chapters Three and Four are needed as the health promoter plans for change in environmental conditions.

The methods presented in Chapter Three included ways to help individuals influence external determinants, such as resisting or coping with norms or barriers, and ways to influence the decision makers who control the resources. We also talked about how the methods directed toward determinants of individual behavior could influence individual agents or gatekeepers at any environmental level. To some extent we have already begun to discuss methods and strategies for influencing health through these higher ecological levels.

However, we realize that this perspective does not fully capture the process of collective action. In dealing with these gatekeeper behaviors, we have not emphasized how these behaviors occur as part of a collective (such as a legislative body, work site, or social network) or how these collectives are systems in their own right with their own regulatory processes. In a collective the whole is greater than the sum of its parts. Clearly, a single legislator's vote does not lead to passage of a law. Law making is a complex process, and much goes on behind the scenes. For example, in the United States, a powerful Speaker of the House sometimes assigns the bills to committees in which they will die; key committee chairs schedule hostile hearings; senators make compromise deals in the construction of bills; opposition party members add fatal amendments; and political party leaders bring their legislators' votes in line.

In this chapter we describe organizational, community, and social change methods that rely on the power and authority vested in organizations, associations of citizens, and government. We examine the methods and strategies at these higher ecological levels used to target collective action at each level that may have an effect on that level or embedded levels (for example, the legislature passes a law limiting minors' access to cigarettes; the company goes tobacco free; a social network supports a first-time mother in quitting cigarettes). These actions may influence the population for risk reduction both directly, as in these examples, or indirectly, as in the legislature's passing a law that companies must reduce emissions of pollutants. When health educators seek to address these upper ecological levels, they often find general methods for community organization and organizational development, but they find less specificity on ways to engage in the process. We attempt to open this black box through a careful review of methods and strategies combined with our earlier discussion of the use of individual-level determinants for persons in specific roles within social systems, for example, a legislator, school principal, or union official.

Figure 4.2 provides an overview of the process by which methods and strategies influence collectivities to provide the products that are external determinants of individual behavior. The products can also be considered as ends in themselves; that is, the particular system has healthy characteristics, in which case the end target, the population's health, would not be considered. However, in general, planners assume, either explicitly or implicitly, that the end result is population health.

Looking at Healthy Environments as Outcomes

Figure 4.1 considers environmental conditions as they relate to health directly or through the path of behavior. Others have looked at the environment as a desired outcome, irrespective of individual health outcomes; and since the 1986 Ottawa Charter, the World Health Organization has focused on healthy settings (Nutbeam, 1998; World Health Organization, 1986). For example, a healthy city could be characterized as one that has health-promoting policy across all sectors (such as a large greenbelt, low population density, recreation facilities, and low unemployment), explicit political commitment to the project at the highest levels, and investment in formal and informal networking and cooperation, focusing on equity and building personal and social competence to deal with issues of importance to the community (Awofeso, 2003; Duhl, 2004; Haglund, Finer, Tillgren, & Pettersson, 1996; Nutbeam & Harris, 1995). A healthy work site would have healthy policies, a health-promoting culture, commitments to self-knowledge and development, respect for individual differences, jobs that foster responsibility and autonomy, safe and healthy working environments, and equitable salaries and promotion opportunities (Chu et al., 2000; Rosen, 1992). A healthy school would have a coherent

FIGURE 4.2. OVERVIEW OF INTERVENTION PROCESS AT HIGHER ECOLOGICAL LEVELS.

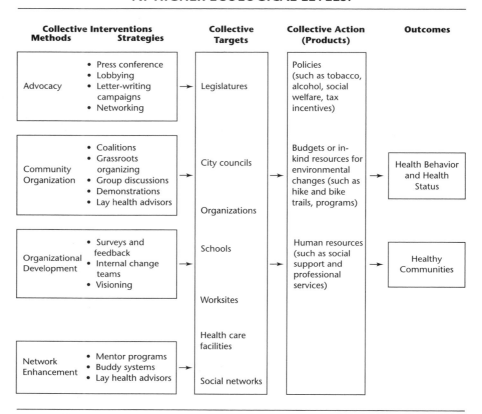

sequential health and physical education curriculum, teacher training, an ethos that supports student and staff well-being, health-promoting policies and practices including those of nutrition and food services, comprehensive health services, counseling, social services, and school-community partnerships, all established with the principles of democracy and equity (Allensworth, Lawson, Nicholson, & Wyche, 1997; Burgher, Rasmussen, & Rivett, 1999; Mukoma & Flisher, 2004; Rowling, 1996). Health-promoting hospitals embrace the aims of health promotion. They have a health-promoting physical environment and organizational structure, a participatory culture, and a focus on health with a holistic approach

(Johnson & Baum, 2001; Nutbeam, 1998; Whitehead, 2004; World Health Organization, 1997). Health-promoting workplaces balance customer expectations and organizational targets with employees' skills and health, extending beyond wellness programs to include broader organizational and environmental issues (Chu et al., 2000). If one starts with the endpoint of environment as an outcome, one uses the same steps of identifying the environmental agents and their behavior and actions, the determinants of the agents' behavior, and methods to change those behaviors.

In health promotion situations in which the environmental condition is the outcome of interest, we suggest that the links through behavior to health and to health directly be considered in the needs assessment (Step 1) and also in the evaluation (Step 6). This will assure program justification at both the outset and in the summative evaluation.

Understanding Power

Understanding power, the probability that an individual or group will determine what another individual or group will do even if it is contrary to the latter's interests, is a crucial concept in order to influence collective action (Orum, 1988). Weber (1947) recognizes three sources of power: authority, charisma, and legitimacy.

Each of the ecological levels has different power structures and methods for the delivery of social influence. In small groups, social influence occurs through interaction and through leadership. The leadership might be shared by members of the group, given over voluntarily to an individual leader by the group, or vested in an individual from a higher authority. At the organization level, the power of authority comes through the organizational hierarchical structure, that is, who is above whom in the organizational chart. Informal power arises from an individual's charisma, from others' satisfaction with a person's previous leadership activities, or from legitimacy, such as being elected or born into a family business. At the community and societal levels, power is "the social capacity to make binding decisions that have major consequences over the directions in which a society moves" (Orum, 1988, p. 402).

J. C. Turner (2005) has developed a social psychological theory related to power, viewing power as an emergent quality of human social relationships. In this view power is the capacity to exert one's will through other people. This can be subdivided into persuasion and control, getting people to do things they are not persuaded of or interested in. Control in turn is subdivided into authority and coercion. In the category of authority, in-group norms have given an authority figure the right to control. Coercion, the attempt to control others against their will, occurs when there is failure to influence others' behavior.

Group identity can unify people so that they influence each other, act as a coordinated body, and thus gain the power of collective action. Social change occurs when a subordinate group develops a distinct identity and its own goals and beliefs and can challenge the power of the dominant group. Persuasion or social influence, a method discussed in Chapter Three, is the chief mechanism for obtaining power, both individually and as a group.

The role of power differs in the three types of social change that J. Rothman (1979) defined. In locality development the democratic town hall process distributes power equally; in social planning the power rests with experts; and in social action, disenfranchised people wrest power from the official power structure. Formal leadership in a community rests with elected and appointed officials to whom community members have given authority to govern. This authority is distributed to the government agencies that carry out federal, state, and local programs. Private organizations, because of their economic power (providing jobs and products), may have even more influence over a community.

Minkler and Wallerstein (1997a, 1997b) have distinguished between the concepts of power with and power over, using a feminist perspective that views power as a limitless resource. They suggest that community building and capacity building are models of power with, whereas empowerment-oriented social action is a model of challenging power over. These two types of community organization lead to community competence, leadership development, and critical awareness.

McCullum, Pelletier, Barr, Wilkins, and Habich (2004) used a three-dimensional framework of power that built on core sociological perspectives. The first dimension, participation in decision making, is at first glance simply a determination of whether community members are at the table. However, the other two dimensions show processes that limit true participation in decision making. In the second dimension, agenda setting, the decision about what issues and decisions are considered, has a bias such that values and beliefs of vested interests determine what is discussed. The third dimension, the shaping of perceived needs, is more insidious. Dominant groups in society frame issues by defining the causes of and solutions for identified problems. Powerless groups have been socialized to accept the frames of reference of the dominant groups and institutions, and they lack awareness of how their ways of looking at the world have been conditioned. Thus, they may adopt values and interests that are not their own but those of the dominant group.

Power is the key to creating change at the higher environmental levels. In planning interventions at higher ecological levels, health educators can bring power to play in several ways. They can identify the agent who has the power to carry out the desired change, choose the change method that is most effective given the position of the agent and the form of power the person holds, and use the form of power that will most effectively influence a change agent. In addition, the health promoter must be conscious of the unintended negative effects of power in his or her work with communities, which can reinforce the status quo and lead to oppression of some groups by others (Hawe & Shiell, 2000).

Empowerment

Empowerment is a process through which individuals, communities, and organizations change their social and political environments. In so doing, they gain a sense of mastery, improved equity, and enhanced quality of life (Minkler & Wallerstein, 1997b). At the individual level, the results of empowerment are psychological, including increased perception of control over one's destiny, political efficacy, and motivation to act (Syme, 1988; M. A. Zimmerman, 1990). This type of empowerment occurs when people take action to gain power and control through organizational and community involvement and to understand their environment critically (see this chapter's discussion of conscientization and social movements) (M. A. Zimmerman, 1995).

At the organizational and community levels, empowerment involves collective problem solving; shared leadership and decision making; and accessible government, media, and resources. M. A. Zimmerman (1990) describes individual-level outcomes as perceived control and behavioral capability to gain power and control and higher ecological-level outcomes as organizational networks, resource acquisition, policy development, evidence of pluralism, and accessible community resources. This is a similar concept to collective efficacy. Defined as "a group's shared belief in its conjoint capabilities to organize and execute the courses of action required to produce given levels of attainments" (Bandura, 1997, p. 477), collective efficacy may be applied to the levels of family, community, organizations, social institutions, and nation. Although related to personal self-efficacy, it is an emergent group-level attribute that is more than the sum of members' perceived personal efficacies. It emerges from the social interdependence of individuals performing tasks and carrying out roles. Specific types of collective efficacy include perceived organizational efficacy (employees' beliefs that their work team or organization can accomplish its goals) and perceived political efficacy (people's beliefs that they can influence the political system). As with personal efficacy, specificity with collective efficacy is important, and collective efficacy should be described and measured for particular behaviors rather than globally. For example, collective efficacy in organizations might be specific to study of the environment for trends, to product development, or to marketing. Political efficacy has subcomponents such as efficacy for voting, fundraising, voter registration, and lobbying.

Collective efficacy has been less well researched than has personal efficacy (Bandura, 1997). However, teachers' collective efficacy has been linked to the academic performance of students in elementary schools; workers' collective efficacy has been linked to the performance of self-managing work teams; and players' collective efficacy has been linked to athletic teams' performance. Perceived protest efficacy (a specific form of political efficacy) along with strong outcome expectations of harm were found to be predictive of people's willingness to protest the placement of a chemical plant in their community (Bandura, 1997).

Change in collective efficacy comes through the same mechanisms that change does in personal efficacy. The most effective way to enhance a community's collective efficacy is through success at accomplishing a particular goal, for example, lobbying the city council to pass a clean indoor-air act for the city. Models of how other communities accomplished similar goals could also enhance efficacy, as might community leaders challenging the community members to take action.

Figure 4.3 extends Figure 4.1 to include the paths by which the health promoter uses methods of change (path a) either to act directly on the environmental agent to influence the environmental condition or to facilitate community empowerment (path b). It also includes the methods by which an empowered community or individuals in a community influence environmental agents to take actions that change environmental conditions (path c) and the paths by which the empowered community may take an environmental action directly (path d). When a community is effective at influencing an agent to take an environmental action or when the community takes that action directly and the environmental condition is changed, we hypothesize that a feedback loop (path e) occurs and results in increased collective empowerment.

In the remainder of this chapter, we discuss theories and provide examples that illuminate environmental change at each ecological level: interpersonal, organizational, community, and society. We present methods by which health promoters facilitate empowerment of social networks, organizations, and communities. These individuals and communities in turn influence the actions that environmental agents take at various levels to create environmental conditions conducive to health.

Interpersonal-Level Theories

Social relationships are the foundation for human existence, and interpersonal-level theories are key to understanding and intervening on relationships.

FIGURE 4.3. MODEL OF ENVIRONMENTAL HEALTH ETIOLOGY AND EMPOWERMENT.

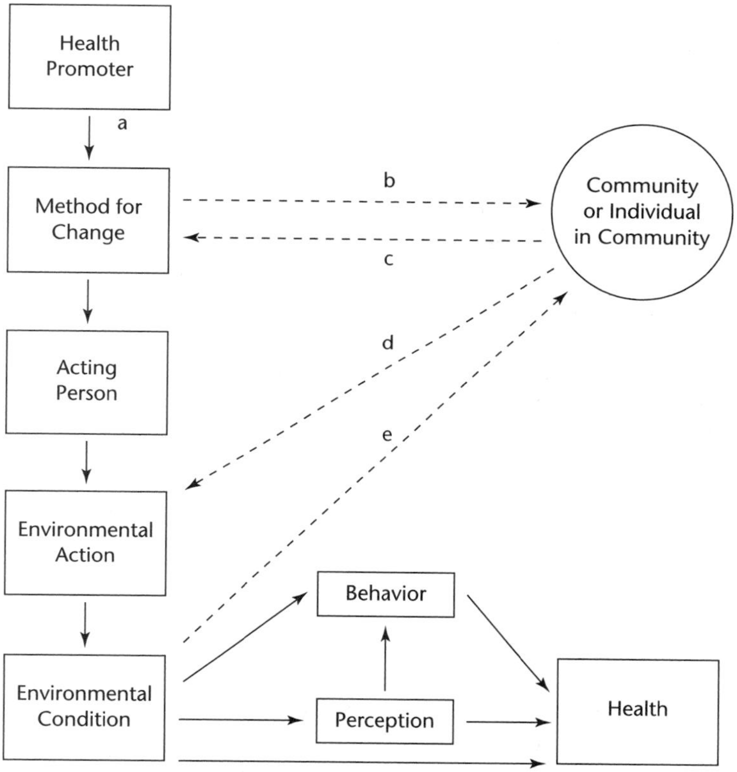

Source: Commers, Gottlieb, and Kok, 2005.

Social Networks and Social Support

Social network is an analytic framework for understanding relationships among members of social systems. Networks are classified as personal, based on the ties an individual has with other persons, or whole network, based on the relationships among a defined group of people. Personal or egocentric networks are particularly useful for the study of social support, whereas the whole-network approach allows the identification of cliques of individuals and the identification of roles, such as occupational positions that extend across networks (boundary spanners).

Networks can be horizontal (peers) or vertical (hierarchy) and can provide a way to understand power relationships in organizations. Community can be understood metaphorically as networks of networks in which the nodes of the larger network comprise smaller-scale networks (B. H. Gottlieb, 1985; Hall & Wellman, 1985; McLeroy, Gottlieb, & Heaney, 2001).

Social networks consist of nodes (individuals, groups, or organizations) that are joined by ties (the relationships among nodes). Networks can be defined by their content—whether they are primarily friendship, kinship, communication, or task-oriented organizational networks. The network also has a structure, including the number of members, the degree of members' similarity to each other, the way they are connected, and their links to other networks. Definitions of key structural properties of social networks are seen in Table 4.1. An individual can play several roles in a network: a group member, a linking agent, or an isolate with few ties to other network members (Fulk & Boyd, 1991). Linking agents are especially important because, as members of multiple networks, they bring information across network boundaries.

The egocentric social network, defined as a person-centered web of social relationships, is the structure through which social support may be provided. Heaney and Israel (2002, p. 187) define *social support* as "aid and assistance exchanged through social relationships and interpersonal transactions." In contrast to other types of interpersonal interactions such as criticism and domination, social support is always something that the sender intends to be helpful. Four main types of social support have been identified: emotional (affective), instrumental (tangible), informational (cognitive), and appraisal (Heaney & Israel). Emotional support includes love, caring, and empathy. Instrumental support includes aid or service, such as babysitting or lending money to a person. Informational support is the giving of information, advice, or suggestions. Appraisal support, a special form of cognitive support, merits its own category; it is self-evaluative information that is important for maintaining one's identity. This information includes constructive feedback, affirmation of beliefs and values, and social comparison (Heaney & Israel; McLeroy et al., 2001).

Different types of social networks are associated with specific types of social support. Small, dense, geographically close, intense networks provide emotional and appraisal support. These networks typically do not have access to the larger society or to information outside the network's domain. On the other hand, large, diffuse, and less intense networks provide more informational support and social outreach. Different types of social support are important at different times in the experience of stressors. For example, with loss of a job, emotional support that the individual is still loved and his or her self is intact is most important at first. Later, the individual needs informational support regarding other job opportunities or

TABLE 4.1. STRUCTURAL AND RELATIONAL PROPERTIES OF SOCIAL NETWORKS.

Structural Properties

Range	The number of network members
Density	The extent to which a network is connected measured by the proportion of direct ties that exist among network members out of all possible ties that could exist among them
Degree	The extent to which a network member has direct ties with other network members
"Boundedness"	The proportion of all ties of network members that stay within the network's boundaries
"Reachability"	The average number of ties required to link any two network members
Homogeneity	The extent to which network members have similar characteristics (such as age, race, sex gender, economic status, and so on)
Cliques	Portions of networks in which all members are tied directly
Clusters	Portions of networks in which all members are not tied directly
Components	Portions of networks in which all members are tied directly or indirectly

Relationship Properties

Strength	The quantity of resources between two network members
Frequency	The quantity of contact between two network members
"Multiplexity"	The number of different types of social support exchanged between two network members
Duration	The length of time a relationship has existed
Symmetry	The extent to which social support is both given and received between two network members
Intimacy	The perceived emotional closeness among two network members

Source: Adapted from A. Hall and Wellman, 1985; B. A. Israel, 1982.

possible career changes. Tangible support such as loans, transportation, or child care may also help people when they are job hunting. In planning for interventions, it is important to distinguish among these types of social support so that support in the social environment is specific to the behavior or health outcome sought.

The extent and nature of social relationships has been linked to health status in a number of studies, and we refer the reader to comprehensive reviews (L. F. Berkman & Glass, 2000; Heaney & Israel, 2002; Hogan, Linden, & Najarian,

2002; House, Umberson, & Landis, 1988; B. A. Israel & Rounds, 1987). The mechanisms underlying this epidemiological finding have been hypothesized to include modeling and reinforcement of positive health-related behaviors, buffering of the effects of stress on health, and provision of access to resources to cope with stress. L. F. Berkman and Glass's comprehensive conceptual model (2000) describes how social-structural conditions such as culture, socioeconomic factors, politics, and social change shape social networks. Social networks in turn provide opportunities for social support, social influence, social engagement, person-to-person contact, and access to resources and material goods. These psychosocial mechanisms affect health through health behavior pathways, psychological pathways, and physiologic pathways.

Social Support Interventions. Hogan, Linden, and Najarian (2002) conducted a comprehensive review of social support interventions for a variety of issues, including cancer, loneliness, weight loss, substance abuse, surgery, and birth preparation. Studies represented three types of interventions: both group and individual interventions, treatment provided by professionals or peers; interventions directed to increasing network size or perceived support; and those directed to building social skills to facilitate creation of support. Of the ninety-two studies with control groups, 83 percent reported at least some intervention benefits. They found support provided by friends, family members, or peers to be beneficial, especially when the support was reciprocal. Training in social support skills was particularly useful. These findings held across individual and group interventions, whether they were led by professionals or peers.

Heaney and Israel (2002) identify four types of intervention to increase social support. First is the enhancement of existing social networks and their linkages. Strategies to increase network density can include activities to bring network members together to get to know one another. Strategies to increase reciprocity include exchange structures such as babysitting or housecleaning exchanges. Norms and incentives for volunteerism and for supporting coworkers, neighbors, and parishioners strengthen social networks. In contrast to the value of radical individualism, a cultural value on cooperation fosters social support.

The enhancement of existing network linkages can be accomplished by training network members in skills for providing support and by training members of the target group to mobilize and maintain their networks. For example, family members may be trained to provide support to individuals who are in programs to stop smoking (S. Cohen & Lichtenstein, 1990; Mermelstein, Cohen, Lichtenstein, Baer, & Kamarck, 1986). A media campaign titled Good Friends Make Good Medicine focused on informing people about the influence of social support on health and encouraging them to connect with their friends and family by phone or in person and to trade favors and share feelings with them (Hersey, Klibanoff, Lam, & Taylor, 1984). In another example of enhancing existing linkages, the STOP AIDS Project in San Francisco worked through existing formal and informal social groups to enhance social support for safe sex as part of its community-organizing strategy. Many groups that the organizers approached were reluctant to provide an organized discussion about AIDS and the role that friends play in encouraging safe sex and discouraging unsafe sex, because the group's goals were unrelated to the project's health and sexual behavior goals. However, organizations as diverse as a gay marching band, a gay Catholic group, and informal social networks participated in the STOP AIDS workshops and discussions (Wohlfeiler, 1997).

At the government and society level, legislation can be enacted to support social networks. Examples of legislation are family leave acts, policies to promote volunteerism, and funding for child and elder care programs (McLeroy et al., 2001). We describe methods for policy change later in this chapter.

The second type of intervention develops new social network linkages through mentor programs, buddy systems, and self-help groups. Groups such as Alcoholics Anonymous, Overeaters Anonymous, and Weight Watchers provide access to new social networks designed to provide cognitive, instrumental, and emotional support for behavioral and life change. Persuasion and encouragement can be given to networks to reach out to incorporate new members. This allows groups to incorporate information from network members who hold membership in other networks.

Third, indigenous or natural helpers have been employed to enhance networks, particularly around health issues. *Natural helpers* are community members to whom other persons turn for advice, emotional support, and tangible aid. Often they agree to become a link between the community and the formal service-delivery system. They may include persons who come into contact with many people in their role, such as hairstylists, shopkeepers, and clergy. They may also be community volunteers and people with similar problems (Eng & Parker, 2002). A recent review of interventions by lay health workers in primary and community health care found that these interventions had promising benefits for immunizations and for improving outcomes for acute respiratory infections and malaria; the interventions had smaller positive effects for breastfeeding and breast cancer screening (S. A. Lewin et al., 2003).

Eng and Parker (2002) note three outcomes of natural-helper interventions addressing different socioecologic levels: improved health practices, improved coordination of agency services, and improved community competence (see Figure 4.4). The intervention inputs described in this figure illustrate how natural helpers function in the social action arenas related to the individual, organizational, and community levels.

FIGURE 4.4. NATURAL-HELPER INTERVENTION MODEL.

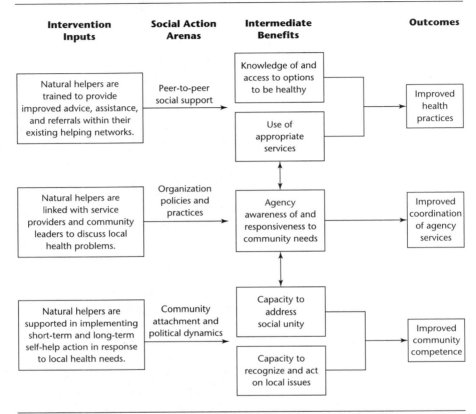

Source: DiClemente, Crosby, and Kegler, 2002, p. 141.

The role of natural helpers is to recruit, train, and support community members to offer social support to members of their networks, to negotiate with professionals for support from the health care system, and to mobilize community resources to sustain support for the health care system (Eng & Parker, 2002). Such helpers have focused on prenatal care (Meister, Warrick, de Zapien, & Wood, 1992), health promotion (Eng & Hatch, 1991), screening for breast and cervical cancer (Eng & Smith, 1995; Lam et al., 2003; C. S. Skinner et al., 1998), stress of urban women with children (E. A. Parker, Schulz, Israel, & Hollis, 1998), and hunger (Eng & Parker, 1994). In Chapter Fourteen, Fernandez and colleagues describe the work of lay health workers, called *promotoras,* in the promotion of breast and cervical cancer screening among migrant farmworkers.

Finally, networks can be enhanced at the community level through participatory problem-solving processes. In the Tenderloin Senior Organizing Project, networks of elderly people residing in single-room occupancy hotels in San Francisco received leadership training and consultation for problem solving and advocacy around such topics as housing policies and security (Minkler, 1997a). Another example is the Health, Opportunities, Problem-Solving and Empowerment Project, in which young Cambodian girls and women living in Long Beach, California, participated in training sessions, team building, and dialogue based on the work of Paulo Freire (1973a, 1973b) (described later in the chapter). The women identified sexual harassment as the issue they wished to address, researched the problem, and conducted a program called Community Forum on School Safety that led to establishment of a community advisory board to work on issues of sexual harassment in the Long Beach schools (Cheatham & Shen, 2003).

Summary of Social Networks and Social Support Theories in Problem Analysis and Intervention Methods.

- Environmental condition: social networks that provide emotional, instrumental, informational, and appraisal support as appropriate for the context
- Agent: social network members, lay health workers
- Behaviors: provision of emotional, instrumental, informational, and appraisal support by the network; mobilizing support for individuals from their networks
- Determinants: knowledge, beliefs and attitudes, self-efficacy, skills; facilitation of policies and culture; availability of self-help groups; network characteristics of reciprocity, intensity, complexity, density, and homogeneity
- Methods: enhancement of existing networks by skills training for providing and mobilizing support; use of lay health workers; teaching of participatory problem solving (see methods for community organization later in this chapter); linking of members to new networks (for example, mentor programs, buddy systems, self-help groups)

Social Capital and Community Capacity

Sociologists refer to the actual and potential resources available to an individual through a network as social capital. Individuals are able to secure benefits through membership in networks—such as those defined by kinship, ethnicity, or friendship—or through other social structures. Portes (1998) points out that such social capital may result not only in positive consequences such as observance of norms, family support, and network-mediated benefits but also in potentially negative consequences such as restricted access to opportunities, constraints on individual freedom, and excessive claims on group members. Researchers' focus on social capital, like that on social support, has been on the positive outcomes of these social networks.

Putnam (1993, 1995) extended the concept of social capital to communities and described it as *civicness*, involvement and participatory behavior. Within health education, L. W. Green and Kreuter (2005, p. 52) have defined social capital as "the processes and conditions among people and organizations that lead to accomplishing a goal of mutual social benefit." High social capital is manifested in high levels of four interrelated constructs: trust, cooperation, civic engagement, and reciprocity (L. W. Green & Kreuter).

Two operational levels of social capital have been described: bonding social capital and bridging social capital (Kreuter & Lezin, 2002; Putnam, 2000; Tempkin & Robe, 1998). Bonding social capital, or the sociocultural milieu, includes residents' identity with the neighborhood and the degree of social connectedness among residents. Bridging social capital, or institutional infrastructure, includes the linking of organizations within a community around a common purpose and outside the community to resources. Bonding social capital has been found to be more uniform among neighborhoods of varying socioeconomic status, whereas bridging social capital was more likely to be found in neighborhoods of higher socioeconomic status and to be linked to neighborhood improvement (Altschuler, Somkin, & Adler, 2004).

Kawachi and Berkman (2000) review the evidence that social capital is related to age-adjusted mortality and self-reported health status. Interpersonal trust, norms of reciprocity, and per capita membership in voluntary association aggregated to the state level has been found to be directly associated with age-adjusted mortality and also, when adjusted for individual-level characteristics, to the likelihood of an individual's reporting fair and poor health. Social capital has also been linked to homicide rates (Lochner, Kawachi, Brennan, & Buka, 2003) and binge drinking (Weitzman & Kawachi, 2000). Although some evidence calls into question the role of social capital in the promotion of health in a cross-national examination (Kennelly, O'Shea, & Garvey, 2003), many researchers agree that it has some role (Kawachi, Kim, Coutts, & Subramanian, 2004).

Bonding and bridging social capital would be expected to be differentially related to the three mechanisms by which social capital is hypothesized to affect health (Kawachi & Berkman, 2000):

- Influence on health-related behaviors through diffusion of healthy behaviors and social control of deviant behavior

- Access to services and amenities
- Psychosocial processes, including affective support and acting as a source of self-esteem and mutual respect

Community capacity is closely related to and inclusive of social capital. It has been defined as the interaction of human capital, organizational resources, and social capital within a community, which can be leveraged to increase community problem solving to improve or maintain community well-being (Chaskin, 2001; Norton, McLeroy, Burdine, Felix, & Dorsey, 2002). Dimensions of community capacity include skills, knowledge, and resources; the nature of social relationships, structures and mechanisms for community dialogue, leadership, civic participation, the value system, and learning culture (Norton et al., 2002). R. M. Goodman and colleagues (1998) have identified several aspects of community capacity. Community participation is the depth and breadth of citizen involvement in defining and resolving needs. Participation is highly interrelated with inclusivity and encouragement by community leaders. Both participation and leadership are predicated on the third dimension of capacity—a collection of skills that includes group process, conflict resolution, collection and analysis of data, problem solving, program planning and evaluation, resource development, policy formulation, and media advocacy. The strength of a community's sense of itself is also a component of capacity. Central to community are the community's ability to analyze its own thinking processes and change efforts; its sense of connection among people and to community rituals; an awareness of previous change efforts and current conditions; and community power—the ability to create change, values, and critical reflection.

Interventions to Build Social Capital and Community Capacity. Interventions to increase social capital can occur at the community level and include community development and participatory problem solving, which we discuss in the following section. In this section we emphasize the importance of linking persons to community organizations, such as churches, social clubs, schools, political groups, and work settings, in which individuals can voluntarily associate with others to address issues of community concern. It is also important for residents to have loose ties outside their primary networks to bring in new information and resources, and interorganizational meetings and coalitions can foster such ties (Steckler, Goodman, & Kegler, 2002). For example, statewide meetings of church associations, nonprofit health agency volunteers, political conventions, and joint neighborhood association meetings allow the opportunity for residents to connect with others with similar concerns and interests, to learn about their activities, and to team up to work together. Democratic management in which "members share information and power, utilize cooperative decision-making processes, and are involved in the design, implementation, and control of efforts toward mutually defined goals" is essential (B. A. Israel, Checkoway, Schulz, & Zimmerman, 1994, p. 152). As noted earlier, Eng and Parker (2002) include improved community competence as an outcome of natural helpers' work with communities in self-help actions, including changing organization policies and practices and health-related environmental factors. (See Figure 4.4.)

The Mpowerment Project, a community-level HIV-prevention intervention, was structured with a core decision-making group of twelve to fifteen gay men of ages eighteen to twenty-nine; a community advisory board of men and women from the AIDS, gay and lesbian, public health, and university communities; and a part-time staff of four young gay men (Kegeles, Hays, & Coates, 1996). An outreach team conducted peer outreach, both formally through visiting locations that young gay men frequented and informally by conversing casually with their friends. Outreach included recruiting men for the project's educational and social activities and informal discussions promoting safer sex. The project is an excellent example of the use of social networks for diffusion of health behavior, shifting of norms, and community capacity building through decision-making control and participation.

Summary of Social Capital Theory in Problem Analysis and Intervention Methods.

- Environmental condition: social capital and community competence
- Agents: social and community networks, members and leaders
- Behaviors: involvement in civic affairs and participation in community organizations
- Determinants: knowledge, beliefs and attitudes, self-efficacy, skills; availability of structures and mechanisms for community dialogue; supportive culture
- Methods: community development and participatory problem solving (see Community Organizing Methods later in this chapter); linking members to community organizations, interorganizational meetings and coalitions; skills training for community participation, and technical assistance

Organizational Change Models and Theories

In this section we introduce several theories explaining organizational change. These theories are used in Intervention Mapping to make changes in policy, culture, and other environmental conditions at the organizational level. They are also used to enable the adoption and implementation of programs in organizations.

We begin with a general discussion of organizational development and the processes that can facilitate change. Then we discuss the stage theory of organizations and diffusion theory.

Organizational Development Theory

Organizational development generally seeks to improve the quality of work life through participatory problem solving, involving organizational diagnosis, structure modification, or human process change. Its origins in applied social psychology can be traced to the action research model that Lewin and his colleagues developed in the 1940s (Bowditch & Buono, 1994). Lewin (1947) proposed that organizations were in a state of quasi-stationary equilibrium in which two sets of forces—those driving for change and those striving for the status quo—were approximately equal. For change to occur, the forces driving for change could increase, or the forces maintaining the status quo could decrease, or both could occur. Lewin advised that decreasing the status quo forces was less disruptive and more effective than was increasing forces for change. He saw the change process as having three phases:

1. Unfreezing
2. Moving
3. Refreezing

Unfreezing reduces the forces that maintain the organization's current behavior, often by providing information showing that the behaviors or conditions that organizational members desire are different from those they currently exhibit. During the moving phase, changes in organizational structures and processes lead to new behaviors, values, and attitudes. In refreezing, organizational norms, policies, and structures are put into place that support the new state of equilibrium (Cummings & Worley, 1993; Lewin, 1947).

Steps from current contemporary organizational development models can be placed within this framework (Brager & Holloway, 1978; Schein, 2004; Steckler, Goodman, & Kegler, 2002). Diagnosis, often conducted using surveys, is equated with Lewin's unfreezing (1947). It includes evaluation of an organization's mission, goals, policies, procedures, structures, technologies, and physical setting; social and psychological factors; desired outcomes; and readiness to take action. Action planning is the selection of change strategies. Criteria for selection include the organization's readiness to adopt a particular strategy, the availability of leverage points on which to intervene, and the skill of the organizational development consultant to conduct the intervention. Intervention, similar to the process Lewin

(1947) called moving, includes the facilitation of problem identification and solving with members of the organization. Group development activities, management building, and structural redesign are among the other intervention elements that can be carried out. Evaluation assesses the planned change effort and the determination of whether additional efforts are needed. Institutionalization, the final step, refreezes the supports for the changes, through written plans, goals, job descriptions, and budgets. Process consultation, or technical assistance, is a relevant method for organizational development and is one of the basic methods for change at environmental levels (see Table 7.10).

Weick and Quinn (1999) make an important distinction between episodic and continuous change. *Episodic change* is discontinuous, infrequent, and intentional. It fits the paradigm of planned change we have just discussed and follows the unfreezing-moving-refreezing sequence. *Continuous change,* on the other hand, views the organization as unstable, with constant modifications in work processes and social practice to meet daily contingencies. In this case, change is seen as a continuous process, a redirection of what is already underway as equilibrium is sought. From an intervention standpoint, the sequence is freezing-rebalancing-unfreezing. *Freezing* is making the processes within the organization visible and describing the patterns. *Rebalancing* involves the reinterpretation, relabeling, and resequencing of patterns, so that there are fewer blockages and barriers to them. Leaders do this by modeling the change and inspiring others with their ideas. The next step in the cycle is *unfreezing,* the resumption of improvisation and learning as the organization continues to meet daily contingencies. The change agent in continuous change is a sense maker who redirects change as opposed to the episodic model's prime mover who creates change (Weick & Quinn, p. 366).

Some organizational development theorists have focused on organizational culture, which is closely aligned with the continuous change model described above. Schein (2004) defines *culture* as a pattern of basic assumptions invented, discovered, or developed by a given group as it learns to cope with its problems of external adaptation and internal integration. For the pattern to be "culture," it must have worked well enough to be considered valid and therefore taught to new members as the way to perceive, think, and feel. Organizational interventions are most effective when they are compatible with the culture, so it is important to understand the culture of the organization in which a health promotion program is being developed and implemented (see also Chapter Five on culturally competent practice).

It is also possible to facilitate changes in organizational culture, although this process is slow and evolutionary. Culture changes with the group's learning and experience over time, as organizational members react to environmental shifts and crises within the organization. Schein (2004) describes the importance of leaders' behavior in shaping organizational culture: what leaders pay attention to; how they react to critical incidents; how they model for and coach others; and what criteria they set for allocating rewards and recruiting and promoting personnel. As seen in Table 4.2, Schein refers to leader behaviors as primary culture-embedding mechanisms. The culture is reinforced by organizational design, structure, and formal statements. In a young organization, leaders create the culture, and the organizational systems reinforce it. In mature organizations the organizational systems become primary and constrain future leaders' behavior.

Organizational Development Interventions. Work-site programs have applied culture change interventions to health issues (J. Allen & Bellingham, 1994; R. Allen & Kraft, 1984). These programs intend for individuals to achieve their personal goals facilitated by the culture, with the condition that the culture allow for individual differences and freedom of choice. The intervention includes assessment of the worksite norms for health-related behaviors such as physical fitness, smoking cessation, stress reduction, nutrition, substance abuse, safety, mental health, and human relations. Employees are also asked what they would like the norms to be. Employees report their perceptions of the health behaviors of organizational members (for example, a worksite norm for people to be a few pounds overweight) and their opinions about worksite support for health-promoting endeavors (for example, whether the organization has facilities for physical activity) (R. Allen & Kraft).

TABLE 4.2. CULTURE-EMBEDDING MECHANISMS.

Primary Embedding Mechanisms	Secondary Articulation and Reinforcement Mechanisms
What leaders pay attention to, measure, and control on a regular basis	Organization design and structure
How leaders react to critical incidents and organizational crises	Organizational systems and procedures
Observed criteria by which leaders allocate scarce resources	Design of physical space, facades, and buildings
Deliberate role modeling, teaching, and coaching	Stories, legends, and myths about people and events
Observed criteria by which leaders allocate rewards and status	Formal statements of organizational philosophy, values, and creed
Observed criteria by which leaders recruit, select, promote, retire, and excommunicate organizational members	

Source: Schein, 2004.

Using document review, participant observation, focus group interviews, and surveys, organizational support factors are then examined. These include modeling; training; rewards and recognition; communication; orientation; relationships and interaction; resource allocation and commitment; confrontation; and rituals, myths, and symbols. Strengths and opportunities for improvement are identified. Examples of findings for a company might include the following observations: that the leader often works out at the company's fitness facility during lunch, that the executive dining room serves alcohol, that new employees are invited to join company-sponsored exercise programs, and that new employee orientation does not include the company health promotion program as a primary benefit but instead focuses on medical coverage and sick leave (J. Allen & Bellingham, 1994).

The facilitators then convene small groups for employees and managers to develop a shared vision of the desired norms and to develop both individual and organizational plans for change. Self-help educational materials, support group programs, periodic work-group discussions, and task forces for promoting health are put into place. A group leader or buddy keeps in touch with the participants. Positive behavioral modeling by participants, especially the organizational leaders, and incentives compatible with the culture are also key components of this intervention. Evaluation, feedback, and goal setting sustain the change (J. Allen & Bellingham, 1994).

Summary of Organizational Development Theory in Problem Analysis and Intervention.

- Environmental condition: health-promoting organizational structures and culture
- Agent: organizational leaders, internal change consultants, and other organizational members
- Agent behaviors: adoption of new policies, practices, structures, cultural beliefs, and norms
- Determinants: outcome expectations, attitudes and beliefs, and resources
- Methods: participatory problem solving through organizational diagnosis and feedback; modeling, team building or human relations training, technical assistance

Diffusion Theory and Stage Theory of Organizational Change

In Chapter Three we discussed individuals' adoption, implementation, and maintenance of health behaviors and other innovations. In this section we discuss organizations' adoption, implementation, and institutionalization of innovations. These innovations may be policies, facilities, or health promotion programs. Obviously, organizations are more complex than are individuals. The organization goes through a process of agenda setting, matching, redefining and restructuring, clarifying and routinizing, all of which involve different organizational members and different levels of authority within the organization (E. M. Rogers, 2003). Other aspects of diffusion theory, however, are similar. Both media and interpersonal channels are used for communicating the innovation to organizational members, and organizations can be categorized with the adoption categories listed earlier. Characteristics of the innovation as described in Chapter Three are also similar. Organizational-level factors such as the organization's goals, authority structure, roles, rules and regulations, and informal norms and relationships must be taken into account (E. M. Rogers, 1983).

Certain organizational characteristics have been found to be associated with innovativeness. However, identifying when these general patterns hold (that is, for what sorts of innovations, under what conditions) is not simple, and we refer the reader to E. M. Rogers (1995) for a summary. With that caveat we can generalize that organizations most responsive to innovations tend to be large and complex and to have leaders who are positive toward change. They tend to have decentralized administration, high interconnectedness and informality, and available organizational resources.

In their work on the establishment of alcohol policy and programs in U.S. government agencies, Beyer and Trice (1978) developed a stage theory of organization change that has been used in health education practice (Steckler, Goodman, & Kegler, 2002). An organization moves sequentially through seven stages as it adopts and institutionalizes a health promotion innovation. Outside consultants may provide technical assistance to this process. The stages, which are more fine-grained that those of E. M. Rogers (2003), are as follows:

1. Sensing unsatisfied demands on the system, noting a problem and bringing it to the surface
2. Searching for possible responses, seeking solutions to the problem
3. Evaluating alternatives, judging potential solutions
4. Deciding to adopt a course of action, selecting one of a number of alternative responses
5. Initiating action within the system, which requires policy changes and resources necessary for implementation
6. Implementing the change, which includes putting the innovation into practice and usually requires some organization members to change their work behaviors and relationships
7. Institutionalizing the change, by including the change in strategic plans, job descriptions, and budgets so that it is a routine part of organizational operations

The key actors involved in change have been found to differ from stage to stage (Huberman & Miles, 1984). Senior-level administrators with political skills are important in the early stages, when a problem is recognized and made public, alternative solutions discussed, and a choice made and initiated within the organization. These administrators are also important at the institutionalization stage. Midlevel administrators are active during the adoption and early implementation stages, in which administrative skills are critical in order to introduce procedures and provide training on the innovation. The people who need to make changes in their practice are the focus of the implementation process. Examples are teachers involved in curriculum innovation or food service workers involved in an innovation in preparing cafeteria food. The focus here is on people's professional and technical skills. Of course, because the agents and behaviors are different at different stages, the determinants change as well. For example, at the decision stage, organizational leaders might be persuaded by an intervention's characteristics, whereas implementation might be determined to a great extent by the skills of the implementers and by feedback and reinforcement to the implementers.

Diffusion Theory and Stage of Organizational Change Interventions. Goodman and colleagues took into account stages in the diffusion of a school district curriculum to stop tobacco use (R. M. Goodman, Smith, Dawson, & Steckler, 1991; R. M. Goodman, Steckler, & Kegler, 1997; D. W. Smith, Steckler, McCormick, & McLeroy, 1995). They used different organizational development interventions at different stages of diffusion. One intervention consisted of holding meetings with senior district administrators to raise their awareness of tobacco use prevention and to encourage them to adopt the project. Another was to help districts address concerns associated with potential adoption of the project combined with intensive training of teachers for curriculum implementation. The project also provided consultation with teachers before and after the training and process consultation with program champions and administrators to address program institutionalization.

Summary of Diffusion Theory and Organizational Change Stage Theory in Problem Analysis and Intervention Methods.

- Environmental condition: innovations, including health-promoting structures and systems and health promotion programs within organizations
- Agent: upper and middle management
- Behaviors: adoption, implementation, and institutionalization of organizational innovations; provision of reinforcement structures for health-promoting behaviors
- Determinants: attitude, outcome expectations, and behavioral capability
- Methods: organizational advocacy, including information, persuasion, and negotiation; and technical assistance; training for implementation; providing cues and reinforcement to agent's behavior

Coalition Theory

Organizations form partnerships to manage their environments. These interactions may be informal and transient or highly structured, with shared decision making and leadership. *Coalitions* have been defined as "an organization of individuals representing diverse organizations, factions or constituencies who agree to work together in order to achieve common goals" (Feighery & Rogers, 1989, p. 1). Community coalitions include a structured arrangement for organizations to work together to achieve a common goal, usually preventing or ameliorating a community problem (Butterfoss & Kegler, 2002). Butterfoss and Kegler have proposed a theory of action for community coalitions (Figure 4.5) that draws on a large body of empirical research. They have generated a set of testable propositions concerning each of the constructs in the theoretical model.

Coalitions develop through specific stages (Butterfoss & Kegler, 2002):

1. Formation
2. Maintenance
3. Institutionalization

FIGURE 4.5. COMMUNITY COALITION ACTION THEORY.

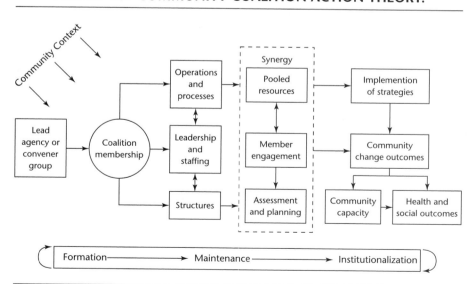

Source: DiClemente, Crosby, and Kegler, 2005, p. 163.

The stages are represented at the base of Figure 4.5. Coalitions recycle through these stages with the recruitment of members, renewal of plans, and addition of new issues. Each stage requires a different set of skills and resources and thus different strategies for training and technical assistance by staff and consultants.

Formation is most successful when a convener or lead agency with linkages to the community provides the resources of technical assistance, material support, credibility, and valuable contacts. The coalition must also include a deeply committed core group that expands to include community gatekeepers and a broad constituency of participants. The coalition should identify strong staff and member leaders who then develop structures, such as formalized rules, roles, and procedures. During this stage open and frequent communication, shared and formalized decision-making processes, conflict management, benefits of participation that outweigh the costs, and positive relationships among members will provide for a high level of member engagement, pooling of resources, and effective assessment and planning.

The key tasks of the maintenance stage are sustaining member involvement; pooling member and external resources; and engaging in assessment, planning, and action to achieve coalition goals. As Figure 4.5 indicates, there is a synergy in these tasks to promote successful implementation of strategies and community-change outcomes. At the institutionalization stage, successful coalitions show improvements in health and social outcomes, as well as capacity that they can apply to other issues.

Coalitions and partnerships are an important method for facilitating *empowerment*, which is broadly defined as influencing conditions that are relevant to people who share neighborhoods, workplaces, or concerns (Fawcett et al., 1995). Fawcett and colleagues describe four primary methods for enabling the empowerment process in partnerships, which could also be seen as participatory problem solving:

- Enhancing experience and competence
- Improving group structure and capacity
- Removing social and environmental barriers
- Increasing environmental support and resources

Strategies to enhance experience and competence include listening sessions and surveys to identify local issues, an inventory of community assets, guidelines for selecting leadership and membership, training on leadership skills, and technical assistance on action planning and early projects. Strategies to improve group structure and capacity include technical assistance with strategic planning, development of an organizational structure, inclusion of key members and volunteers, and financial development. For removing social and environmental barriers, suggested strategies include focus groups, social marketing to promote adoption of new programs, and training in conflict resolution. Strategies to increase environmental support and resources include information and feedback about community change; development of ties to existing community sectors, organizations, and groups; opportunities for networking; and the promotion of policies and resource allocations. Participatory problem solving, such as the process described earlier, is a basic method for change at environmental levels (see Table 7.11).

Summary of Coalition Theory in Problem Analysis and Intervention Methods

- Environmental condition: high-functioning health promotion coalition
- Agents: leaders of organizations for formation of coalitions; coalitions themselves for implementation, maintenance, and action
- Behaviors: coalition formation, implementation, maintenance, and action
- Determinants: motivation to collaborate, organizational capacity, models of coalitions, barriers to collaboration, community capacity, and community resources
- Methods: participatory problem solving, technical assistance, skills training for leadership and conflict management, and interlinking organizations and networks

Community-Level Theories

Communities may be based on geography; on gender, ethnic, or cultural identity; or on an issue such as the environment, animal rights, or public health. A shared reality or identity is key to the construct (Labonte, 1997). In this section we come back to social norms and then discuss conscientization and several models of community organization, all aimed at empowering people in their lives and in the lives of their communities (Minkler & Wallerstein, 1997a). After that we turn to models of community organization from the United States, beginning with a description of J. Rothman's classic models of community organization (1979) and next discussing the approach of Minkler and Wallerstein (1997a, 1997b), who extend earlier models to include an explicit focus on community strengths and capacity.

Social Norms Theories

Social norms, that is, expectations of behavior that others in the social group hold for a person, are a property of a community. They are the social rules that specify what is appropriate or inappropriate in a particular situation. Norms are the external determinant that is the basis for perceived social influence, the individual-level variable we discussed earlier. They are transmitted to individuals through the process of socialization. Socialization occurs primarily in childhood through the family and then is continued through institutions such as churches, voluntary associations such as Boy Scouts, and schools (Smelser, 1998). Note that theories at the individual and interpersonal level describe the perception of social norms (see Chapter Three); here we describe the norms themselves and try to identify methods that may change these norms.

Interventions to Change Social Norms. Mass media portrayals of role models and reinforcement have been used to shift social norms. A combination of education and entertainment has been used to transmit social norms and culture (Bouman, Maas, & Kok, 1998; Steckler et al., 1995). In various formats, including soap operas, popular music, films, and comic books, popular characters have modeled health behaviors. For example, in Nigeria family planning was introduced in a popular television series in which characters began to use family planning and were reinforced or were socially punished for resisting the practice of family planning. Evaluation showed that family planning clinic visits increased threefold, and about half the new clients mentioned the television show as a referral source (see E. M. Rogers, 1995).

Behavioral journalism uses mass media role-model stories of community members and advice from experts to increase adoption of behaviors. News stories, talk shows, feature stories in newspapers, and cartoon-style newsletters have been used as media vehicles. The media materials use models who are perceived as attractive and similar to members of the at-risk population; and these models give their reasons for adopting the new behavior, demonstrate skills used or acquired in adopting the behavior, and state the perceived reinforcing outcomes they received. Potential models are interviewed with questions designed to elicit this information in their own words. The distribution of role-model stories in a campaign may address different stages of change. Behavioral journalism has also been combined with use of a community network of volunteers who cue people to watch the television documentary stories. Community volunteers also model behaviors for their contacts and reinforce their contacts' stated intentions or demonstrated targeted behaviors. These methods increase the visibility of behaviors of opinion leaders and early adopters, increasing the speed of adoption of the behaviors within the population (McAlister, 1991; Pulley, McAlister, Kay, & O'Reilly, 1996; A. G. Ramirez et al., 1999).

Mobilizing social networks is another method used to influence social norms. For example, in a natural-helper model intervention, J. A. Kelly and colleagues (1992) trained respected and popular patrons of gay bars to adopt protective sexual practices and persuade acquaintances to follow their example. This intervention led not only to a change in individual behavior but to increased norms supportive of protective behavior.

Summary of Social Norm Theories in Problem Analysis and Intervention Methods.

- Environmental condition: social norms
- Agent: community members and opinion leaders at various levels
- Behaviors: supporting the health-promoting behavior
- Determinants: all determinants at the individual level, and availability of models
- Methods: role modeling in mass media, entertainment-education, behavioral journalism, and mobilization of social networks

Conscientization

Paulo Freire's work (1973a, 1973b) in liberation education has formed the basis for empowerment models (Wallerstein, Sanchez-Merki, & Dow, 1997). Individuals in small groups are led through a consideration of their own realities and the constraints they experience to an understanding of the social forces underlying the problem and their responsibility to act.

Critical consciousness, or conscientization, links individual and community-level empowerment and is a key method for strengths-based community organization. Using the context of developing literacy in his country, Freire described the method by which critical consciousness emerges. Educators began the process by being with the people in a local community; by discovering the way they talked about daily life, that is, the words and phrases they used; and by observing the way they lived. Generative words were then selected for their social meaning and also to represent all phonemes in the language. The educators continued to divide and reintegrate these codes, or representations of the life of the people, to develop their interventions' program content. Program participants then discussed these codes, which might be pictures, songs, or words, through a questioning process, in cultural circles, or in learning groups, framing the discussion in terms of the participants' lives and the root causes of the conditions of their lives. This reflection on root causes gave rise to a political and social understanding that was accompanied by action to transform this reality. Literacy was an instrument of this struggle. The final step of conscientization was the understanding that oppressive reality is a process that can be overcome. This understanding results in praxis, the unity between a person's understanding and actions (Freire, 1973; Gadotti, 1994).

Freirian Methods in Health Education. The Freirian method has been applied in health education to such areas as women's health; smoking, drug, and alcohol prevention; sexuality and sexual harassment; homelessness; environmental health; occupational health; and health of the elderly (Cheatham & Shen, 2003; D. T. Goodman, 1998; McFarlane & Fehir, 1994; Minkler, 1997; Rudd & Comings, 1994; Wallerstein & Sanchez-Merki, 1994; Wang, 2003; Wang & Burris, 1994; Wang, Yi, Tao, & Carovano, 1998). The codes for discussion varied among these projects. For example, Wang and colleagues used photographs taken by rural Chinese women of their everyday activities; of community residents in Flint, Michigan; and of residents of a homeless shelter in Ann Arbor, Michigan (Wang, 2003). Photonovels for environmental health (*A Working Neighborhood: What Does It Take?*), smoking prevention (*Decisions, Decisions*), and occupational health (*Workers Take Action: Fighting Asbestos in the Building Trades*) were developed by participants in the three programs described by Rudd and Comings (1994) through dialogue about the issues to explore root causes, development of a story line, and design and production of the books. Triggers for discussion in the Adolescent Social Action Program were stories that students would listen to from hospital patients and jail residents who had problems related to drug and alcohol abuse, violence, unsafe sex, and other risky behaviors. Other triggers included role-plays, students' life stories, videotapes, collages, and photographs (Wallerstein et al., 1997). Codes developed by Cherokee parents were short paragraphs describing the gap between what was needed and what was being done to help people in such diverse areas as healthy sexual decision making, culturally sensitive programming for Native American youth, teen pregnancy, and cultural traditions as guidelines for living (D. T. Goodman, 1998).

These projects all rely on participatory analysis using critical reflection and dialogue. Questions to encourage a critical stance, described by Shaffer (1993) and used by Wang (2003), include the following: "What do you see here? What's really happening here? How does this relate to our lives? Why does this problem, concern or strength exist? What can we do about it?" (Wang, 2003, p. 196). Issues, themes, and theories emerge that inform action.

The cycle of reflection-action-reflection continues into the policy realm. The rural Chinese women presented their concerns to provincial policymakers (Wang et al., 1998); adolescents have been involved in peer education, participating in a statewide youth leadership group for policy development and carrying out service projects (Wallerstein et al., 1997); and low-income elderly residents of hotels have formed building tenants' associations, achieved better living conditions, and received compensation for lack of services (Minkler, 1997). However, a sustained effort is required for action and advocacy to be demonstrated. In the project by Rudd and Comings (1994), the completion of the photonovels for environmental health, smoking prevention, and occupational health was the major outcome of the interventions. The photonovels were disseminated to other groups, who found them to be credible and used them to increase their intention to act. However, the participants who developed them did not engage in active advocacy (Rudd & Comings).

From their work with the Adolescent Social Action Program, which focused on alcohol and substance abuse prevention, Wallerstein and Sanchez-Merki (1994) have identified three stages through which an individual passes from apathy to a social responsibility to act (Figure 4.6). The first stage involves individuals beginning to care about the problem, each other, and their ability to act in the world. This stage is accomplished through dialogue and self-disclosure in small groups and through the use of questioning. At the next stage, individual responsibility to act, as well as individuals' self-efficacy to talk and help others increases as a result of engaging in participatory and caring dialogue with community members who have experienced problems with alcohol or drugs. The final stage, social responsibility to act, involves critical thinking about the social forces that underlie the problem and a commitment to change both self and community. This three-stage transformation results in individual and community empowerment.

FIGURE 4.6. STAGES OF RESPONSIBILITY TO ACT.

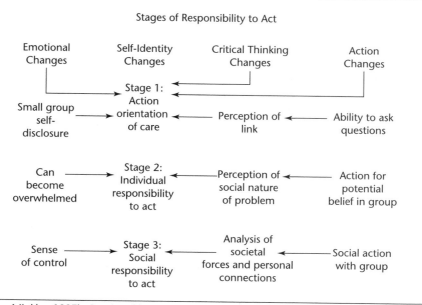

Stages of Responsibility to Act

Source: Minkler, 1997b. Reprinted by permission of Oxford University Press.

Summary of Conscientization Theory in
Problem Analysis and Intervention Methods.

- Environmental condition: community empowered to confront larger social and political environments
- Agent: community groups, especially marginalized populations
- Behaviors: to become politically and socially active
- Determinants: understanding of the root causes of problems and collective self-efficacy
- Methods: reflection-action-reflection, nonjudgmental small group discussion of learning materials, question posing, and self-disclosure

Community Organization

Building on the three types of social change identified by Bennis, Benne, and Chin (1969), Rothman (1979) developed three models of community organization: locality development, social planning, and social action.

Locality development uses normative-reeducative change, which involves raising consciousness about the underlying causes of problems and identifying strategies for action. It is heavily process oriented, with an emphasis on consensus, cooperation, and development of a sense of community. This model is most akin to the community development tradition in health education. Social planning, based on rational-empirical change, uses information derived from empirical research. It is heavily task oriented, with an emphasis on expert (technical) assistance as a means to solve problems. Social action is based on coercive change and seeks to redress imbalances of power. It relies on conflict methods of change such as demonstrations and boycotts, and the change agent is both an activist and a partisan. The skillful organizer assesses the context of the community and of the problem at hand and mixes and matches the change models (Rothman, 1979).

Minkler and Wallerstein (1997a, 1997b) extend Rothman's work (1979), presenting a typology of community organization based on change method (consensus vs. conflict) and view of the community (needs-based vs. strengths-based). In their typology, diagrammed in Figure 4.7, earlier models of community organization—both community development and social action—are viewed as needs-based, centering on the organizer helping the community. Current community organization practice is seen as centered on the community, building on community strengths and assets. The form of practice differs with whether consensus or conflict is the change strategy. Community-building approaches use consensus and inclusiveness, a concept of power as power with, whereas empowerment-oriented social action uses conflict and challenges power over. Both types of community

FIGURE 4.7. COMMUNITY-ORGANIZING AND COMMUNITY-BUILDING TYPOLOGY.

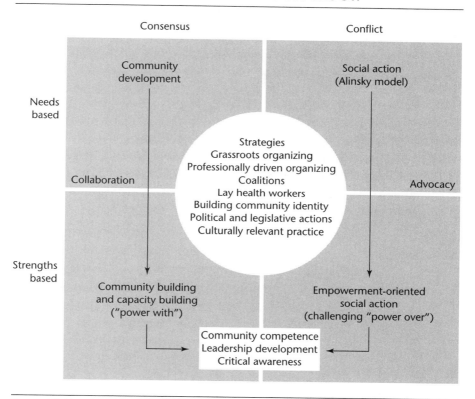

Consensus

Conflict

Community development

Social action (Alinsky model)

Needs based

Strategies
Grassroots organizing
Professionally driven organizing
Coalitions
Lay health workers
Building community identity
Political and legislative actions
Culturally relevant practice

Collaboration

Advocacy

Strengths based

Community building and capacity building ("power with")

Empowerment-oriented social action (challenging "power over")

Community competence
Leadership development
Critical awareness

Source: Minkler and Wallerstein, 1997a.

change are directed toward increased community competence, leadership development, and critical awareness within the community. Methods and strategies in their typology include participatory problem solving, grassroots organizing, professionally driven organizing, coalitions, lay health workers, development of community identity, political and legislative actions, and culturally relevant practice.

Important methods for the community-building approach for health educators engaged in this process are participation and relevance, that is, starting where the people are. The health educator should work with the community to identify issues, assess networks, and map community assets (Heitzmann & Kaplan, 1988; Kretzmann & McKnight, 1993; McCallister & Fischer, 1978). Furthermore, health educators should generally practice health education in a culturally competent manner whereby they are more likely to hear the real community discourse (Ladson-Billings, 1995).

Community participation is a core method of community work and is one of the bases of the Healthy Cities movement (World Health Organization, 2002a). It has been defined as "a process by which people are enabled to become actively and genuinely involved in defining the issues of concern to them, in making decisions about factors that affect their lives, in formulating and implementing policies, in planning, developing and delivering services and in taking action to achieve change" (World Health Organization, 2002a, p. 10). Community participation achieves a number of objectives, including increasing democracy, combating exclusion of marginalized and disadvantaged populations, empowering people, mobilizing resources and energy, developing holistic and integrated approaches, achieving better decisions and more effective services, and ensuring the ownership and sustainability of programs. Theorists see community participation as falling along a continuum or ladder from low (no community control) to high (community has control) as can been seen in Table 4.3. Health promoters using community organization methods must decide whether the issue and context make aiming for the highest levels of community participation appropriate. Table 4.3 divides the participation continuum into four categories, from low to high community participation, information, consultation, participation and empowerment; and it provides examples of objectives and techniques for each category. Community organizers may have a greater challenge in engaging people at the higher levels, but they should not settle for a lower level simply because using the more passive processes of providing information and consultation is easier (WHO, 2002).

Community Participation Interventions. Yoo and colleagues (2004), working primarily within a locality development framework, used the social ecology evaluation model developed by R. M. Goodman (2000) as the basis for a method of community empowerment and described its use with four community groups. The facilitation process, which could also be defined as participatory problem solving, involved six steps: entrée into the community, issue identification, prioritization of issues, strategy development (in which the social ecological model was used to construct the group's own model of the issue), implementation with action plans and feedback, and transition (in which responsibility was transferred from the facilitators to community leaders and an iterative process of action planning using the model continued). Three of the community groups carried out all six steps of the process. Factors related to success of the project were the sound conceptual framework that was clearly understood and applied, consistent well-attended community meetings, available community organization support staff, open communication, focused community leaders, a community network, and regular debriefing among facilitators. Challenges that Yoo and colleagues noted were limited space, time, money, and data;

TABLE 4.3. CATEGORIES OF COMMUNITY PARTICIPATION WITH EXAMPLES.

Level of Involvement	Categories of Participation in Official Organizations				
	Information	Consultation	Participation	Empowerment	
Low	Organization decides on all matters itself, without community consultation (except when legally required to do so). Example techniques: public notices, minutes of meetings	Organization provides information in a limited manner with the onus often placed on the community to respond. Example techniques: public meetings, surveys, recruitment through leaflets	Organization invites communities to draw up proposals for organization consideration. Example techniques: citizens' panels, nominal group process, Delphi and other ways to prioritize issues	Organization delegates limited decision-making powers in a particular area or project, such as tenant management organizations and school boards. Example technique: application of participation techniques with low political support to delegate power	
Medium	Organization tells the public what it wants to tell them, not what the public wants to know. Example techniques: press releases, newsletters, campaigns	Organization introduces a customer-oriented service, customer care policy, or a scheme for complaints or comments. Example techniques: comment cards, one-on-one interviews	Organization solves problems in partnership with communities. Example techniques: stakeholder groups, formal partnerships, interactive planning	Organization is obligated to provide a service but chooses to do so by facilitating community groups and other agencies to provide that service on their behalf. Example technique: application of participation techniques with moderate political support to delegate power	
High	Organization provides information the community wants and needs. Example technique: written plans, discussion papers, exhibitions of development plans, guidance notes for conservation area development	Organization actively discusses issues with communities prior to taking action. Example techniques: citizens' panels, district circles, focus groups, opinion meters, user panels, customer satisfaction surveys, stakeholder groups	Organization allows communities to make their own decisions on some issues, such as management of community halls. Example techniques: application of participation techniques with high political support to delegate power	Organization devolves substantial decision-making powers to communities, such as tenant management organizations. Example technique: application of participation techniques with high political support to delegate power	

Source: Adapted from World Health Organization, 2002, p. 15.

slow process on action steps; difficulty attracting community participation; lack of promotion of the project in the community; and unexpected situations that required a response.

One community group was to repair homes structurally damaged by the Sewage and Water Board (S&WB) during a major construction process. This group identified, through a facilitated process, the interrelated conditions at each ecological level that it wished to change:

- Homes damaged by S&WB (individual and family level)
- The community not working together with individuals with damaged homes (community level)
- S&WB policy not clear to the community (organizational level)
- Time limitations on filing claims (policy level)

The group then determined the desired outcomes and the methods and action plans by which they would achieve these changes. The group had representatives of the S&WB, a lawyer, and police representatives speak at a community forum on issues related to the processes, policies, laws, and safety issues related to the situation. They worked with a member of the city council who advocated for them with the S&WB. They videotaped the homes and went en masse to city hall to ask for redress. They were successful in extending the time limitation on filing claims and on getting the S&WB inspectors to come to homes on a timely basis (R. Goodman, personal communication, March 15, 2005; Yoo et al., 2004).

In another example the Contra Costa County Health Services Department in California, through its Healthy Neighborhoods Project, worked with the El Pueblo neighborhood, a public housing development, to identify and train neighborhood health advocates in health, tobacco use prevention, and nutrition using Freirian popular education methods. The advocates were also trained in aspects of community organization, including door-to-door interviewing, community asset mapping, cross-cultural communication, and media and policy advocacy. Using the health department coordinator as a facilitator and broker for resources, the neighborhood health advocates assessed the capacities of residents and residents' perceptions of their community and organized a community mapping day, on which trained adult and youth volunteers mapped the neighborhood's positive and negative physical and institutional features. The group presented its findings at a community forum, and residents who attended developed an action plan and organized the painting of a mural by local children to show the residents' vision for the community (el-Askari et al., 1998).

To achieve the top priority of installation of speed bumps to slow traffic and reduce drug dealing, an El Pueblo residential council talked with the police chief, lobbied the city council, spoke at public meetings, organized demonstrations, and involved the media. These actions resulted in a consensus decision by the housing advisory commission to approve the speed bumps. Better street lighting and increased police patrol, two other priorities, were also accomplished. Residents also organized to have a billboard that advertised cigarettes removed from the neighborhood and to have a community-based organization offer healthy cooking classes (el-Askari et al., 1998).

Following its initial successes, the El Pueblo residents' council became larger, better organized, and more representative of the residents. Members began to visit other San Francisco Bay Area public housing residents' councils to share their experiences. The council then wrote and received funding for three grants: a tenant opportunities grant to establish computer classes, job training classes, and job search workshops; a drug elimination effort; and a youth sports grant. Over the course of the project, success motivated residents to take leadership roles in addressing other issues and led to a strong sense of control. Residents reported increased energy and life satisfaction, and strong social ties developed. Residents also began involvement in broader policymaking initiatives, such as the county's public and environmental health advisory board (el-Askari et al., 1998).

The two examples clearly show both the health promoter's methods in working to facilitate empowerment in the communities and the communities' methods to achieve the environmental conditions they wanted. As residents achieve success, they increase their collective self-efficacy and empowerment. The latter, however, is contingent on social identity, such that reflection on the action taken results in meaning that the action is legitimate and that one's social identity is active and powerful (Drury & Reicher, 2005).

Social Action. Social action organizing, according to Rothman (1979), has as its goal the shifting of power relationships and resources from the haves to the have-nots. Social action as a method achieves change by crystallizing issues and organizing people to take action. Historical examples of this type of community organization practice have included method organizing; the civil rights movement; the United Farm Workers movement; community action programs; and the work of the Students for a Democratic Society, the Student Non-Violent Coordinating Committee, the Black Panthers, the Brown Berets, and La Raza Unida (Alinsky, 1969, 1972; Fisher, 1997). Methods include boycotts, demonstrations, and strikes.

Social Movements. The study of social movements overlaps considerably with community organization and advocacy that challenges power over. It offers insights for understanding the processes of change at the community level. *Social movements* have been defined "as collectivities acting with some degree of organization and continuity outside of institutional or organizational channels for the purpose of challenging or defending extant authority, whether it is institutionally or culturally based, in the group, organization, society, culture or world order of which they are a part" (Snow, Soule, & Kriesi, 2004b, p. 11).

We briefly discuss key insights from studies and theories of social movements particularly relevant to health education practice and refer the reader to other sources (Snow, Soule, & Kriesi, 2004a, 2004b) for fuller elaboration. Resource availability increases the likelihood of collective action, and resources have been inequitably distributed historically, geographically, and socially. Resources have at times been redistributed by the state; by organizations such as foundations, religious organizations, corporations, and movement-mentoring organizations; and by individuals through financial donations and endorsements. Five categories of resources have been distinguished (Edwards & McCarthy, 2004):

- Legitimacy and other moral resources
- Cultural resources such as knowledge about how to accomplish specific tasks and tactics
- New and appropriable social organizational resources, including infrastructures, social networks, and organizations
- Human resources, including human capital
- Material resources, such as monetary resources, property, office space, equipment, and supplies

The mobilization of these resources is a key issue for the emergence of social movements.

Framing is the process of assigning meaning and interpretation to relevant events and conditions in order to mobilize potential constituents, gain bystander support, and demobilize antagonists. Frames focus attention on what is relevant in a situation, create a set of meanings or narratives as to what is going on there, and serve a transformative function for both individuals and groups. Transformation can include altering the meaning of objects and one's relationship to them, including reconfiguring one's biography, and transforming routine grievances into injustices in the context of collective action (Snow, 2004). This construction of meaning can be viewed as a "politics of signification" (Snow, p. 384), in which social movements, governments at all levels, other authority structures, the media, and interested stakeholder groups seek to establish, among contested frames, the dominant meaning ascribed to persons, experiences, objects, and events. The mass media arena is especially important, as it serves as a public forum, is assumed by all players to have persuasive influence, and signals and diffuses changes in cultural codes, such as language used for framing an issue (Gamson, 2004).

These collective (as opposed to individual) frames are formed within a cultural context, using deeply held cultural values, such as justice, self-reliance, and rights. The culture shapes the framing process; the framing process in turn can shift culture. Movements focused on moderate change act on commonly shared meanings with the available culture, whereas attempts at radical social change require a critique of the current cultural understandings with which many people may not resonate. Thus, the appeals must be different and, for radical change, go beyond cognitive persuasion to embodiment and action. For example, during the civil rights movement, African Americans used facilities that had been designated for "whites only" (W. Williams, 2004). Social movements use tactics such as persuasion, facilitation, bargaining, and coercion. These have been characterized as either nonconfrontational or insider tactics (such as leafleting, letter-writing campaigns, lobbying, boycotts, lawsuits, and press conferences), and confrontational or outsider tactics (such as sit-ins, demonstrations, vigils, marches, and blockades). Protest tactics may be characterized as conventional (such as lobbying), disruptive (such as boycotts or demonstrations), or violent (such as bombings) (V. Taylor & Van Dyke, 2004).

Advocacy. Advocacy is a primary method used in community organizing, whether sharing power with or challenging power over. Advocacy is one of the basic methods for change at environmental levels (see Table 7.11). This method addresses many of the processes that social movement theorists have discussed. *Advocacy* has been defined as "the set of skills used to create a shift in public opinion and mobilize the necessary resources and forces to support an issue, policy, or constituency" (Wallack, Dorfman, Jernigan, & Themba, 1993, p. 27). Advocacy ensures that the rights of disenfranchised individuals are protected, that institutions work the way they should, and that legislation and policy reflect the interests of the people. It addresses attitudes and policies at all levels from organizational, through community and state, to the national arena. In public health advocacy, efforts are made to change community conditions, often pitting consumers against large industry and pitting citizens against city hall. Community activism is rooted in democratic principles and practices; and though it is often viewed as synonymous with social action, it includes cooperation as well as confrontation. Examples of advocacy groups include local and national groups participating in social movements—such as those for the environment, environmental justice, and tobacco control—and citizen groups that have come together to support issues of importance in their communities. Advocacy groups have different tactics. For example, some are confrontational, such as ACT UP (an AIDS-awareness activist group); others are research based, such as the League of Women Voters (Altman, Balcazar, Fawcett, Seekins, & Young, 1994; Wallack et al., 1993).

It is important that health promoters choose tactics and activities that fit the type of community organizing, the issue, and the community. Groups must decide the way in which they intend to accomplish goals, and those activities will likely change over time in response to reactions to actions taken and to shifting external forces. Altman and colleagues (1994) list the following approaches to advocacy: coalition building, community development, coordination, education, networking, public awareness, and policy or legislative change. They suggest the principles of presence, generosity, shaping, escalation, accuracy, and honesty to enhance tactical efforts (see Table 4.4). These principles should underlie action, regardless of whether the action flows from a social action, community development, or social planning perspective.

Another basic element in advocacy is framing the issue. The issue must be framed in terms that the advocacy group puts forward. For example, the tobacco industry might say, "Smoking is a matter of personal choice," whereas a public health advocacy group would say, "People smoke because they are addicted." The tobacco industry might say, "Smoking bans discriminate against smokers," whereas the advocacy group would say, "Nonsmokers have the right to breathe clean air" (Altman et al., 1994, p. 61).

Altman and colleagues (1994) divide advocacy strategies into three categories: research and investigation, encouragement and education, and direct action. In research and investigation, the advocacy group conducts studies of the issue to

TABLE 4.4. PRINCIPLES UNDERLYING EFFECTIVE TACTICS.

Principle	What to Do
1. Presence	Remind people of the issue by doing something about it frequently.
2. Generosity	Praise others for their strengths and actions to gain good will and to reinforce their actions.
3. Shaping	Reward small steps of those who change toward your goals.
4. Escalation	Continue to mobilize more people and increase the intensity of the tactics if the first efforts are unsuccessful.
5. Accuracy and honesty	Be scrupulously accurate to maintain credibility and to keep opponents from successfully arguing against the issues raised.
6. Consistency	Distribute praise and criticism fairly. If one group is criticized for its position, other groups should be treated the same way.

understand it as fully as possible by gathering data on public opinion, obtaining information about the opposition and its strategies and tactics, and acting as a watchdog of target organizations. The advocacy group can also request accountability by formally asking responsible parties for the reasons behind a decision of concern to them, by documenting complaints with evidence, by organizing consumer service audits, and by demonstrating the financial benefits of acting on their issue.

Strategies for encouragement and education include giving personal compliments and public support to reinforce other people's actions, arranging celebrations and publicizing them, developing a detailed proposal for addressing the problem being focused on, and establishing contact with the opposition organization even to the extent of influencing its decision-making processes. The advocacy group can also prepare fact sheets on the issue (and on the group) to maintain consistency and continuity in public relations, offer public education through mass media and presentations to community groups, and counter attacks by explaining the group's point of view.

Interventionists can use direct action strategies to make the group's presence felt, mobilize public support, and use the system (Altman et al., 1994). Strategies to make the group's presence felt include postponing action until the issue has matured, establishing alternative programs or finding another source to provide the service, establishing lines of communication with the opponent's traditional allies, criticizing unfavorable actions (first privately and then publicly if there are no results), expressing opposition publicly, reminding those responsible, making complaints (first informally, then formally), and lobbying decision makers. Ways to mobilize public support include sponsoring a conference or public hearing; conducting a letter-writing campaign, a petition drive, or a ballot drive; registering voters; and organizing public demonstrations. For using the system, the advocacy group might file a formal complaint; seek enforcement of existing laws and policies; lobby for new laws, policies, or regulations; use other resources such as a negotiator, mediator, or fact finder to work with opponents; and initiate legal action if that proves to be the only way to address the issue. Altman and colleagues also describe strategies to use if efforts to work within the system fail. These include arranging a media exposé, overwhelming an unworkable system (for example, by arranging unmanageable requests for service), organizing a boycott, and using passive resistance.

Advocacy can lead to counteradvocacy by opponents, who may deflect the issue or shift the focus of attention away from the responsible party. The opponents may also delay, deny, and discount the importance of the problem or of the advocacy group's legitimacy. Deception, dividing the advocacy group by co-opting leaders or splitting moderate and militant members, appeasing the group with short-term benefits, discrediting the advocacy group, and destroying the group are all techniques designed to silence the advocates. If those tactics don't work, opponents may make a deal that falls short of the advocates' goals. Altman and colleagues (1994) suggest that advocates turn negatives into positives in response to the opposition's tactics; groups can go public with the opponent's tactics, frame the debate on the advocate's terms, keep the opponent off balance by being unpredictable, and know when to negotiate. Table 4.5 presents a list of twenty rules of etiquette drawn from the experiences of a number of advocates and summarized by Altman and colleagues as guidelines for advocacy.

R. Fisher and Kling (1991) see contemporary community-based social action as blending social action with community development and social planning. Strategies used include building coalitions across constituency groups and integrating community politics more closely with electoral activity (R. Fisher, 1997). These

TABLE 4.5. GUIDELINES FOR EFFECTIVE ADVOCACY.

1. Accentuate the positive.
2. Plan for small wins.
3. Begin by assuming the best of others.
4. Do your homework and document your findings.
5. Take the high ground.
6. Reframe opponents' definitions of the issue.
7. Keep it simple.
8. Be passionate and persistent.
9. Be willing to compromise.
10. Be opportunistic and creative.
11. Be fearless in the face of intimidation.
12. Maintain focus on the issues.
13. Make it local and keep it relevant.
14. Be broadly based and nonpartisan from the beginning.
15. Develop an independent public identity.
16. Try to stay within the experiences of individuals in your group.
17. Whenever possible, go outside the experience of your opponent.
18. Make your opponents live by their own rules.
19. Tie advocacy group efforts to related events.
20. Have a good time.

Source: Altman, Balcazar, Fawcett, Seekins, and Young, 1994, pp. 27–35.

theorists believe that policy advocacy is not sufficient, that groups must win and hold power through elected office. Fisher develops the argument that a major focus must be on challenging the ideology of privatization and free enterprise that serves the needs of international capital rather than those of low- and moderate-income people. This challenge should be mounted through legislation to protect public sector services and public life. Finally, community organizers must bring together people across different agendas and different cultural and identity-based groups to organize around common grievances with a commitment to "human solidarity, mutual responsibility, and social justice" (p. 65).

Media Advocacy. Wallack and his colleagues (1993) have developed the approach of media advocacy, a set of strategies for using the media to promote public health. They recognized that the mass media, particularly television, provide a forum for surfacing and discussing issues, and setting the agenda for policymakers and the public. Media advocacy seeks to influence the selection and presentation of topics by the media in order to set and achieve a public health agenda.

Media advocacy is based on three steps:

1. Setting the agenda (framing for access)
2. Shaping the debate (framing for content)
3. Advancing the policy

In framing for access, the goal is to get the media to select the story. Framing for content involves shifting the view of health from the individual to the social level and dealing with the complexity of health and social problems so that a public health perspective defines the debate. Advancing the policy is framing the content so that it reaches the key decision makers whom the advocacy group is trying to influence.

To gain access the health promoter needs to understand the various access points of each of the major media outlets. For television these points are news, public affairs, entertainment, editorials, paid advertising, and public service advertising; for newspapers they are the front page, sports, lifestyle, arts, comics, business, editorial section, letters to the editor, and paid advertising. The media advocate needs skills in determining where and how to place the particular issue within the media. Media advocacy strategies focus on earned media (that is, not paid, such as news and talk shows) and paid placements rather than on public service announcements, in which control over the placement and framing of the story is lost. One can achieve news coverage by targeting journalists who are interested in health issues and providing them with accurate information and story ideas. Creating news and piggybacking onto breaking news are also strategies.

Elements of newsworthiness include linking the story to the anniversary of an event, a breakthrough, a celebrity, a controversy, injustice, irony, a local point of view, a milestone, a personal angle, and a seasonal theme (Wallack et al., 1993, p. 98). By monitoring the media, a health promoter can understand which reporters are covering which topics and what the current community concerns are.

To give the public health perspective, the health promoter can frame an individual problem as a social issue, shifting the primary responsibility away from blaming the individual. For example, the advocate can shift the subject from teen drinking to the promotion of alcohol and include a solution with an approach to policy. Story elements to be developed include compelling images, powerful symbols, and social math to show the extent of the problem (for example, in a year "enough alcohol was consumed by college students to fill 3,500 Olympic-size swimming pools, about 1 on every campus in the United States" (Wallack et al., 1993, p. 108). It is important to use voices of people who are credible because of their experiences but who are deeply involved in the policy aspects of the issue. For example, a college president at a campus on which a death has occurred due to binge drinking who has worked with the college board of trustees to change rules about student alcohol use might be a good source for a campaign about student alcohol use. Using sound bites of fewer than ten seconds to summarize the issue is a valuable skill for the health promoter to learn.

Wallack and colleagues (1993) also provide practical advice for developing media goals and objectives, pitching the story to journalists, developing media kits, and giving interviews. Their summary rules for working with reporters are to be honest, help the press better understand the issues, only comment on issues that you know about, and remember that everything you say is on the record (Wallack et al., p. 141).

Summary of Community Organization Theories in Problem Analysis and Intervention Methods.

- Environmental condition: community with high capacity for problem solving
- Agent: community leaders and members
- Behaviors: taking action to change community conditions related to health
- Determinants: motivation to act, collective efficacy, political efficacy, and community structures that are facilitating
- Methods: participatory problem solving; organizing (grassroots organizing and professionally driven organizing); forming coalitions; using lay health workers; advocacy (information, persuasion, negotiation); framing to shift perspectives; media advocacy to build community identity, political and legislative actions, and culturally relevant practice; participation and community mapping; ad-

vocacy (research, encouragement, and direct action); turning of negative into positive responses; media advocacy (framing for access, framing for content, and advancing the policy)

Societal and Governmental Theories

For the societal level, we examine theories that relate to public policy and its development.

Public Policy

Public policy is "a guide to action to change what would otherwise occur, a decision about amounts and allocations of resources, made at any level of government" (Milio, 2001, p. 622). Health policy is directly related to public health and health services. Other public policies directed to issues such as economics, housing, or public safety also have much potential to influence health. Milio (1981) views economic policy as acting directly on people's biophysical and socioeconomic environments and indirectly through various areas for public policy, such as environmental safety, energy, income maintenance, and health and human services delivery (see Figure 4.8). This framework shows policy as a determinant of health behavior and of health.

Public policy sets options for organizations and for individuals, both directly and indirectly through organizations. According to Milio (1981, p. 83), policy components should make "the creation and maintenance of healthful environments and personal habits the easiest—the 'cheapest' and most numerous—choices for selections by governmental units and corporations, producers and consumers, among all the options available to them." Policy instruments include direct spending, such as grants and contracts and the production of goods and services; regulation and monitoring; and fiscal incentives such as subsidies, taxation, and tax deductions.

Policy formation is a cyclical process, occurring within a system open to the environment (Longest, 2002; Themba & Minkler, 2003). In a rational or economic decision-making model, a policymaker would select the most efficient alternative to maximize the most valuable output. However, policy formation is much more complex than that, with many stakeholders and interest groups with varying power and diverse ideologies, insufficient information about policy problems and solutions, and unique contexts for specific issues. Theorists have endeavored to isolate key constructs and their relationships in this process to create hypotheses that can be tested (Jones, 2003). We will discuss several of these theories in the context of a model developed by Longest.

FIGURE 4.8. PUBLIC SOCIOENVIRONMENTAL POLICY THAT SHAPES AMERICAN ENVIRONMENTS.

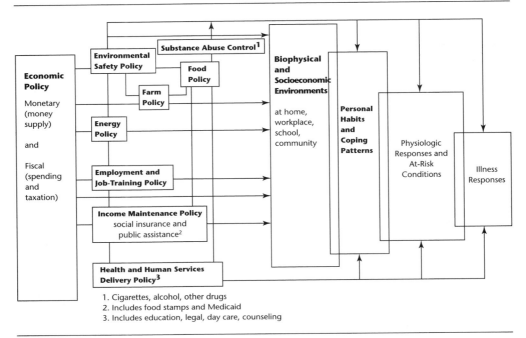

1. Cigarettes, alcohol, other drugs
2. Includes food stamps and Medicaid
3. Includes education, legal, day care, counseling

Source: Milio, 1981.

Longest (2002) has identified three intertwined phases of the policy process: policy formulation, policy implementation, and policy modification. Policy formulation includes setting the policy agenda and the development of legislation. Policy implementation includes activities associated with rule making that guide operationalization and implementation of a policy. Policy modification is feedback from individuals, organizations, and interest groups to policy formulation and policy implementation. These phases and their components are displayed in Figure 4.9. Health advocates and activated communities have opportunities to influence the policy process at each phase.

The policy process involves the movement from "policy primeval soup" (Kingdon, 2003, p. 116) to the development of legislation. Three theories—Agenda Building, the Policy Window Theory, and the Advocacy Coalition Framework—are especially useful in understanding how this process occurs (Cobb & Elder, 1983; John, 2003; Kingdon, 2003; Sabatier, 2003).

FIGURE 4.9. A MODEL OF THE PUBLIC POLICYMAKING PROCESS IN THE UNITED STATES.

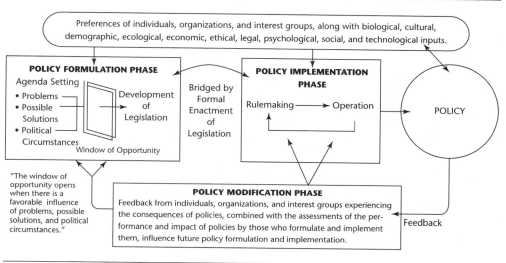

Source: Longest, 2002, p. 115.

Agenda-Building Theory. Agenda setting is the process of moving an issue to the systemic and institutional agenda for action. The systemic agenda contains issues that politicians see as meriting public attention and as being within the legitimate jurisdiction of existing governmental authority. The institutional agenda contains issues that are available for the active and serious consideration of political decision makers. Cobb and Elder (1983) propose three models for agenda building:

- Outside-initiative model
- Inside-initiative model
- Mobilization model

In the outside-initiative model, public support for an issue and the idea that the issue requires action that falls within governmental authority bring the issue first to the systemic agenda and then, with continued public pressure, to the institutional agenda. In the inside-initiative model, the initiative comes from within the government system and does not involve the larger public; it often moves quickly from the systemic agenda to the institutional agenda. In the mobilization model, policy proposals are developed within government, and then support is sought among the public for formal policy passage and successful implementation. When an issue is on the systemic agenda, politicians are more likely to place it on the institutional agenda if it has high and long-term social relevance, is not technical or technocratic, and is unique. These criteria suggest how advocates should frame the policy and messages concerning it.

Methods to influence policy development depend on which model best describes a process and where in the process an issue is. In the outside-initiative model, public support is needed to bring the issue to the systemic agenda. For public health issues, the methods of grassroots organizing, media advocacy, and professionally driven organizing use the media to show the importance of the issue and its effects on people, the urgency of the problem, and the power and legitimacy of the groups wishing to address the issue. Earlier in this chapter, we discussed the strategies and tactics for community organization and advocacy to generate public support.

In the inside-initiative model, the initiative comes from within the government system and moves from there to the institutional agenda without involving the larger public. Here, the advocacy work is much more behind the scenes. Health advocates form relationships with legislative staff members, persuade them of the importance of the issue, and show how the issue fits with their legislator's agenda. Supplying information that is accurate and well timed to the legislative staff member's needs as the issue moves through the policy process enables the legislator's staff to get the issue into play. This process does not require large-scale community mobilization and media, because the issue is likely floating close to the systemic agenda. Here, individual policy entrepreneurs may be as effective as organized community groups. Policy entrepreneurs use the methods we discussed earlier (for example, persuasive communication, value discussions, and presentation of facts) to get policymaking insiders to place the issue on the systemic and institutional agendas.

In the mobilization model, policy proposals are developed within the government, and then support is sought among the public for passing the policy and implementing it successfully. In this instance, government insiders use the media and community forums to inform and persuade the public of the importance of the issue in order to mobilize broad-scale support for the policy proposal. The methods are similar to the dual-channel methods (that is, mass media and interpersonal communication) that we discussed earlier in this chapter.

Issues have a life cycle, and an understanding of the stages and their determinants allows the advocate to move an issue forward more effectively. Cobb and Elder (1983) identified five stages in the cycle:

1. Issue awareness
2. Issue recognition
3. Issue resolution
4. Issue realignment
5. Issue dormancy

In the issue awareness stage, groups and individuals begin to discuss problems and potential issues. For an issue to be recognized, a policymaker must decide that the issue should be addressed. Issues are more likely to be recognized if they are defined broadly, have a large social impact, have long-term implications, are not too technical and complex, and are not routine. Interest-group characteristics are also important. The group's ideology and values must arouse enough tension concerning the problem for the potential issue to emerge. The more powerful the group is (in terms of size and legitimacy) and the more committed it is to the issue, the more likely it is to influence the policy. Time is important as well. Too rapid an emergence can lead to a crisis in which policymakers are unprepared; some issues require time to ripen. But too long a period can lead to loss of interest by the public.

De Leeuw (2000) raises the important question of who determines which policy is to be formulated. She suggests that the social planning model underlies traditional hierarchical policy formulation in which government sets policy. In comparison, locality development and social action community processes are most relevant to current policy agenda-setting models. The individuals or organizations that best use these processes set the policy. Social entrepreneurs such as academicians, nongovernmental organizations, and community activists who value social justice and seek innovative solutions for social problems can have a significant impact on policy.

A group that wishes to get its issue on the policy agenda must gain media attention as well as the support of opinion leaders and political leaders. Media advocacy provides a framework and set of tools for a community group to use to influence policy (Wallack et al., 1993). The three steps of media advocacy are setting the agenda, or framing it for access to the media and thus to specific opinion leaders; shaping the debate, or framing the content to highlight social definitions and solutions to problems; and advancing the policy by articulating the solutions and placing pressure on policymakers. We discussed methods for media advocacy in the previous section on advocacy for community change.

Policy Windows Theory. Kingdon (2003) has also investigated how issues reach systemic or governmental agenda status, inserting an element of chance that explains the fluidity and rapid change of the policymaking process. He views this process in terms of three streams: politics, problems, and policies. The political stream includes changes in administration, party platforms, elections, and national mood regarding government. The problem stream includes issues within the various policy sectors, such as global warming, the national debt, health care costs, teenage pregnancy, specific diseases, and poor housing infrastructure. Policy solutions, such as pollution controls, universal health insurance, school-based clinics, or cooperative housing, "float around in or near government, searching for problems to which to become attached or political events that increase their likelihood of adoption" (p. 112). Events and ideas in these streams move along independently until there is a change in one stream, such as a change in government, emergence of a large problem, or advocacy of new policies. At this point a window between the streams opens up so that a problem may enter the political stream or a policy may become linked to a problem. The role of the policy advocate is to create, monitor, and capitalize on these opportunities.

Policy advocates or entrepreneurs promote their proposals and the associated problems and facilitate coupling between the streams, linking problems, policies, and political opportunities together when the windows are open. Characteristics of effective policy advocates are recognized authority; visibility; strong political, communication, and negotiation skills; ability to engage in strategic planning; creativity; relative independence in resources and structure; and persistence (Duhl, 1990; Kingdon, 2003; Milio, 1988).

In policy advocacy, as in many other arenas, timing is everything; and opportunity knocks for those advocates who are prepared. Much of the success in placing issues on the systemic and institutional agendas and in achieving policy enactment comes from an understanding of when to act and how to frame the issue. Kingdon's notion of policy windows (2003) provides a framework for timing. Kingdon says that policy is placed on the agenda when the windows between the three streams of politics (including elections, party platforms, and national mood regarding government), problems (all the issues within different policy sectors, including health, housing, economic sectors), and policy solutions (such as school-based clinics and universal health insurance) open so that the policy can be put forward. For example, newly elected officials may focus on certain problems, for which prepared advocates who have networked with the right gatekeepers can present their solutions. Community advocacy groups can work with each of the streams. For instance, they can support candidates for elected office or influence party platforms, build community demand to address particular problems, and develop and promote well-researched and persuasive policy proposals.

Laumann and Knoke (1987) point to the importance of organizations in the policy development process. They argue that influential organizations that have specific national policy interests and fluid resources and that are embedded within communication and resource-exchange networks are the main actors in the national policy process. These organizations are typically corporate entities, such as trade associations, professional societies, labor unions, corporations, public interest groups, government bureaus, and congressional committees. The policy process begins when one or more of these organizations recognizes a condition as a problem or an issue and alerts other organizations to it. The interested organizations then generate options, often as solutions in search of issues. The alternative options are then narrowed to get the policy option onto the governmental agenda for consideration. Each step is a product of negotiation and advocacy.

Powerful corporate entities representing industries such as health insurance, pharmaceuticals, processed foods, and tobacco take positions opposed or aligned with those of health promoters. Developing and maintaining strong entities on behalf of public health, such as public health professional associations, associations representing public health officials, and citizens' groups, and carefully creating alliances where appropriate with corporate groups are strategies necessary in order to represent health promotion in the policy development process.

After policy is enacted into law, it must be operationalized; and advocates, especially strong interest groups, seek to influence this process through lobbying and other forms of influence. Especially important are long-standing working relationships between those implementing policy and leaders of affected organizations and interest groups. These relationships are marked by the exchange of information and expertise. For complex policies that may affect a number of interest groups, advisory committees and task forces may be set up to help develop the proposed rules. Gaining a seat on these bodies allows for direct input to the process (Kingdon, 2003; Longest, 2002).

According to Longest (2002), the success of the operational implementation of the policy rests on the fit between the implementing organizations and policy objectives and on the amount of resources (for example, authority, fiscal, personnel, information and expertise, and technology) the organization has. The competence of agency managers related to strategy, leadership, collaboration, and conceptual and technical knowledge and skills are key. Implementation problems are certain to arise, and management must be able to address these challenges.

The policymaking process is cyclical, and most health policies are the result of modifying previous policies. Policy modification occurs when stakeholders incorporate feedback from policy implementation and consequences into the policy formulation and policy implementation phases. Rules and practices may be changed or the law may be amended, typically in an incremental fashion. Feedback comes both from the groups affected by the policies, especially key interest groups, and from those who formulate and take charge of implementation. Pressure to change can be both external, from individuals, organizations, and interest groups, and internal, through oversight by the legislative, executive, and judicial branches. Evaluations of policy implementation and outcomes of policy are often crucial to decisions regarding modification.

Advocacy Coalition Framework. Sabatier (2003) describes work he and colleagues have done on their Advocacy Coalition Framework to focus attention on policy subsystems, the set of actors who follow and seek to influence public policy in a given area across a time frame of a decade or more. Actors can be elected and agency officials at all levels of government, interest-group leaders, researchers, and important journalists who cover the issue. The actors engage in coordinated activity such as advocacy coalitions based on deep and unchangeable shared basic values, causal assumptions, and problem perspectives in the particular policy arena, along with more changeable secondary beliefs about how to implement the policy core. A small number of coalitions within a particular policy subsystem compete, promoting conflicting strategies, and policy brokers within the subsystem attempt to find a reasonable compromise to reduce this conflict so that policy can be enacted.

Stable factors such as a society's perception of the issue area, distribution of natural resources, cultural values, social structure, and basic legal structure constrain the options available to the actors. For example, the U.S. cultural values of individualism and capitalism limit the policy options that can be advocated. Dynamic events such as socioeconomic conditions and technology, large changes in governing coalitions, and decisions and impacts from other subsystems alter the constraints and opportunities of the subsystem actors. The AIDS epidemic can be viewed as an outside event that enabled the harm-reduction coalition to overthrow the well-established abstinence coalition in the drug policy subsystem in Western Europe (Kubler, 2001). Bleach kits and needle exchange programs became policy options.

The Advocacy Coalition Framework provides guidance for carrying out policy advocacy. The framework rejects the notion that there are coalitions of convenience of actors motivated by short-term self-interest. Instead, core beliefs or ideology create a stable lineup of allies and opponents. Advocacy coalitions will negotiate on the secondary beliefs, including decisions on administrative rules, budgets, interpretation of statutes, and information about the problem, before shifting on the fundamental policy core. Because of this, the core attributes of a governmental program are unlikely to change as long as the coalition that instituted that program remains in power; a perturbation from outside the policy subsystem is necessary for change to occur. In comparison to Kingdon's Policy Window Theory (2003), the Advocacy Coalition Framework sees the policy solution stream as much more integrated with the political stream because of the foundation of core normative and policy beliefs (Sabatier, 2003).

The importance of political ideology in public health has been increasingly recognized (J. E. Cohen et al., 2000). Particularly important has been the tension between the views that government has the duty to protect its citizens' health and that individuals have the right to make their own choices. Ideological arguments on both sides have been made regarding pasteurization of milk, fluoridation of public water supplies, use of motorcycle helmets, and tobacco control. Review of newspaper coverage of tobacco issues in the United States from 1985 to 1996 showed that the tobacco industry framed the issue around the core values of freedom, fairness, free enterprise, and autonomy. Tobacco-control advocates, on the other hand, framed the issue around the value of health (Menashe & Siegel, 1998). J. E. Cohen and colleagues (2000) have suggested that ideological arguments be used to benefit tobacco control. They and others suggest that advocates use the perspective of the New Right, including its laissez-faire approach, its retreat from state intervention in economic and social affairs, and its belief in market forces; advocates should also use the values of freedom, fairness, and free enterprise to frame the argument for tobacco control (J. E. Cohen et al.; McKinlay & Marceau, 2000). This would avoid challenging normative core beliefs so that the focus can be on changing tobacco policy. With regard to framing the issue, freedom could include freedom from the influence of the tobacco industry and from the addiction of tobacco; fairness, treating bar and restaurant workers the same as workers who have protection from secondhand smoke; and free enterprise, that the tobacco industry seeks government tax breaks, trade advantages, and protection of its proprietary information.

Summary of Policy Theories in Problem Analysis and Intervention Methods.

- Environment: health-promoting public policy
- Agent: policymakers
- Behaviors: enactment of health-promoting legislation, regulation, and policy
- Determinants: motivation and behavioral capability, barriers
- Methods: policy advocacy (information, persuasion, and negotiation), tailoring to policy initiation model, timing for policy windows

PART TWO

INTERVENTION
MAPPING STEPS

CHAPTER FIVE

INTERVENTION MAPPING STEP 1: NEEDS ASSESSMENT

Reader Objectives

- Establish a planning group that includes potential program participants and plan the needs assessment
- Conduct the needs assessment using the PRECEDE model (Green & Kreuter, 2005) to analyze health and quality of life problems and their causes and to decide on priorities
- Balance the needs assessment with an assessment of community capacity
- Link the needs assessment to evaluation planning by establishing desired program outcomes

The purpose of this chapter is to enable the reader to perform a needs assessment and to invite and facilitate participation by those who will be affected by the resulting program. Intervention Mapping or any other health education program planning must be based on a thorough assessment of community capacity and needs. This assessment encompasses two components:

1. An epidemiologic, behavioral, and social perspective of an at-risk group or community and its problems
2. An effort to begin to understand the character of the community, its members, and its strengths

In the first part of the chapter, we discuss the preassessment, which includes putting a together work group for intervention development, the first step of which is needs assessment. We touch on essential elements of encouraging participation, including work-group management and culturally competent practice. The preassessment also includes choosing or creating an organizing framework for the assessment; for this purpose, we present the PRECEDE model (L. W. Green & Kreuter, 2005).

Conducting the needs assessment includes the following tasks:

1. Choosing methods and data sources
2. Describing the population and context for the assessment
3. Describing problems including health and quality of life and their behavioral and environmental causes
4. Describing community strengths and capacities

We present this material in three sections. First, we present methods for describing the population and its health and quality of life problems and the causes of these problems. Next, we turn to methods of data collection; and finally, we talk about assessing community strengths. Postassessment includes setting priorities and setting program objectives, activities we cover in the chapter's last two sections.

Perspectives

Our perspectives in this chapter highlight the importance of needs assessment as a part of intervention planning and encourage a focus on community strengths.

Needs Assessment as Part of Intervention Planning

In the first edition of this book, we included a discussion of needs assessment as a process in preparation for intervention development. This presentation might have inadvertently given the impression that the needs assessment is optional. Nothing could be further from the truth. An effective program must address a real problem or need. In this edition, therefore, we include needs assessment as the first step of Intervention Mapping.

Assessment of Both Needs and Strengths

A *needs assessment* is a systematic study of the discrepancy between what is and what should be in a group and situation of interest (Gilmore & Campbell, 1996). Gilmore and colleagues (Gilmore, Campbell, & Becker, 1989; Gilmore & Campbell, 1996) suggest that planners not worry too much about the difference between need and perceived need for three reasons: (1) Needs are always changing in character and quantity; (2) needs are always interpreted by someone; and (3) the needs that people report are an important source of information. Needs assessments should include opinions of the stakeholders or those with a vested interest in the problem and its solution as well as a factual description of the problem and its causes (Witkin & Altschuld, 1995). Because the definition of something as a problem is a value-laden social construction, the labeling of something as a problem should always include the perspective of those with the condition (Suarez-Balcazar, 1992). Suarez-Balcazar and colleagues (1992) suggest that problem identification in intervention research should include the following principles:

1. Avoid blaming the victim
2. Involve community participants
3. Examine the environmental causes of problems

Sometimes the literature calls a needs assessment that is done for the purpose of contributing to the development of a program by the term *formative research* (Kraft, Beeker, Stokes, & Peterson, 2000; Sorensen et al., 2004; Newes-Adeyi, Helitzer, Caulfield, & Bronner, 2000). Formative research can also refer more specifically to a type of pretesting program materials (Chapter Eight).

In the case of health problems, a needs assessment seeks to understand what is compared to what is more desirable in terms of quality of life and health status as well as those factors that influence health or health risk, such as behavior and environment. Needs assessments of health problems include an analysis of the physiological risk factors and behavioral and environmental risks to health, even when the actual health problems have not yet manifested. For example, cardiovascular disease is a health problem; high-fat levels are a physiological risk factor; eating high-fat foods is a behavioral risk; and poor access to healthy diet is an environmental risk factor. Finally, health-related needs assessments include study of the determinants of behavior and environmental contributors to health problems or health risks. By *determinants*, we mean those factors that have been found to be associated with the at-risk behavior or the environmental condition. The implication for intervention is that determinants are causally related to the conditions. However, even though the logic is causal, the empirical evidence most often is not (see Chapter Two).

The study of a community from the perspective of capacity, or resources and strengths, rounds out the assessment (Curtis & Jones, 1999; Fawcett, 1991; Fawcett et al., 2000; Goeppinger & Baglioni, 1985; R. M. Goodman, Steckler, Hoover, & Schwartz, 1993; Issel & Searing, 2000; Kretzmann & McKnight, 1993; McKnight & Kretzmann, 1997). Studying the strengths of a community can help the health educator keep in mind a community's unique character and its ability to plan its own interventions. An attitude of partnership between health professionals and community members can help to prevent a top-down or outsider planning approach (Minkler & Wallerstein, 1997a, 1997b). For example, a class at a school of public health began an assessment of a community that had many health problems. This minority area had originated as a community where few city services were available. Community residents and planners worked together to understand needs in a context of both current and historical community pride, entrepreneurship, and leadership. Despite a host of urban problems, inconsistent support from the city, and deficits in health services, the community maintained a strong African American culture that had begun attracting new resources. From a perspective of health needs, the community had a certain profile; and from a capacity perspective, it had another look entirely.

Furthermore, a focus on community competencies and resources from the outset of program planning directs attention to the need for enhancement of capacity in the program development and implementation. All too often, health education and other social programs, especially research and demonstration efforts, have entered communities, only to leave them unchanged when funding ended (R. M. Goodman & Steckler, 1989). Programs that aim to enhance capacity from the start of planning can make this scenario less likely to develop.

Collaborative Planning and the Preassessment Phase

⊃ *The first task in the Step 1 needs assessment is to establish a planning group that includes potential program participants and plan the needs assessment.*

This task includes two important elements: (1) establishing and working with a planning group and (2) planning the needs assessment. Prior to discussing how to select members for the planning group and what methods to use for managing group process, we provide an in-depth discussion of cultural competence and the ways that practitioners can prepare themselves to work effectively with community members from cultures other than their own. Then we address the technical task of planning the needs assessment. We use the PRECEDE model, a population-based epidemiologic planning framework, to guide data collection and analysis (L. W. Green & Kreuter, 2005).

Cultural Competence

The very first process in beginning health promotion practice in general, and any one project in particular, is to consider the community and its cultural groups and subgroups. Often, health educators work with groups of people who are members of a cultural group different from themselves. In the United States, Healthy People 2010 (U.S. Department of Health and Human Services, 1998) highlights the health disparities among racial and ethnic groups, with particular emphasis on eliminating those disparities in infant mortality, cancer screening and management, cardiovascular disease, diabetes, HIV/AIDS, and childhood and adult immunizations. For example, in comparison to whites, infant mortality rates are 2.5 times higher for African Americans and 1.5 times higher for Native Americans. The prevalence of diabetes in Hispanics is nearly twice that of whites (U.S. Department of Health and Human Services). In order to address these and many other priority health issues effectively, health educators must be able to develop culturally appropriate programs. Health educators who wish to look beyond their geographic borders and work in international settings must become immersed in the culture in which they are working. Furthermore, culture is not an issue of ethnicity alone. Ethnicity is but one of several group designations that act to define enduring aspects of a group culture.

Triandis (1994) states that, in observing other cultures, we humans see the world through a lens of who we are rather than seeing the world as it is. Under this condition health educators must learn to see the other culture as clearly as possible in order to create programs that are culturally competent. If culture is to society what memories are to an individual (Triandis, citing Kluckhohn, 1954), then a culturally competent program is one that uses those memories for the empowerment of the individual and the community. A culturally relevant program is one that uses culturally appropriate images and themes to make a program attractive and appealing to a group, thus affecting attention and comprehension.

Culture can be defined as the implicit and explicit guidelines that individuals inherit as members of a particular group. These guidelines tell people in that culture how to "view the world, how to experience it emotionally, and how to behave in it in relation to other people, to supernatural forces or gods, and to the natural environment" (Helman, 1990, pp. 2–3). The more cultures differ from one another, the higher the cultural distance is; and the less likely it is that people from those different cultures will attach the same meaning to words, gestures, and symbols. Witte and Morrison (1995) have described the specific impact of cultures on health communications, including how different cultures explain disease. Ethnomedical systems can be described as either personalistic, naturalistic, or Western scientific. Personalistic systems view supernatural spirits or people as causing disease. Naturalistic systems describe health in impersonal terms of equilibrium, for example: hot and cold, active and passive. Western medicine seeks analytical and physiological explanations and cures for disease. Closely related to these explanatory systems are cultural concepts regarding the mind-body connection and the roles of religion and the family. Those concepts, because they mediate how people conceptualize and manage health and illness, are an important context for health education. Pasick (1997), for example, mentions *fatalismo*, a concept of fatalism that can influence health behaviors such as cancer screening. A woman considering mammography might say, "Why find the cancer if it can't be cured?"

Exploring Personal Ethnocentrism. Triandis (1994) describes personal ethnocentrism as an individual's sense of slight superiority in response to stories from other cultures and boredom at the expectedness of stories from one's own culture. Because of this boredom, such individuals do not seek to understand their own viewpoint or explore their own culture. Stereotyping can occur in the incubator of ethnocentrism if individuals begin to ascribe similar attributes to all members of a group. For example, to suggest that all members of the Hispanic culture believe in *fatalismo* is at best simplistic and at worst stereotyping. Do all members of this hugely diverse group express a belief in *fatalismo*? How much variation is there among members of the group who do ascribe to this belief? Do members of other cultures ascribe to this belief, and are these beliefs manifested in a way similar to those in Hispanics?

Human beings have much in common as well as much that differs between cultures. In addition, individuals within a culture have many differences from each other. Stereotyping can obscure both of these facts. A superficial effort to draw on elements of another culture in an educational situation may only exacerbate a tendency to stereotype (Rios, McDaniel, & Stowell, 1998). Rios and colleagues recommend taking a cultural plunge into another culture with concurrent efforts at self-awareness regarding both one's own culture and one's response to the host culture.

D. C. Locke (1986, 1992) offers the following set of questions as a guide in a first step at developing cultural self-awareness:

- What is my cultural heritage? What was the culture of my parents and grandparents? With what cultural group do I identify?
- What is the cultural relevance of my name?
- What values, beliefs, opinions, and attitudes do I hold that are consistent with the dominant culture? Which are inconsistent? How did I learn these?
- How did I decide to be a [health] educator? What cultural standards were involved in the process? What do I understand to be the relationship between culture and [health] education?
- What unique abilities, aspirations, expectations, and limitations do I have that might influence my relations with culturally diverse individuals?

Rios and colleagues (1998) argue that the development of a culturally competent educator begins from hostility or denial; progressing through awareness, integration, acceptance, respect, and valuing; and finally arriving at commitment to social justice. Borkan and Neher (1991) describe a seven-stage developmental progression:

1. Fear or mistrust
2. Denial of cultural differences
3. Feelings of superiority over other cultures
4. Minimization of cultural differences
5. Cultural acceptance and respect
6. Empathy
7. Multiculturalism

This growth process requires active motivation to explore personal reactions and can be aided by writing field notes and journal entries during cross-cultural encounters. In addition, learning another language provides an invaluable opportunity for cultural insight.

Beginning to describe one's own culture can be a start to liberation from ethnocentrism. For a practitioner in the United States, the list by R. M. Williams (1970) of themes of U.S. Anglo-Saxon culture may be of interest. Williams identifies the following themes:

- Achievement and success: rags-to-riches stories
- Activity and work: busy people who stress work as a worthy end in itself
- Humanitarian mores: sympathy for the underdog, offering spontaneous help
- Moral orientation: situations judged in terms of right or wrong
- Efficiency and practicality: getting things done
- Progress: things will get better
- Material comfort: the good life
- Equality
- Freedom
- External conformity: of dress, housing, recreation, and manners
- Science and secular rationality
- Nationalism, patriotism, and democracy
- Individual personality
- Racism and related group superiority

Exploring Another Culture. Only the person who becomes more aware of his or her ethnocentric lens can effectively explore another culture. D. C. Locke (1992) suggests scrutinizing the following ten cultural elements to begin exploring another culture:

- Degree of acculturation
- Poverty
- History of oppression
- Language and the arts
- Racism and prejudice
- Sociopolitical factors
- Child-rearing practices
- Religious practices
- Family structure
- Values and attitudes

Triandis (1994) presents a different structure for looking at cultures. He describes the cultural syndromes of individualism versus collectivism, complexity versus simplicity, and tightness versus looseness. In an individualist culture such as that of the United States, the wishes of the individual have a very high priority, whereas in a collectivist culture, the group and its needs are paramount. In a tight culture, there is considerable agreement about norms of correct behavior. Understanding elements of these syndromes may be very helpful for health educators. Characteristics of individualism and collectivism have some specific implications. For example, the role of the group may influence the content of health education messages. If the focus in a culture is doing what the group wants, the message may be directed differently than it would be in a culture in which the emphasis is on the individual. The strong influence of norms and role-relevant goals in collectivist cultures makes for greater interdependence and embeddedness of social behavior. It may be much more difficult for someone of a collectivist culture to participate in health behavior that differs from the group's.

Work-Group Membership

All health promotion program development and evaluation should be based on broad participation of community members, perhaps through development of a work group (Hunt, Lederman, Potter, Stoddard, & Sorensen, 2000; B. A. Israel et al., 2003; Krieger et al., 2002; Minkler, Thompson, Bell, Rose, & Redman, 2002; Sullivan et al., 2003; Yoo et al., 2004). A work group might best be composed of stakeholders who have an interest in the health problem, the program, or its outcome. Community participants can be unaffiliated residents, community organizations, staff members who work with community members, and managers or leaders from community organizations (Krieger et al., 2002). In a discussion of environmental health promotion, Kreuter, De Rosa, Howze and Baldwin (2004) describes community participation as particularly important for "wicked problems . . . wherein stakeholders may have conflicting interpretations of the problem and the science behind it, as well as different values, goals and life experiences. Accordingly, policy makers, public health professionals, and other stakeholders who grapple with these problems cannot expect to effectively resolve them by relying solely on expert driven approaches to problem solving" (p. 441).

Another way of looking at work-group participation is as a linkage system (Orlandi, 1986, 1987; Orlandi, Landers, Weston, & Haley, 1990). In the development of programs, there may be a resource system (developers), an intermediate user system (implementers), and an end-user system (participants or intervention groups). For successful development and implementation, a planner must develop a linkage among these three systems. The development of this linkage system should begin as early in the project development as possible, optimally in project-funding development and needs assessment. Stakeholders in the linkage system may come from government organizations, health care systems, professional organizations, third-party payers, media, voluntary health agencies, academic institutions, organizations that represent the at-risk group, community-based organizations, and others. The linkages can be defined on a continuum. At one end is minimum involvement with the health educator accessing the community and the implementers for information or consultation; at the other is a full partnership model in which the community members are the planners, and the planning becomes a part of the intervention, as in a community empowerment model (E. B. Fisher, Auslander, Sussman, Owens, & Jackson-Thompson, 1992; E. B. Fisher et al., 1994; Hugentobler, Israel, & Schurman, 1992).

Principles of collaboration include the following (Krieger et al., 2002; L. W. Green & Kreuter, 2005):

- Community involvement from the beginning of the project
- Equally shared influence on the direction and activities of the project
- Community participation in objective selection, implementation, and evaluation
- Respect of the values, perspectives, contributions, and confidentiality of everyone in the community
- Time and resources devoted to group function
- Compensation for community participants
- Concern with sustainability of projects, including long-term community benefit and development of community capacity

Members of the group with the health risk or problem are an important group of stakeholders. The philosophy of health education is built on the principle of self-determination, an individual's governance of his or her own behavior (Allegrante & Sleet, 2004). Health education has a history of community participation in program development including acknowledgment that people have both the right and the responsibility to participate in planning for their own health (World Health Organization, 1978). Participation increases the probability that health improvement goals will be achieved, that listening to people and freely sharing information will improve their participation and consensus, and that feedback on the progress of programs they have planned increases trust in the process (L. W. Green, 1986; L. W. Green & Kreuter, 2005; Hunt, Lederman, Potter, Stoddard, & Sorensen, 2000; M. W. Kreuter, Lezin, Kreuter, & Green, 1997; Macaulay, et al., 1999). Many examples exist of community members participating in all aspects of planning, from documenting needs (Wang & Burris, 1994) to developing program materials (Rudd & Comings, 1994) and implementing programs (Eng & Young, 1992; Ovrebo, Ryan, Jackson, & Hutchinson, 1994).

Membership in the linkage system may need to be reassessed and enhanced at various times in the program development process. (We discuss this further in Chapters Seven through Nine.) Whatever the level of participation, the health promoter cannot be sure at any given moment that the resource system fully represents the end users. Health promoters should make continual efforts to represent the community. Even when health planners work in a mode of collaborative community participation that is as pure as possible, they should never assume that they understand the community; understanding is a process. Therefore, health planners must keep asking whether they know whom the intervention is meant to affect, and they must continue to build relationships based on listening and sharing in order to move to ever-higher levels of understanding. They must also be sure that they access various members of communities, not simply those who have been recruited to be part of the resource team; health planners must be sure that they are not working only with information that is filtered by members of the planning group.

In addition to at-risk population partnerships, health educators must build linkages with the intermediate users or program implementers. Even though the intermediate users are not usually the focus of the needs assessment, they may be one important source of information about both the problem and the community. These key informants may have very different perspectives on a problem than do the potential program recipients (Rossi, Lipsey, & Freeman, 2004). For example, in planning health services for the homeless, physicians, workers at homeless shelters, and members of the city council may all be important key informants;

but they are likely to have different viewpoints. That key informants or potential program implementers are not the focus of the needs assessment may seem self-evident. However, the person who works with a health problem, rather than the individuals who have the health problem, may be the first contact for the health educator—the physician or nurse for a chronic disease, the emergency medical service for injuries, the HIV counselor for AIDS. The perspective of this care provider or expert can overwhelm the assessment picture if the health planner does not take care to maintain balance between the views of the provider and the clients. We discuss the concept of implementers or intermediate users in more detail in Chapter Nine, which covers adoption and implementation.

Work-Group Management

Once a work group is put together, it must be managed for project productivity. Group management is an important skill, for which planners will need to pursue resources in addition to this book, including training to learn and practice group skills. To get started, the group will need to define members' responsibilities, choose a basic structure, and decide how the group will make decisions (Centers for Disease Control & Oak Ridge Institute for Science and Education, 2003). Groups may work as a whole or break into a variety of working and advisory groups. Early tasks will be working with the group members to define structure, organize and agree to tasks, and propose a timeline.

Having stakeholders work together is a good way to bring a variety of perspectives and a great deal of knowledge to creating a health promotion program. It also allows stakeholders to nurture feelings of ownership of the program. Another major reason to create a multiperspective work group is the group's contribution to developing culturally competent programs. The intended recipients and implementers of a program are best able to interpret the needs and perspectives of various cultural groups. As we further discuss in Chapter Eight, the respectful give-and-take of ideas is a major contributor to cultural competence.

However, working in a group to create an effective program requires good group management by the leader of the group as well as by each individual member. According to Johnson and Johnson (2003), effective groups are characterized by communication that is active and two-way, as well as distributed among group members rather than to and from group members and the leader. Leadership and responsibility for group function is also distributed, including group generation of goals and agendas. Furthermore, goals should be fluid and reflect both individual and group needs. Group cohesion is advanced through high levels of problem-solving competence, inclusion, affection, acceptance, support, and trust.

D. W. Johnson and F. P. Johnson (2003) also argue that avenues to power and methods of decision making are other important aspects of a group. Effective groups are likely to have power and influence that are equalized and shared as well as being based on ability and information (rather than, for example, position). In addition, decision-making procedures should be predominantly consensus and should match the various situations the work group encounters.

Every group, whether the members recognize the need or not, has three types of functions (Bradford, 1976):

- Project tasks
- Group maintenance
- Team building

Project tasks are whatever must be accomplished to do the group's work. However, unless the relationships among group members, feelings of inclusivity, group norms, predictability of procedures, and issues of participation and trust are addressed through group maintenance and team building, the work of the group may suffer.

We now address some group management processes in each of these three categories with the recognition that activities in the categories occur simultaneously (Bradford, 1976). For example, good process for accomplishing tasks goes a long way to developing group cohesion and trust. Table 5.1 describes processes that can be practiced to develop a work group that matures to a team capable of producing a better program than any one team member could create alone. The set of individual communication behaviors in the table is from D. W. Johnson and F. P. Johnson (2003), whereas the group management behaviors are from Bradford (1976), Sampson and Marthas (1990), and Toseland and Rivas (2005).

The list in Table 5.1 does not include processes for diagnosing and dealing with group problems, and we encourage the reader to delve more deeply into and pursue in-depth training in group management to attain these skills. The motivation for practicing these skills must include the beliefs that individual group members bring unique types of intelligence, perspective, information, and skill to a program development situation and that the application of these diverse contributions strengthens the program. Group management is built on listening to others' ideas with a willingness to review and make transparent for group review one's own assumptions about the health problem and its solutions (Senge, Kleiner, Roberts, Ross, & Smith, 1994). With this as a starting place, processes in Table 5.1 can lead to a productive work group.

TABLE 5.1. GROUP MANAGEMENT.

Process	Description
Communications	
"Owns" statement	Using first-person singular pronouns (*I* or *me*)
Completeness and specificity	Clearly stating all necessary information, including frame of reference, intention in communicating, and assumptions
Congruence	Making verbal and nonverbal communication congruent
Redundance	Using more than one channel of communication (written, oral, graphic) to clarify meaning
Requesting feedback	Asking for information about how a communication is being understood
Frame of reference	Making the communication appropriate to the receiver's frame of reference
Expressing feelings	Describing feelings by name, action, or figure of speech
Describing behavior	Describing other's behavior without evaluating or interpreting
Task Functions	
Developing the agenda	Listing, setting priorities, and time budgeting are usually most effective if set as a group process.
Initiating	Beginning a discussion includes both substantive offerings (such as the background of an issue) and methodological offerings (such as a suggestion to begin by brainstorming).
Information seeking and information giving	The goal is to elicit pertinent information from members by asking for information, keeping issues from closing prematurely, encouraging members to speak, and creating an environment where neither people nor ideas are rejected.
Opinion giving	Allowing opinions to be freely given and valued by the group as coming from the members' experience is important. Groups should sort out opinion from fact or information.
Elaboration	Asking for elaboration on a partially stated idea to promote hearing and use of members' contributions
Coordinating	Joining together two or more ideas (that might seem disparate at first) brought up by different members
Partializing	Pointing out the fine differences in two ideas that might seem the same at first glance
Evaluating	Evaluating what needs to be done so that ideas—not individuals—are evaluated. Sometimes discussion should be structured so that ideas are first listed without evaluation (brainstorming).
Structuring	Deciding and facilitating the ways in which a group can work, such as using subgroups or completing some assignments outside of the group

TABLE 5.1. GROUP MANAGEMENT, Cont'd.

Process	Description
Energizing	Moving a group through a "stuck" point by a revision in structuring, humor, a novel idea, the expression of feeling, a short break, or feedback
Summarizing	Summing up the points, progress, and needs of the group should be done orally in the meeting and in meeting notes, summaries, and action items after the meeting. (Note: meeting "minutes" for work groups should usually be written as summaries that include brief discussion items, points of consensus, points of disagreement, and action items. They usually should not be written as word-for-word presentations of meeting content.)
Synthesizing	Making connections between meanings expressed in the group

Maintenance and Team-Building Functions

Gatekeeping	Keeping the door open for the less talkative members of the group
Encouraging	Encouraging members to participate in the group
Harmonizing Consensus seeking	Seeking common goals or common ground in a conflict
Giving and receiving feedback	Feedback should be shared with the whole group by giving a direct, specific, descriptive, immediate description of the impact of group or individual communication.
Standard setting	Setting and revisiting group norms around efficiency, fairness, and open communication
Processing	Setting aside the final minutes of a meeting for reviewing how the work progressed and how it can be improved

---

Box 5.1. Mayor's Project

Looking in on the health educator from Chapter One, we see her meeting with her boss, the department head. The two are struggling with how to get the planning group started. The health educator is worried that, although the mayor handpicked the planning group, it is not representative enough of the neighborhoods in which the group wants to focus its violence project. The planning group may not include all of the project's stakeholders. The health educator wants permission to add interested community members to the planning group during the needs assessment.

Health educator: Adding more community people will be good for the group, good for planning, and politically good for the mayor.

Department head: Yes, but too large a committee is too hard to handle.

Health educator: These will be the people who understand the problem first-hand. But they are also the people who will ensure the implementation of whatever program we come up with. Besides, people who don't feel included can sabotage our efforts.

Department head: OK, I'll get the mayor's approval, but I trust you to really manage this group. Better review your group skills books. Make sure your group leadership is not rusty. I don't have to tell you how anxious the mayor is to see something happening. I know, I know! You say we have to do a needs assessment. I'm convinced, but is that going to give us the visibility we need? Can we just think of how to do this in such a way that it is clear to everyone that we are doing something?

Health educator: Yes, I've been thinking about this. We need both qualitative and quantitative evidence about this problem. We also need information from our own community as well as from studies conducted elsewhere. We need information about violence and its context, but we also need a real feel for the strengths of these communities.

What if we could make the complexity work for us in two ways? Let's break the group into teams. Some people will go after the scientific literature. We have some talented library researchers on the team. Another group will get out into the community and talk to people. That will keep us visible. It also will help us balance our examination of needs and strengths. We'll structure short reports based on our needs-assessment model and present them to the mayor as we go along.

Department head: That sounds good. Now that we have that settled, let's get started.

Planning the Needs Assessment

Before delving into assessment, the planner and the work group will need to plan how to assess the health problem or need (Witkin & Altschuld, 1995). One of the first tasks will be for the work group to figure out what it already knows about the problem and the community and what further information the work group needs. To help us guide the assessment, we use a modified PRECEDE model. A population-based epidemiologic planning framework that is also ecological in its perspective, the model directs planners to determine health problem characteristics such as morbidity, mortality, disease risk, and burden of disease in various population groups (L. W. Green et al., 1994; L. W. Green & Kreuter, 2005). The model prescribes an analysis of causation of health problems at multiple levels and the consideration of multiple determinants of health-related behavior and environment. For example, health problems such as coronary artery disease have both behavioral risk factors, such as eating high-cholesterol foods, and environmental causes, such as the unavailability of exercise facilities. The several editions of the PRECEDE model clarified and amplified the important role of both social and physical environment in the causation of health problems (L. W. Green & Kreuter, 1991, 1999, 2005). It has been used as the basis for health education planning in hundreds of programs (cf., Bartholomew, Koenning, Dahlquist, & Barron, 1994; Bartholomew, Seilheimer, Parcel, Spinelli, & Pumariega, 1989; Chiang, Huang, & Lu, 2003; Farley, Otis, & Benoit, 1997; Gielen, McDonald, Wilson, Hwang, Serwint, Andrews, et al., 2002; Goodson, Gottlieb, & Smith, 1999; Green & Frankish, 1994; Maiburg, Hiddink, van't Hof, Rethans, & van Ree, 1999; Mann, 1994; Mann, Lindsay, Putnam, & Davis, 1996; Mercer et al., 2003; Paluck, Green, Frankish, Fielding, & Haverkamp, 2003; S. M. Taylor, Elliott, & Riley, 1998; S. M. Taylor, Elliott, Robinson, & Taylor, 1998; Welk, 1999; Williams, Innis, Vogel, & Stephen, 1999). When developed in the 1970s, the PRECEDE model was not intended to guide the health education field through all of the steps of intervention but to lead the field to a more outcome-based approach to planning (L. W. Green, personal communication, February 26, 1997).

The logic model we use (Figure 5.1) is derived from the PRECEDE model (Green & Kreuter, 2005). Planners develop the model from right to left, usually beginning with descriptions of quality-of-life and health problems. (When completed the model is read from left to right as a causal model of the health and quality of life problems.) Lessening these problems should be the intention of a health education or promotion intervention. For example, if premature mortality and morbidity from cardiovascular disease are the health problem, loss of productive years and the burden of heart disease begin to define the quality-of-life issues for society and the individual. Next, the planner must support these relationships with data and begin to find evidence of behavioral and environmental causes.

Next, moving to the left in the model, the behavioral analysis typically includes what the at-risk individuals do that increases their risk of experiencing the health problem. In the case of secondary and tertiary prevention, the analysis investigates what individuals do that increases the risk of disability or death from a health problem they already have.

The environmental analysis includes conditions in the social and physical environments that influence the health problem directly or through its behavioral

FIGURE 5.1. LOGIC MODEL FOR NEEDS ASSESSMENT.

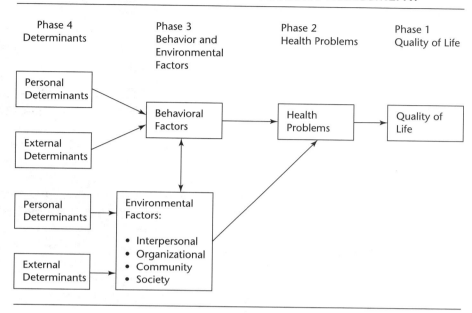

causes. In most analyses of health problems, the environment plays a significant and modifiable role in causing the problem either directly, such as air pollution in lung disease, or indirectly through behavior, such as availability of condoms and the social norms to use them in safer sex.

We modified a diagram by Richard and colleagues (1996) in Chapter One (Figure 1.1) to depict individuals embedded in multiple, interacting levels of environment. When this concept is transferred to the needs assessment, it is apparent that each of the levels of environment (interpersonal, organizational, community, and societal) can influence both individual behavior and any lower level of environment. In an example of teen alcohol use, peers' reinforcement of teenagers' alcohol use would be in the interpersonal level of the environment; lack of policy concerning alcohol use at high school parties would be in the organizational level; social norms for teen drinking, in the community level; and laws restricting sales to and possession by minors, in the societal level.

Many environmental factors are determinants of the behavior of the at-risk group. These determinants are external to the individual. For example, reinforcing and enabling factors, which are included in educational and ecological assessment in the PRECEDE model as determinants of behavior can also be viewed as environmental factors. Enabling factors are described in the PRECEDE model as characteristics of the environment that either facilitate or hinder health-promoting behavior. Reinforcement, events that occur after a behavior that make the behavior more or less likely to reoccur, is also very important to behavior change. This category may include punishment, an event that occurs after an action that makes the reoccurrence less probable.

The next phase of the logic model is an analysis of the personal determinants of behavior and environmental factors. Because the evidence for these determinants is usually correlational rather than causal, these determinants are somewhat hypothetical. Personal determinants reside at the individual level. They include L. W. Green and Kreuter's (2005, p. 14) predisposing factors, "a person or population's knowledge, attitudes, beliefs, values, and perceptions that facilitate or hinder motivation for change," with the addition of existing skills.

The original PRECEDE model had a separate depiction of nonbehavioral factors such as the natural history of disease (L. W. Green, Kreuter, Deeds, & Partridge, 1980). These were nonmodifiable factors that nevertheless should be considered in needs assessment because they may influence factors that are themselves modifiable. In the current PRECEDE model, genetics is in the model as a factor that is not yet modifiable but may be quite important in understanding the health problem and various affected groups (L. W. Green & Kreuter, 2005).

Where to Enter the Needs-Assessment Model

A consideration in completing the needs assessment is where to begin: with the quality of life in the community? With health problems or risks? With behavioral or environmental risks? Health promotion planners are sometimes unable to enter the model through assessment of quality of life issues because agencies that employ the planners are funded, at least in part, with categorical funds designated for one disease or risk (for example, cardiovascular disease or lung disease). We often are directed to look at needs and problems in terms of the funding or employer's specific focus. The health educator who works for a cancer agency focuses on cancer. The health educator who works for an AIDS agency focuses on HIV. These are health problems, and health educators have entered the assessment model at the level of health. Perhaps, though, the health educator works for the American Cancer Society or the American Lung Association on a tobacco project. The health educator in these instances has entered the assessment model at the level of behavior. It is perfectly legitimate to begin in the middle of the assessment model with a behavioral or environmental risk so long as there is strong epidemiologic evidence for the causal relation between the risk and one or more health problems.

Some planners will be entering the needs assessment with wide parameters for the issues on which they are empowered to work, even as wide as license to work with the community as a whole to designate health and quality-of-life needs and choose issues on which to work. These planners will begin by assessing quality-of-life indicators or by working with the community to determine priority health issues. Many other planners will have an assigned task that is related to a specific health problem, health-risk behavior, or environmental problem. No matter where a health educator begins the needs assessment, he or she will need to cover all the model's phases, including the relation of health to quality of life. The emphasis on covering all levels of the model regardless of where health educators begin is based on the assumption that health and behavior are instrumental values, that they are valuable because of their relation to other values. Health is related to quality of life; behavior and environment are related to health.

Beginning with Quality of Life. Some planners work with a community to conduct a broad assessment beginning with quality of life and moving through health, behavior, environment, and determinants. Once quality-of-life issues are described for a community, health educators move to health and describe health problems related to the quality-of-life issues they have documented. Because they will have uncovered a wide range of quality-of-life issues, they will have a long list of health problems to prioritize. Once they choose the health problem or problems that will be the focus of their work, they can also narrow down the quality-of-life factors that are specifically tied to the health problem or problems that are priorities. Then they can move to the left (see Figure 5.1) and analyze behavior, environment, and determinants that are all related to the same health problem.

For example, a health educator is working with a group of homeless and precariously housed teens. She conducts a survey with youth who congregate at certain hangouts in a neighborhood of about ten square blocks in a large inner city area. The health educator conducts individual interviews and observations; and she relies on agency, city, and state data for her quantitative data set. She finds that the quality-of-life issues for these youth include lack of family and other social support, alienation, lack of role models and life goals, fear of HIV/AIDS, depression and hopelessness, fear of violence and aggression, and victimization. In terms of health, they have a high prevalence of unwanted pregnancy, sexually transmitted infections (STIs), and HIV. She also finds drug addiction, malnutrition, and disordered sleep. Based on the prevalence estimates in the literature and the youth's priorities, she narrows the health problem that she will work on to violence and victimization. Then she works to the right in the PRECEDE model through quality of life, this time as it relates only to violence, and to the left to behavior and determinants, again as they predict violent acts and the probability of becoming a victim.

Beginning with a Health Problem. If health educators begin with a specific health problem, they then move to the right in the needs assessment to include an analysis of the impact of the health problem on the quality of life in the at-risk population before moving on to study the behavioral, environmental, and determinant factors that contribute to the health problem. Let's suppose that the health educator from our previous example is working with the same population. This time, however, she is working for an AIDS agency. Her supervisor convenes a meeting during the first week to clarify her job description. The supervisor says that the health educator should work not only on HIV prevention among homeless youth but also focus on the risk factor of multiple sexual partners. As the health educator begins her needs assessment, she is confused; she thinks that the HIV-prevention focus suggests that she is beginning on the health level, but she heard her supervisor mandate an emphasis on a certain risk behavior, sexual intercourse with multiple partners. She wonders if she is beginning with behavior. After thinking for a while, she enters the model with data on the health problem. She reasons that if she starts with health, then she frees herself to consider risk factors other than multiple sexual partners.

The health educator begins her assessment with HIV transmission and AIDS in the population of youth between the ages of eleven and twenty-one years who are living on inner-city streets. She uses data from the Centers for Disease Control (CDC) to find the U.S. prevalence rates of HIV in this age group. She then looks at local figures for HIV incidence and prevalence that she obtained from the city health department and at figures from other cities with comparable groups of street youth. Once she has a picture of HIV transmission as a problem in this group, she works forward to the implications of HIV for quality of life and backward to behavior, environment, and determinants. When she analyzes behavior, she finds that having multiple sexual partners is one factor but that other important factors are condom use and needle sharing. When the health educator reports her needs-assessment data to her supervisor, she is able to present all the risk behaviors and gain support to work on them. She is not limited by her supervisor's original bias.

Beginning with Environmental or Behavioral Risk. Another option is to begin with specific behavioral risk factors, such as unsafe sexual behavior, or an environmental condition, such as polluted drinking water, and move to the right in the model to include the impact of these factors on health and quality-of-life indicators for the population. The health educator will look at determinants of the risk behavior or environmental condition. In our example of the person working with street youth, where might the health worker begin the needs assessment if she were working for an agency concerned with the risky behaviors of early sexual intercourse, intercourse with multiple partners, and intercourse without the protection of a condom? The educator would probably go to the literature to establish estimates of these behaviors in similar populations. She might also use survey techniques to establish estimates of these behaviors in her population and qualitative methods, such as ethnographic interviews and focus groups, to understand the context and meaning of the behaviors to the youth. She then would move to establishing the relation of these behaviors to health problems and quality of life and, finally, to determinants of the behaviors.

Conducting the Needs Assessment

➲ *Conduct the needs assessment using the PRECEDE model (Green & Kreuter, 2005) to analyze health and quality of life problems and their causes and to determine priorities.*

Describing the Population at Risk and Environmental Context

The designation *population at risk* refers to a group with a definable boundary and shared characteristics that have or are at risk for certain health and quality-of-life problems or that have health problems and are at risk for the sequelae. To lay the foundation for intervention, planners should also be concerned with the environmental context of the at-risk group. The environment may contribute directly to the health problem, as in the case of drinking contaminated water causing diarrhea. Or it can be a more indirect influence, such as the contribution of social networks to the continuation of smoking. We suggest four levels of analysis of the environmental context:

- Interpersonal
- Organizational
- Community
- Societal

These levels are similar to the ones proposed by Richard and colleagues (1996). We have added the interpersonal level in order to facilitate thinking about intervention, and we have incorporated the supranational level into our societal level for the same reason.

Organizations are "systems with a formal multi-echelon decision process operating in pursuit of specific objectives. Schools, stores, companies, and professional associations are a few examples" (Richard et al., 1996, p. 320). Communities in

Richard's description require a geographical area comprising persons and organizations. Locus is the most commonly cited characteristic of community (MacQueen et al., 2001; Mattessich & Monsey, 1997). A geographic community is more than a physical space. It is a social place shared by individuals in units such as families, neighborhoods, and clubs and by organizations such as civic groups, churches, local media, and local government (J. McKnight, 1995). Groups within a geographic boundary, such as a city, village, or town, usually share a sense of living or working in a location as well as some common elements of values, culture, norms, language, and problems of health and quality of life (Institute of Medicine, 2002b). Members of these geographic communities will have perceptions of boundaries, appropriate representatives, and concerns or problems (Sullivan et al., 2003).

However, we include in communities other groups that exhibit relationships and experience a sense of community among the members of a group whose members may or may not share physical boundaries (Chavis & Wandersman, 1990; Fellin, 1995; Kraft, Beeker, Stokes, & Peterson, 2000; McMillan & Chavis, 1986). In addition to geopolitical boundaries, there are demographic boundaries (for example, socioeconomic status, gender, age, and family structure) and demographic-ethnic boundaries (for example, Latino, European American, African American, and Dutch of Surinamese origin). There are also groups with shared characteristics, such as persons with a certain disease or those served by the same agency. For example, a double minority (defined by race and by sexual orientation) participant in the study by Kraft and colleagues (2000) described community as about being with people you identify with and feel similar to because they have the same values, beliefs, and habits. A community may also be a group coming together for a cause or political agenda (Eng & Parker, 1994). Also, more recently, people with shared characteristics link together in Internet communities without regard to geographic proximity (Hospers, Harterink, van den Hoek, & Veenstra, 2002; Hospers, Kok, Harterink, & de Zwart, 2005; Ross, Tikkanen, & Mansson, 2000). Societies are larger systems that possess means to control several aspects of the lives and development of their constituent systems. They also are more self-contained than are communities. Examples of societies are provinces, states, and countries (Richard et al., 1996). We also include in this environmental level multinational organizations such as the European Union.

Often, in an assessment of a health problem, the relatedness in a population at risk may be that all the members have a risk factor or health problem in common, for example, cystic fibrosis, cardiovascular disease, or AIDS. Sometimes these individuals come together in organizations for mutual support—the Multiple Sclerosis Society, Mothers Against Drunk Driving, and so on. Of course, the population may be defined by a combination of variables, such as adults with cystic fibrosis who are English speaking and living in North America or as adolescents age thirteen to sixteen who live in the inner city and are at risk for HIV and other STIs. The important issue is that the populations are well defined during the assessment process (Gilmore & Campbell, 1996; Gilmore, Campbell, & Becker, 1989; Soriano, 1995; Witkin & Altschuld, 1995).

The broad scope of the environmental context of health problems suggests not only complex causation of health and illness but also the need for health education and promotion intervention on a variety of levels and at a variety of venues (for example, work sites, schools, communities, and health care organizations). However, we do not believe that these different types of communities and program sites need a substantively different type of planning process. They do need a systematic planning process that allows for the incorporation of their unique qualities.

An important task in performing a needs assessment is to describe the individuals who are the potential recipients of the health promotion intervention. There may be several groups in a comprehensive multilevel program, and the recipients of program benefits may not necessarily be the population at risk. They could be environmental agents, such as the health care provider in a case of chronic disease management, or organizations and government in a case of primary prevention policy. An intervention often targets multiple groups, some of whom are populations at risk and others that influence the environment. The at-risk population always is the intended recipient of program benefits such as risk reduction or improvements in health status or quality of life. The need to define an intervention group means a programmatic need for an epidemiologically and demographically defined population in order to plan effective programs and to measure their effects on health and quality of life. Precisely defining the various groups who will benefit from the program enables the planner to know both the numerator, the people who actually participate in the program, and the denominator, the population for whom the program is intended (Glasgow, Vogt, & Boles, 1999).

Health Problems and Quality of Life

A population at risk is a group of people who have a significant probability of developing a health problem or of experiencing morbidity or death from a health problem they already have (Rossi et al., 2004). For example, overweight individuals who do not already have diabetes can be part of a population at risk for diabetes. Preventing diabetes in this group would be a primary prevention objective. Among those with diabetes, secondary and tertiary prevention objectives are possible: preventing morbidity and mortality from the conditions.

Most health educators begin a needs assessment with some idea of both a health risk or problem and the population groups that have it. They use concepts from epidemiology, the study of the occurrence and distribution of diseases and their risk factors in populations, to further define both the nature of the health problem and the population that is the focus of the needs assessment in a somewhat interactive process. The basic questions for this process are the following:

- What is the problem?
- Who has it?
- What are the incidence, prevalence, and distribution of the problem?
- What are the demographic characteristics of the population that faces the problem or is at risk for the problem?
- Is there a community? What are its characteristics, including its resources and strengths?
- What segments of the population have an excess burden from the health problem?
- Where can the groups at risk, especially groups at excess risk or excess burden, be reached by a program?

Not only does the health educator need to understand the health problem, but he or she must also understand how it is exhibited in the particular population of interest and what the health problem or risk means to those who have it. In the process of needs assessment, the health educator will constantly be working to develop understanding of the groups for whom the program should be a priority. Dimensions of health problems include disability, discomfort, fertility, fitness, morbidity, mortality, and physiological risk factors (L. W. Green & Kreuter, 2005). To discover dimensions of the health problem, mostly quantitative data sources are used; whereas to understand the problem's meaning and its quality-of-life effects, qualitative methods may be the most revealing. Dimensions of quality of life include effects of illness on both individual and societal indicators such as cost of health care, absenteeism, work or school performance, activities of daily living, isolation and alienation, discrimination, happiness and adjustment, self-esteem and employment (to name a few).

The first step is to describe demographically who has the health problem and for whom it represents an excess burden. However, the health educator will also need to fully explore the cultural group or groups represented in the priority population beyond a simple description by race or ethnicity (Kreuter, Lukwago, Bucholtz, Clark, & Sanders-Thompson, 2003).

Rates and Risk. A number of risk concepts and statistics are helpful in the process of describing the health problem. The discussion here is a very brief introduction to thinking about the health problem with rates and ratios, and we refer the reader to texts in epidemiology (Friis & Sellers, 2004; K. J. Rothman, 2002; Rothman & Greenland, 1998). The extent of the health problem is usually described as a rate so that comparisons among groups and geographic areas and judgments of the importance or seriousness of the problem can be made. A rate is the number of events (people with a problem) over a period of time per population of one thousand or one hundred thousand. A rate can be incidence, the new cases of a problem in a certain time period, or prevalence, the number of existing cases. Usually, both types of rates are needed to fully understand a problem. The number of new cases divided by the number of persons at risk per unit time is the crude incidence rate (Kelsey, Whittemore, Evans, & Thompson, 1996).

The importance of rates is that they can be compared across group characteristics and geographic areas to answer questions such as this: Is this an important problem in a specific community? Is it more or less prevalent in this community than in other communities? Is it more prevalent than in communities that are demographically similar? Many factors influence rates of a problem. In order to sort out the true extent of a problem in a population, rates may need to be adjusted by demographic variables such as age and gender. Rates are often reported as age-specific and can be weighted to match the age distribution in the population of interest (Kelsey et al., 1996).

Another important concept is that of the probability or risk of developing a disease over time. The term *risk* is often used to refer to the average risk for a group of people. Because it is a probability, risk is sensitive to the period of time over which observations are made. For example, the risk of developing lung cancer for a smoker increases as the period of observation lengthens.

An Asthma Example. Two of this book's authors began working on the needs assessment for asthma in the Houston metropolitan area, entering the PRECEDE model with the health problem of asthma in children and then exploring the quality-of-life issues surrounding asthma. (See Figure 5.2.) We entered a partnership with the Houston Independent School District because the district administration was concerned that children of elementary school age had high rates of asthma and symptoms that interfered with schoolwork and attendance. We asked: What is the prevalence of asthma in the United States and in our local community? Does the prevalence vary between children of various ages and race ethnicity groups? We also wanted to know whether any groups had an excess burden from the disease. First, we reviewed the literature and found that asthma is an important public health problem in the United States, affecting 20.3 million people (Mannino, Homa, Akinbami, Moorman, Gwynn, & Redd, 2002). The highest prevalence is among African Americans (8.3 percent) followed by whites (7.5 percent) and Hispanics (5.8 percent). Other subgroups with high prevalence rates are children (age zero to seventeen years) with a prevalence of 8.7 percent.

Next, we wanted to know how the children in the Houston Independent School District (urban and primarily low income and ethnic minority) compared to other children in the United States in terms of their risk of morbidity from asthma. Was asthma more or less of a problem in Houston as compared to the rest of the United States? We surveyed 21,835 children of elementary school age and the parents of 10,454 children who reported symptoms (Sockrider et al., 2005; Tortolero, Bartholomew, et al., 2005). The overall prevalence of a parent response suggesting possible asthma was about 10 percent for the entire population. The prevalence of asthma in African American children was significantly higher than in the other groups. Parents reported that 1,788 children had a current diagnosis, and only 6 percent of those were found to have report of diagnosis or active medication reported to the school nurse. This prevalence of possible asthma is similar to that reported by other recent studies of urban low-income areas (for example, N. M. Clark et al., 2002; Gerald et al., 2002; Yawn, Wollan, Kurland, & Scanlon, 2002).

Next, we wanted to understand the impact of asthma on the children and their families. We asked: How does asthma affect the quality of life of children, for example, their activities of daily living such as school attendance and participation in normal activities of childhood? We also wanted to know how asthma affects parents and how asthma contributes to societal indicators such as cost of health care. We found that asthma prevalence rates do not fully illustrate the burden of asthma on individuals, families, and communities. Asthma exacerbations are the leading cause of hospitalization and emergency room visits in the United States (Mannino et al., 2002). The CDC estimates that 23.6 percent of children with asthma have activity limitations (Mannino et al., 2002). Asthma also affects a child's functional status with an average of twenty days of restricted activity and ten school absences per year (Newacheck & Halfon, 2000). Lieu and others (2002) found that 27 percent of children with asthma had missed school within a two-week period. Eleven percent of the children who missed school had missed more than three days of school during the same period. In comparison with their non-Hispanic white peers, slightly higher proportions of Latino and black children with asthma had missed more than three days of school in a two-week period. A study by Fowler, Davenport, and Garg (1992) showed that 42 percent of children with asthma missed more than six days per school year, compared to 12 percent of children without asthma. They also found that Hispanic children with asthma were more likely to suffer grade failure than were Hispanic children without asthma (23 percent vs. 16.7 percent).

Asking About the Causes of Health Problems

Risk factors are those behaviors or environmental conditions that affect the health of populations. The most commonly used measure of the association between exposure to a risk factor and development of a related health problem is relative risk

FIGURE 5.2. ASTHMA PRECEDE MODEL.

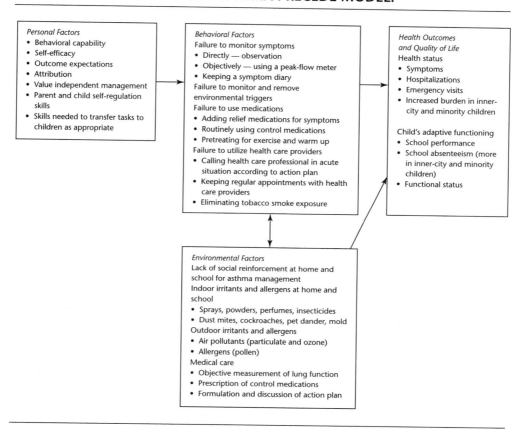

Personal Factors
- Behavioral capability
- Self-efficacy
- Outcome expectations
- Attribution
- Value independent management
- Parent and child self-regulation skills
- Skills needed to transfer tasks to children as appropriate

Behavioral Factors
Failure to monitor symptoms
- Directly — observation
- Objectively — using a peak-flow meter
- Keeping a symptom diary
Failure to monitor and remove environmental triggers
Failure to use medications
- Adding relief medications for symptoms
- Routinely using control medications
- Pretreating for exercise and warm up
Failure to utilize health care providers
- Calling health care professional in acute situation according to action plan
- Keeping regular appointments with health care providers
- Eliminating tobacco smoke exposure

Health Outcomes and Quality of Life
Health status
- Symptoms
- Hospitalizations
- Emergency visits
- Increased burden in inner-city and minority children

Child's adaptive functioning
- School performance
- School absenteeism (more in inner-city and minority children)
- Functional status

Environmental Factors
Lack of social reinforcement at home and school for asthma management
Indoor irritants and allergens at home and school
- Sprays, powders, perfumes, insecticides
- Dust mites, cockroaches, pet dander, mold
Outdoor irritants and allergens
- Air pollutants (particulate and ozone)
- Allergens (pollen)
Medical care
- Objective measurement of lung function
- Prescription of control medications
- Formulation and discussion of action plan

or rate ratio (Kelsey et al., 1996). *Relative risk* is the incidence of the problem in those exposed to the risk factor divided by the incidence of the problem in those not exposed to the risk factor. Another useful statistic is the risk ratio or comparison of probabilities of developing the disease when one is not exposed to the risk factor and when one is exposed (the probability of disease when not exposed divided by the probability of disease when exposed). The risk ratio is particularly applicable when the period of time over which a health problem might develop is fixed, such as the risk of the birth of a low-weight infant.

Another frequently used measure of association is the odds ratio, which is defined in terms of exposure rather than in terms of disease (probability of exposure in the presence of disease divided by the probability of exposure without the presence of disease over the probability of exposure with lack of disease divided by the probability of lack of exposure with lack of disease) (Kelsey et al., 1996).

Behavior of the At-Risk Group. Some behaviors of the at-risk group may be causally related to the health problem. For example, a huge body of epidemiologic evidence shows smoking to be associated with both a variety of cancers and cardiovascular disease. Furthermore, as the number of cigarettes smoked increases, the association with cancer (for example) increases. This is a dose-response relationship, and is a higher level of epidemiologic evidence. In another example, behavioral risks for HIV transmission include intravenous drug use and unprotected sexual intercourse. When the prevalence of the health problem (or death from the health problem) and the prevalence of risk factors and the relative risk of acquiring the health problem (or mortality from the health problem) are known for a population group, estimates can be made of the proportion of the health problem (or mortality) that is attributable to each risk, the attributable fraction (the risk for the exposed minus the risk for the unexposed divided by the risk for the exposed) (Kelsey et al., 1996).

Environment. Even though it may be intuitive to think in terms of the behavior of the at-risk group first, the physical and social environment should be a major focus in a needs-assessment study. For example, in a study of the social and physical environments related to nutrition and physical activity of middle school students, Bauer, Yang, and Austin (2004) found aspects of the interpersonal environment of the students (interactions with peers and teachers) that may be related to physical activity and particularly participation in gym class. They also explored the organizational environment related to the accessibility of food in the school cafeterias and snack carts. In a related example, quite a lot of research is occurring regarding the impact of the built environment and the social environment on physical activity (Brownson et al., 2004). E. A. Parker, Baldwin, Israel, and Salinas (2004, p. 492) focused on the indoor air environment in their efforts to decrease morbidity from asthma, stating that "Oftentimes, reduction or mitigation of exposure requires a change in behavior of an individual exposed or of a policy maker who can enact laws to reduce the exposure."

It may help to think of environmental factors that influence health directly through disease-causing exposures or indirectly by influencing health-related behavior. These factors can be understood further by ecologic levels as we have depicted in the PRECEDE-based logic model in Figure 5.1. Schulz and Northridge (2004) propose three levels of environmental determinants of health:

1. The fundamental or macro level, including macrosocial factors such as historical conditions and the economic order along with inequalities such as the distribution of material wealth

2. The intermediate or meso or community level, including aspects of both the built environment such as parks and the social context such as community capacity

3. The proximate or micro or interpersonal level, including characteristics such as working and housing conditions and social integration and support (Figure 5.3)

Another way of looking at environment is to examine exposure categories (Kelsey et al., 1996):

- Biologic, for example, vectors, presence of reservoirs, population density, and food sources
- Familial, for example, size, presence of diseases, age distribution, housing, nutritional environment and behavioral characteristics

FIGURE 5.3. ENVIRONMENTAL LEVELS AND THEIR IMPACT ON HEALTH.

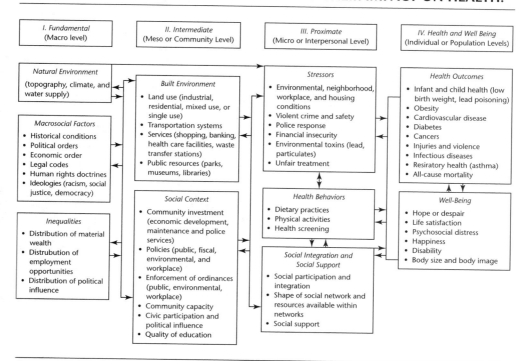

Sources: Schulz and Northridge, 2004; Schulz, Williams, Israel, and Lempert, 2002; Northridge and Sclar, 2003.

- Chemical, for example, substances in the air, water, soil, housing, and workplace
- Physical, for example, climate, radiation, sound, temperature, and the built environment
- Psychosocial, for example, stressful life events and social support systems
- Socioeconomic, for example, poverty and health care accessibility

Behavior and Environment in the Asthma Example. The planners in the asthma example (Figure 5.2) continued to review the literature to understand the behavioral and environmental factors related to asthma exacerbations and disability. In the behavioral category, lack of use of both relief medications and controller medications is a problem (Bauman, Wright, Leickly, Carin, Kurszon-Moran, Wade, et al., 2002; A. B. Becker, 2002; Burkhart, Dunbar-Jacob, Fireman, & Rohay, 2002; Wraight, Cowan, Flannery, Town, & Taylor, 2002), as is failure to monitor and protect against environmental triggers (Cabana et al., 2004; Joseph, Adams, Cottrell, Hogan, & Wilson, 2003).

However, as we moved to the analysis of environmental factors, we were intrigued to discover that families cannot use medications when they are not prescribed by their children's health care providers! Appropriate health care for asthma includes a partnership between family and provider, objective assessment of lung function for diagnosis and monitoring, prescription of relief medication, prescription of controller medication for persistent asthma, and provision of an asthma action plan with instructions for routine care and management of exacerbations (National Heart, Lung, and Blood Institute, 1997). Despite the distribution of national evidence-informed guidelines more than a decade ago, good medical care for pediatric asthma is often lacking (Diette, et al., 2001). For example, the U.S. and international guidelines recommend that all children with moderate to severe asthma use daily maintenance medications, preferably inhaled corticosteroids. Despite these recommendations, rates of inhaled anti-inflammatory medication continued to be low to moderate from both patient report and pharmacy records even for those individuals using large amounts of inhaled beta agonists (medications for symptoms and exacerbations) (R. J. Adams et al., 2001; Buchner, Carlson, & Stempel, 1997; Butz, Eggleston, Huss, Kolodner, & Rand, 2000; Eggleston et al., 1998; D. C. Goodman, Lozano, Stukel, Chang, & Hecht, 1999).

Another reason for concern is that asthma treatment differs in minority populations as compared to non-Hispanic whites, including fewer prescriptions for anti-inflammatory medication (Diette et al., 2001; Eggleston et al., 1998; Legorreta et al., 1998and less access to beta agonists and nebulizers at home (Finkelstein et al., 1995; Krishnan et al., 2001). African American and Hispanic American children of all asthma severity levels may be medically undertreated (Eggleston et al., 1998).

Again, we wanted to explore some of these factors in our local area. In the asthma project named Familias y Escuelas Junta para Controllar Asma, Families and Schools Together to Control Asthma (Familias) (Fernández, Bartholomew, Lopez, Tyrrell, Czyzewski, & Sockrider, 2000; Fernández, Bartholomew, Sockrider, Czyzewski, Abramson, Linares, et al., 2000), the planners discovered, through focus groups, observations, and interviews, that parents have some difficulty obtaining a diagnosis for their children's lung problems, an important asthma management behavior located in the environmental analysis in the needs assessment for Hispanic families. (See Chapter Fourteen.)

Determinants of Behavioral and Environmental Risks

The next part of the needs assessment is to ask questions about what factors cause or in some way modify the behavior of the risk group. Here, the planner asks why: Why do members of the at-risk group behave in ways to increase their risk of a health problem? As we described in Chapter Two, we refer to these factors as personal determinants because, from an intervention development perspective, causation is implied. We would not intervene on a variable that was not affecting the behavior of the at-risk individual. On the other hand, the reality is that we are usually just using the core processes to build a case for the strength of association of the determinants with the behavioral factors.

In an example of asking questions about determinants in a needs assessment, Partin and Slater (2003) sought to uncover key barriers to mammography use. Using a telephone survey, the most important barriers they found were the following:

- Women state that it is hard to find time to have a mammogram.
- Women disagree that mammograms give peace of mind.
- Women say that they only go to the doctor when they are sick.
- Mammography sites do not have reminder systems.
- Screening guidelines are incorrectly stated.

Note that the first three barriers are personal determinants and the last two are environmental factors that limit mammography use.

Determinants in the Asthma Example. We first asked the question: Why do parents and children often not manage asthma? When we began our asthma work, for example, there was some evidence in the literature of social cognitive theory variables as answers to the question of why. For example (Figure 5.2), many parents and children do not have the necessary asthma-specific skills, self-regulatory skills, self-efficacy, or behavioral capability (N. M. Clark, 1989; N. M. Clark,

Rosenstock, et al., 1988; Clark & Starr-Schneidkraut, 1994; Creer, 1990; Wigal et al., 1993). They also may not attribute asthma control to an internal locus (versus a powerful other, that is, a physician). In our local work with Hispanic families, we also found that they may not understand asthma as a chronic disease, may rely on home remedies and indigenous healers, and may have difficulty achieving a diagnosis of the child's problems—all factors that could lead to failure to manage asthma (Lopez, 2004).

Sources of Needs-Assessment Data

Most needs assessments require multiple data sources because they are answering multiple questions and they are often seeking various perspectives on the answers. Witkin and Altschuld (1995) suggest the following considerations for deciding on data sources:

- Consider the groups and individuals that may be respondents for the assessment. Different groups have different needs for data collection modalities.
- Usually multiple sources are needed, and they should be providing different types of information.
- Consider feasibility including cost, time, and other constraints.
- Consider the degree of interaction desired with respondents and other participants such as stakeholders and the needs-assessment team.

Data sources will primarily be chosen by the questions being asked in the assessment and the data that can be used to answer them. Sources of data to address needs assessments for health promotion include archival or secondary data and primary data collected from individuals and groups. The latter types of data can be either interactive (for example, focus groups, community forums, and nominal group process) or noninteractive (such as surveys, key informant interviews, and mailed Delphi surveys).

In doing the asthma needs assessment, the team found that the scientific literature contained considerable information about health and quality-of-life issues. Other questions, such as local impact, required data collection through surveys, observations, focus groups, and interviews.

Some environmental factors such as health care providers' actions would require a survey of providers. Determination of the factors such as assessment of city zoning policy would require simply a review of existing city regulations; and assessment of the availability of hiking and biking trails in a town could be done using a map and an observational strategy. Typically, behavioral and attitudinal data are collected by self-report using written or telephone surveys. The human and monetary resources required vary among the different methods of data collection, and this may limit the techniques used in the needs assessment. Finally, the needs assessor's philosophy of participation and empowerment through assessment will lead to the selection of methods. Freirian question-posing methods and participatory analysis, which we discussed in Chapter Four, would both provide data and change the consciousness of community members who were involved (Freire, 1973a, 1973b; Wang, 2003).

We briefly present some of the more common needs-assessment methods but also refer the reader to texts that present needs-assessment techniques in detail (Aday, 1996; Gilmore & Campbell, 1996; L. W. Green & Kreuter, 2005; Wholey, Hatry, & Newcomer, 1994; Witkin & Altschuld, 1995).

Secondary Data

Archival or secondary data are collected for a purpose other than the needs assessment. Many governmental, health, social service, and education agencies collect data describing health problems and demographics that can be useful to the needs assessor. These can be census-type data, in which the goal is to describe every event or person, for example, birth and death records; or they can be survey-type data, in which an attempt is made to capture a representative sample of the population of interest.

Secondary sources can be local, regional, national, or international. They can be obtained directly from the agency responsible for collection and analysis or from a library. For example, local health departments collect census data such as birth and death records. National agencies such as the CDC collect a variety of data on disease incidence and prevalence as well as survey data regarding disease risk. The Internet makes acquiring data from agencies at all levels very easy. Table 5.2 presents examples of sources of secondary data and their Web addresses.

Primary Data from Individuals

We provide two brief examples of data collection from individuals and refer the reader to primary sources on survey research. Table 5.3 indicates the variety of methods of primary data collection from individuals. Written and telephone surveys are the most often used, with Internet surveys gaining in popularity. These use structured forms or protocols that employ a variety of scales and response modes and are relatively easy to administer. Key issues are the validity and reliability of items and scales, appropriate sampling to represent the population, and the ability to achieve high response rates (Aday, 1996; Dillman, 2000; Witkin & Altschuld, 1995).

TABLE 5.2. EXAMPLES OF SECONDARY DATA SOURCES FOR NEEDS ASSESSMENT.

Type of Data	Example Sources	Web Address
Demographic	U.S. Census	http://www.census.gov/
	European census information	http://www.hist.umn.edu/~rmccaa/ipums-europe/enumeration_forms.shtml.htm
	Statistical Abstracts of the U.S.	http://www.census.gov/statab/
Health and vital statistics	National Vital Statistics Report (NVSR)	http://www.cdc.gov/nchs/products/pubs/pubd/mvsr/mvsr.htm
	Morbidity and Mortality Weekly Report (MMWR)	http://www.cdc.gov/mmwr/
	National Center for Health Statistics	http://www.cdc.gov/nchs/
	Guide to Federal Statistics	http://www.fedstats.gov/
	Guide to U.S. Government Statistics	http://www.library.vanderbilt.edu/romans/fdtf/
	Behavioral Risk Factor Surveillance Survey (BRFSS)	http://www.cdc.gov/brfss/
	Centers for Disease Control and Prevention (CDC)	http://www.cdc.gov/
	World Health Organization (WHO) World Health Statistics	http://www.who.int/en/
	WHO Weekly Epidemiological Record	http://www.who.int/en/
	U.S. Department of Health and Human Services	http://www.hhs.gov/

Risk factors	Behavioral Risk Factor Surveillance Survey (BRFSS)	http://www.cdc.gov/brfss/
Environmental data	Environmental Protection Agency	http://www.epa.gov/
	Access to Air Pollution Data	http://www.epa.gov/air/data/idex/html
Local and regional health data	Health Departments (such as Texas, Houston)	http://www.dshs.state.tx.us/
		http://www.houstontx.gov/health/
Sources for cancer (as an example of disease)	Texas Cancer Registry (provides access to cancer incidence and mortality rates in Texas from 1997–2001)	http://www.dshs.state.tx.us/tcr/data.html
	National Cancer Institute	http://seer.cancer.gov/
		http://seer.cancer.gov/about/activities.html

Interviews. Interviews can be highly structured (much like a survey) or unstructured, using a general guide outlining the set of issues to be addressed. Unstructured interviews have the advantage of allowing the respondent opportunities for free expression, with attitudes more likely to be revealed, but the method requires skilled interviewers and qualitative data analysts. As with surveys, it is important to determine the purpose of the interview and select the sample. Mall intercept interviews, in which potential respondents are approached in public places, are frequently used for structured interviews with convenience samples. Key informants can supply information about needs, barriers, and previous programs (Witkin & Altschuld, 1995).

Ethnographic Methods. Ethnographic methods from anthropology provide a particularly key role in describing marginalized settings and hard-to-reach populations, such as drug users, persons engaging in HIV-risk behaviors, or homeless persons (R. Parker & Ehrhardt, 2001; Tross, 2001). Ethnographic methods include participant observation, in-depth interviews, focus groups, and analysis of written textual materials; and they are focused on the description of a culture through the experiences and perspectives of persons in their own language and on their own terms. Scrimshaw and colleagues have developed rapid assessment techniques based on anthropological methods that have been applied in the planning and evaluation of a variety of international programs in such areas as nutrition and primary health care, reproductive health, AIDS, epilepsy, hunger, water and sanitation, and emergency relief (Scrimshaw & Hurtado, 1987, 1992).

Primary Data from Groups

Using groups to collect needs assessment data has recently gained significantly in popularity among health promoters and other planners. We present three examples here to give a flavor of data collection with groups. We discuss Freirian question posing, using various triggers for discussion (Freire, 1973a, 1973b; Wallerstein, Sanchez-Merki, & Dow, 1997; Wang, 2003) in Chapter Four. Community meetings, focus groups, nominal group-process groups, electronic chat groups, and many other small group venues and methods are available for determining community members' perspectives on health and quality-of-life problems as well as the causes of those problems (Gilmore & Campbell, 1996; Witkin & Altschuld, 1995). We describe data collection from three types of groups.

Planning Groups. One of the first places to look for information is from the group or groups that planners have developed to help them through the program development work. This is usually some combination of a work group and various advisory groups. Both types of groups can contribute to defining the problem

TABLE 5.3. PRIMARY SOURCES OF EVIDENCE FOR BEHAVIOR AND ENVIRONMENT.

Data Collection from Individuals

Ethnographic interview and observation

Critical incident technique (as part of a survey or interview)

Key informant interview (or survey)

Survey (mail, in-person, telephone, internet)

Interview

Data Collection from Groups

Noninteracting

    Mailed Delphi technique

Interacting

    Community forum

    Focus groups

    Nominal group technique

    Freirian question posing

    Delphi technique

    Natural groups and planning groups

    Photovoice

and understanding the community if they include a variety of types of community members, including those with the problem. Levy and colleagues (2004) describe a needs-assessment process in two Chicago communities affected disproportionately by diabetes and heart disease. The needs assessment began with providing structure for the planning activities by creating four work groups, each concerned with a different subject: risk factors and programs, quality of clinical care, policy and advocacy, and data and evaluation. "Planning council members included individuals from different racial and ethnic backgrounds with professional expertise across a broad spectrum of fields such as public health, medicine, nursing, community organizing, and evaluation. Representatives from the American Diabetes Association and the American Heart Association were on the planning council. Community members also participated, including persons affected by the targeted health conditions, local business people, and religious leaders" (p. 60). The planning council reviewed data from all components of the needs assessment and provided critical information and analysis.

Focus Groups. Focus groups are a data-gathering technique that health promotion has borrowed from marketing (Gilmore & Campbell, 1996). Focus groups, led by moderators who refer to interview guides with seven to ten questions, are often used in health promotion, most profitably as a part of a multimethod approach to needs assessment or program development (Goldberg, Rudd, & Dietz, 1999; Nakkash et al., 2003; Sorensen et al., 2004). The goal of a focus group is to stimulate discussion among six to twelve fairly homogenous persons to ascertain opinions and attitudes related to the topic of interest. Kreuger (1994) describes processes in planning and conducting focus groups:

Development of a focus group guide

Recruitment of participants

Discussion including introductions, facilitation, and recording

Transcription

Analysis

The number of focus groups to conduct is based on a variety of considerations: determining whether saturation has been reached and no additional themes are forthcoming, ensuring that different segments of the community are represented, and allowing the opportunity to ask new questions that emerge during earlier focus groups. For example, Beeker, Kraft, Southwell, and Jorgensen (2000) stratified their groups on colon cancer screening by both age and gender. Young, Gittelsohn, Charleston, Felix-Aaron, and Appel (2001) held focus groups related to the behavior of interest: exercisers, nonexercisers, people who successfully lost weight, and people who did not successfully lose weight. Fernandez and colleagues used a multimethod phased approach to needs assessment in the Familias program (Fernández, et al., 2000; Fernández, et al., 2000; Lopez, 2004). The team conducted three phases of focus groups with Hispanic mothers, in addition to observations at clinic appointments and interviews with key informant health care providers. The first phase of focus groups was to address general health and health care concerns; the second was to focus on asthma; and the third was to recruit more parents who worked outside of the home because the first two sets of groups overrepresented new immigrants.

Nominal Group Process. Often in group interactions not all members are able to participate equally. The more vocal individuals can color the results of an interactive group process such as a focus group or town hall meeting until their ideas take prominence (Dewar, White, Posade, & Dillon, 2003). One of this chapter's authors previously worked as health education director for a large hospital. Eliciting ideas from planning group members was often hampered by the norms at the hospital that enforced a strict hierarchy: physicians at the top, administrators in the middle, and other care providers at the bottom. Physicians talked most in planning meetings and were not challenged when presenting needs-assessment or program ideas. This was a perfect situation for a group method that can equalize contributions.

Nominal group technique (NGT) (Carney, McIntosh, & Worth, 1996; Delbecq, 1983; Delbecq, Van de Ven & Gustafson, 1975; Ginsburg, Menapace, & Slap, 1997; Miller, Shewchuk, Elliot, & Richards, 2000) is a partially interactive process for group data collection that creates boundaries to equalize contributions by group members. A facilitator poses a question to groups of five to seven members, who silently write individual answers to the question. For needs assessment, the question might be something like, "In this neighborhood, what health threat concerns you the most"? They then give answers to the question one at a time, round-robin style. The facilitator groups the answers, using a board or Post-It notes. After clarification of the listing of answers, group members make preliminary rankings, which they record and discuss. A second vote is taken, yielding a final prioritization (Gilmore & Campbell, 1996). A more formal approach to this process, concept mapping, uses multidimensional scaling and cluster analysis to develop a visual display of themes or categories (W.M.K. Trochim, 1989; W. M. Trochim, Cook, & Setze, 1994; W. M. Trochim, Milstein, Wood, Jackson, & Pressler, 2004).

Delphi Survey. The Delphi survey (named for the Oracle at Delphi in ancient Greece, who was thought to predict the future) is a paper-and-pencil process. It may be conducted with up to fifty participants, who complete two to four rounds of surveys that lead to clarification and consensus regarding such aims as determining goals and objectives, establishing priorities, educating a respondent group, exploring alternatives and gathering information (Moore, 1994; Witkin & Altschuld, 1995).

Geographic Methods

Geocoding links data such as demographics, social and health indicators, and physical structures (for example, health facilities) to individual data that has been aggregated over an area by using codes for street addresses or census tract numbers to denote geographic locations (Witkin & Altschuld, 1995). For example, the immunization bureau in a large city with lower than average immunization rates wanted to plan interventions to improve its performance. The immunization bureau staff mapped the children known to be underimmunized and were able to then look at groups by demographics as well as by health indicators, availability of services, and other important information for understanding what might be determining the low uptake of immunization.

Community Landscape Asset Mapping (CLAM) is a survey to determine community-level factors that may influence health behaviors (Levy et al., 2004). The survey is done by observation to identify four aspects of landscapes: ecological, materialistic, consumption, and therapeutic (Curtis & Jones, 1999). In the needs assessment of neighborhoods on the west side of Chicago, Levy and colleagues (2004) used a modified version of CLAM to assess community and policy influences on health. The survey team noted vacant lots, streets, police presence, street lighting, and smoking in restaurants. Because they were particularly interested in factors related to cardiovascular disease and diabetes, they observed restaurants and grocery stores. The authors note the importance of including community residents in debriefing meetings with the survey teams to fully understand the data.

The Needs Assessment as a Risk Model

So far, we have discussed the PRECEDE model as a risk model: a model of health and quality-of-life problems and their causes. In the next chapter, we move to a health-promoting model and ask what needs to change in the behavior of the at-risk group or the environmental agents in order to create a health-promoting situation. For example, in work on asthma, cystic fibrosis, and arthritis, we have often talked about health-promoting self-management models that are couched in terms of health-promoting behavior and environment (Bartholomew et al., 1989; Bartholomew et al., 1994; Bartholomew et al., 1996; Bartholomew, Koenning, Dahlquist, & Barron, 1994). In other words, we analyzed what patients and families as well as their environments would have to do in order to manage disease and minimize the health and quality-of-life consequences of a chronic illness. To use the PRECEDE model for planning self-management programs for chronic health conditions such as asthma, we ask what at-risk or ill individuals could do to decrease their risk of the health and quality-of-life problems related to the illness. Any problem can be analyzed in this positive direction, but, for most issues of health risk, we suggest understanding the risk model first and then making the transition to a health promotion model. Much can be learned from fully understanding a causal model of a health problem before translating the problem behavior and environment (and their determinants) into health-promoting factors. In cardiovascular disease, for example, one of the risk factors is sedentary lifestyle, and one health-promoting behavior is to increase exercise. Of course, the determinants of increasing exercise are different from the determinants of sedentary lifestyle, and understanding the determinants of the latter will help us understand some of the barriers to exercising. This analysis might not occur if we began directly by looking only at the health-promoting behavior. This process of translating the negative behavior and environment into the positive must be completed as we begin the process of Intervention Mapping.

In Intervention Mapping, the planner is faced with choosing what should be changed from an array of behavioral and environmental factors. The planner must decide whether the environmental factors are important to the problem and whether they are changeable in the scope of the program mandate. Having chosen the environmental factors, the planner must discover the agents at each level for each environmental change objective. These agents are the people (and the social or organizational roles assigned to them) who are in positions to change the environment. In another example, this one concerning adolescents taking sexual risks, parents might be in a position to change something about the adolescents' immediate environment, such as the amount of unsupervised time at home (related to the opportunity to have sexual intercourse).

The MATCH model presents the environment in this way, where environmental levels are chosen for intervention whether or not they have been directly implicated in causation of a health problem (Simons-Morton, Greene, & Gottlieb, 1995; Simons-Morton, Simons-Morton, Parcel, & Bunker, 1988). Environmental agents often are not responsible for the original environmental condition, but they can create change. For example, legislators or city council representatives may not be responsible for violence that occurs in unsafe streets or parks, but they might be able to change the environment of their cities. They are leverage points for citizen efforts to change the parks and streets, thereby reducing the probability of violent acts in these environments.

Community Capacity

➲ *Balance the needs assessment with an assessment of community capacity.*

Community-Based Health Promotion

McLeroy, Norton, Kegler, Burdine, and Sumaya (2003) describe a typology of communities as they pertain to community-based health promotion interventions. The term *community-based* often refers to the community as a setting for interventions that McLeroy and colleagues suggest are usually oriented toward changing individuals' health behavior. In this category communities may function most like intervention hosts. A second model of community-based interventions has a very different meaning—one of the community as the target for change. For example, community indicator projects use community data to encourage change in communitywide policy, institutions, and services (Coulton, 1995). A third model is community as a resource of community ownership and participation in health promotion programs to ensure sustained program success. Finally, McLeroy and colleagues describe community as agents of adaptation that through their many institutions meet the needs of community members.

McLeroy and colleagues (2003) argue that the latter three models for understanding community enable health promotion outcomes to be broadened from changing individual behavior to changing community capacity. They suggest that an understanding of a community's capacity can lead to a better match with health promotion interventions and can shift intervention strategies to broader community-building approaches.

In Chapter Four we discussed the theoretical base for community capacity and social capital. In this section we will look at the assessment of characteristics of the community, with a particular focus on the strengths of a community. A healthy community has been described as one that is continually creating and improving resources in its physical and social environments that enable people to mutually support each other in performing all the functions of life (Hancock & Duhl, 1986). Community capacity assessment examines the community's social and physical infrastructure related to community problem solving and development, as well as the policy and physical environments that facilitate health-promoting behaviors.

Assessing Community Capacity

Goodman and colleagues (1998) participated in a process to identify and define the dimensions of community capacity and examined the linkages across the dimensions. They found ten dimensions:

- Citizen participation
- Leadership
- Skills, including group process, conflict resolution, community assessment, problem solving, program planning, intervention design and implementation, evaluation, resource mobilization, and advocacy
- Resources internal and external to the community, including social capital
- Social and interorganizational networks
- Sense of community
- Understanding of community history
- Community power (power with)

- Community values
- Critical reflection

Each of these had subdimensions that would be part of operationalizing the construct. Study authors point out the challenge of measuring the constructs and suggest that the list be used in dialogue within the community as community members assess and address their community's capacity.

Others have suggested methods of assessment such as key informant interviews, focus groups, surveys, documentation of participation logs, meeting minutes, program plans, and sociograms. Labonte and Laverack (2001) describe a spider-web mapping technique based on ordinal rankings that provide visual representation of the domains of community capacity. They review various researchers' methods to obtain these rankings by community informants and health promoters through an interactive process. Singer and Kegler (2004) determined the reliability of network analysis data from organizations participating in a community intervention to prevent lead poisoning to assess interorganizational relationships, one dimension of community capacity.

Mapping Community Capacity. Capacity assessments go hand in hand with participatory community development. Table 5.4 shows the differences between a needs and an assets approach to community enhancement. In asset mapping, local people and organizations explore the problems and resources in their communities and develop strategies to solve the problems together. The process is internally focused, not relying on the advice of outside experts, and relationship driven, with all participants working together as a team (Beaulieu, 2002).

TABLE 5.4. CONTRASTING THE "NEEDS" VS. "ASSETS" APPROACH TO COMMUNITY ENHANCEMENT.

Needs	Assets
Focuses on deficiencies	Focuses on effectiveness
Can result in fragmentation of responses to local needs	Can build interdependencies
Makes people consumers of services; can build dependence	Identifies ways that people can give of their talents
Residents have little voice in deciding how to address local concerns	Seeks to empower people

Source: Beaulieu, 2002, p. 4.

McKnight and Kretzmann (1997) suggest mapping three types of resources:

- Resources located in the community and under its control
- Assets within the community but largely controlled by outsiders
- Resources originating outside the neighborhood and controlled by outsiders

The community's most accessible assets are those resources located in the community and largely under its control. These include individuals' assets, such as individual capacities, personal income, gifts of labeled people (such as the physically challenged), individual local businesses, home-based enterprises, and assets of organizations and associations. The latter include citizens' associations as well as organizations of businesses, financial institutions (for example, the Gameen bank in Bangladesh and the South Shore Bank in Chicago), cultural organizations, communications organizations, and religious organizations. Kretzmann and McKnight also include a protocol for assessing personal capacity in areas such as construction, office equipment operation and repair, food preparation, transportation, and child care (Kretzman & McKnight, 1993). Many other domains of individual competence can be imagined, including leadership, group process, problem solving, and participation skills.

The second type of resources includes assets located within the community but largely controlled by outsiders. Kretzmann and McKnight consider these to be secondary building blocks. They are divided into private and nonprofit organizations, public institutions and services, and other physical resources. Institutions of higher education, hospitals, and social service agencies fall in the first category. Public institutions and services include public schools, police, libraries, fire departments, and parks. Physical resources include unused land and buildings as well as programs to conserve and recycle energy and waste.

Finally, there are resources originating outside the neighborhood and controlled by outsiders. All public expenditures are considered to be investments in development, although often they are used for maintenance of individuals without work and of impoverished neighborhoods. These are welfare expenditures, public capital improvement expenditures, and public information.

The community-planning process should involve representatives of internally located and controlled assets to take full advantage of participants' interests and strengths. Following this mobilization of internal community resources, the next step is to build bridges to outside resources (McKnight & Kretzmann, 1997).

Measuring Social Capital. Social capital has often been measured by questions about reciprocity, trust, and civic participation (Lochner, Kawachi, Brennan, & Buka, 2003; Veenstra, 2002). For example, Veenstra created a social capital index to measure associational and civic participation and the density of associational life, combining information on voting behavior, social involvement, and the number of community organizations within each health district. In another example, Kennelly, O'Shea, and Garvey (2003) measured membership in voluntary organizations and whether unpaid work was done for the associations. They created the variables of density of association membership and density of unpaid work. Greiner, Li, Kawachi, Hunt, and Ahluwalia (2004) used the Community Involvement Module of the Kansas Behavioral Risk Factor Surveillance System (BRFSS) to measure two constructs. The first was an overall rating of a community as a place to live. The other measured community involvement in coalitions or civic groups focused on local problems.

In a brief review of the measurement of social capital, Baum and Ziersch (2003) suggest that a more sophisticated measurement of social capital would keep the sources (that is, networks and values) distinct from the outcomes (that is, the types of resources available through the sources). They also suggest qualitative consideration of social capital to examine the contexts in which social capital works and the complexity of the concept. Recently, the World Bank has developed an assessment tool that includes both qualitative and quantitative components (Grootaert & van Bastelaer, 2002).

Measuring Policy and Physical Environment As we pointed out earlier, the policy and physical environment are important external determinants of health-promoting behaviors and characteristics of healthy communities. Several indicators examine these elements within different community sectors. The School Health Policies and Programs Study assessed the physical education and activity, health services, mental health, social services, food service, school policy, and environmental components of school health programs at the school, district, and state levels, using computer-assisted personal interviews (Jones, Brener, & McManus, 2003). The CDC (2004) has developed a self-assessed school health index for schools to use to assess their programs.

The Texas Department of State Health Services (2004, 2005) has adapted the CDC's school health index for work sites and communities. The work-site instrument addresses the presence of a work-site plan; policies on physical activity, nutrition, and tobacco use; health care coverage, access to screening services, and health promotion interventions. The community index includes indicators of community accessibility to walking; access to physical activity facilities; access to healthy food through restaurants, grocery stores, and farmers' markets; and the presence of health promotion programs in work sites and schools.

Handy, Boarnet, Ewing, and Killingsworth (2002) have looked at measurement of aspects of the built environment that have been related to physical activity. These include density and intensity, land-use mix, street connectivity, street scale, aesthetic qualities, distribution of activities, and transportation across a region. An example of a checklist based on such aspects is that of the National Center for Bicycling and Walking (2002). It includes items within the categories of transportation; land use and development; schools; parks, recreation, and trails; and safety, security, and crime prevention. These measurements are still undergoing refinement for use by researchers. However, their use by a community group can result in identification of issues and assets and be a very useful tool for planning. Survey items for measuring environmental supports for physical activity have also been developed (Brownson et al., 2004; Kirtland et al., 2003).

Setting Priorities

Setting priorities in a needs assessment is an iterative process, occurring throughout the assessment as well as after data analysis at the assessment's end. Setting priorities about health problems and populations of interest begins when one determines in the preassessment what groups and problems to study. As health planners ask questions and gather information during the assessment, they make various decisions about the continuing focus. For example, the asthma needs assessment came to be focused on schoolchildren. In the stroke-project example at the end of this chapter (and continuing through the chapters that describe Intervention Mapping steps), planners made a decision to focus only on stroke treatment (secondary and tertiary prevention) rather than on prevention of stroke (primary prevention). On what basis should these health planners make such priority decisions?

Criteria for Decisions About Priorities

Witkin and Altschuld (1995) suggest a number of factors that influence priorities. One is the magnitude between what is and what could be. For example, in the stroke project, the needs-assessment team discovered that the rate of drug therapy for acute stroke in the United States was only about 1 to 2 percent. The rate could be much better, maybe four to five times the current rate. The difference between the current status and what was desirable and possible was great. A related criterion is the difference in burden from a problem among groups. Once a problem becomes a focus, priorities may narrow to certain groups due to a heavier burden or to a health inequality or inequity.

A set of practical issues also influences the decision. These are the potential difficulty in ameliorating the needs, the consequences of ignoring the needs, and the possible costs of implementing a solution (Witkin & Altschuld, 1995). Political and other social factors also affect the ultimate priorities and the decision-making process. These include community values, the context of priorities (that is, the local, regional, national, and international priorities), public and leader expectations, available interest and expertise, momentum, and availability of funding and human resources.

Relevance and Changeability

Once the health planner has decided on the health problem(s) and population(s) and completed the analysis of behavioral and environmental causes, further decisions are made. In Chapter Two we defined *relevance* as the strength of the evidence relating a determinant and the behavior or environmental factor we want to change, and we defined *changeability* as the strength of the evidence that the proposed change can be realized by an intervention. L. W. Green and Kreuter recommend rating the importance (that is, relevance) and changeability of behaviors and environmental conditions using findings from the needs assessment. Behaviors and environmental conditions that are both more relevant and more changeable will be a high priority for program focus; factors that are more relevant and less changeable may be a priority for innovative programs for which evaluation is crucial. Factors that are less relevant but more changeable may be deemed as lower priorities except to demonstrate initial change to encourage community support and program participation. Behaviors that are both less relevant and less changeable should not be a focus for intervention. This analysis should be carefully done so that factors that are very relevant but hard to change are not neglected.

Implications for Evaluation

⮫ *Link the needs assessment to evaluation planning by establishing desired program outcomes.*

The last task in performing a needs assessment is to relate the needs assessment to the future evaluation of the resulting program by establishing objectives regarding health and quality-of-life program outcomes. L. W. Green and Kreuter (1991) state that "objectives are crucial: they form a fulcrum, converting diagnostic data into program direction" (p. 118). Both in funding agency requests for proposals and in the literature, references to the terms *goals, objectives,* and *program aims* do not share common definitions. The words have different meanings to different users. Therefore, we have carefully defined several types of objectives to Intervention Mapping. They work for this purpose and may be generalizable to other planning. However, we strongly advise the reader always to find out what others mean when they use the terms and to respond with objectives as required by the requester, especially when the other is an employer, a funding agency, or a reviewer. The important issue is not what these planning tools are called but what information they contain.

For use in the Intervention Mapping framework, we define *program goals* as general or broad statements of the desire to reduce the gap between the current status and the optimal status of a situation; this is distinct from an objective, which is stated in terms that are operationally defined and can be measured (Rossi, Freeman, & Lipsey, 1999). The first objectives encountered in this book are written from the needs assessment to address desired program effects on health and quality of life.

Writing Objectives for Health and Quality-of-Life Outcomes

At the end of the needs assessment, we want to have program outcomes: what the overall program is meant to accomplish. Table 5.5 presents all of the types of objectives the planner will use in Intervention Mapping. The ultimate outcomes are usually related to health or quality-of-life. If health and quality-of-life program outcomes can be accomplished in a typical program and evaluation time frame, then those become the specified outcomes. If the time frame is too long for program effects on health and quality of life to be measurable within the program time frame (as, for example, in a program concerned with HIV or cardiovascular disease), then the planning group can make a decision to define the program outcomes in terms of behavior or environment.

Health and quality of life are most often the desired program outcomes. Health outcomes are stated as indicators of health status, such as morbidity, mortality, incidence, prevalence, disability, and physiological risk factors. These include a statement (with a strong verb) of what will change in a specified population, by how much, and by what period of time. The amount of expected change and the time frame must be empirically justifiable. For example, the health educator working with street youth established objectives related to the incidence of sexually transmitted infection (STI) in her population. She set an objective of a 10 percent decrease in the incidence rate of these STIs in the first two years of the program based on other intensive work with this population reported in the literature. She stated her health objective as follows: The program will reduce the incidence rate of STI infection 10 percent in the population during the first two years of the program. Some programs also seek to improve quality of life, and Green and Kreuter (2005) list many examples of quality-of-life indicators, including employment, crowding, absenteeism, achievement, alienation, discrimination, happiness, and self-esteem. Some of these factors are defined at the societal level and may change

TABLE 5.5. TYPES OF OBJECTIVES.

Type of Objective	Definition	Stage of Planning Process Where Occurs
Health outcomes	These are derived from the needs assessment and are usually in terms of reducing problems in health that were documented in the needs assessment. What will change? By how much? Among whom? By when?	Step 1: End of needs assessment
Quality-of-life outcomes	These are derived from the needs assessment and are usually in terms of reducing problems in quality of life that were documented in the needs assessment. What will change? By how much? Among whom? By when?	Step 1: End of needs assessment
Health-related behavior outcomes	These come from the specification of behaviors of the at-risk group that the health promotion intervention will address. What will change? By how much? Among whom? By when?	Step 2: Matrices of change objectives
Health-related environmental outcomes	These come from the specification of environmental change that the health promotion intervention will address. What will change? By how much? Among whom? By when?	Step 2: Matrices of change objectives
Performance objectives	These are in the left-hand column of the matrices. They address what the at-risk group members or environmental agents must do to accomplish the health-related behaviors or environmental conditions.	Step 2: Matrices of change objectives
Change objectives	These are in the cells of the matrices. They are the combination of the performance objectives with their determinants.	Step 2: Matrices of change objectives
Performance objectives (adoption, implementation, sustainability)	These are in the left-hand column of the adoption, implementation, and sustainability matrices. They address what the program adopters and implementers must do to use and continue the program.	Step 4: Planning for adoption, implementation, sustainability
Change objectives (adoption, implementation, sustainability)	These are in the cells of the adoption, implementation, and sustainability matrices. They are the combination of the performance objectives with their determinants for program adoption, implementation, and sustainability.	Step 4: Planning for adoption, implementation, sustainability

only over long periods of time, whereas others are more individual and can be measured in the time periods more typical for program evaluation. Another point about indicators of quality of life is that they often are constructs that require operational definition and sometimes psychological or sociological measurement instruments. For example: How does one define and measure happiness? How does one define and measure crowding?

At the end of the needs assessment, the planner sets outcome objectives related to health and quality of life. In the next chapter (Intervention Mapping Step 2), the planner decides what needs to change regarding behavioral and environmental outcomes. Because of the time required for change to occur, this level of outcome is sometimes described as the main outcome instead of health or quality of life. This is acceptable when there is an empirically documented link between the behavior or environment and the health outcome. For example, someone working in tobacco control among youth might have outcomes regarding smoking rates and access to tobacco that can be measured in the short run rather than health outcomes regarding incidence of cardiovascular disease and cancer that could only be observed after many years. Behavioral and environmental outcomes are also stated as what must change, by how much, and by when. The program outcome for the street youth included reduction of the rate of unprotected sexual intercourse by 30 percent in the first year of the program.

Other Objectives in Intervention Mapping

In Chapter Six we present three additional types of objectives. First, the planner will specify desired health-related behavior and environmental conditions. Next, the planner will further specify these desired changes into performance objectives; and finally, he or she will merge the performance objectives with their determinants to form change objectives, the most immediate targets of a program. Performance objectives and change objectives recur in Step 4 to address planning for program adoption, implementation, and sustainability (Chapter Nine).

Box 5.2. Stroke Project

The T.L.L. Foundation Temple Stroke Project is an example of an application of Intervention Mapping to develop a successful intervention (Morgenstern et al., 2002, 2003). We present this example step by step at the end of each Intervention Mapping step (Chapters Five through Ten). We organize the example by the tasks that we present in the chapter.

⊃ *Establish a planning group that includes potential program participants and plan the needs assessment.*

Community Partnership

The T.L.L. Temple Foundation Stroke Project was focused in Angelina, Nacog-doches, and Shelby counties in east Texas. The program was funded by the T.L.L. Temple Foundation, which asked that we conduct the intervention in its community. We began by hiring a local health educator from one of the two midsize towns in the area, and putting together a program planning group. Our team included health educators, behavioral scientists, and neurologists from an academic medical center about one hundred miles from our project area and community members concerned with stroke. We had participation from persons who had suffered a stroke (including the mayor of one of the towns); representatives of community organizations with some interest in stroke; community media gatekeepers including English- and Spanish-language newspapers, radio stations, and television stations; and health care providers who treat stroke. During intervention development, the team met bimonthly in the Lufkin city hall conference room.

Logic Model of the Problem

The health educator and behavioral scientist on the team helped the group choose the PRECEDE model (L. W. Green & Kreuter, 1999; 2005) as the organizing framework for our needs assessment, and we began immediately putting everything we already knew about stroke in our community into the model. We began with the project assumption that we were entering the model at the health problem. We defined the health problem as excess morbidity and mortality from untreated stroke.

Although the U.S. Food and Drug Administration (FDA) approved intravenous recombinant tissue plasminogen activator (rtPA) as the only treatment for acute ischemic stroke in 1996, only a small minority of patients (about one to two percent) receive this treatment, which can significantly improve stroke outcomes (National Institute of Neurological Disorders and Stroke rtPA Stroke Study Group, 1995). Treatment must begin within three hours of symptom onset. Despite some risk of intracranial hemorrhage, the studies of rtPA suggested that the use of the treatment resulted in at least a 30 percent relative benefit in reducing disability from stroke. Consensus statements from the American Heart Association (H. P. Adams et al., 1996), the American Academy of Neurology (American Academy of Neurology, Quality Standards Subcommittee, 1996) and the American College of Chest Physicians (Albers, Easton, Sacco, & Teal, 1998) supporting the use of IV rtPA have been published. Despite the published data, consensus statements, and guidelines, the problem persists that only a very small minority of acute stroke patients currently receive IV rtPA for acute ischemic stroke

FIGURE 5.4. PRECEDE LOGIC MODEL.

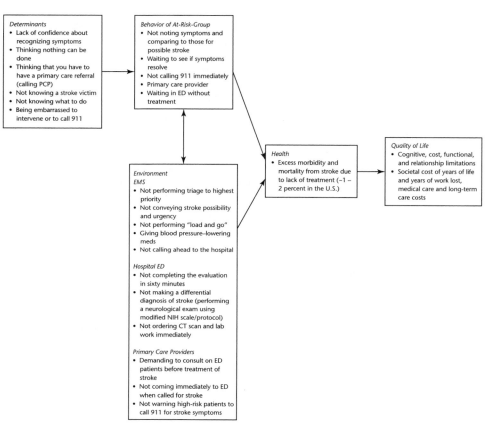

Determinants
- Lack of confidence about recognizing symptoms
- Thinking nothing can be done
- Thinking that you have to have a primary care referral (calling PCP)
- Not knowing a stroke victim
- Not knowing what to do
- Being embarrassed to intervene or to call 911

Behavior of At-Risk-Group
- Not noting symptoms and comparing to those for possible stroke
- Waiting to see if symptoms resolve
- Not calling 911 immediately
- Primary care provider
- Waiting in ED without treatment

Environment
EMS
- Not performing triage to highest priority
- Not conveying stroke possibility and urgency
- Not performing "load and go"
- Giving blood pressure–lowering meds
- Not calling ahead to the hospital

Hospital ED
- Not completing the evaluation in sixty minutes
- Not making a differential diagnosis of stroke (performing a neurological exam using modified NIH scale/protocol)
- Not ordering CT scan and lab work immediately

Primary Care Providers
- Demanding to consult on ED patients before treatment of stroke
- Not coming immediately to ED when called for stroke
- Not warning high-risk patients to call 911 for stroke symptoms

Health
- Excess morbidity and mortality from stroke due to lack of treatment (~1 – 2 percent in the U.S.)

Quality of Life
- Cognitive, cost, functional, and relationship limitations
- Societal cost of years of life and years of work lost, medical care and long-term care costs

in the United States. Based on this beginning problem definition, we started the PRECEDE model and continue the description of its development below.

> *Conduct the needs assessment using the PRECEDE model (Green & Kreuter, 2005) to analyze health and quality of life problems and their causes and to decide on priorities.*

Needs Assessment Methods

In order to flesh out the needs-assessment model, we reviewed the literature, held focus groups and interviews, led discussions with our planning group, and conducted a community telephone survey.

We addressed two questions with a review of the stroke literature. We needed to be able to estimate stroke in our intervention community. The questions were the following:

1. What is the prevalence of the health problem, both stroke and untreated stroke?
2. What factors are associated with lack of treatment for stroke and delay in presentation to emergency room with stroke symptoms?

We conducted two focus groups of seven persons with stroke and significant others and four interviews of patients and significant others. Our work group served as an ongoing source of information about the intervention community. As mentioned, we had many community stakeholders in stroke including two persons who had suffered a stroke. The purpose of the qualitative data collection was to explore recognition of stroke symptoms, activities in response to symptoms, and emotions and attitudes toward the stroke experience.

We conducted a community telephone survey to address the question of what attitudes predict a rapid and assertive response to stroke symptoms in our intervention community. Variables measured in the survey are included in Table 5.6. We used random-digit dialing to conduct 106 interviews.

We met with administrative representatives of the five hospitals and three emergency medical services (EMS) in the intervention community to assess the capacity of the hospitals to treat stroke in the emergency room.

Describing Health Problems, Quality of Life, and the Populations at Risk

The intervention was located in the sponsoring agency's community. The community was far enough from Houston, the largest nearby metropolitan area, that referral for acute stroke care was prohibitive without an initial stop at a local hospital. The intervention community contained five hospitals in Angelina, Nacogdoches, and Shelby counties, Texas. In 1998 the intervention community comprised an estimated 160,833 residents (77 percent non-Hispanic white) (Population Projections, 1998) The incidence of stroke in the United States is about seven hundred thousand per year or about 2.6 per thousand. The mortality rate is about 38.5 percent in males and 61.5 percent in females. Persons aged seventy-five and above are at the highest risk of stroke. In the counties in which we were working, we could expect about 418 strokes per year. To our knowledge, only one person had ever been treated with rtPA in the intervention community.

Stroke results in decrements of quality of life in the sufferer and family including, for example, loss of cognitive functioning, loss of financial and physical independence, and costs for medical care. Our focus groups and interviews highlighted the community view of stroke as something that results in terrible

TABLE 5.6. STROKE PROJECT COMMUNITY SURVEY VARIABLES.

Variable	Definition and Measurement
Knowledge of symptoms	Signs of stroke in a friend
Knowledge of what to do	"Exactly what would you do in the face of the symptoms you just described?"
Self-efficacy	Confidence in ability to call 911, get appropriate emergency department (ED) care
Perceived norms	What a person thinks known associates would do related to stroke
Barriers	Calling the doctor first (before going to the ED)
	Family members do not take medical problem seriously
	Waiting before doing anything about a medical problem
	Calling insurance first
	Calling a primary care doctor
	Being embarrassed or afraid to act for a friend
	Being embarrassed or afraid to act for self
Outcome expectations	A person with stroke can be treated and get better.
Behavioral intentions	Intention to provide assertive support to get stroke treatment
	Intention to call 911
	Intention to wait
Ethnicity	Caucasian Non-Hispanic, Hispanic, African American
Gender	Male or Female

impairment of quality of life. One respondent reported: "I don't ever want to be like that, just let me die." Further, all respondents had known someone with a stroke who suffered significant impairment and restrictions of activities of daily living.

Describing Behavior of At-Risk Individuals

Moving to the left in the PRECEDE model (Figure 5.4), we asked the question: What is the behavior of the lay person at risk that contributes to morbidity and mortality from stroke? The literature review indicated delay in arriving at the hospital and arriving at the hospital in a personal car rather than an ambulance (that is, not calling 911) were related to lack of treatment (Alberts, Bertels, &

Dawson, 1990; Bratina, Greenberg, Pasteur, & Grotta, 1995; Feldmann et al., 1993; National Institute of Neurological Disorders and Stroke, 1997). The community survey and focus groups (to be discussed later), though intended to explore determinants of behavior, suggested new risk behaviors such as waiting to see whether symptoms resolve and calling the primary care doctor before proceeding to the emergency department.

Describing Determinants of Slow Response to Stroke

Moving again to the left in the PRECEDE model (Figure 5.4), we concentrated on the determinants of delay in stroke treatment. The literature suggested that several factors related to less delay in response to stroke symptoms include exhibiting recognizable symptoms and being accessible to someone who can do the recognizing. Factors that may have been associated with recognizable symptoms were greater severity, occurrence during the day on a weekday, the fact of living with someone, and employment (Alberts et al., 1990; Azzimondi et al., 1997; Fogelholm, Murros, Rissanen, & Ilmavirta, 1996). Calling 911 and arriving at the hospital by ambulance have been noted by many investigators as factors related to decreased time to hospital arrival and faster evaluation once in the hospital (Barsan et al., 1993; Bratina, Greenberg, Pasteur, & Grotta, 1994; Menon, Pandy, & Morgenstern, 1998;. Not waiting to consult with a primary care provider may also be important (Fogelholm et al., 1996). Knowledge of symptoms and ability to recognize stroke symptoms were also found to be related to faster arrival (Alberts et al., 1990; Feldman et al., 1993; Fogelholm et al., 1996; Williams, Bruno, Rouch, Marriot, & Mas, 1997) Symptoms that are more recognizable because the problem becomes quickly a stable deficit are also related to decreased time to the hospital (Feldmann et al., 1993).

The results of our community study also contributed to the understanding of variables related to delay in care for stroke. Although approximately 79 percent of people responded to an open-ended question that they would call 911 for stroke symptoms, there were several barriers: lacking knowledge of symptoms, having to call the insurance carrier first, and having to call the primary care provider first.

We performed three regression analyses on the survey data (on the intention to act assertively, the intention to call 911, and the intention to wait without responding). The following factors predicted intention to act assertively:

- Being male
- Being minority
- Knowing a stroke victim
- Not tending to wait a while
- Having self-efficacy

For intention to call 911, predictors were the following:

- Being male
- Being minority
- Knowing what to do
- Having self-efficacy
- Not having to call the doctor first (in males but not in females)
- (Not) having family and friends who do not take the problem seriously (in males but not in females)

   For intention to do nothing in the presence of stroke symptoms, predictors were the following:

- Being female
- Being an older minority
- Feeling embarrassment
- Needing to call the doctor first
- Having less self-efficacy
- Having less knowledge of symptoms

Focus groups and interview results uncovered the following themes related to responding to stroke symptoms to get care:

- Lacking recognition of stroke symptoms
- Thinking there is no hope for stroke victims ("Just let me die")
- Having problems with primary care referrals ("Just wait until Monday")
- Being reluctant to take action for self or others
- Not calling 911
- Calling primary care doctor
- Waiting to see whether symptoms would resolve

Describing Environmental Causes of Lack of Treatment

For the stroke project, the hospital emergency department (ED) and the emergency medical services (EMS) are the organizations that have the agents able to make change in stroke treatment. The agents are a variety of health care providers and administrators such as medical directors and chairs of the critical care committees. Stroke patients can receive treatment only if the community ED is prepared to give acute stroke therapy and if the ED conducts a neurological examination and specific radiologic and laboratory tests within a certain time frame. Likewise, the ED can perform its function in the chain of events only if the EMS transports the individual quickly and contributes to a speedy evaluation (National Institute of Neurological Disorders and Stroke, 1997).

Even though the literature suggests that a major cause of lack of treatment for stroke was delay time in getting to the hospital and thus missing the three-hour treatment window, it is apparent that some delays occur in the medical workup once patients arrived at the ED (Albers et al., 2000) and that some physicians are resistant to treatment with rtPA (Caplan, Mohr, Kistler, & Koroshetz, 1997).

Although it was originally a part of the intervention development rather than of the needs assessment, we held meetings with hospital critical care committees, ED medical staff, and EMS in each of the three counties. These meetings documented the failure of ED staff to work up patients for or deliver rtPA. The themes that emerged from the ED meetings were the following:

- The supposed ownership of patients by community physicians ("We can't treat them because they are patients of primary care physicians or community neurologists").
- What about side effects (bleeds)?
- We don't have a protocol.
- We don't have rtPA on the ED formulary.
- It takes too long to work up a patient.
- We don't believe it will make much of a difference.

The themes that emerged from the meetings with community EMS were the following:

- No reason to transport at highest priority if the hospital doesn't triage at highest priority
- Failure to call hospital en route
- Expectation that the hospital will do nothing

The ED physicians did not talk about lack of skill for neurological workup or inability to establish time of onset of the stroke, but these are high-level neurological skills that we included in the needs assessment based on the experience of the planning team.

⊃ *Balance the needs assessment with an assessment of community capacity.*

In addition, the interviews confirmed that all hospitals had some basic capacity to treat stroke. A neurologist was on staff in four of the five community intervention hospitals. The hospitals had twenty-four hour EDs and protocols for emergent head CT scan imaging. All three communities had full 911 EMS.

⊃ *Link the needs assessment to evaluation planning by establishing desired program outcomes.*

Outcome Objectives for the Stroke Project

Looking at the needs-assessment model (Figure 5.4), we determined that outcome objectives of health should include the following:

- Over the two years of the intervention, increase the proportion of eligible patients who receive rtPA to 50 percent at the five hospitals in the intervention community.
- Over the two years of the intervention, increase the proportion of all stroke patients who receive rtPA to 5 percent in the intervention community.

We were ultimately interested in decreasing disability from stroke. However, we did not quantify this objective, and we used treatment as a proxy objective.

CHAPTER SIX

INTERVENTION MAPPING STEP 2: PREPARING MATRICES OF CHANGE OBJECTIVES

Reader Objectives

- State expected change or program outcomes for health-related behavior and environmental conditions
- Subdivide behavior and environmental conditions into performance objectives
- Select important and changeable personal and external determinants of behavior and environmental conditions
- Create a matrix of change objectives for each level of intervention planning (individual, interpersonal, organizational, community, and societal) by crossing performance objectives with determinants and writing change objectives

The basic tool for Intervention Mapping is the matrix of change objectives. Change objectives state what needs to be achieved in order to accomplish performance objectives that will enable changes in behavior or environmental conditions that will in turn improve the health and quality-of-life program outcomes identified in Step 1.

In this chapter we explain how health educators use the findings from the needs assessment and other information to specify intended change in individual health-related behaviors and environmental conditions at the interpersonal, organizational, community, and societal levels. Next, performance objectives are stated for behaviors and for environmental conditions at each ecological level. These performance objectives describe exactly what the at-risk population members and the agents or influential people at each environmental level need to do in order to accomplish improvements in health outcomes.

The matrices in this chapter are created by the intersection of the performance objectives with determinants of behavior and environmental conditions. These matrices form the critical foundation for intervention conceptualization and program development, steps that we explain in Chapters Seven and Eight. The matrices contain the change objectives that the program will target in order to influence change in determinants and accomplishment of performance objectives. This chapter describes in detail the principal components of matrices and guides the reader to use the core processes and the information from the needs assessment to create sound matrices. The final product of Step 2 of the Intervention Mapping process is a set of matrices that specifies the immediate objectives for a health education or promotion program to accomplish.

Box 6.1. Mayor's Project

The mayor's planning group had done a great job on the needs assessment. Many of the members commented that they had no idea that the problem of violence was so complex. Looking at the theories helped them to delve into some of the root causes of violence among the youth in their neighborhoods. They were practically bubbling over with enthusiasm, and they were sure that they were ready to talk about intervention.

Participant A: Now that we know better what some of the factors are that are related to violence, let's go after them.
Participant B: I could call the school district tomorrow, because surely we will want to intervene there.
Participant C: Yeah, and what about that Communities in Schools Group?
Participant D: We could . . .

The health educator sat quietly for a moment getting up the courage to tell them the truth. They had completed only the first phase of their planning. Things were likely to get more complex before a coherent planning framework could emerge. Finally, the health educator said: "Let's back up for just a minute. There are some other things we have to do before we can talk about intervention."

Amid the moans and groans, she told the group about the building blocks of matrices.

Perspectives

In this section we highlight the importance of continuing with the ecological perspective on program development and of building the program logic model.

Continuing with the Ecological Framework

The perspective for this chapter is the continued use of an ecological framework for the planning of interventions for a health promotion program. Causation of health problems is a web of factors that occur at multiple levels. Some influences external to the individual work through the behavior of the at-risk individuals, such as the effects of advertising on the smoking behavior of adolescents (Biener & Siegel, 2000; Pierce, Choi, Gilpin, Farkas, & Berry, 1998; Pierce, Gilpin, & Choi, 1999; Pollay et al., 1996; Schooler, Feighery, & Flora, 1996; L. Turner, Mermelstein, & Flay, 2004), whereas others, such as air quality (Kilburn, 1998), work directly on health. These levels of causation are represented in this chapter's matrix products.

The Logic Model for Program Effects

The logic model for planning in Step 2 of Intervention Mapping (shown in Figure 6.1) is similar to the logic model for the needs assessment except that the focus is on program effects rather than on needs or problem assessment. It begins, however, with the health and quality-of-life outcomes to be achieved by the health promotion program on the right side of the model. This was the last task in Step 1 and forms the basis for continued planning in Step 2. Working to the left in the model, the program planner states the behaviors and environmental conditions in terms of what is necessary to achieve the health and quality-of-life outcomes. The process for creating a matrix of change objectives is based on the assumption that the needs assessment identified behaviors or environmental conditions that are causes of health or quality-of-life outcomes. The next assumption is that development of certain more favorable behavioral or environmental conditions will lead to better health and improved quality of life. Thus, the first task in creating a causal pathway for influencing change is to specify the behavioral and environmental objectives that the health promotion program seeks to accomplish.

The next link in the model is the specification of performance objectives for obtaining the behavioral and environmental outcomes. *Performance objectives* are statements of what a program participant will do or of how an environmental condition will be modified (including who will create the change). They can be a somewhat complex list of steps or actions in preparation for performing the health

FIGURE 6.1. LOGIC MODEL OF CHANGE.

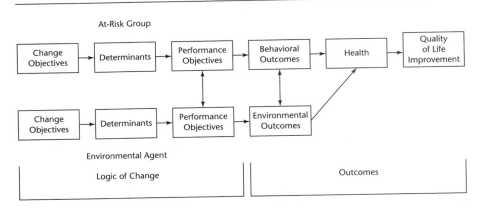

promoting behavior or environmental change. Performance objectives are then examined in light of the determinants of behavior and environmental conditions to generate change objectives. Change objectives specify what needs to change in the determinants of behavior or environmental conditions in order to accomplish the performance objectives.

Thus, the logic for the pathways of program effects starts with the health promotion program addressing the accomplishment of the change objectives that will lead to changes in the determinants of the behavioral and environmental outcomes. Changes in the determinants will influence achievement of the performance objectives, which will enable accomplishment of the behavioral and environmental outcomes. Finally, if the program obtains behavioral and environmental outcomes, health and quality-of-life outcomes will improve.

Behavioral and Environmental Outcomes

➲ *The first task in Step 2 of Intervention Mapping is to state what health behaviors and environmental conditions need to change to improve health and quality-of-life outcomes.*

The needs assessment (see Chapter Five) should provide a clear statement of behavior and environmental conditions linked to a health problem. However, before creating a logic model for an intervention, the health educator needs to reexamine the behavior and environmental conditions in order to define them in terms of what the health education or promotion program is intended to accomplish. What health-promoting behaviors and healthy environmental conditions will be the focus of the program? For example, a behavioral cause of lung cancer is smoking, but the behavioral outcome for an intervention could be either not starting to smoke or quitting smoking (U.S. Department of Health and Human Services, 1994). Likewise, the environment can stimulate or support smoking, but an intervention would have to address a specific part of environmental change, such as advertising campaigns by tobacco product manufacturers (Gilpin, Distefan, & Pierce, 2004; M. J. Lewis, Yulis, Delnevo, & Hrywna, 2004; Pierce et al., 1998; Pollay et al., 1996; Schooler et al., 1996). Well-defined behavioral and environmental outcomes will, in the next task, lead to a better specification of program objectives.

Identifying Health-Related Behaviors of the At-Risk Group

Many types of health-related behaviors can be the focus of the health education and promotion intervention. The needs assessment often identifies behavior related to increased risk, but intervention development requires restating the behaviors as either reducing risk or promoting health. For example, one of the risk behaviors for HIV infection is having unprotected sexual intercourse. For the purpose of designing a health promotion intervention, this risk behavior can be restated into two health-promoting behaviors: (1) using condoms when having sexual intercourse and (2) choosing not to have sexual intercourse when not protected. In this case the objectives of the Intervention Mapping process would be directed at obtaining and improving the performance of these two behaviors (Begley, Fourney, Elreda, & Teleki, 2002).

When thinking of behavioral change, planners can focus on different types of behaviors. As a matter of fact, one of the difficulties in planning health education programs is confusion over what is meant by the term *behavior*. Examples of types of behavior are risk reduction, health promotion, screening and early detection, compliance or adherence, and self-management.

Risk-Reduction Behaviors. Epidemiologists look at risk factors as a way of understanding causes of disease and factors associated with higher prevalence and incidence of disease in different populations. For example, documented cardiovascular disease risk factors include hypertension, hyperlipidemia, lack of exercise, genetics, stress, and smoking (Kannel, D'Agostino, Sullivan, & Wilson, 2004; Labarthe, 1998; Labarthe, 1999; Luepker, 1998; Shekelle et al., 1981). The underlying assumption is that, if an intervention can reduce the prevalence of the risk factors, it can reduce the prevalence of the disease (depending on how closely they are linked). The difficulty in designing interventions based on these risk factors is that they are not all clearly behavioral causes of the disease. There is a mixture of physiological and behavioral risks. The first task is to sort out what behavior is related to morbidity and mortality. For example, heart disease is associated with hyperlipidemia (a physiological risk), which is strongly influenced by diet (a behavioral risk) (Bayne-Smith et al., 2004; Frank, Vaden, & Martin, 1987; Labarthe, 1998, 1999; Smalley, Wittler, & Oliverson, 2004). Thus, risk behaviors, as opposed to risk factors, are defined as actions, such as eating certain foods that have been demonstrated to increase directly the risk of disease or disability. An intervention can be approached from a population perspective, in which it is designed to reduce the prevalence of the risk behavior within a defined population; or it can be approached from an individual perspective, in which it is designed to help the individual stop (or not start) the risk behavior. Because of the addictive nature of some behaviors, for example, smoking, the goal is the elimination of the behavior, not just a reduction. For other behaviors, for example, fat intake, the goal is a reduction. However, some behaviors that contribute to fat intake, such as cooking with saturated fat, might be eliminated altogether. The desired impact of a health education program on risk behaviors is to reduce or eliminate the practice and prevalence of these behaviors.

Health-Promoting Behaviors. A health-promoting behavior is, in some cases, the opposite of a risk behavior. For example, if eating high-fat food were the risk behavior, then eating low-fat food would be the health-promoting behavior. In contrast, some behaviors, such as getting immunizations, wearing a bicycle helmet, wearing a seat belt, or using a condom, are health promoting because they protect against a potential risk (D. L. Kelly, Zito, & Weber, 2003). Increasing the practice of health-promoting behaviors can be viewed as an action taken to enhance health or provide protection.

Often health education and health promotion are directed to primary prevention (preventing a health problem before it occurs). However, the same principles of intervention can apply to secondary prevention (reducing the consequences of a disease or slowing its progress). Secondary prevention is especially important for diseases in which early signs or symptoms are not apparent. When symptoms are not present or not easily detectable by laypeople, screening is necessary to identify individuals at high risk for the disease or to detect the disease process early so that appropriate medical treatment can be started to prevent more severe illnesses or mortality (U.S. Preventive Services Task Force, 2004). For example, mammography is used to screen for changes in the breast to detect breast cancer in the early stages, when treatment has the best chance of effectiveness (Alcoe, Wallace, & Beck, 1990; Hurley & Kaldor, 1992; Smart, Hendrick,

Rutledge, & Smith, 1995). Other recommended tests are the Pap test for cervical cancer (R. A. Smith, Cokkinides, & Eyre, 2003), self-exam and clinical skin exam for skin cancer (Saraiya et al., 2004), and four different recommended tests for colorectal cancer (Pignone, Rich, Teutsch, Berg, & Lohr, 2002; Tilley et al., 1999; Walsh & Terdiman, 2003). Tests for blood pressure and blood cholesterol levels are examples of screening tests for elevated risk for cardiovascular disease (Abel, Darby, & Ramachandran, 1994; Labarthe, 1998; Ohkubo et al., 1997; Thompson, Pyke, & Wood, 1996). Screening tests are also used to detect infectious diseases such as sexually transmitted infections (STIs) and HIV (Janssen et al., 2001, 2002; U.S. Preventive Services Task Force, 2004) and genetic diseases such as Tay-Sachs disease (Natowicz & Prence, 1996) and cystic fibrosis (Brock, 1996; Livingstone, Axton, Mennie, Gilfillan, & Brock, 1993).

Screening and early detection range from self-administered tests to complicated medical procedures, but almost all require some behavior by the person at risk. Participation in screening requires an individual's decision and action. Health education programs can influence individuals to make decisions to participate. In general, interventions are usually designed to motivate individuals to participate in self-administered screening or to seek out and attend screening procedures by health professionals (Craun & Deffenbacher, 1987; Hou, Fernandez, & Parcel, 2004). The exact nature of the behavior is specific to the screening method and the purpose of the screening. Some screening involves a onetime behavior (that is, going to a health care facility and having blood or other specimens taken to be examined by a laboratory or health care professional). Other screening procedures, such as breast self-examination, are repeated and require skills, reliable procedures, and long-term maintenance (Agars & McMurray, 1993).

Some screening procedures, such as genetic testing and prostate cancer screening with a prostate specific antigen test (PSA), are controversial in that there are no agreed-upon guidelines for screening (American Urological Association, 2000). Instead, there are recommendations for informed decision-making processes (with or without the provider) to determine whether or not to have the test (Briss et al., 2004; Myers et al., 1999; Rimer, Briss, Zeller, Chan, & Woolf, 2004). In these cases the behavioral goal is making an informed decision rather than engaging in screening. Thus, intervention strategies must target the type of behavior necessary to make the screening effective.

Adherence and Self-Management Behaviors. Patient education, a specific type of health education, can help individuals who are receiving health care for a diagnosed health problem not only to adhere to the prescribed therapy but also to understand the disease and treatment better (Alewijnse, Mesters, Metsemakers, & van den Borne, 2002). With most forms of medical therapy, the patient is usually expected to follow through with the recommendations of the health care provider. The extent to which the patient follows through with the recommended action is referred to as a level of adherence (Brawley & Culos-Reed, 2000). The field has moved from the term *compliance* to the term *adherence* to avoid the implication that the patient is being told what to do without having any involvement in the decision. For example, if a patient were instructed to take antibiotic medication three times a day for ten days, full adherence would mean taking the right dose at the right time each day for ten days. Studies have shown that, for most recommended follow-up procedures, adherence is incomplete (DiMatteo & DiNicola, 1985; Rapoff, 1999; Riekert & Drotar, 2000; Sackett & Snow, 1979). Thus, the goal of health education interventions in this case is to improve adherence behavior.

Often the behavior required for follow-up to medical care is much more complex than simply adhering to a set of instructions, especially in the case of chronic illnesses for which management of the condition requires the patients or their families to take continuing action at home or elsewhere outside of health care facilities (Brug, Schols, & Mesters, 2004; D'Angelo, 2001). Good disease management depends on making judgments to take action based on changing physiological conditions and life situations. For example, someone with diabetes must manage the disease by balancing the intake of food, expenditure of energy, and medication (Glasgow et al., 1992). This type of behavior is referred to as self-management because monitoring, decision making, and action must be made independently of the health care provider (Creer, 2000a, 2000b; Clark, Janz, Dodge, & Sharpe, 1992; Clark et al., 1997; Dodge, Janz, & Clark, 2002; N. M. Clark & Zimmerman, 1990; Gibson et al., 2003). The goals for self-management may include increasing the performance of the behavior as well as improving the quality of the behavior, for example, helping the patient become better at decision making and problem solving (Cameron & Leventhal, 2003; N. M. Clark et al., 1997).

Stating Behavioral Outcomes

Behavioral outcomes should be stated in terms of the behaviors to be accomplished as a result of the health education or promotion program. The following statements are examples of health-related behavioral outcomes:

- Reduce total fat intake to 30 percent of calories.
- Increase eating of low-fat foods to include five servings of fruits and vegetables per day.
- Use condoms correctly and consistently when having sexual intercourse.
- Monitor symptoms of asthma to detect early changes in status of illness.

Later in this chapter, we present the matrices from a recently conducted project called Sun Protection Is Fun (Project SPF). Funded by the U.S. National Cancer Institute, Project SPF developed and tested an intervention to prevent skin cancer by reducing preschool children's exposure to ultraviolet rays (Tripp, Herrmann, Parcel, Chamberlain, & Gritz, 2000). Children are the at-risk group for the project, and parents and preschool day-care center staff are additional intervention participants because they are part of the interpersonal and organizational environment of the children and can play a role in protecting children from sun exposure and early damage to the skin. These environmental agents also help to establish children's behavioral patterns and habits for sun protection. Because of the children's age, they can take only limited action by themselves to achieve protection from the sun and to reduce the amount of exposure to ultraviolet rays. Therefore, most of the focus of Project SPF is on the behavior of others in the children's environment and on environmental change at the interpersonal and organizational levels (see example of environmental conditions later in this chapter). The project team stated the health-promoting behaviors for the child that will likely be brought about by changes in the child's environment this way:

- Remain indoors or in full shade during peak sun times of 11:00 A.M. to 3:00 P.M.
- Wear sunscreen with a sun protection factor (SPF) greater than fifteen when outdoors.

Identifying Environmental Conditions

In the needs assessment, environmental factors are identified as social or physical conditions that influence risk behavior (thus acting as indirect causes of the health problem) or that cause the health problem directly. The needs-assessment process should lead to an identification of environmental conditions that influence the risk behavior or the health problem and to a prioritization of conditions according to their importance and changeability (see Chapter Five). When planners conduct an environmental analysis, they realize that they must consider each level of the environment as embedded in and having reciprocal influences with the higher levels (L. Richard, Gauvin, Potvin, Denis, & Kishchuk, 2002).

Interpersonal Environment. Humans are embedded in social systems. Families are the primary influence for socialization of children and continue to have an effect on behavior throughout life. As children grow older, peer groups become more important, beginning with playmates and continuing with friends, neighbors, coworkers, and members of organizations with which they affiliate (such as churches, social clubs, and service groups). Certain individuals may hold special influence by the role they play, such as teachers, coaches, religious leaders, or health care providers.

Social support is a protective factor for health outcomes that researchers have studied extensively (Ganster & Victor, 1988; Heaney & Israel, 2002; Hogan, Linden, & Najarian, 2002; House, Umberson, & Landis, 1988; McLeroy, Gottlieb, & Heaney, 2001). The types of support that individuals may receive from their social networks include emotional support, information or advice, material support, maintenance of social identity, and social outreach (Heaney & Israel, 2002; Israel, 1982; Jacobson, 1986; McLeroy et al., 2001). Social support may influence health through several pathways. There is considerable evidence that it buffers the effects of stress through the processes of cognitive appraisal of stress and coping (L. F. Berkman & Glass, 2000; Heaney & Israel, 2002; Hirsch & DuBois, 1992; House et al., 1988; Rhodes, Contreras, & Mangelsdorf, 1994). The environment may provide modeling and reinforcement for the practice of specific health behaviors (Cohen et al., 1988; Epstein & Wing, 1987), and it may also directly influence physiological health, including immune function and blood pressure (Earp & Ory, 1979; Kiecolt-Glaser, McGuire, Robles, & Glaser, 2002; Morisky, DeMuth, Field-Fass, Green, & Levine, 1985; Seeman, 2000; Uchino, Holt-Lunstad, Uno, Betancourt, & Garvey, 1999). The presence or absence of supports from important others within the individuals' immediate interpersonal environment may have an influence on the performance of the health behavior as well as on the health outcomes.

The Child and Adolescent Trial for Cardiovascular Health, known as the CATCH program, a school-based intervention program to prevent cardiovascular disease among children in elementary school, is an example of how program planning can focus on instrumental support of children's health behaviors by parents and school staff (C. L. Perry et al., 1990, 1997). Developers intended the CATCH program to influence children's diet, physical activity, and tobacco-use behavior. The school program addressed change at the individual level for the students and change at the organizational level to modify environmental conditions in the school to be more favorable and supportive of healthy eating and physical activity. In addition, the CATCH program planners hypothesized that parental support for the children eating low-fat food and being physically active would be an important environmental factor; they therefore evaluated the added effectiveness of a program component that addressed support from the children's parents. The focus of the family component of CATCH was not on the diet, physical activity, or smoking behavior of the parents but more directly on how they could support their children's healthy behavior (Nader, Sellers, Johnson, Perry, Stone, et al., 1996).

In another example of interpersonal environment, the Watch, Discover, Think, and Act asthma program targeted the behavior of physicians in prescribing anti-inflammatory medication to children, providing an asthma action plan, and reinforcing the child and family's management efforts (Bartholomew, Gold, et al., 2000; Bartholomew, Shegog, et al., 2000). The program developers also focused on the supportive behavior of parents, school nurses, and teachers with regard to self-management (see Chapter Twelve). In a subsequent asthma program developed to accompany Watch, Discover, Think, and Act, the focus of the intervention was on the parent's behaviors (an important person in the interpersonal environment of a child with asthma). This program, called Families and Schools Together for Asthma Management (or Familias) (Fernandez, Bartholomew, Lopez, et al., 2000; Fernandez, Bartholomew, Sockrider, et al., 2000; Lopez, 2004) focused on increasing parent asthma management behavior among Hispanic parents and began with the identification of specific parental behaviors that influence management of childhood asthma. The Familias project is fully described in Chapter Fourteen.

The following statements are examples of specific parent behaviors from Familias that represent an important component of the child's interpersonal environment:

- Obtain a diagnosis of asthma from a health care provider
- Reduce the child's exposure to triggers
- Manage the child's symptoms
- Take the child for regular medical care

Organizational Environment. Organizational environments include elements such as norms, policies, practices, and facilities (Oldenburg, Sallis, Harris, & Owen, 2002; Steenhuis, Van Assema, & Glanz, 2001). For example, policies can exert strong control over behavior, as in work-site bans on smoking, which have been shown to reduce the number of cigarettes that workers consume in a workday (Brownson, Eriksen, Davis, & Warner, 1997; Eriksen & Gottlieb, 1998). In other examples, combinations of preventive health care policies and health care facility characteristics such as service hours can determine whether workers obtain care. The availability of corporate exercise facilities and the personnel practices of management may each have an impact on workers' physical activity. In the school asthma management project, the planning team assessed the physical environment of the schools to identify potential triggers for asthma symptoms (Tortolero et al., 2002).

The CATCH program also provides examples of addressing environmental conditions at the organizational level. CATCH addressed the organizational practices of cafeteria food preparation and physical education teaching. In addition, the program addressed policies regarding tobacco use on school grounds and during school-sponsored activities. Organizational-level change was needed to make it easier for children to eat healthy food, be physically active, and avoid exposure to tobacco use.

In Project SPF the unavailability of sunscreen, the lack of shade on the playground, and the time schedule for outside play are organizational conditions that contribute either directly to increased risk of exposure or indirectly by making the protective behaviors more difficult to perform. These conditions are under the control of the center directors, who may be influenced by parents, teachers, or voluntary health agencies to take steps to decrease children's risk of skin cancer.

Community Environment. The community environment contains conditions that affect the health of populations, either through behavior or directly. Examples of these conditions include availability of work and income, the quality and quantity of housing, health care, availability of recreational resources, smoking and other health ordinances, law enforcement, judicial practices, and treatment resources for social problems such as child abuse, violence, and drug addiction. Further, community environment issues deal with social capital and the capacity of the community to form and maintain problem-solving relationships (R. M. Goodman et al., 1998; Kreuter & Lezin, 2002; Minkler & Wallerstein, 1997a, 1997b; Norton, McLeroy, Burdine, Felix, & Dorsey, 2002). Examples of supportive environments that communities have achieved through health promotion projects include protecting communities against diesel fuel particulates (Kinney, Aggarwal, Northridge, Janssen, & Shepard, 2000; Northridge et al., 1999), protecting children from the hazard of high unbarred windows from which they could fall (Schulz & Northridge, 2004), and establishing a runaway house for young people in Finland (Haglund, Finer, Tillgren, & Pettersson, 1996).

Society. The societal level focuses on legislation, enforcement, regulation, and resource allocation as well as policies, programs, and facilities of large political and geographic groups. Societal influences often function through governments, which may be at the local, state, national, or international level. For example, legislation that influences tobacco use includes minors' access laws, clean air acts, and tobacco excise taxes. These laws, along with lawsuits against tobacco companies by states and individuals, have been pivotal to the success of the tobacco control movement (Wisotzky, Albuqureque, Pechacek, & Park, 2004; Warner, 2001; Lynch & Bonnie, 1994; Task Force on Community Preventive Services, 2001). State and federal agencies, including those for health, human services, education, agriculture, transportation, and food and drugs, originate regulations, policies, and programs that affect health status. Societal influences may work on individual behavior, such as the America Responds to AIDS campaign of the CDC (Gentry & Jorgensen, 1991), or directly on the physical environment, such as regulations for road construction in New Zealand (Haglund et al., 1996). They may also work through organizations, for example, by allocating resources to set up drug-free schools (Brandon, 1992; Fox, Forbing, & Anderson, 1988). Healthy Cities projects have focused on intersectoral policy development that aims to create supportive environments for health and to integrate health into the economy, culture, and life of the community (Awofeso, 2003; Goumans & Springett, 1997).

Stating the Environmental Outcomes

Intervention Mapping guides planners to consider those environmental factors in the needs assessment that require change and to state clearly the desired environmental outcome that the health promotion program is to achieve. For example, if the needs assessment finds a lack of low-fat food options at school that contributes to schoolchildren's high-fat diets, one of the desired outcomes can be stated as follows: increase the availability of low-fat foods offered in school lunch and breakfast programs to include options with less than 30 percent of calories from fat at every meal. Accomplishment of this environmental outcome would result in more low-fat food options being available in the school cafeteria and would make it easier for children to select and eat low-fat foods.

Project SPF illustrates how both behavior and environmental conditions need to be addressed to accomplish the program objectives. Young children who attend day-care and preschool education programs spend an average of six to eight hours a day at these centers during the time of day when exposure to the sun is likely to be the most intense and most harmful. The project planning team stated the health-promoting environmental outcomes for parents and preschools that the intervention needed to address as follows:

- Apply SPF 15+ to children before their exposure to the sun
- Reapply SPF 15+ sunscreen to children when no longer effective (every 1.5 to 2 hours, or after swimming or profuse sweating)
- Dress children in protective clothing such as hats, sleeved shirts, long shorts, and sunglasses
- Direct children to play in shaded areas

An assessment of preschools identified three environmental conditions at the organizational level that either contributed directly to increased risk of exposure or contributed indirectly by making the protective behaviors more difficult to perform. These conditions were the unavailability of sunscreen, the lack of shade on the playground, and the time of day of scheduled playtime. The following environmental conditions at the organizational level were stated for Project SPF:

- Provide SPF 15+ sunscreen in the preschools and day-care centers for staff to apply to children
- Increase the amount of shade in the play areas
- Schedule activities so that children are not outside during peak sun hours

Peformance Objectives

⤸ *The second task in Intervention Mapping Step 2 is to subdivide behavioral and environmental outcomes into performance objectives.*

Once the program planners have defined the program's behavioral and environmental outcomes, they write performance objectives for each of them. The use of performance objectives is not new, nor is it unique to health education. For example, therapeutic outcomes are sometimes stated in performance terms at the individual client level, and, on an organizational level, quality assurance defines a standard of performance to maintain certain levels of service or production. In education, performance objectives usually reflect academic performance (Bloom, 1956; Gagne, Briggs, & Wagner, 1992). In the area of training, participants must perform at a criterion level in order for a program to be successful. Although the term *performance objectives* may not be applied exactly the same way in each of these examples, they are used to further delineate behavioral and environmental program outcomes.

Performance Objectives for Behaviors

When first considered, behavioral outcomes usually are broad conceptualizations: Stop smoking. Don't drink and drive. Exercise aerobically thirty minutes per day. Eat less than 30 percent of calories from fat. These injunctions do not have sufficient detail on which to base an intervention. Therefore, we use performance objectives to clarify the exact performance expected from someone affected by the intervention. To determine the performance objectives for behavior, planners ask: What do the participants in this program or the environmental agents need to do to perform the behavior or to make the environmental change stated in the behavioral or environmental outcomes? Performance objectives enable planners to make a transition from a behavior or environmental condition to a detailed description of its components. For example, eating a low-fat diet is a health-promoting behavior, but many subbehaviors or components make up that broader behavior. To perform the behavior, an individual would need to take many actions, including the following: read labels, select low-fat food, prepare low-fat food, and avoid the use of fat additives. These subbehaviors, specified by action words, become the performance objectives. They are used to refine, focus, and make more specific what the program participants must do as a result of the intervention.

The performance objectives also help ensure the appropriateness of the program's behavioral expectations. For example, eating low-fat food might have a different set of performance objectives for schoolchildren than for an adult with a high risk for cardiovascular disease. In another example Graeff, Elder, and Booth (1993) describe an intervention focused on mothers' hand washing in Guatemala. These researchers suggest that the experts often disagree about the components of ideal performance in terms of what is really necessary to have a health impact. They describe lengthy discussions by experts about how many times the hands should be rubbed, whether fingernails should be cleaned, and whether each fingernail should be washed separately. The experts' disagreements are arguments for (rather than against) good behavioral specification. Health educators have less chance of changing a behavior if they do not know precisely what it is. In the program that Graeff and colleagues described, the project team defined the ideal hand washing as a set of discrete steps that the mothers would perform at various times: they would wash hands after using the latrine, before and after preparing food, before eating, before giving food to an infant, after changing a diaper, before entering the home, before going to bed, and before touching the cooking or drinking water. Unfortunately, the original performance objectives for this project required the mother to bring an extra jug of water into her home every day and spend one hour a day washing her hands. The original objectives were impractical; they were later extensively modified to include addition of an environmental change to make the entire process less consuming of both time and water.

Some branches of education, such as curriculum and instruction, sometimes make little distinction between learning objectives and performance objectives. Both usually are specified in cognitive or affective (rather than behavioral) terms, and the terms for these types of objectives are sometimes used interchangeably (Gronlund, 1978; Mager, 1984). Intervention Mapping makes a clear distinction. Most cognitive and affective performance is related to the determinants of behavior and is considered part of change objectives, which are described later in this chapter. Planners can distinguish performance objectives from change objectives by thinking of the performance objective as an observable subset of the behavior and a change objective as what the priority population must learn or change in order to meet or maintain the performance objective.

Changing health-related behaviors and environmental conditions usually requires complex multistep processes. These processes, described as performance objectives, are what has to be done to accomplish the change. The specification of performance objectives helps program planners to sequence the behavioral learning process when the learner needs to learn one part before another and to include all necessary supports for the behavior. For example, Table 6.1 illustrates how to break down the behavior of using condoms correctly and consistently when having sexual intercourse into subcomponents, which are the performance objectives.

TABLE 6.1. PERFORMANCE OBJECTIVES FOR CONSISTENTLY AND CORRECTLY USING CONDOMS DURING SEXUAL INTERCOURSE.

1. Buy Condoms
   1.1. Locate condom displays in drug or grocery store
   1.2. Choose condoms that are product tested
2. Carry condoms or have condoms easily available
   2.1. Carry condoms in wallet or purse for no longer than a month
   2.2. Carry or store condoms in place that is not susceptible to extreme temperatures
3. Negotiate the use of a condom with a partner*
   3.1. State mutual goals such as pregnancy or AIDS prevention
   3.2. State clearly intention of using a condom as a prerequisite for intercourse
   3.3. Listen to partner's concerns
   3.4. Pose solutions to partner's concerns that reference mutual goals and personal requirements
4. Correctly apply condoms during use
   4.1. Use a water-soluble rather than petroleum-based lubricant
   4.2. Use a new condom for each occurrence of intercourse
   4.3. Follow instructions on package insert for use
   4.4. Follow instructions on package insert for disposal
5. Maintain use over time

*Example of using theory to specify performance objectives. This uses negotiation theory as described by R. Fisher and Ury, 1991.

Performance Objectives for Environmental Conditions

The process for writing performance objectives for changing environmental conditions parallels the process for writing performance objectives for health behaviors. The condition stated in the environmental outcome must be broken down into its component parts. For example, at the organizational level, one can break down the environmental outcome "School lunch and breakfast provide meals that are no more than 30 percent of calories in total fat content" into the following performance objectives for environmental change agents:

- Food service directors will modify menus so that foods have 30 percent or fewer calories from fat.
- Food service directors will modify purchase order specifications to reduce the fat content of vendor-prepared food to 30 percent or lower.
- Nutritionists will modify recipes to reduce the fat content by replacing fat with bouillon or water for boiling or "frying."
- Nutritionists will replace dessert recipes that call for fat with recipes that substitute fruit and grains.
- Cooks will modify cooking practices to reduce the fat content of prepared foods by chilling foods, removing the fat, and then reheating to serve.

The basic question to ask to determine performance objectives for changing environmental conditions is: What does someone in the environment need to do to accomplish the environmental outcome? This general question addresses who is doing the action to accomplish the objective, because the agent may be different for each of the performance objectives. This question is somewhat different from the question asked about performance objectives for the health-related behavior, because the health behavior question assumes a reference to the behavior of the at-risk population. Environmental change usually requires people outside the at-risk population to take action to modify the environmental conditions.

Exactly who will be taking the action to accomplish the performance objectives will depend on the agent in the environment who has control over or can influence a modification in the environmental conditions. This agent might be, for example, family members, policymakers, lawmakers, resource controllers, or service providers. In the beginning of the planning process, it may be difficult to identify specific people to include in the performance objectives for modifying an environmental condition. We suggest starting with whatever information may be available about the agent and stating the "who" in terms of general groups of people or appropriate positions of responsibility, that is, roles or agents that may be able to accomplish the performance objective. As work on the intervention progresses, the health educator can figure out specifically who, in terms of either roles or individuals, will perform the modification in the environmental condition.

Project SPF provides a good example. The performance objectives listed in Table 6.2 were constructed to enable modification of the environmental conditions. At the interpersonal level of the environment, the focus was primarily on the behavior of the parents and preschool staff to protect children from sun exposure. The sun-protective behaviors of parents and preschool staff were fairly simple. However, the stated performance objectives added specificity that enabled the program planners to more effectively communicate the essential components that the intervention should address.

TABLE 6.2. ENVIRONMENTAL PERFORMANCE OBJECTIVES FOR THE SPF PROJECT.

Interpersonal Environment

Behavior 1: Apply sunscreen with a sun protection factor (SPF) of 15+ to children before exposure to the sun

  1.1. Parents and preschool staff apply sunscreen at least thirty minutes before going outside.

  1.2. Parents and preschool staff spread sunscreen evenly.

  1.3. Parents and preschool staff cover all exposed areas head to toe.

Behavior 2: Reapply SPF 15+ sunscreen to children when no longer effective

  2.1. Parents and preschool staff carry sunscreen on outdoor outings.

  2.2. Parents and preschool staff reapply sunscreen after more than two hours of continued exposure to sun.

  2.3. Parents and preschool staff reapply sunscreen after swimming or profuse sweating.

Behavior 3: Dress children in protective clothing (hats, sleeved shirts, long shorts, and sunglasses)

  3.1. Parents and preschool staff ensure protective clothing is with child at day care.

  3.2. Parents and preschool staff ensure protective clothing is worn before going outside.

  3.3. Parents and preschool staff ensure protective clothing stays on child when outside.

TABLE 6.2. ENVIRONMENTAL PERFORMANCE OBJECTIVES FOR THE SPF PROJECT, Cont'd.

Behavior 4: Direct children to play in the shade

4.1. Parents and preschool staff locate shaded areas.

4.2. Parents and preschool staff plan activities for shaded areas.

Behavior 5: Reduce unnecessary sun exposure

5.1. Parents and preschool staff limit time children spend in the sun.

5.2. Parents and preschool staff avoid peak sun hours.

Organizational Environment

Behavior 6: Provide SPF 15+ sunscreen in the day care centers for staff to apply to children

6.1. Preschool directors purchase or obtain sunscreen with an SPF of 15+.

6.2. Preschool teachers modify daily schedules to allow time to apply sunscreen to children.

Behavior 7: Increase the amount of shade in the play areas

7.1. Preschool directors decide to prioritize increasing the amount of shade in play areas used by preschoolers.

7.2. Preschool staff will assess the adequacy of the current natural and structural shaded areas and determine ways to increase shade.

7.3. Preschool directors assess available resources for accomplishing changes to increase shade.

7.4. Preschool directors and/or governing board will seek additional resources to accomplish changes to increase shade.

7.5. Preschool directors determine structures to implement based on ranking of effectiveness and feasibility.

7.6. Preschool directors seek feedback from teachers and staff.

7.7. Preschool directors garner administrative approval for proposed changes.

Behavior 8: Schedule activities so children are not outside during peak sun hours

8.1. Preschool teachers will determine which outdoor activities fall within peak sun hours.

8.2. Preschool teachers will modify schedules to keep children indoors during peak sun hours.

8.3. Preschool directors approve and communicate the modified schedule.

Core Processes for Writing Performance Objectives

How to break down a health-related behavior or an environmental condition into subparts is not always apparent and may require additional thinking and information. The core processes presented in Chapter Two serve as guides for writing performance objectives as applied in the following steps.

The starting place is to formulate a question. For health-related behavior, the question is: What do the participants of this program need to do to perform the health-related behavior? For environmental conditions, the question is: What does someone in the environment need to do to accomplish the environmental condition? The answers to these questions form a provisional list of performance objectives. Often the initial list is a logical sequence of smaller steps that are necessary to perform the behavior or achieve the environmental condition.

Next, the planner reviews the research and practice literature to determine whether the performance objectives on the initial list are consistent with what the literature reports as essential subparts of the behavior or environmental condition. The review results in revisions, deletions, or additions to the initial list.

Sometimes theory provides a rationale for performance objectives. For example, a self-management approach to behavior change can help the planner develop performance objectives, especially for complex behavior (Bandura, 1986; Barlow, Wright, Sheasby, Turner, & Hainsworth, 2002; Creer, 2000a, 2000b; Gibson et al., 2003; Scheier & Carver, 2003; Zimmerman, 2000). In that case the subprocesses of self-control, self-monitoring, comparison to a personal standard, self-evaluation, and reward would become performance objectives as they relate to a specific behavior. Often these processes are expanded to include goal setting, implementation intentions, monitoring and appraisal, problem identification, solution identification, action, and evaluation (N. M. Clark, 2003; N. M. Clark & Zimmerman, 1990; Gollwitzer, 1999; Abraham, Sheeran, & Johnston, 1998; Janis & Mann, 1977; Lazarus, 1993; B. J. Zimmerman, Bonner, Evans, & Mellins, 1999). Behavior change for establishing a healthier diet, for instance, might be approached with specific dietary advice, such as choosing low-fat cheese or abstaining from snacks, but such a list of specific behaviors would be long and impractical. A self-regulatory approach might look quite different from a list of specific dos and don'ts. It might include the following:

- To monitor one's own food intake
- To compare intake to personal goals based on guidelines for a healthy diet
- To decide if discrepancies exist

- To make a detailed plan of implementation intentions and take action to improve dietary behavior
- To evaluate the action's effects
- To recycle to self-monitoring

The specific actions needed would vary by person and setting.

Health educators may find it useful to consider the self-regulatory process when designating health-promoting behaviors for the self-management of chronic disease. For example, in a pediatric asthma self-management program, Bartholomew and colleagues (Bartholomew, Gold, et al., 2000; Bartholomew, Shegog, et al., 2000) conceptualized both asthma-specific behaviors (for example, taking control medications) and self-regulatory behaviors (for example, monitoring for symptoms of asthma) in their performance objectives (see Chapter Twelve). For the Familias project, Fernandez, Bartholomew, Lopez, and colleagues (2000) described specific performance objectives using self-regulatory constructs for parents' management of their child's asthma.

Another example of the application of a self-regulatory approach to health behaviors can be found in HIV-prevention programs. Table 6.3 presents a comparison of performance objectives for condom use. Schaalma and colleagues (see Chapter Eleven), working with adolescents and focusing specifically on condom use, decided on seven specific performance objectives. Van Kesteren, Hospers, Kok, and van Empelen (2005), however, working with HIV-positive gay men and focusing on safe sex in a broader framework of sexual health—which is a more complex behavior—applied a self-regulatory approach.

Other theories that have been used to create performance objectives are negotiation (Fisher & Ury, 1991), coping (Lazarus, 1993; Lazarus & Folkman, 1991) and relapse prevention (Marlatt & Gordon, 1985). In the Cystic Fibrosis Family Education Program (CF FEP), Bartholomew, Sockrider and colleagues (1993) used coping theory to delineate performance objectives for the self-management of cystic fibrosis. Applying work by Lazarus (1993) that suggests that coping is situation specific, should be judged by its effectiveness, and depends on accurate appraisal of situations and flexibility in problem-solving alternatives, the cystic fibrosis project team specified the coping objectives in Table 6.4.

Finally, the planner will review the list of performance objectives and reduce the list to essential objectives needed to perform the behavior or achieve the environmental condition. This step is important because each performance objective is the basis for further work. Each will be linked with determinants to form change objectives. Nonessential (interesting but not necessary) performance objectives will expand the subsequent planning and potentially diffuse the intervention's focus.

TABLE 6.3. COMPARISON OF PERFORMANCE OBJECTIVES.

Adolescent Condom Use (Schaalma, Kok, Poelman, & Reinders, 1994)	HIV+ Men Who Have Sex with Men (MSM) Safe Sex (Van Kesteren, Hospers, Kok, and van Empelen, 2005)
1. Make an adequate decision on future condom use to prevent human immunodeficiency virus (HIV) infection	1. (MSM) Self-observe sexual behavior and compare sexual behavior to standard of safer sex
2. Buy condoms	2. Identify when a problem exists
3. Carry condoms regularly	3. Implement solutions:
4. Communicate about condom use with potential sex partners within the context of both one-night stands and regular dates	3.1. Decide to use nonpenetrative sexual techniques
5. Use condoms correctly and consistently	3.2. Decide to use condoms for anal sex
6. Maintain condom use in teenage years	• 3.2.1. Purchase condoms
7. Use condoms in relations that are perceived as steady	• 3.2.2. Carry condoms or have condoms easy available
	• 3.2.3. Negotiate condoms for anal sex
	• 3.2.4. Use condoms correctly and consistently
	• 3.2.5. Maintain use over time
	4. Implement selected coping strategies
	5. Evaluate actions and return to monitoring

Validating Performance Objectives

The planner may also need to collect new data to determine the validity of performance objectives. What do potential participants in the program actually do, or say they do, when performing the behavior? Data may also be collected from service providers, key informants, or persons who may implement the program (Averch, 1994).

To validate performance objectives, the planners obtain additional information by questioning and observing both members of the intervention groups and the service providers. The CF FEP illustrates the process of asking service providers to validate performance objectives (Bartholomew et al., 1993). Program planners sent the draft of performance objectives for cystic fibrosis (CF) self-management to a panel of five physicians who specialize in the treatment of CF and five behavioral scientists experienced at working with CF patients. The panel

TABLE 6.4. PERFORMANCE OBJECTIVES USING COPING THEORY.

Members of a family of a child with Cystic Fibrosis (CF) use coping strategies to manage CF-related problems:

1. Recognize need to cope with CF

   1.1. Accept CF as the medical diagnosis (including genetics, prognosis, variable course)

   1.2. Acknowledge potential extent of the physical effects of CF

   1.3. Acknowledge that disease-related problems can occur at any time

   1.4. Recognize need for adjustment by child and family to demands of self-care

   1.5. Accept the occurrence of emotional distress to the child and family as a periodic consequence of CF

2. Appraise situations for potential CF-related problems

   2.1. Identify sources of stress

   2.2. Identify personal and family signs of stress

   2.3. Estimate likelihood of undesirable outcomes from stressful situations

3. Generate multiple coping alternatives, including categories of action, stopping action, information-seeking, and thinking or feeling about things differently

   3.1. Acknowledge the value of using a variety of coping strategies (flexibility)

   3.2. Generate alternatives to solve problems, including strategies of seeking information and social support

   3.3. Generate alternatives to ameliorate emotional distress, such as seeking distraction and social support and practicing anxiety management

4. Use selected alternatives from coping strategies generated

   4.1. Use a variety of strategies to solve problems

   4.2. Use a variety of strategies to ameliorate emotional distress

5. Evaluate effectiveness of coping strategies used

   5.1. Judge whether problem has been solved

   5.2. Judge whether new problems have been created through application of coping strategies

   5.3. Judge whether emotional distress has been reduced

   5.4. If coping strategy not judged effective, return to appraisal was asked to rate the importance of each performance objective in contributing to the health and quality of life of a child with CF. Following a revision of the objectives based on the experts' ratings and comments, the performance objectives were sent to all the directors of CF treatment centers in the United States. About 50 percent of the directors returned the questionnaire, which was sufficient to enable the program planners to revise the performance objectives. Although conducting the validation did take some time and resources, the program planners could continue with the intervention development process confident that their performance objectives were in line and consistent with a wide consensus regarding CF care.

Another way to identify or validate performance objectives is to obtain a review and feedback from community representatives. Through focus groups or interviews, potential program participants can be asked whether the performance objectives fit with their views of how they would go about performing the health-related behaviors. Feedback from individuals who have had experience with the health behavior or the environmental condition can be very helpful. For example, in planning a smoking-cessation program, talking with both those who have quit smoking and those who have had difficulty quitting can give the planner ideas of how to construct performance objectives.

An often overlooked but in some cases essential source of information about performance objectives is direct observation of the health behavior or environmental condition. For some health problems, there may be a limited amount of information, experience, or documentation of how the related health behavior is performed or how environmental conditions break down into component parts. Observation of performance in natural settings as well as in simulated settings can be very helpful. For example, program planners developing a nutrition improvement program for schoolchildren can spend time in the school cafeteria observing how children select, trade, modify, and eat or don't eat food. Observations may be done by program planners or by participant observers who are interviewed by or report on their experiences to the program planners. The needs-assessment phase of the Familias program included direct observation of the patient visit with the medical provider. Data collectors described the interaction between the provider and parent and child and gathered information that informed the development of performance objectives for parents and providers (Lopez, 2004).

Performance objectives may also be validated by predicting health-related behaviors from the performance objectives specified within the target population. This approach is illustrated by a study conducted by van Empelen and Kok (2005) to examine the role of preparatory performance in explaining condom use among adolescents. For writing the performance objectives, they relied on experts and theoretical and empirical evidence. Several theories explain that the decision to act is a very important step in getting people to act. However, making the decision to act is not enough. Thus, for young people to use condoms, they should first make the decision to use condoms. The AIDS risk-reduction model has suggested that it is also important that people engage in supportive acts to reduce HIV risk. Empirical evidence could be derived from Sheeran, Abraham, and Orbell (1999), who showed, by means of a meta-analysis, that people are more likely to use condoms when they have condoms available and are discussing condoms. Finally, young people may not maintain condom use. Misovich, Fisher, and Fisher (1997) showed that young people are more likely to use condoms in casual than in steady relationships; but their work also showed that a relationship is rather quickly defined as a steady relationship.

Thus, from the evidence available, van Empelen and Kok (2005) derived young people's performance objectives:

1. They decide to use condoms.
2. They buy condoms.
3. They have condoms available at all times.
4. They discuss condom use with their partner.
5. They use condoms.

In order to encourage maintenance of condom use, it was also important to ensure that adolescents would use condoms with partners in both casual sex and steady sex.

To validate these performance objectives, a prospective survey study was carried out among four hundred secondary school students. The research team focused on the sexually active students and derived that condom use with steady sex partners could be explained by the decision to use condoms with steady sex partners (operationalized as intention) (van Empelen & Kok, 2005). Secondly, they showed that this relationship was mediated by buying and carrying condoms and communicating condom use with steady sex partners. Thus, the results suggested that performance objectives are valuable in explaining condom use among steady sex partners. Moreover, the researchers showed that consistent condom use was negatively related to the quitting of condom use and that people who are using condoms in steady sexual relations are also likely to maintain condom use over a longer period of time. A further examination of the sequence of performance objectives indicated that the decision to use condoms predicted the buying of condoms, which in turn predicted the carrying of condoms, which finally predicted actual condom use. Although communication also increased the likelihood of condom use, the carrying of condoms did not predict communication about condom use.

When focusing on condom use with casual sex partners, van Empelen & Kok (2005) did not find the predicted sequence of performance objectives. Actual condom use with casual sex partners was predicted only by the decision to use condoms, not by the additional performance objectives. Does this mean that they are not important? Not at all. First of all, the data showed that adolescents simply do not prepare themselves for sexual encounters. Second, and possibly because of the lack of anticipation and preparation for possible casual sexual encounters, young people were more willing to engage in unsafe sex. Thus, although the researchers were not able to validate the sequence of performance objectives in the case of casual sex, they were able to show that the lack of such performance objectives enhances risk-taking behavior (that is, not using condoms).

Finally, the study showed that intended condom use did predict actual condom use and condom buying, but not carrying, whereas buying predicted carrying (van Empelen & Kok, 2005). Thus, it seemed that there was a logical sequence of performance objectives.

In summary, the study showed that performance objectives can be validated by asking the target population what they actually do regarding the performance objectives and then determine how the actual performance predicts behavior. Not being able to validate the sequence of performance objectives may, however, also give valuable information, in the sense that performance objectives that professionals find important may not be ones that a priority population recognizes. In this case, the intervention should include those performance objectives and provide the rationale for the at-risk population. This brings us to the third task in Intervention Mapping Step 2, selecting important determinants that may facilitate change (van Empelen, Kok, Schaalma, & Bartholomew, 2003).

Personal and External Determinants

⮌ *The third task in Step 2 is to select important and changeable determinants of the health behavior and environmental conditions.*

Determinants are those factors that have been found to be associated with the performance of the behavior or environmental condition and that can be hypothesized to mediate the behavior of the at-risk group or modification of the environment by the responsible agent. The needs assessment, completed in Step 1, may provide important information on determinants, but more refinement is usually necessary. The writing of the performance objectives adds specificity to the health behaviors and environmental conditions and may help narrow or expand the list of possible determinants. A matrix of change objectives is created by entering the performance objectives into the left column of the matrix and entering the personal and external determinants across the top of the matrix. Because each selected ecological level has a separate matrix, additional decisions will be necessary to assign determinants to each matrix. Determinants may be duplicated in more than one matrix. Basically, if a determinant can be considered an important influence for accomplishing one or more of the performance objectives, it should be included in the matrix.

Those factors that rest within individuals (people at risk or agents in the environment) and are subject to their direct control or influence are referred to as personal determinants. These factors can be changed or influenced by interventions that involve individual learning. Personal determinants usually include cognitive factors (such as knowledge, attitudes, beliefs, values, self-efficacy, expectations) and capabilities, such as skills.

Those factors that rest outside the individual and influence health behavior or environmental conditions are referred to as external determinants. These factors may be social influences (such as norms, social support, and reinforcement) or structural influences (such as access to resources, policies, and organizational climate). The individual is not able to control these factors directly; therefore, change in these determinants is not likely to be accomplished by an individual learning process.

The question arises among students of Intervention Mapping: "What is the difference between an environmental factor and an external determinant?" If the planner looks at the needs assessment logic model, it should be clear that environmental factors are potential determinants of the behavior of the at-risk group and directly of health. Some of these factors are quite important and will require development of their own matrices so that the determinants are adequately analyzed. These important factors should be intervened upon directly with guidance from the environmental matrices. Others are factors that the at-risk group can be taught to manage or change and will be analyzed on the at-risk group matrices as external determinants.

The needs assessment should provide a good starting list of determinants in answer to these questions:

- Why would a person perform a particular behavior?
- Why would a certain environmental agent make an environmental modification?

However, the needs assessment often uncovers more about variables associated with the health problem and the risk behavior and condition. Therefore, this step requires the careful consideration of determinants of the health promoting behavior and environmental conditions.

To answer the questions the planning group first creates a provisional list of answers. To refine or add to this provisional list, the health educator can follow the core processes outlined in Chapter Two. In reviewing the literature, the planner begins with studies regarding the issue at hand (van Empelen, Schaalma, Kok, & Jansen, 2001). Next is the review of theoretical constructs that have been used to explain the health behavior or environmental condition of interest or related behaviors or conditions. Finally, the planner undertakes a review of the literature on general theories that include some of the identified determinants as constructs within those theories (Kok, Schaalma, Ruiter, van Empelen, & Brug, 2004; Murphy & Bennett, 2004). For example, if the review of the literature identified self-efficacy as a possible determinant of the behavior, then going to the literature on Social Cognitive Theory (SCT) for which self-efficacy is a central construct would be useful (Bandura, 1986). A review of the general theory may suggest other constructs that might be considered as important determinants of the health behavior.

The needs-assessment and the literature reviews provide the planner with informed or hypothesized relationships of factors to the health behavior or environmental conditions. Determinants on the provisional list should be well supported by the literature, and the planner should retain only those with the strongest relation to the behaviors. The planner may want to organize the review by levels of evidence and many published systematic reviews give good explanations of how the strength of the evidence was judged and can serve as models.

Planners often need to collect data from the at-risk groups and environmental agents to identify additional determinants and to understand how determinants manifest in a particular group. Qualitative methods, such as focus groups or interviews, can be helpful in generating new ideas for determinants or in verifying some of the findings from the research literature. Quantitative data collection, using questionnaires that measure the determinants and the health behavior and environmental conditions of interest, can be especially helpful in judging the strength of the association between determinants and behavior or environmental conditions. With both types of data collection, planners can estimate the presence or absence of the determinant, as well as its importance for influencing change. For example, in designing an AIDS-prevention program for adolescents, knowledge about the seriousness of AIDS may at first be viewed as an important determinant of risk-reduction behavior. However, formative research may show that adolescents already know about AIDS. Therefore, it is unlikely that an intervention to increase knowledge about AIDS will have much of an effect on that group's behavior. Another way to judge whether a determinant is important is to measure the determinant in population subgroups: those who practice the behavior and those who do not. For example, if children who eat five servings of fruits and vegetables daily have a high self-efficacy for the behavior and those who eat only two servings of fruits and vegetables daily have a low self-efficacy for the behavior, then self-efficacy is likely to be an important determinant.

Eventually, the planner must refine the list of determinants. A long list of determinants is not practical for program development. Determinants that have weak evidence of association or no logical or theoretical interrelatedness are unlikely to be useful foci for an intervention. Therefore, careful analysis of the determinants at this stage improves planning results at later stages. To conduct this analysis, planners can start by rating each determinant in terms of relevance (that is, strength of association with the behavior or environmental condition) and changeability (that is, how likely it is that health education or promotion intervention is going to influence a change in the determinant).

As much as possible, the basis for rating relevance and changeability should be based on evidence from the research literature. Sometimes, the literature will not adequately discuss a proposed determinant, and the planner will need to collect data from the at-risk group and from others in the field. In addition, decisions to retain or delete determinants may be based entirely on a theoretical or conceptual basis when data are not available. For example, the evidence may be strong for one determinant (such as self-efficacy), but the literature may provide little evidence to support the relevance of a related factor (such as outcome expectations). However, the theoretical literature suggests that these two constructs are interrelated, and for some behaviors it may be important to address both with intervention strategies (Bandura, 1986, 1997). There may be situations in which the literature provides little evidence for a hypothetical determinant, but you may find literature that supports the importance of a determinant for a similar behavior. For example, you may not find evidence to support the relationship between perceived risk and use of clinical breast examination, but there may be literature that supports the importance of this determinant for mammography screening.

Matrix of Change Objectives

⊃ *The fourth task in Step 2 is to create the matrices. Related to this task are the processes of selecting intervention levels and differentiating the population.*

Performance objectives and determinants are the building blocks of matrices. Matrices are simple tables, formed by entering the performance objectives on the left side of the matrix and determinants along the top (see the matrices for Project SPF in Tables 6.5 and 6.6). Change objectives are entered into the cells formed at the intersection of each performance objective and determinant. Conceptually, a matrix of program objectives represents the pathways for the most

TABLE 6.5. MATRIX FOR AT-RISK CHILDREN IN THE SPF PROGRAM.

Performance Objectives (Children)	Personal Determinants				External Determinants		
	Attitudes	Skills and Self-Efficacy	Knowledge	Outcome Expectations	Cues	Reinforcement	Norms
PO.1. Cooperate with sun protection practices by parent or preschool staff	A.1. Express positive feeling toward being protected from the sun			OE.1. Describe how cooperating will keep skin healthy	C.1. Parents and daycare teachers provide cues for cooperating with sunscreen application.		N.1.a. Preschool directors post pictures and guidelines for sun protection. N.1.b. Children in the school talk to each other, parents, and teachers about sun protection.
PO.1.1. Stand still for application	A.1.1. Express positive attitude toward being a helper		K.1.1. Explain how standing still allows sunscreen to be put on evenly			R.1.1. Parents and daycare teachers praise the child for standing still and getting good coverage of sunscreen.	
PO.1.2. Dress in covering clothes for playing outside						R.1.2. Parents and daycare teachers praise the child for dressing in covering clothes.	
PO.1.3. Leave on clothes and hat	A.1.3.a. Feel positive about protective clothes A.1.3.b. Like sun hat			OE.1.3. Expect to be safe from the sun and healthy when wearing protective clothing	C.1.3. Hat and clothes hang by preschool door and home door.	R.1.3. Parents and daycare teachers praise the child for leaving hat and covering clothes on while in the sun.	N.1.3. Family and playmates wear protective clothing.

PO	SE		OE	C	R	N
PO.2. Remind parent or pre-school staff to practice sun protection on behalf of the child					R.2. Parents and daycare teachers praise the child for reminding the adults about sunscreen.	N.2.1. Teachers talk about how good it is for children to remind parents about health issues in general and sunscreen in particular.
PO.2.1. Tell adult that can't go outside without sunscreen	SE.2.1.a. Demonstrate telling an adult about the need for sunscreen SE.2.1b. Express confidence that can tell an adult about sunscreen		OE.2.1.a. Describe expectation that an adult will help with sunscreen if reminded OE.2.1.b. Describe expectation that even coverage by an adult will help every part of the skin stay healthy	C.2.1. Parents and teacher place sun protection preparation "station" by door.	R.2.1. Parents and daycare teachers to praise child for standing still and getting good coverage of sunscreen	
PO.2.2. Bring sunscreen to adult	SE.2.2. Demonstrate bringing sunscreen to adult		OE.2.2.a. State that an adult will help with sunscreen if reminded OE.2.2.b. State that even coverage by an adult will help every part of the skin stay healthy	C.2.2. Parents and teacher to place sun protection preparation "station" by door.	R.2.2. Parents and teachers praise the child for bringing sunscreen to adult as part of preparation for playing outside.	
PO.2.3. Come to adult for reapplication				C.2.3. Parents and teacher place sun protection preparation kit in tote bag.	R.2.3. Parents and daycare teachers praise the child for coming when called for sunscreen.	

TABLE 6.6. SAMPLE OF ROWS FROM MATRIX FOR ORGANIZATIONAL ENVIRONMENTAL CHANGE IN SPF PROGRAM.

Performance Objectives (Preschool Directors)	Personal Determinants					External Determinants	
	Perceived Norms	Attitudes	Skills and Self-Efficacy	Knowledge	Outcome Expectations and Perceived Susceptibility	Climate and Management Support	Reinforcement
PO.1. Decide to prioritize increasing the amount of shade in outdoor areas used by preschoolers	PN.1. Recognize sun protection and shade adequacy as concerns for preschool administration	A.1. Describe assuring shade as positive			OEPS.1.a. Describe children as susceptible to skin cancer caused by lack of shade OEPS.1.b. Argue that increasing shade will decrease risk	CMS.1. Managers express concern for need for shade.	R.1. Managers and parents notice staff providing shade and praise them.
PO.2. Assess adequacy of current natural and structural shaded areas and determine ways to increase shade	PN.2. Recognize that peers are taking action to assess shade		SSE.2.a. Demonstrate ability to assess shade SSE.2.b. Express confidence in ability to assess shade			CMS.2. Managers make time and resources available to conduct assessments.	
PO.3. Assess available resources for accomplishing changes to increase shade	PN.3. Talk about other preschool administrators as seeking resources for sun protection			K.3. State cost of change in terms of money, personnel, and time		CMS.3. Managers share information on current resources with director.	R.3. Managers and parents provide help for seeking additional funding.

PO.	SSE.	K.	CMS.
PO.4. Obtain additional resources to accomplish changes to increase shade	SSE.4. Demonstrate contacting community organizations about funding	K.4. Identify sources for seeking funding	CMS.4.a. Directors and managers maintain open communication. CMS.4.b. Managers listen to suggestions from director and staff for use of resources.
PO.5. Seek construction consultation and determine structures to implement based on ranking of effectiveness and feasibility	SSE.5. Express confidence in ability to rank structural changes	K.5. Identify features that make options for shade more effective and feasible	
PO.6. Seek feedback from teachers and staff			CMS.6. Staff members express support for plans to increase shade.
PO.7. Garner administrative approval for proposed changes	SSE.7. Express confidence in ability to discuss changes with management		CMS.7. Managers express support for plans to increase shade.

immediate changes in motivation and capability to influence health behavior and environmental conditions. Thus, each element of the matrix is interrelated, and collectively the elements are a logic model for the change process.

Selecting Intervention Levels

A separate matrix is constructed for each level of intervention for which program planners have written performance objectives. The final number of matrices of program objectives is different for each program and is influenced by the problem's complexity, the span of the program across levels, and the population's diversity. To select intervention levels, program planners ask: At what levels of intervention is it necessary to attain the performance objectives? For example, Project SPF was developed for the organizational setting of preschools, and the project team identified only a few performance objectives for children (that is, at the individual level). Most of the emphasis was on parents, teachers, and administrators, who were to create environmental changes to reduce children's exposure to the sun. Therefore, the intervention also addressed interpersonal and organizational levels; and planners created matrices for the individual, interpersonal, and organizational levels. Had the needs assessment identified important community or governmental factors influencing young children's sun exposure, then these levels would also have been reflected in the performance objectives.

For the Familias asthma management program, the focus was on the child's interpersonal environment, including parents and providers. Performance objectives for the individual level (child) and organizational level (school) had largely been addressed with the previous project, Watch, Discover, Think, and Act (Bartholomew, Gold, et al., 2000; Bartholomew, Shegog, et al., 2000). The Familias program developed performance objectives and matrices for parents and providers (Table 6.7).

Differentiating the Intervention Population

Planners may also need to create separate matrices for subgroups at any level of intervention (most often at the individual or at-risk group level). To differentiate a population means to describe two or more subgroups in which membership affects performance objectives or determinants of the health-related behavior or environmental condition. Differentiating a population often occurs simultaneously with writing performance objectives or exploring determinants because of the question that guides differentiation: Are either performance objectives or determinants substantially different for subgroups?

The rationale for differentiating a population is the basic understanding that populations are made up of individuals and groups with different characteristics and needs, all of which must be considered in relation to a health problem and to a health promotion program. The greater these differences, the less likely that a single intervention focus will fit everyone in the intervention population. Differentiating subgroups within the group leads to separate matrices for the program objectives so that planners can conduct a parallel planning process. The decision to differentiate the population should be very carefully considered because each differentiation into two or more subgroups will expand the details of the planning process and potentially increase the program's complexity and costs. If identified differences in the subpopulations are not great, planners can often accommodate them within the program with a few variations of the intervention strategies to address differences.

Some of the variables that may be important to consider in the differentiation of a population are the ones that were mentioned in the needs assessment. They include age and gender, geographic location, socioeconomic status, education, and cultural group. Resnicow, Baranowski, Ahluwalia, and Braithwaite (1999) describe the importance of understanding the impact of elements of culture on health behaviors and their determinants; the cultural group can often be a basis for differentiation. In addition, using stage theories and models such as child development, adult development, stages of change models (DiClemente & Prochaska, 1998; Prochaska & DiClemente, 1984), and stages of organizational change (Scheirer, Allen, & Rauch, 1987; Steckler, Goodman, & Kegler, 2002; Trice, Beyer, & Hunt, 1978; Zaltman & Duncan, 1977) to differentiate populations will in many cases enhance a planner's ability to develop change objectives that successfully define the program change for a group.

Differentiation by developmental stage offers a good example. To formulate performance objectives for the CF FEP, planners asked: What should the child with cystic fibrosis be able to do to manage the disease? (Bartholomew et al., 1991, 1993). Because children in the CF population spanned the range of four through eighteen years, the planners asked how the performance objectives would be different for the developmental stages represented by preschoolers ages four through six, school-age children ages seven through eleven, and adolescents ages twelve through eighteen. Having different objectives for different age groups was important because the behavioral, cognitive, emotional, and social capabilities of children at these various stages of development are so different that the children could not be expected to carry out similar activities to manage their chronic illness (Eiser, Patterson, & Tripp, 1984; Johnson et al., 1982).

Another reason to differentiate within a population is that determinants, the variables that lead to performing behaviors or to making environmental modifications, may be different for subgroups even when the performance objectives are the same. For example, peer norms may strongly influence a smoker in the

TABLE 6.7. SELECTED CHANGE OBJECTIVES: ASTHMA IN HISPANIC CHILDREN—PARENT MATRIX.

Manage Asthma Problem (Family Members)	Behavioral Capability	Personal Determinants		Outcome Expectations
		Skills and Self-Efficacy (for Dealing with Competing Advice)	Skills and Self-Efficacy	
Get a Diagnosis of Asthma				
Identify Problems (Watch and Discover)				
PO.1. Observe child for pattern or details of symptoms	BC.1. Describe possible symptoms of asthma	SSECA.1.a. Express confidence in telling others about good asthma management SSECA.1.b. Demonstrate telling others that good asthma managers believe that getting diagnosis of asthma is important for the child's health	SSE.1.a. Express confidence in identifying symptoms and environmental conditions SSE.1.b. Demonstrate identifying symptoms and environmental conditions	OE.1. Expect that getting a diagnosis of asthma when needed is the first step toward better health for the child
PO.2. Discover that symptoms are recurrent	BC.2. Analyze the pattern of symptoms over time		SSE.2. Express confidence in noticing symptoms	OE.2. Expect that by noticing and describing symptoms over time they will be able to get better health care for the child
PO.3. Discover conditions under which child has these symptoms	BC.3.a. Identify where the child spends time and note symptoms BC.3.b. Draw a relation between symptoms and exposure	SSECA.3. Express confidence in being able to get friends and family to help watch for symptoms and discover exposure patterns	SSE.3. Express confidence in linking symptoms to exposures	OE.3. Expect that by noticing and describing symptoms over time they will be able to get better health care for the child
PO.4. Question whether this is asthma	BC.4.a. Describe asthma as a chronic disease whose symptoms are sometimes better and sometimes worse BC.4.b. Describe asthma as a disease that can be controlled	SSECA.4.a. Talk to friends and family about asthma as a chronic disease whose symptoms are sometimes better and sometimes worse SSECA.4.b. Talk to friends and family about asthma as a disease that can be controlled		OE.4.a. Expect that when the doctor and the parent agree on the nature of the illness, they will work together better to provide care for the child OE.4.b. Expect that asthma can be treated and that symptoms will be controlled

Think (Generate Solutions)

PO.5. Identify current provider or other low-cost provider who gives good asthma care	BC.5.a. List low-cost and no cost doctors BC.5.b. Identify characteristics of good treatment for asthma	SSECA.5.a. Express confidence in telling others about the importance of identifying a good asthma doctor SSECA.5.b. Demonstrate telling others that good asthma managers think that it is important to locate an asthma doctor and to be assertive SSECA.5.c. Express confidence in telling others about what is good asthma care SSECA.5.d. Demonstrate telling others the characteristics of good asthma care	SSE.5.a. Express confidence in calling to ask about insurance eligibility and payment SSE.5.b. Express confidence in evaluating doctors	OE.5. Believe if they go to good asthma doctor, it will result in diagnosis and better care
PO.6. Identify possible health insurance or benefits	BC.6. Explain how to figure out what they are eligible for			OE.6. Believe if they follow steps to obtain insurance the child's health will benefit

Act (Take action to solve the problem)

PO.7. Make appointment with provider			SSE.7. Demonstrate finding an appropriate provider and making an appointment	OE.7. Expect that if they go to the doctor they will be treated with respect
PO.8. Tell doctor about symptoms	BC.8. State symptoms	SSECA.8.a. Express confidence in telling others about asthma management SSECA.8.b. Demonstrate telling others that good asthma managers tell their doctor about symptoms in detail	SSE.8. Demonstrate describing asthma symptoms	OE.8. Expect that taking record of symptoms to a doctor visit will result in a diagnosis that is important in child's health

TABLE 6.7. SELECTED CHANGE OBJECTIVES: ASTHMA IN HISPANIC CHILDREN—PARENT MATRIX, Cont'd.

Personal Determinants

Manage Asthma Problem (Family Members)	Behavioral Capability	(for Dealing with Competing Advice)	Skills and Self-Efficacy Skills and Self-Efficacy	Outcome Expectations
PO.9. Ask doctor about the possibility of asthma and ask the doctor to define the severity	BC.9. Define asthma and severity categories	SSECA.9.a. Express confidence in telling others that good managers manage asthma assertively SSECA.9.b.Demonstrate telling others that good asthma managers assertively ask doctor about asthma diagnosis and its severity	SSE.9. Demonstrate asking about asthma and severity and feel confident about all the above	OE.9. Expect that asking doctor about diagnosis and severity is important to result in better treatment and outcomes

Manage Asthma Problems

Identify Problems (Watch and Discover)

PO10. Observe child for specific symptoms	BC.10.a. Describe symptoms and episodes of asthma BC.10.b. Explain that asthma is an ongoing inflammation (not the final result of a series of illnesses or only asthma when the child has bad symptoms/exacerbation) BC.10.c. Discuss that early symptoms should be treated BC.10.d. Describe asthma as a disease with chronic symptoms and periodic exacerbations BC.10.e. Identify which symptoms can be asthma BC.10.f. Explain how to use the symptom chart to keep track of asthma	SSECA.10.a. Express confidence in managing the opinions and advice of others SSECA.10.b. Demonstrate telling others that good asthma managers believe that monitoring of child's symptoms benefits the child's health	SSE.10.a. Express confidence in monitoring symptoms and episodes SSE.10.b. Demonstrate keeping track of symptoms and episodes SSE.10.c. Express confidence in being able to recognize symptoms SSE.10.d. Demonstrate noting symptoms SSE.10.e. Express confidence in distinguishing between asthma symptoms and non-asthma–related symptoms	OE.10.a. Expect that if symptoms are monitored, asthma can be managed OE.10.b. Expect that identifying symptoms of asthma will enable better communication with physicians

PO.11. Identify severity of symptoms	BC.11.a. Describe early symptoms BC.11.b. Describe how to determine if symptoms are worsening in severity BC.11.c. Explain that asthma is an ongoing inflammation (not the final result of a series of illnesses or the worst exacerbation)		SSE.11.a. Express confidence in discerning mild symptoms SSE.11.b. Express confidence in discerning when a child is developing more severe symptoms	OE.11.a. Expect that by noticing worsening symptoms, they can prevent a bad exacerbation

Generate Solutions (Think)

PO.12. Identify medication for symptoms	BC.12.a. List prescribed medicines and treatments for symptoms BC.12.b. Describe early symptoms as something that must be treated	SSECA.12.a. Express confidence in telling others about using an action plan SSECA.12.b. Demonstrate telling others that good asthma managers provide appropriate medication and treatment according to action plan	SSE.12.a. Express confidence in identifying medicines for different symptoms SSE.12.b. Demonstrate identifying appropriate medicines and treatment for different symptoms	OE.12.a. Expect that if they give medicine it will not harm the child OE.12.b. Expect that if they give appropriate medicines and treatment the child's asthma can be controlled
PO.13. Identify medications for control	BC.13.a. List medicines for control (every day to keep symptoms from appearing) BC.13.b. Describe how control medicine works and that it will not stop working if given every day	SSECA.13.a. Express confidence in telling others about managing inflammation SSECA.13.b. Demonstrate telling others that good asthma managers give medicine to control inflammation even when there are not symptoms		OE.13.a. Expect that if they give appropriate medicines and treatment the child's asthma can be controlled OE.13.b. Expect that when given every day the medicine will continue to work and control symptoms
PO.14. Talk with doctor about home remedies PO.14.1. Balance home remedies with physician-prescribed medication	BC.14.a. Describe the treatments that they use for asthma BC.14.b. Ask the physicians for advice about which treatments are okay to use with the prescribed asthma medicines	SSECA.14.a. Express confidence in telling others about balancing home remedies with medications SSECA.14.b. Demonstrate telling others that good asthma managers provide prescribed medication along with some home remedies	SSE.14.a. Express confidence in taking time to manage asthma SSE.14.b. Demonstrate taking time to manage the child's asthma	OE.14. Expect that the doctor will be respectful of their attempts to treat asthma with home remedies

TABLE 6.7. SELECTED CHANGE OBJECTIVES—ASTHMA IN HISPANIC CHILDREN—PARENT MATRIX, Cont'd.

Manage Asthma Problems

Manage Asthma Problem (Family Members)	Behavioral Capability	(for Dealing with Competing Advice)	Skills and Self-Efficacy Skills and Self-Efficacy	Outcome Expectations
Take Action to Solve Problem (Act)				
PO.15. Get action plan and discuss with doctor	BC.15. Describe how to use action plan	SSECA.15.a. Express confidence in telling others about getting an action plan SSECA.15.b. Demonstrate telling others that good asthma managers provide appropriate medication and treatment according to action plan	SSE.15.a. Express confidence in following an action plan SSE.15.b. Demonstrate following an action plan	OE.15. Believe that if they discuss and follow action plan they can manage the child's asthma
PO.16. Follow an action plan	BC.16.a. Explain how to give medicines BC.16.b. Explain what to do when symptoms are becoming worse	SSECA.16.a. Express confidence in telling others that action plans are necessary SSECA.16.b. Demonstrate telling others that good asthma managers think action plan is necessary to manage child's asthma	SSE.16. Interpret fear and concern as a signal to act	

precontemplation stage of change for cessation, whereas lack of skills for quitting might have a higher impact on the behavior of a smoker in the preparation, action, or maintenance stages of change. Furthermore, if the determinants are different, then the theoretical methods chosen to influence the determinants may be different. For example, some research suggests that determinants of condom use among high school students vary according to experience with sexual intercourse using condoms (Schaalma, Kok, Poelman, & Reinders, 1994). Adolescents who had previous experience with condoms had more negative attitudes about the effects of condoms on pleasure. Self-efficacy for buying and having condoms was higher, but self-efficacy for negotiating condom use with a partner was lower. Experience with condom use was correlated with age and having a steady relationship, and when people had a steady relationship, intention to use condoms was lower. Based on this knowledge of determinant difference related to experience, program planners might choose to develop different matrices of objectives and include program strategies and messages for these different intervention groups.

Both performance objectives and determinants may be different for subgroups. In Project Parents and Newborns Developing and Adjusting (PANDA) (Chapter Thirteen), an intervention to help pregnant women who had stopped smoking refrain from returning to smoking after the delivery of the baby, the planners differentiated the population of women by stage of change: precontemplators, contemplators, and action and maintenance stages. The planners hypothesized that the women, although they had stopped smoking, were not all in the action stage of change. Considerable evidence indicated that most of the women during pregnancy had not used the processes of change that would enable them to remain nonsmokers. Therefore, performance objectives and determinants were defined for each group according to stage of change. For example, precontemplators needed to move to contemplation of remaining smoke free; and to do this, they had to shift their decisional balance to being more negative about smoking. Those women in the action stage needed to apply processes to remain in action, for example, stimulus control, removing items that stimulate smoking from their environments. The PANDA example also illustrates the point that the development of separate matrices does not imply the need for separate programs, but it does imply the need for program methods to address the different change objectives from each of the matrices.

Similar to differentiation, segmentation refers to grouping the population by variables (such as preferred communication network) that will influence the message's effectiveness (Lefebvre & Flora, 1988, 1992; Lefebvre, Lurie, Goodman, Weinberg, & Loughrey, 1995; Lefebvre & Rochlin, 1997; Leviton, Mrazek & Stoto, 1996; Ling, Franklin, Lindsteadt, & Gearon, 1992; Maibach, Rothchild, & Novelli, 2002). The variables used by marketers and communicators to segment a population in service of message development may imply underlying differences in determinants, but these differences may not be explained as they are in Intervention Mapping.

Differentiation is based on subpopulations, whereas tailoring is a technique of individualizing intervention messages based on certain measured characteristics of the individual (Campbell, DeVellis, Strecher, Ammerman, DeVellis, & Sandler, 1994; Kreuter & Strecher, 1996; Skinner, Strecher, & Hospers, 1994; Strecher, 1999; Strecher, Bishop, Bernhardt, Thorp, Cheuvront, & Potts, 2000; Strecher, Greenwood, Want, & Dumont, 1999; Strecher, Wang, Derry, Wildenhaus, & Johnson, 2002). Tailored health promotion materials are any combination of information and behavior change strategies intended to reach one specific person based on characteristics that are unique to that person, related to the outcome of interest, and derived from individual assessment (Kreuter, Farrell, Olevitch, & Brennan, 2000). Tailoring may be done on the basis of differences in behaviors or determinants, and it may be done at a later stage of program development on characteristics that did not lead to differentiation and the creation of different matrices. Tailoring and segmentation are very important for development of intervention strategies and programs, but they do not imply the need for separate matrices in Step 2. They can be done later and are discussed again in Step 4 (Chapter Eight).

In summary, differentiating the population leads to separate matrices of program objectives for each group. The matrices are used to guide program planning to design interventions appropriate for each subgroup. The result may be a separate program for each group or a single program with multiple components, methods, or strategies that can accommodate differences among groups.

Constructing Matrices and Change Objectives

At this point the planner has made a preliminary decision about the number of matrices for the project, based on population differentiation and levels of environmental change. For each behavioral outcome objective and environmental outcome objective, the planner enters the performance objectives down the left side of a matrix and the determinants across the top. The next task is to assess each cell of the matrix to judge whether the determinant is likely to influence accomplishment of the performance objective. It is unlikely that each of the determinants will be an important influence for every performance objective. Because change objectives are needed for those cells in which the determinant is likely to influence accomplishment of the performance objective, this task can be a review and elimination process. One way that the planner accomplishes this task is to look at each cell, decide whether change in a particular determinant is necessary for the performance objective, put an X through unimportant cells, and then write change objectives for the cells that remain.

The planner writes change objectives for both the personal and the external determinants. The question that leads to formation of a change objective for personal determinants is: What needs to change related to the determinant for the program participants to do the performance objective? For example, Table 6.8 shows a cell in which the performance objective "purchase condoms" is paired with the determinant of "knowledge." The question used to address this cell can be worded this way: What needs to change related to knowledge in order for the participants to be able to purchase a condom? Answers to this question lead to the following change objectives:

Explain how to buy or obtain a condom

List places where condoms can be purchased or obtained free

Compare different types of condoms and features to improve effectiveness

These change objectives become the targets for program methods and strategies to increase knowledge. In another example that uses the same performance objective (purchase condoms), a focus on the cell connected with the determinant of self-efficacy leads to the question: What needs to change regarding self-efficacy in order for program participants to purchase condoms? This question yields the following change objectives:

Express confidence in ability to go into a store and buy a condom

Express confidence in ability to deal with embarrassment when buying a condom

These examples show that change objectives are stated with strong verbs. Table 6.9 includes words to help with this task (Caffarella, 1985). Change objectives begin with a verb that defines the action. The action is followed by a context or condition in which the performance objective is likely to occur, and the change objective ends with a restatement of the essential action from the performance objective. The purpose of stating a change objective in this manner is to make as specific as possible what change in the determinant needs to be achieved to accomplish the performance objective. Planners who write change objectives with an action verb, context, and performance have a clear direction to the next steps in the Intervention Mapping process: selecting intervention methods and translating methods into learning strategies.

Change objectives for personal determinants are essentially the same as the learning objectives that are typically used in curriculum development for educational programs. In fact, in the first edition of this book, we called them learning

TABLE 6.8. EXAMPLES OF CELLS FROM A SIMULATED MATRIX: CONSISTENTLY AND CORRECTLY USING CONDOMS DURING SEXUAL INTERCOURSE.

Performance Objectives (Adolescents)	Personal Determinants			
	Knowledge	Skills and Self-Efficacy	Outcome Expectations	Perceived Norms
PO.1. Purchase condoms	K.1. Explain how to buy or obtain a condom	SSE.1.a. Reflect confidence in ability to go into a store and buy a condom SSE.1.b. Express confidence in ability to deal with embarrassment when buying a condom		PN.1. Explain that peers go into stores and buy condoms
PO.1.1. Locate condom displays in drug or grocery store	K.1.1. List places where condoms can be purchased or obtained free			
PO.1.2. Choose condoms that are product tested	K.1.2. Compare different types of condoms and features to improve effectiveness			
PO.2. Carry condoms or have condoms easily available	K.2. List private, effective places to keep condoms	SSE.2. Express confidence that can find a private, safe, accessible place for condoms	OE.2. Describe how having condoms easily available will result in more routine condom use	PN.2. State that peers have condoms easily available
PO.2.1. Carry condoms in wallet or purse for no longer than a month	K.2.1. Describe how long condoms can be kept without increasing risk of breakage			PN.2.1. State that peers make sure condoms are not carried too long

PO.2.2. Carry or store condoms in place that maintains correct temperature	K.2.1. State safe temperatures for storing condoms and compare temperatures where planning to store condoms		OE.2.2. Expect that if stored properly condoms will work to prevent disease and pregnancy	PN.2.2. State that peers store condoms at safe temperatures
PO.3. Negotiate the use of a condom with a partner	K.3. List the steps of successful negotiation		OE.3. Describe personal beliefs that negotiation will lead to positive experience where both partners are satisfied and result in condom use	PN.3. Explain that peers talk to their partners about condom use
PO.3.1. State mutual goals such as pregnancy or AIDS prevention		SSE.3.1. Summarize mutual goals as would be said to a partner	OE.3.1. State belief that discussing mutual goals will result in condom use	
PO.3.2. State clear intention of using a condom as a prerequisite for intercourse		SSE.3.2. Advocate clear intention to not have sex without a condom	OE.3.2. Expect partner to maintain relationship in face of intention not to have sex without a condom	
PO.3.3. Actively listen to partner's concerns	K.3.3. Describe components of active listening	SSE.3.3. Demonstrate actively listening to partner's concerns	OE.3.3. Describe how condom use protects against STIs and HIV	
PO.3.4. Pose solutions to partner's concerns that reference mutual goals and personal requirement		SSE.3.4. Express confidence in ability to do each step of negotiation		

TABLE 6.9. LIST OF ACTION WORDS
FOR WRITING PERFORMANCE OBJECTIVES.

accept	develop	outline
adopt	differentiate	persuade
advocate	discriminate	plan
analyze	draw	prepare
arrange	evaluate	prescribe
approve	execute	produce
appraise	explain	purchase
bargain	express	question
calculate	fill out	rank
care	forecast	recall
change	formulate	recognize
choose	generate	reflect
classify	identify	remove
categorize	inform	research
challenge	install	resolve
chart	interview	review
compare	judge	select
conduct	justify	sort
construct	label	specify
contrast	list	state
cooperate	locate	study
check	manipulate	take
defend	modify	tell
define	name	translate
demonstrate	operate	use
describe	organize	write

Source: Caffarella, 1985.

objectives, but we decided to simplify our terminology in the second edition and use the term *change objectives* for both personal and external determinants.

For external determinants, change objectives define what needs to be changed in determinants that are external to the individual to accomplish the performance objective. For example, a planning group addressing smoking prevention in adolescents has identified from the research literature that peer norms are an important external determinant of smoking behavior (van den Bree, Whitmer, & Pickworth, 2004). The behavioral outcome for the program is "choosing not to smoke." One of the performance objectives for choosing not to smoke is "Resist peer pressure to smoke a cigarette." When the external determinant of peer norms intersects the performance objective, the following examples of change objectives can be formulated and used to guide the design of intervention methods and strategies:

> Peers demonstrate resisting pressure to smoke.
>
> Peers desist from pressuring others to smoke.

Project SPF can be used here to illustrate the writing of change objectives for external determinants at the interpersonal level of environmental change. One of the environmental outcomes is this: Teachers will apply sunscreen to children at least thirty minutes before going outside. Here is a sample performance objective intersecting the external determinant cues to create change objectives:

> Child asks for sunscreen.
>
> Fellow teachers remind teacher to apply sunscreen to children.
>
> Teachers place sun protection supplies by the classroom door.

Examples of matrices for the SPF program are provided in Tables 6.4 and 6.5. Table 6.6 also contains an example for a portion of the parent matrix developed for the Familias asthma management program.

Clarifying External Determinants and Environmental Conditions

Neither external determinants nor environmental conditions are likely to be under the control of individuals at risk for the health problem. Such determinants and conditions are controlled by external agents, for instance, peers for social support, teachers for reinforcement, managers for organizational climate, decision makers for policies, and gatekeepers for access to resources. As a result, change objectives for external determinants are formulated by referring to an external agent who will act: peers will give support, teachers will reinforce, and managers will support the innovation. A logical relation exists between external determinants and environmental conditions. If the planner very carefully and exhaustively analyzes the environment, not many external determinants are left for the individual's behavior because they are part of the specified environmental change and related performance objectives. But if the environmental analysis proves insufficient (in hindsight), some very relevant external determinants may show up after the fact.

The earlier example about school lunches identified "Availability of low-fat alternatives in the schools" as an environmental factor, with this performance objective: "Food service directors will modify menus to include more low-fat food." As a result, the planning team members who created this matrix did not need the external determinant of availability for the individual student's behavior. However, if they had not identified availability as an environmental condition, they might have perceived later that availability is indeed a relevant external determinant of students' food choices. Thus, their change objective (not their performance objective) would then be this: "Food service directors will modify menus to include more low-fat food."

The school lunch example illustrates the importance of making judgments in using Intervention Mapping as a planning tool (Hoelscher, Evans, Parcel, & Kelder, 2002). In some cases leaving an external determinant as a determinant and using change objectives as the program objectives will fit well with planning the program. In other cases the external determinant is such a strong environmental influence that it makes sense to elevate it to an environmental condition and address it in greater detail with performance objectives and related determinants. Intervention Mapping does not offer a cookbook approach; planning groups must continuously make judgments about where external determinants fit best in the matrix structure.

One way that planners can use to decide where to place an external determinant is to look at the intervention's main emphasis. Can the change objective be taken care of in the program (for example, the food service director as one of the implementers), or does part of the program need to be directed at an environmental condition (for example, the food service director as an environmental agent)? Notice that in both cases the planning team has to follow the Intervention Mapping process of analyzing determinants of the behavior, selecting methods and strategies, and developing an intervention (such as training). The difference is that in the first case, the team does this process as part of anticipating implementation (Chapter Nine), and in the second case the team does it with the intervention program component that targets environmental conditions.

Another example illustrates the use of the external determinant of reinforcement. In the asthma self-management program Watch, Discover, Think, and Act (Bartholomew, Gold, et al., 2000; Bartholomew, Shegog, et al., 2000), the planning team identified reinforcement as an external determinant for the child's performance objectives. The question team members asked themselves was, Should we address reinforcement in the intervention component for children, or should we create a program component for an environmental agent who will provide the reinforcement? The team could, for instance, have decided to develop a computer program that would reinforce the child after successful self-management behavior. In that case the team members could have taken care of the change objective in the computer program. They could also have decided to have the asthma specialist give the reinforcement to the child. In that case, because they knew how difficult it is to change specialists' behavior, they might have wanted to direct a substantial part of their intervention to this environmental agent. Therefore, they would need to develop a matrix focused on the child's interpersonal environment that included the specialist's behavior as an environmental factor. They would then have to formulate specific performance objectives, define personal and external determinants, and choose specific change objectives to complete the environmental level matrix.

When health educators treat a change objective as something that can be handled through the at-risk groups as a small part of the program, they leave the change objective where it is: in the cell that intersects the performance objective with external determinant. When they decide the change objective is a bigger issue, they add a new item to the list of environmental conditions: the external determinant now becomes an environmental condition. Then the planners add new performance objectives, determinants, and change objectives (Gottlieb et al., 2003). The planners, of course, need to think about personal and external determinants of these new performance objectives, which may lead to a repetition of this whole process at a higher level. For instance, food service directors may be seriously restricted by regulations, or specialists may be seriously restricted by time. This shift to higher levels, however, soon reaches a point at which the determinants are outside the health educator's scope to plan and execute appropriate programs.

External determinants may present another challenge. Sometimes individuals can actually do something about external determinants. When the social norm is negative, planners might want to change the social norm, but they could also try to increase the individual's resistance to that norm (Evans et al., 1978). When physicians do not take enough time to explain expected treatment behaviors to patients, for example, health educators might want to change the physician's behavior, but they could also try to prepare the patients to ask certain questions. When the external determinants are very difficult to change, a health educator's only alternative may be an indirect approach that addresses personal determinants and change objectives of the individual or the agent. An example of this situation is tobacco advertising. The local group planning a smoking prevention program for adolescents may not be able to get the tobacco companies to alter their marketing to young people; the group can, however, create objectives for adolescents to resist the messages of tobacco advertising (CDC, Tobacco Information and Prevention Source, 1999; Choi, Ahluwalia, Harris, & Okuyemi, 2002; D'Onofrio, Moskowitz, & Braverman, 2002; Gilpin et al., 2004; Maziak, Rzehak, Keil, & Weiland, 2003). A word of caution is in order: program planners must be careful not to place individuals in situations that make them responsible for environmental conditions that are not in their control and not to raise unrealistic expectations that individuals can influence these conditions without interventions occurring at other levels of the environment.

Environmental Agents and Program Implementers

Another potential source of confusion for program planners is the distinction between using agents in the environment to make environmental changes and using them to implement components of an intervention program. For example, in a school-based program such as CATCH, the cardiovascular disease prevention program for children, teachers may be both agents to change the environmental conditions and program implementers. A component of the intervention in the CATCH program was directed at performance and change objectives for ensuring that children have scheduled time during the school day to engage in moderate physical activity. This was part of the school's environmental change program. In addition, the teachers implemented the physical education program that enabled the children to be physically active at school. A training program helped to prepare the teachers to implement the physical education program. Program implementation is not part of planning done in Step 2 but is addressed in Step 5, following a similar set of tasks with the focus on implementation outcomes rather than health behavior or environmental change outcomes. If planning leads to environmental change that focuses on implementation of a component of the program for the at-risk population or agents to change environmental conditions, then it should be addressed in Step 5.

Creating a Matrix for Program Revision

We often hear people say: "Let's not reinvent the wheel." When they say this about program planning, they typically mean: if a program already exists that addresses a health problem and it has been shown to be effective, why start from scratch to develop a new one? This is a perfectly reasonable question, and program planners would be wise to consider existing programs before investing time, money, and resources to develop a new program. An obvious starting point is to access the evidence that the program is effective in achieving the program objectives and health and quality-of-life outcomes.

If they find evidence of program effectiveness, then the planning group should determine whether the existing program is a good match for both the context and the potential program participants. To determine a match, the planning group will need detailed information on the behavioral and environmental outcomes, performance objectives, determinants, and change objectives for the existing program. If the existing program used Intervention Mapping, then an examination of the matrices used in developing the program can provide the detailed information. If the program under consideration was not developed using Intervention Mapping, then we suggest that the planning group attempt to reconstruct matrices for the existing program. The planning group can then assess the matrices for the existing program to determine how they will address the needs for the new target population.

Unless the populations and context for the original program and the new application are very similar, it is likely that even with a close match of the existing program matrices with the needs assessment, the planning group will need to modify the existing program for the new target population. The planners can adapt the existing program by adding to or modifying the behavioral and environmental conditions, performance objectives, and determinants and modifying the matrices for change objectives (De Stevens & Van Oost, 2001). These modified matrices can then be used to guide the planners in making changes in methods and strategies for a program adapted to the new target population.

A good example is a program called Safer Choices 2 (Tortolero, Markham, et al., 2005). Safer Choices is a theory-based, multicomponent program that was extensively evaluated and shown to be effective in reducing sexual risk-taking behavior in youth (Basen-Engquist et al., 2001; K. Coyle et al., 1996; K. Coyle et al., 1999; K. Coyle et al., 2001). The program planners for Safer Choices 2 wanted to adapt Safer Choices to a new target population: at-risk youth attending alternative schools.

Tortolero, Markham and colleagues (2005) first did a thorough needs assessment for youth attending alternative schools. This included a review of the relevant literature, collection of new data using a survey administered to alternative school students, and qualitative data from focus groups of alternative school youth. Using the findings from the needs assessment, the planners then applied the steps and tasks of Intervention Mapping to adapt the original Safer Choices program to a new target population. They dropped one of the behavioral outcomes and added another. They wrote new performance objectives to better meet the needs of the new target population, and they added additional determinants based on the findings from the needs assessment. These changes led to the need to create new matrices of change objectives that served to guide the planners in modifying the methods and strategies used to make up the Safer Choices 2 program. Table 6.10 provides a list of question the planning group used to apply Intervention Mapping to the adaptation of an existing program.

TABLE 6.10. USING THE INTERVENTION MAPPING STEPS TO ADAPT A PROGRAM FOR A NEW POPULATION.

Step 1: Needs Assessment

- What new cultural or other population issues are present?
- What new environmental issues must be considered?
- What is the community capacity of the new population?

Step 2, Task 1: Review Behavioral Outcomes

- Which behavioral outcomes need to be added for the new population?
- Which behavioral outcomes need to be deleted as inappropriate?
- Which behavioral outcomes need to be deleted or adapted as impractical?

Step 2, Task 2: Specify Performance Objectives

- Which performance objectives should be deleted as irrelevant?
- Given the new or revised behavioral outcomes,
  - Which performance objectives need to be added?
  - Which performance objectives need to be revised?

Step 2, Task 3: Specify Determinants

- Which determinants were used in devising the original program?
- What is the supporting evidence for those determinants?
- Does the evidence indicate that the determinants are relevant to the new population?
- Which determinants should be deleted or revised?
- Which determinants need to be added for the new population?
- Which determinants need to be added for the new performance objectives?

Step 2, Task 4: Develop Proximal Program Objectives

- For each determinant of each performance objective, what are the change objectives of the existing program?
- Given the changes in determinants and performance objectives,
  - Which change objectives should be deleted?
  - Which change objectives should be revised?
  - Which change objectives should be added?

Step 3, Part 1: Identifying Theoretical Foundation

- Which behavioral theory is associated with each determinant in the original program?
  - Which of these theories is relevant to the new population?
  - Which of these theories is appropriate for the new determinants?

TABLE 6.10. USING THE INTERVENTION MAPPING STEPS TO ADAPT A PROGRAM FOR A NEW POPULATION, Cont'd.

- Which part of the theoretical foundation should be discarded?
- What should be added to the theoretical foundation of the revised program?

Step 3, Part 2: Selecting Methods and Strategies

- Are the methods and strategies of the original program effective for the new population?
- Are they feasible given the new study design?
- Are they practical given the new community context?
- Given that methods and strategies are specific to change objectives,
  - Which methods or strategies should be deleted?
  - Which methods and strategies should be revised?
- Looking at the new change objectives and the relevant theories,
  - Which methods can be expanded to cover new change objectives?
  - Which new intervention methods or strategies need to be added?

Step 4: Developing Program Content

- Comparing the content of the original intervention with the revised change objectives,
  - Which change objectives are well covered by existing content?
  - Which change objectives are partially addressed by existing content?
  - Which change objectives require new content?
- Looking at the program content,
  - What content should remain the same?
  - What content should be adapted or deleted?
  - What content should be added?

Step 5: Adoption and Implementation

- Is the new population comparable to that targeted by the original intervention?
- If not, how does this affect the ability to replicate the intervention with fidelity?
- Does the new community context present new practical or logistical issues?
- If so, how must adoption and implementation be adapted?

Step 6: Evaluation

- What is the evaluation model required for this population and setting?
- Are the original indicators and measures the most relevant and useful for the new community context, population, behavioral outcomes, and performance and change objectives?
- If not, which new indicators and measures of impact variables are needed?
- What are the appropriate process measures for this population and setting?

Implications for Program Evaluation

Each task in Step 2 produces information that is used to guide the program evaluation (see Chapter Ten). In the first task, the planners specified the behavioral and environmental outcomes that the program would address. For program evaluation these outcomes are measured to determine the impact of the program on behavior and environmental conditions (Abbema, Van Assema, Kok, De Leeuw, & De Vries, 2004; Hou, Fernandez, Baumler, & Parcel, 2002).

In the second task, the planners further delineated the behavioral and environmental conditions by writing performance objectives. These performance objectives help to define the critical components and necessary prerequisites for the performance of the behavior and environmental conditions. As part of the program evaluation, questions can be asked to determine whether program participants did the performance objective, which provides valuable information to better understand a program's effectiveness. For example, if the behavior was performed, then responses to questions about the performance objectives help the evaluators to know the relative importance of the objectives to the behavior's performance. If the behavior is not performed, then the responses to questions about the performance objectives may help to explain why the program did not have an effect on behavior and may provide important information to guide revisions of the program. In some cases the performance objectives help to define the behavior or environmental condition and can be used to construct evaluation questions to measure the behavior. For example, eating a low-fat diet so that less than 30 percent of calories are from fat can not be effectively measured without more specific questions about what and how much was eaten, which can be guided by performance objectives such as "Drink low-fat milk instead of whole milk."

In the final task in Step 2, the planners create matrices for change objectives that the intervention program will address. These matrices can also be used to guide the development of measures to evaluate the most immediate impact of the program. The design of the program is intended to address the change objectives, as the first effect in the logic model of change (see Figure 6.1). Accomplishment of the change objectives is intended to influence changes in the personal and external determinants of the performance objectives. For impact evaluation the evaluator will want to know whether the program was successful in influencing changes in the determinants. The change objectives in the cells of the matrices can be used to help guide the development of instruments to measure the determinants. For example, to develop a knowledge instrument, the change objectives for knowledge constitute the critical knowledge needed to accomplish the performance objectives. Planners can thus use the change objectives for knowledge to construct questions to ask the participants in order to measure their knowledge before and after participating in the intervention program. This same principle can be applied to the construction of items to measure other determinants, such as self-efficacy, subjective norms, attitudes, and beliefs.

It is most difficult to evaluate the effectiveness of a health promotion program if the planners have not clearly stated the program's objectives and outcomes. Step 2 of Intervention Mapping provides the program evaluators with clearly stated behavioral and environmental outcomes, performance objectives, and change objectives that can guide the program evaluation (Tripp et al., 2003).

Box 6.2. Stroke Project

⮑ *The first task in Step 2 is to state what health behaviors and environmental conditions need to change.*

Following from the needs assessment for the T.L.L. Temple Stroke Project introduced in Chapter Five, the health-related behavior outcome for the at-risk group was to arrive at the hospital within several minutes after experiencing symptoms of stroke. The environmental outcome was to provide acute stroke therapy for all eligible patients (those who arrived at the hospital with time for a work-up within the three-hour window and for whom recombinant tissue plasminogen activator (rtPA) was not contraindicated).

⮑ *The second task is to subdivide behavioral and environmental outcomes into performance objectives.*

The performance objectives for the at-risk group, that is, the individual experiencing symptoms and the bystander, are included in Table 6.11.

The performance objectives for the environment were conceptualized at the organizational level and included objectives for the emergency department (ED) of the five local hospitals, the three emergency medical services (EMS), and the community primary care physicians. Tables 6.12, 6.13, and 6.14 present these objectives.

TABLE 6.11. COMMUNITY (BYSTANDER) PERFORMANCE OBJECTIVES.

PO.1. Note symptoms and compare to those of possible stroke

PO.2. Call 911 immediately (do not call primary care provider for triage)

PO.3. Insist on rapid care from the emergency medical service (EMS) (transport at highest level)

PO.4. Ask about treatment for stroke and rapid care in the emergency department (ED)

TABLE 6.12. EMERGENCY DEPARTMENT PERFORMANCE OBJECTIVES.

PO.1. ED physicians and teams complete stroke evaluation in sixty minutes.

    PO.1.1. Triage nurses have patient seen by the physician in ten minutes.

    PO.1.2. ED physicians notify the designated ER stroke team within fifteen minutes.

PO.2. ED stroke teams send lab work STAT (HCT, platelets, glucose, PT, PTT) and get it back.

PO.3. ED physicians and stroke teams make rapid differential diagnosis of stroke (use modified NIH scale and protocol).

PO.4. ED stroke teams perform pulse oximetry, attach cardiac monitor, and perform EKG.

PO.5. ED stroke teams obtain accurate onset time of stroke symptoms.

PO.6. ED stroke teams ensure patient receives CT scan within twenty-five minutes and notifies on-call radiologist.

PO.7. Radiologists and stroke teams read the CT scan immediately (within forty-five minutes of arrival).

PO.8. ED stroke teams rule out contraindications.

PO.9. ED stroke teams manage diagnosed stroke.

    PO.9.1. ED staff members insert an IV in each arm if not done by EMS.

    PO.9.2. ED physicians administer rtPA within sixty minutes.

    PO.9.3. ED physicians treat blood pressure appropriately.

    PO.9.4. ED physicians give appropriate dose of rtPA; infuse properly; document time (do not give heparin or coumadin).

TABLE 6.13. EMS PERFORMANCE OBJECTIVES.

PO.1. Dispatchers triage to highest priority of transport.

PO.2. Dispatchers convey stroke possibility and urgency to responders.

PO.3. Responders perform "load and go."

PO.4. Responders call ahead to the hospital.

PO.5. Responders encourage family member or witness to accompany to the hospital.

PO.6. Responders interview patient and witness to determine symptom onset.

PO.7. Responders deliver patient with IV in both arms (perform in ambulance).

TABLE 6.14. PRIMARY CARE PROVIDER PERFORMANCE OBJECTIVES.

PO.1. Receptionists and nurses tell the person with the possible stroke to call 911.

PO.2. Primary care providers identify high-risk patients for stroke and tell patients about their stroke risk, possible symptoms, and instructions for calling 911.

PO.3. Primary care providers educate office staff regarding how to recognize stroke and what to tell patients (such as to call 911 immediately).

⮑ *The third task in Step 2 is to select important and changeable determinants of the health behavior and environmental conditions.*

Based on the needs assessment (Chapter 5, Stroke Project), the planning group brainstormed possible determinants. The planners worked first on the lay performance objectives and then on the health care provider objectives. The brainstormed preliminary list was limited because the information in the literature included mostly knowledge and behavioral determinants of treatment, such as arriving at the ED within a short time after symptoms arise and arriving by ambulance. Therefore, the planners modified the preliminary list using theoretical constructs from SCT and the Theory of Planned Behavior (TPB), the two theories that matched most closely the preliminary ideas from the needs assessment. The work on the determinants is presented in Tables 6.15 and 6.16.

TABLE 6.15. WORK ON HYPOTHESIZED DETERMINANTS OF COMMUNITY MEMBERS' RESPONSE TO STROKE.

Preliminary List	Final List
Confidence in recognizing symptoms	Self-efficacy (for recognizing symptoms and for intervening)
Thinking something can be done for stroke	Outcome expectations
Thinking that you don't have to have a primary care referral or call a primary care provider	Knowledge (symptoms, calling 911, not calling primary care provider)
Knowing a stroke victim	Perceived social norms
Knowing what to do	Social norms
Not being embarrassed to intervene or to call 911	Barriers

TABLE 6.16. WORK ON HYPOTHESIZED DETERMINANTS OF HEALTH CARE PROVIDERS' RESPONSE TO STROKE.

Preliminary List	Final List
Understanding of rtPA clinical trial results	Skills (for neurologic exam, determining last time seen normal, and ruling out hemorrhagic stroke)
Not thinking that primary care providers and neurologists want to be consulted before patient is treated	Self-efficacy
Not worrying about hemorrhage	Outcome expectations
Protocol in ED	Knowledge
rtPA on formulary	Perceived social norms
Skills in ruling out hemorrhagic stroke	Social norms
Skills in determining last time seen normal	Barriers
EMS expectation that hospital will respond urgently	Reinforcement
Confidence that workup times can be lowered	
Expectation that rtPA will produce better outcomes	

⊃ *The fourth task in Step 2 is to create the matrices.*

The planners created separate matrices for the at-risk group, that is, the community, and three different health care provider groups, the EDs, the EMSs, and the primary care providers. The matrices are shown in Tables 6.17, 6.18, 6.19, and 6.20.

TABLE 6.17. COMMUNITY (BYSTANDER) MATRIX FOR RESPONSE TO STROKE.

Performance Objectives (Persons in Proximity)	Personal Determinants				External Determinants	
	Skills and Self-Efficacy	Knowledge	Perceived Social Norms	Outcome Expectations	Social Norms	Barriers
PO.1. Note symptoms and compare to those of possible stroke	SSE.1. Express confidence in recognizing stroke symptoms	K.1.a. Recognize stroke symptoms: numbness, weakness, ↓vision, ↓ speech, ↓walking, tingling, vertigo, headache K.1.b. Describe all adults at risk for stroke	PSN.1. Recognize that others in the community take symptoms of stroke seriously	OE.1. Expect that identifying symptoms signifying stroke can improve outcome	SN.1. Community demonstrates assertiveness in responding to stroke symptoms.	B.1.a. Primary care physicians remind high-risk patients about symptoms. B.1.b. Primary care policy advises patients to go directly to emergency department (ED) via emergency medical service (EMS).
PO. 2. Call 911 immediately (does not call primary care provider for triage)	SSE.2. Express confidence in describing symptoms of stroke	K.2.a. Recall what to say to operator ("I believe someone is having a stroke, and they need to go to the ED right away.") K.2.b. Describe stroke as a brain attack with the same urgency as a heart attack	PSN.2. Recognize that others in the community call 911 for stroke	OE.2. Expect that by acting assertively can get prompt stroke treatment and possibly minimize damage	SN.2. Community demonstrates assertiveness in response to stroke symptoms by calling 911.	B.2.a. Primary care policy states to advise patients to go directly to ED via EMS. B.2.b. Primary care doctors remind high-risk patients about symptoms.

TABLE 6.17. COMMUNITY (BYSTANDER) MATRIX FOR RESPONSE TO STROKE, Cont'd.

Performance Objectives (Persons in Proximity)	*Personal Determinants*				*External Determinants*	
	Skills and Self-Efficacy	Knowledge	Perceived Social Norms	Outcome Expectations	Social Norms	Barriers
PO.3 Insist on rapid care from EMS (transport at highest level	SSE.3. Express confidence in insisting on priority care	K.3. Describe stroke as a brain attack with the same urgency as a heart attack	PSN.3. Recognize that others in the community are assertive about stroke	OE.3. Expect that EMS and ED will respond to assertiveness with appropriate patient care	SN.3. Community demonstrates greater assertiveness by asking for rapid transport.	B.3. Primary care policy advisers to go directly to ED via EMS.
PO.4. Ask about treatment for stroke and rapid care in the emergency department	SSE.4.a. Express confidence in asking about treatment and insisting on priority care SSE.4.b. Express confidence for insisting on CT scan	K.4.a. Describe what to do in ED: ask for CT scan; tell last time normal K.4.b. State that stroke requires rapid workup to allow for treatment to prevent damage	PSN.4. Recognize that others in the community are assertive about stroke	OE.4. Expect that EMS and ED will respond to assertiveness with appropriate patient care	SN.4. Community demonstrates greater assertiveness by asking for evaluation and treatment.	B.4. Primary care physician does not demand or imply need to see the patient before treatment.

TABLE 6.18. EMERGENCY DEPARTMENT MATRIX FOR RESPONSE TO STROKE.

Performance Objectives (ER Staff Members)	Personal Determinants				External Determinants	
	Knowledge	Outcome Expectations	Skills and Self-Efficacy	Perceived Social Norms and Standard of Care	Reinforcement	Barriers and Resources
PO.1. Emergency department (ED) physicians and team complete stroke evaluation in sixty minutes. PO.1.1. Triage nurses have patient seen by the physician in ten minutes. PO.1.2. Physicians notify the designated ER stroke team within fifteen minutes.	K.1.(1.1,1.2)a. Describe three-hour window for stroke treatment K.1.(1.1,1.2)b. Describe study results from rtPA trials K.1.(1.1,1.2)c. Describe the urgency of assessment to treatment window	OE.1.(1.1,1.2)a. Describe probability that treatment with rtPA will improve outcome OE.1.(1.1,1.2)b. Expect that community neurologists and primary care doctors want patient's stroke to be managed without consultation		SN.1.(1.1,1.2)a. Describe that professional associations include rtPA in guideline documents SN.1.(1.1, 1.2)b. Describe that other EDs are changing practice to provide acute treatment for stroke SN.1.(1.1, 1.2)c. Describe other EDs in the U.S. as lowering their workup time for stroke	R.1.(1.1, 1.2). ED shares graphs of times at baseline and after interventions are initiated.	BR.1.(1.1, 1.2)a. Create designated stroke team BR.1.(1.1., 1.2)b. ED defines protocol with standing orders for CT, lab work, venous access, oxygen, electro-cardiogram, cardiac monitoring, chest radiograph, and blood glucose level. BR.1.(1.1., 1.2)c. Create flow chart of team protocol
PO.2. ED-designated stroke teams send lab work STAT (HCT, platelets, glucose, PT, PTT) and get it back STAT.					R.2. ED shares successes with lab.	BR. 2. ED nurses, staff physicians, radiologists, CT techs, pharmacy and lab have STAT workup protocol for stroke.
PO.3. ED physicians and stroke teams make rapid differential diagnosis of stroke (use modified NIH scale and protocol).	K.3. Describe diagnostic protocol—aspects of history and physical and studies—that will allow differential diagnosis	OE. 3. Expect that community neurologists and primary care doctors want patient's stroke to be managed without consultation	SSE. 3. Demonstrate using modified NIH protocol for diagnosis			BR. 3. ED nurses, staff physicians, radiologists, CT techs, pharmacy, and lab have STAT workup protocol for stroke.

TABLE 6.18. EMERGENCY DEPARTMENT MATRIX FOR RESPONSE TO STROKE, Cont'd.

| Performance Objectives (ER Staff Members) | Personal Determinants | | | | External Determinants | |
	Knowledge	Outcome Expectations	Skills and Self-Efficacy	Perceived Social Norms and Standard of Care	Reinforcement	Barriers and Resources
PO.4. Perform pulse oximetry, attach cardiac monitor, and perform EKG	K.4. Describe monitoring protocol					
PO.5. Designated ED stroke teams obtain accurate onset time of stroke symptoms.	K.5. Describe the process of obtaining onset time	OE.5. Describe that determining stroke onset time can make the difference between having treatment success and complications	SSE.5.a. Demonstrate interview to determine onset time SSE. 5.b. Increase confidence in performing interview			
PO.6. Designated stroke teams ensure patient receives CT scan within twenty-five minutes and notify on-call radiologist.					R.6. EDs share successes with radiology.	BR.6.a. EDs call CT technician when EMS calls. BR.6.b. EDs involve trained CT technician and radiology in protocol development.
PO.7. Radiologists and designated stroke teams read the CT scan immediately (within forty-five minutes of arrival).	K.7. Describe CT scan contraindications for rtPA		SSE.7.a. Demonstrate interpreting CT scan for hypodensity greater than one-third of MCA SSE.7.b. Correctly use CT to verify time of onset SSE.7.c. Express self-efficacy for reading CT scan		R.7. ED shares successes with radiology.	

PO.8. Designated stroke teams rule out contraindications.	K.8. Describe the necessity to rule out hemorrhagic stroke prior to acute treatment				BR.9.a.(1-4). Correct formulary and logistical issues for the delivery of rtPA (such as have rtPA in hospital formulary and available; have rtPA protocol; have hemorrhage protocol) BR.9.b.(1-4). Engage pharmacy in protocol development
PO.9. Designated stroke teams manage diagnosed stroke. PO.9.1. Insert an IV in each arm if not done by EMS PO.9.2. Administer rtPA within sixty minutes PO.9.3. Treat blood pressure appropriately PO.9.4. Give appropriate dose of rtPA; infuse properly; document time (do not give heparin or coumadin)	K.9.a.(1-4). Describe rtPA orders and dosing K.9.b.(1-4). Discuss trial results and adverse side effects of rtPA administration K.9.c.(1-4). Discuss rationale for giving standard treatment if BP above 210/125 and excluding from rtPA K.9.d.(1-4). Discuss rationale considering rtPA and lowering if BP above 210/125	OE.9.a.(1-4). Expect that stroke patients (especially those with moderate presenting disability) can recover function with acute treatment OE.9.b.(1-4). Expect that community neurologists and primary care doctors want patient's stroke to be managed without consultation	SSE.9.a.(1-4). Demonstrate administration of rtPA SSE.9.b.(1-4). Express confidence in the ability to administer rtPA SSE.9.c.(1-4). Demonstrate management of blood pressure	R.9.(1-4). EDs share patient recovery stories.	

TABLE 6.19. EMERGENCY MEDICAL SERVICE MATRIX FOR RESPONSE TO STROKE.

| Performance Objectives (Emergency medical service (EMS) Personnel) | Personal Determinants | | | | External Determinants | |
	Knowledge	Skills and Self-Efficacy	Outcome Expectations and Previous Experience with Stroke	Perceived Social Norms	Barriers and Resources	Reinforcement
PO.1. Dispatchers triage to highest priority of transport.	K.1. Recognize symptoms of stroke	SSE.1.a. Demonstrate recognition and labeling of symptoms SSE.1.b. Demonstrate interviewing informant about symptoms	OE.1. Believe that the outlook for stroke has improved dramatically with the approval of rtPA	PSN.1. Recognize that dispatchers around the country are making these same kinds of changes to make stroke more like heart attack and trauma	BR.1. EMS medical directors and staff members change departmental policy to increase urgency of stroke transport.	R.1.a. Emergency department (ED) staff members administer stroke therapy. R.1.b. Responders are told when patients have a good outcome from receiving acute treatment.
PO.2. Dispatchers convey stroke possibility and urgency to responders.	K.2. Recognize change in departmental protocol regarding transport of stroke	SSE.2. Participate in the development of the departmental protocol for stroke	OE.2.a. Describe that the outlook for stroke has improved dramatically OE.2.b. State probability of receiving stroke treatment is improved when patient is transported at the highest level of priority	PSN.2. Recognize that dispatchers around the country are making these same kinds of changes to make stroke more like heart attack and trauma	BR.2. Change departmental policy to increase urgency of stroke transport	R.2.a. ED staff administer stroke therapy. R.2.b.Responders are told when patients have a good outcome from receiving acute treatment.
PO.3. Responders perform "load and go."	K.3.a. Recognize symptoms of stroke K.3.b. Describe change in departmental protocol regarding transport of stroke	SSE.3. Participate in the development of the departmental protocol for stroke	OE.3.a. Describe that the outlook for stroke has improved dramatically with the approval of rtPA OE.3.b. State probability of receiving stroke treatment is improved when patient is transported at the highest level of priority	PSN.3. Recognize that responders around the country are making these same kinds of changes to make stroke more like heart attack and trauma	BR.3. Change departmental policy to increase urgency of stroke transport and to specify on-site and in-ambulance protocol	R.3.a. ED staff members administer stroke therapy. R.3.b. ED staff members tell responder when patients have a good outcome from receiving acute treatment.

PO	K	SSE	OE	PSN	R
PO.4. Responders call ahead to the hospital.	K.4. Describe the steps the ED team takes to prepare ahead for STAT workup		OE.4. Recognize that the hospital has changed protocol to treat stroke	PSN.4. Recognize calling ahead as part of standard of care for transport of stroke patients	
PO.5. Responders get family or witness to accompany to the hospital.	K.5.a. Describe the importance of having a witness to establish the last observation of baseline K.5.b. Recognize that ED personnel will need to verify time of onset before giving rtPA		OE.5. Describe probability that rtPA (medication that can only be given in a small time window) reduces disability from stroke		
PO.6. Responders interview patient or witness to determine symptom onset.	K.6.a. Describe the importance of establishing the last observation of baseline K.6.b. Recognize that ER personnel will need to verify time of onset before giving rtPA	SSE.6. Demonstrate ascertainment of stroke symptom onset with good interviewing technique			
PO.7. Responders deliver patients prepared for treatment.		SSE.7. Demonstrate in-transport management of stroke patient		PSN.7. Recognize that other EMS follow standard of care for in-transport stroke management	R.7. ED stroke teams react with urgency.
PO.7.a. Responders deliver patients with IVs in both arms (perform in ambulance).	K.7.a Describe the way rtPA is given and the ED time constraints				

TABLE 6.19. EMERGENCY MEDICAL SERVICE MATRIX FOR RESPONSE TO STROKE, Cont'd.

| Performance Objectives (Emergency medical service (EMS) Personnel) | Personal Determinants | | | | External Determinants | |
	Knowledge	Skills and Self-Efficacy	Outcome Expectations and Previous Experience with Stroke	Perceived Social Norms	Barriers and Resources	Reinforcement
PO.7.b. Responders deliver patient having drawn blood.	K.7.b. Recognize that the ER will need HCT, platelets, glucose, PT and PTT before acute stroke treatment can be given					
PO.7.c. Responders deliver patient having managed fluids and glucose.	K.7.c. Recognize the importance of good stroke management prior to acute treatment					
PO.7.d. Responders refrain from giving blood pressure–lowering medications.	K.7.d. Describe the effect of blood pressure on ischemic stroke					

TABLE 6.20. PRIMARY CARE PROVIDER MATRIX FOR RESPONSE TO STROKE.

	Personal Determinants				External Determinants	
Performance Objectives (Health Care Staff Members)	Skills and Self-Efficacy	Knowledge	Perceived Social Norms	Outcome Expectations	Social Norms	Barriers
PO.1. Receptionists and nurses tell the person with the possible stroke to call 911.	SSE.1. Express confidence in recognizing stroke symptoms	K.1.a. Recognize stroke symptoms: numbness, weakness, ↓ vision, ↓ speech, ↓ walking, tingling, vertigo, headache K.1.b. Describe all adults at risk for stroke	PSN.1. Recognize that others in the community take symptoms of stoke seriously	OE.1.a. Expect that identifying symptoms signifying stroke can help patient improve outcome OE.1.b. Expect that advising immediate transport to emergency department (ED) can help improve outcomes	SN.1. Primary care practices advise patients to get immediate transport to ED.	B.1. Primary care physicians teach staff about stroke and telephone protocol policy to advise to ED via emergency medical services (EMS).
PO2. Primary care providers identify high-risk patients for stroke and teach them about their risk, how to identify symptoms, and how to call 911.			PSN.1. Recognize that other primary care providers in the community educate patients	OE.2.a. Expect that by acting assertively can get prompt stroke treatment and possibly minimize damage OE.2.b. Expect that talking to patients about stroke risk will result in faster response	SN.2. Community providers demonstrate interest in stroke treatment.	
PO.3. Primary care providers educate office staff regarding signs of stroke and communication with patients (such as telling them to call 911).	SSE.4. Express confidence in being able to educate office staff on stroke protocol		PSN.4. Recognize that others in the community are assertive about stroke	OE.4. Expect that EMS and ED will respond to assertiveness with appropriate patient care		

INTERVENTION MAPPING STEP 3: SELECTING THEORY-INFORMED INTERVENTION METHODS AND PRACTICAL STRATEGIES

Reader Objectives

- Review program ideas with the intended participants and use their perspectives when identifying methods and strategies
- Use core processes to identify theoretical methods that can influence change in determinants and identify the conditions under which a given method is most likely to be effective
- Choose theoretical methods for the program
- Select or design practical strategies for applying the methods to the intervention program
- Assure that the final strategies (still) match the change objectives

A *theoretical method* is a general technique or process for influencing changes in the determinants of behaviors and environmental conditions. A *practical strategy* is a specific technique for the application of theoretical methods in ways that fit the intervention population and the context in which the intervention will be conducted. For example, a change objective for an intervention might be to increase adolescents' self-efficacy to resist social pressure to use drugs. For the change objective of increasing self-efficacy, theoretical methods might include modeling, skill training, guided practice with feedback, and reinforcement. One strategy for modeling could be a videotaped step-by-step demonstration by adolescents of how to resist peer pressure in situations they commonly encounter. In another example, an environmental condition of adolescent drug use could be the availability of drugs for sale in neighborhoods where adolescents live, with a performance objective that the mayor would get police to actively enforce laws against neighborhood drug dealers. A change objective for this might be to increase the mayor's positive outcome expectations, for example, that this enforcement will save children's lives, be popular with constituents, be positively received by powerful groups in the city, and increase tourism to the city. The primary theoretical method for this could be advocacy, which includes methods of information, persuasion, negotiation, and coercion. One strategy might be for influential neighborhood activists to hold a breakfast meeting with the mayor, neighborhood constituents, and key city opinion leaders. The activists might present detailed case histories of neighborhood teens, along with pictures of open drug dealing on the street. If the mayor does not respond to this strategy, the group might undertake media advocacy with an exposé story with calls for action by the mayor on the local television channel as additional strategies.

Methods and strategies form a continuum that extends from abstract theoretical methods through practical strategies to organized programs with specified scope, sequence, and support materials. For instance, skills training is a theoretical method; a step-by-step instruction from a videotape with guided practice would be a practical strategy to deliver the skills training; and a program would include descriptions of when and how the training would be delivered and supported. The difference between theoretical methods and practical strategies can be confusing. Modeling is more a method than a strategy; role-model stories are both a method and a strategy; and demonstrations are more a strategy than a method. The point is that methods should always be considered, and strategies should never be devoid of the effective component—the method. Yet methods are easy to overlook because health educators most often think in terms of concrete program components, such as a videotape or a brochure.

In this chapter we show how to choose methods from theory and the literature. These methods will be the basis of intervention components to modify performance and change objectives for behavior and environmental conditions of the at-risk population and environmental agents. The planner's challenge is to cover all of the objectives while creatively translating methods into strategies. Planners use methods and strategies from all intervention levels (individual, interpersonal, organizational, community, and societal) to match determinants. An intervention at higher system levels may have direct or mediated influence on lower (embedded) levels and may be the intervention of choice to change individual behaviors. For example, a media campaign may influence individuals to change their behavior directly or may influence a change in public or organizational policy. Also, interventions at levels beyond the individual may operate directly to change characteristics of that system (that is, family, organization, community). As shown in Figure 7.1, planners choose methods and strategies to influence change objectives. Change objectives describe the desired changes in the determinants of performance objectives for health behavior and environmental conditions, at the individual and at higher environmental levels. Modeling may change individual health behavior, but it could also be applied to influence the behavior of decision makers in organizations required to make changes in the environment. For example, persuasive communication could be applied to influence the behavior of politicians to take action that would change environmental conditions.

In this chapter we present various methods for different determinants starting with methods for determinants that are related to change in the individual health behavior of the at-risk group. Then, we discuss methods for changing determinants at environmental levels, which are more specifically appropriate for groups, organizations, communities, and public policy. We describe only a sample of methods that can be used to address change objectives and refer the reader to social science texts, particularly those with explicit applications to health education (Bracht & Kingsbury, 1990; R. J. DiClemente, Crosby, & Kegler, 2002; Glanz, Lewis, & Rimer, 2002; Maibach & Parrott, 1995; McGuire, 1985; Minkler, 1997a, 1997b).

FIGURE 7.1. LOGIC MODEL OF CHANGE WITH METHODS AND STRATEGIES.

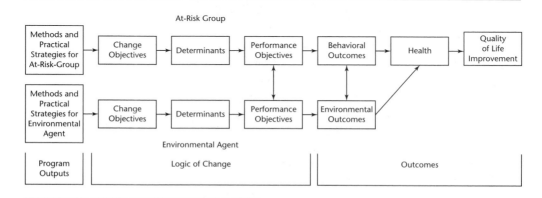

Perspectives

Our perspectives in this chapter concern the importance of ensuring that programs contain theoretical methods that are capable of producing the planned change at the planner's desired ecological level.

The Case of the Missing Methods

The causal chain from objectives to methods to strategies is not often reported in the health education literature, and without this description, it is impossible to review the theory and evidence base for what the planners have chosen to include in the intervention. Most publications on health education interventions, often evaluation studies, lack clear information about what the authors actually expected to cause a change. They often present the strategy and the program, for example, a tailored letter to encourage mammography or a videotape to teach breast self-examination. But they may not be explicit about what methods they used in the letter or how the videotape actually teaches or motivates the screening behavior. Tailoring can be considered a general method, but the letter must use specific theoretical methods that would, according to the theory, "cause" a woman to obtain a mammogram. Did the researchers use persuasion, modeling with vicarious reinforcement, a cue to action, or some other method? In another example, researchers might write that they used nonsmoking contracts to stimulate resistance to smoking, but they do not mention the theoretical method of commitment on which the strategy was presumably based—a method that would include, in order to be effective, making a public commitment. We want to stress here that all program components must contain methods as well as strategies.

One source of confusion about methods may be that the same concept, such as modeling or reinforcement, can be used to describe both determinants and methods. The double use of these concepts is actually an interesting part of theories, because it means that the theory explains both behavior and behavior change. The difference for health promoters is that modeling as a determinant refers to what happens in the actual situation, whereas modeling as a method will be part of a well-designed program. For instance, with respect to condom use, modeling that occurs in the television shows and movies that adolescents see may be negative, whereas health educators may use positive role models in their interventions to compensate for negative role models in the media (Kok, Schaalma, De Vries, Parcel, & Paulussen, 1996).

Translating methods into strategies demands a sufficient understanding of the theory behind the method, especially the theoretical parameters that limit the effectiveness of the theoretical process (Kok, Schaalma, Ruiter, van Empelen, & Brug, 2004). Modeling is a strong method but only when certain parameters are met, for instance, reinforcement of the modeled behavior. People do not just behave in the desired manner because a model shows that behavior; they follow the model when the model is reinforced for that particular behavior and when they expect to be reinforced in a similar way. Reinforcement may be in terms of outcomes or of social rewards. Translating the method modeling to a practical strategy includes taking care that in the actual program, from the perspective of the program participants, the model is reinforced. When we describe translating methods into strategies, we will give more detail on this process and provide examples.

Methods at Different Levels of Intervention

There are two basic differences between descriptions in the literature of behavioral change methods and those of methods for changing environmental conditions. One difference is that theories that focus on individual behavior change are more likely to be process theories (that is, closer to what we call methods), whereas theories regarding environmental change are more likely to be implementation theories (that is, closer to what we call strategies) (Porras & Robertson, 1987; Steckler, Goodman, & Kegler, 2002).

The second difference is in the way knowledge is garnered regarding the application of different types of theories to health education. In individual behavior change, there has been a somewhat deductive approach: program planners extract behavioral science theoretical change constructs and then apply them to health. This approach to theory application is not theory testing; it is still a theory-of-the problem approach, but in its philosophy it resembles theory testing. On the other hand, social change activities—people doing things such as community organization and coalition building—have been reported in the literature as case examples. This is not a process of applying a construct in a community, and sometimes it is not possible to determine whether these activities are methods or strategies and whether theoretical constructs are involved in the applications. Possibly this approach to intervention is more inductive, intervening with a strategy without naming the method. Where possible in this chapter, we label the methods inherent in community-oriented strategies. However, we do not force the upper ecological levels into theoretical constructs when none seems applicable. If the literature reports mostly strategies, then we report strategies. Sometimes we speculate about methods, or we label something as a method. Health educators should consider what method is used in a social change strategy so that they can be clear about what aspect of an intervention is expected to produce what change.

Ideas About the Program

⤵ *The first task in Step 3 is to review program ideas with intended participants and use their perspectives when identifying methods and strategies.*

Intervention Mapping stimulates the planner to follow the steps of conducting the needs assessment, developing the matrices for performance and change objectives, selecting theoretical methods that are translated into practical strategies, and then creating the actual intervention program. However, most planners already have some idea of a program that may reach the desired program objectives. It is, in fact, important to keep in mind that elaborating on theoretical methods will eventually lead to a program. The idea behind the Intervention Mapping steps is not to keep planners from thinking of programs but to help them to develop programs that have a solid theory and evidence base. Planners must find a balance between preliminary ideas for programs on the one hand and theory- and evidence-informed decisions for methods, strategies, and programs on the other hand. For example, mass media campaigns may be useful for changing social norms but probably not for increasing self-efficacy and skills. Fear-arousing messages may be popular with the representatives of the at-risk population and intermediates, but they often are not effective in influencing change and performance objectives.

On the other hand, evidence-informed methods and strategies may not be easily applicable in the actual context of the program or the potential participants in the program. For instance, peer education is often cited as an effective method for change, but peer education is not appropriate in all contexts and cultures. In Chapter Eleven Schaalma and Kok explain that peer education for HIV prevention among adolescents in Dutch schools was not acceptable to Dutch teachers because peer education is not part of their normal routine.

The first task in this step is to review program ideas with the intended participants and use their perspectives when identifying methods and strategies. The linkage group, which was established in the first step of Intervention Mapping, should include both members of the potential program participants and possible program implementers. While working on this step, the program planners should review the representation in the linkage and program planning groups so that they have a good forum for balancing existing ideas on strategies and programs, theoretical and empirical input on methods, and limitations and potentials of the program context. Establishing an appropriate linkage group and adding relevant program users during the planning process is an essential condition for the resulting program's effectiveness.

Identifying Theoretical Methods

The next task is to use core processes to identify theoretical methods that can influence change in determinants and identify the conditions under which a certain method is more likely to be effective.

Theoretical methods are general techniques or processes for influencing changes in determinants of behaviors of the at-risk group or environmental agents. To match a method with a change objective, the linking concept is the determinant involved. For example, take the change objective: adolescents (the population) demonstrate skills (the determinant) in communicating with a partner about condom use (the performance objective). The method to reach this objective can be found by looking at methods for the determinant: skills. Of course, within the various methods for skills training, the planner will need to consider the population and the performance objectives. Adolescents can be reached through the schools, but teachers may have ideas on what skills training methods they would want to apply with the topic of condom use.

To get from the matrices with change objectives as a result of Step 2 to the selection of methods in Step 3, planners reorganize the change objectives by determinants. They make a list of all change objectives that have to do with increasing knowledge, another list of all change objectives that have to do with changing outcome expectations, and so forth. Methods will then be matched to the determinants; there may be multiple methods for a determinant as well as multiple objectives for a method. For example, modeling is often used for various skills-related change objectives, but for training some skills, it may also be necessary to use guided practice. In the HIV-prevention program for Dutch adolescents, the risk perception and awareness change objectives were matched with a number of methods, as presented in Table 7.1.

Table 7.1 shows three change objectives for two performance objectives, as well as four methods for changing awareness and risk perception. The planners of this intervention elected to personalize risk for all three objectives, because that is a very broad and effective method. They also decided to apply all four methods for the third objective, because they found that objective to be especially rel-

TABLE 7.1. OBJECTIVES AND METHODS FOR CHANGING AWARENESS AND RISK PERCEPTION.

Determinant: Awareness and Risk Perception

Change Objectives	Methods
Performance objective: plan condom use	
• Recognize that human immunodeficiency virus (HIV) and sexually transmitted infections (STIs) are related to behavior, not to risk group	Personalize risk
• Recognize the possibility of finding oneself in situations in which infection is possible	Personalize risk Scenario-based risk information
Performance objective: use condoms with regular partner	
• Describe own sexual behavior as serial monogamous rather than monogamous	Scenario-based risk information Fear appeals Personalize risk Loss frame

evant for this target group: many adolescents see themselves as monogamous, whereas in fact they are serially monogamous, resulting in multiple sex partners.

Methods can be applied at any ecological level; however, as we have seen, methods at the higher levels often take a different form than do similar methods at the individual level. Persuasive communication with individuals in a counseling context is different from political advocacy in a meeting between politicians and a lobbying group or in a meeting between company managers and union representatives. The determinant may be the same (that is, outcome expectations), but the content and the vehicle for delivering a selected method are different. Therefore, we present methods for individual change by determinant, and we follow up with methods at environmental levels that are directed at the same determinant but for a higher environmental level.

From the Sun Protection Is Fun (SPF) project (see Chapter Six), we describe two change objectives for attitude change, one at the individual level and one at the organizational level (see Table 7.2). Modeling is a useful method for attitude change and can easily be applied with the children. Of course, reinforcement of the model is an essential parameter; we will come back to parameters later in this chapter. Persuasive communication can be applied with both the children and the preschool director, but the content will be different: What are new and strong arguments for the children are different from what are new and strong arguments

TABLE 7.2. OBJECTIVES AND METHODS AT VARIOUS LEVELS.

Determinant: Attitude Change

Change Objectives	Methods
Individual level performance objective: child wears protective clothes and hat	
• Feels positive about protective clothes	Modeling Persuasive communication
Organizational level performance objective: preschool director provides shade in outdoor areas	
• Describes enduring shade as positive	Shifting perspective Persuasive communication

for the directors. In this case the directors are responsible for the protection of the schoolchildren, so shifting perspective may be a very effective method to change the attitudes of preschool directors. They have to realize how their behavior influences the health of these children, in addition to considering economic or financial concerns related to providing shade structures, for example. If that method were not effective, planners could move to methods for other determinants, such as social pressure by stimulating parents to write letters to the school board.

External Determinants and Environmental Conditions: The Agent's Role

In Chapter Six we explained how to specify behavioral outcomes and environmental outcomes and translate them into performance objectives of the at-risk population and the environmental condition. Each performance objective has an actor, either an at-risk person or a change agent in the environment. The performance objectives are influenced by determinants, and the change objectives at the individual level and at the environmental level form the most immediate objectives for a program (see Figure 6.1). The methods and strategies that we introduce in this chapter are directed at those change objectives. Many performance objectives have personal and external determinants. If the needs assessment is done carefully, most of the external determinants for the performance objectives for the at-risk individual have become part of the specified environmental change and related performance objectives. Only those few external determinants that are part of the environment but can be dealt with without an extensive analysis (and matrix) remain on the matrix of the at-risk group.

Neither external determinants nor environmental conditions are likely to be under the direct control of the individuals at risk for the health problem. They are controlled by external agents, such as peers, teachers, managers, decision makers, and gatekeepers. Therefore, change objectives for external determinants and for environmental outcomes are formulated by referring to an environmental agent. Moreover, there may be various environmental levels: interpersonal, organizational, community, and societal levels. In project SPF, there are matrices at the at-risk individual, interpersonal, and organizational levels: children, parents, teachers, school directors, and school management. The planning team focused on change objectives at all these levels and considered methods such as skills training for parents and organizational advocacy for school management.

In another example, smoking by adolescents is influenced by personal determinants but also by a supportive school environment. When the school environment is not supportive enough, the health promoter will want to change this external determinant by urging the school management to develop and implement a nonsmoking school policy. So the focus of the health promoter will shift in this instance to the behavior of agents related to the school. Perhaps the school management, school board, superintendent, or parents could be persuaded to implement a nonsmoking policy. The health promoter might use methods of persuasive communication and modeling to influence the school management's decision-making process. However, there are external determinants for the school management's decision making as well, in the form of state and national regulations related to nonsmoking policies in schools. When those regulations are lacking, the health promoter might want to change this external determinant by urging the Ministry of Education and the Ministry of Health or their U.S. counterparts to declare stricter rules banning smoking in schools. The health promoter will use the method of political advocacy to influence this policymaking process. Figure 7.2 offers a schematic representation of this chain of events. Even the government will be influenced by external factors, such as public support. Again, the health promoter may want to influence citizens to advocate for school policies that ban smoking, by applying methods from the community level.

Note that this example illustrates two assumptions about effectiveness and evidence. The first assumption is that the environmental outcome will actually promote the health-promoting behavior, that is, that establishing a school ban on smoking will decrease the onset of and increase the cessation of students' smoking. In Step 2 (Chapter Six), the planner will have paid attention to making sure that an evidence base exists for this assumption. The second assumption is that there is evidence that the method will actually change the agent's behavior. We presented evidence for various individual and higher-level methods used to

FIGURE 7.2. SCHEMATIC REPRESENTATION OF THE SHIFT FROM EXTERNAL DETERMINANTS TO ENVIRONMENTAL FACTORS.

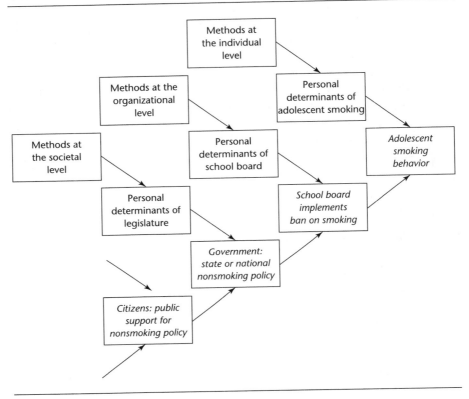

change determinants of the agents' behavior, such as persuasive communication or parental advocacy, in Chapters Three and Four.

To summarize, to select methods for external determinants, the first thing to do is to find out who may be in a position to make the expected change. Sometimes persons at risk for the health problem may be able to cope with the external determinant themselves, for instance, in the case of peer pressure by improved skills to resist peer pressure. Sometimes the health promotion planner can take care of an external determinant, for instance, by providing cues for the behavior as part of the program. However, most of the time, external determinants are under the control of an environmental agent. The plan then has to identify the performance objectives for the agent that will actually change that external determinant or environmental condition. The health promoter then applies methods for influencing the determinants of the agent's performance objectives. Notice that determinants, including personal determinants, often have different content at various ecological levels, depending on the environmental agent's role. The adolescent's outcome expectations (for example, that not smoking will result in more clean smelling breath and clothes) differ from the school management's outcome expectations about implementing a nonsmoking policy (for example, that parents will appreciate the school's having a nonsmoking policy), and those are different still from the government's outcome expectations about declaring a national nonsmoking policy for schools (that is, constituents will support a stricter policy). Therefore, methods directed at the same type of determinant, such as outcome expectations or skills, will be different for various environmental levels. That is why later in this chapter we describe methods for change organized by environmental level: interpersonal, organization, community, and society.

Core Processes

Two of the core processes presented in Chapter Two are essential for identifying and selecting methods: reviewing existing empirical evidence in the literature and reviewing theories of change. With the topic approach to finding and using theory, the health educator goes back to the literature on the problem. If the problem is drug abuse, for example, the health educator discovers what methods others have used to influence resistance to social pressure. Unfortunately, much of the literature is vague about methods and more forthcoming about practical strategies. The health educator can then use the construct approach, with the change objective stated as "Resist social pressure to use drugs," and find theoretical methods specifically about resisting social pressure to use drugs, resisting social pressure to other risk behaviors such as smoking, and resisting social pressure in general. The health educator may find that this literature cites theories on conformity and nonconformity and on social comparison. The health educator may also use the general theories approach to explore those theories that address behavior change in general (for example, Social Cognitive Theory (SCT) and discover what those general theories have to offer about accomplishing this particular objective. In Chapter Two we provided a detailed example of the application of the core processes to the selection of methods for influencing drug users' HIV-preventive behavior.

There may be several methods for one objective as well as one method for multiple objectives. In cases in which available information is extremely sparse, such as reducing fear for social contact with people with AIDS, planners may have to develop more insight on appropriate methods through a third core process: additional research with the intervention group (Dijker, Kok, & Koomen, 1995).

Methods Selection

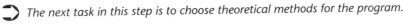 *The next task in this step is to choose theoretical methods for the program.*

To complete this task, planners must be sure to distinguish between theoretical methods and practical strategies and ensure that all program components contain methods. They also must consider preliminary ideas on the program in light of information from theory and evidence. In this section we describe the various ways that work groups can select methods and strategies. After making the preliminary selection, groups should evaluate each method on relevance and changeability. We then describe general methods and those specific to the most relevant determinants for behavior change, along with their parameters or considerations for their use. We then turn to general environmental change methods and those directed specifically to social norms, social support, social networks, organizations, community, and policy with considerations for their use. This review facilitates the health promoter's consideration of a variety of methods when deciding which methods would be best to change a determinant in the context of the at-risk population, environmental agents, and program setting.

Box 7.1. Mayor's Project

When we drop in on the mayor's work group, we hear the group deliberating on what to do next. The one person who had used Intervention Mapping previously is quite comfortable continuing in a somewhat linear process.

Participant A: OK, now we just group the learning and change objectives at each ecological level by determinants. Then we discuss what methods could change that group of objectives. You see, the whole process at this point is driven by the determinants.

Participant B: What? I thought we had already dealt with the determinants. Now we are back at the matrices with the change objectives?

Participant A: Yes, that's right. It's just that the determinant part of the matrix—the determinant grouping—guides this process.
[Many in the mayor's group groan.]

Participant C: I am so tired of tables. I just cannot think this way anymore. Isn't there any other way of doing this? I have so many ideas about this program, and I've managed to keep my enthusiasm through this entire Intervention Mapping process to this point. But to tell the truth, if I have to do one more table, I might lose all of my creative program ideas.

Participant D: I feel the same way. And on top of that, I don't understand the difference between a method and a strategy. It seems to me that this is just one more set of unnecessary vocabulary words that get in the way of really being creative about a program. Furthermore, throughout the planning process, I have been asked to hold on to my program ideas. When do I get to stop holding on? Is that now?

The mayor's health educator listens to her colleagues and recommends that they all close their Intervention Mapping notes and put away their matrices. The group structures the next hour as a brainstorming session. Brainstorming had worked well for this group in the past, and they liked generating ideas without censure or correction. The health educator draws a line down the board and labels one side Methods and the other side Strategies. The group takes one determinant at a time, and with that set of change objectives, it thinks about what method would affect those objectives. How would they produce change? Each time someone comes up with something, the group decides whether it is a theoretical way to change the determinant—a method—or a programmatic idea about how to deliver methods—a strategy. The health educator records the ideas in the appropriate columns.

Work Style

People have different work styles; work groups do too. In selecting methods and strategies, health educators may take any of several routes based on their experience with theory and practice. Some will move carefully from objectives to methods and then to strategies. Others will move from objectives to strategies and then back to the underlying method. Still others will brainstorm methods and strategies simultaneously. For example, one health educator may think of commitment as a theoretical method for increasing self-efficacy of adolescents to remain nonsmokers. He or she would then brainstorm about practical strategies to apply that method. Another health educator may think of a nonsmoking contract as a strategy for improving self-efficacy and then find out from the literature that the underlying theoretical method is commitment. During that process the health educator might also find alternatives to a nonsmoking contract that may have the same or even better results. What is essential in these different routes is that methods are identified, and the parameters of the methods—the conditions under which the methods are shown to be effective—are kept in mind during the translation from method to strategy and to program. For example, the health educator who likes the idea of a nonsmoking contract should be aware that commitment is only effective as a method for increasing self-efficacy when the act of commitment has been made public. Therefore, contracts that individuals make in private settings may have positive effects as reminders, but they do not have the strong effect of public commitment.

There is no reason why planners cannot start with strategies and then think about theoretical methods. However, the essential question here is: Why would the particular strategy work? For every creative idea, there needs to be a theoretical process describing why the expected effects are going to happen. For instance, health educators working with gay men who chat on the Internet to meet others for dating and sex decided to use a guide with illustration of an attractive gay man to lead the user through a web-based program for HIV prevention. The potential participants had very clear but different preferences for the choice of guides from six options. Most men selected one guide and stayed with him when they returned to the site. Why would this strategy be expected to work? The guides and the municipal health service that produce the site were both seen as sources of information. Research on persuasive communication (a method for attitude change) suggests that theoretically relevant source characteristics are attractiveness and expertise (parameters for the method). These characteristics function is primarily to be the source of the information. In this case, giving the men the choice of their own guide helped to improve the effectiveness of the persuasive messages on the Web site. Of course, the quality of the arguments in the messages is equally important. Guides who are chosen for their attractiveness but who are then found to lack good arguments will probably have little impact on the users of the Web site.

Having found methods from the list of theoretical methods or from consideration of the process behind preliminary ideas, planners should select methods for their program by evaluating all the suggested methods on relevance and changeability. *Relevance* is the strength of the evidence for the relation between the determinants this method addresses and the behavior or environmental condition we want to change using this method. *Changeability* is the strength of the evidence that the proposed change can be realized by this specific method in this specific setting. Selected methods should have relatively high scores on both relevance and changeability. For an elaborated example, see Table 2.7 on methods for changing risk perception and social influence for an HIV-prevention program for drug users. See also Table 11.6 for an application in an HIV-prevention program for schools.

Methods for Changing Behavior

In this section we describe theoretical methods for behavior change. The first part presents methods geared to changing determinants (for example, attitude, skills) of the at-risk individuals. We then move to methods for change in determinants of agents within the environment. For instance, attitude change of an individual could be facilitated by persuasive communication. Attitude change of a politician who serves as a gatekeeper for policy change could also be facilitated by persuasive communication. However, the content and the vehicle of the messages would be quite different in the two cases. The content varies by the role of the agent, and the vehicle is tailored to the power involved, for example, power over and power with in organizations and community.

The following section summarizes methods for change for the determinants of individual behavior. However, it is very difficult to imagine a health promotion intervention setting that is not embedded in some kind of social or physical structure. A child with asthma is in an environment with parents, nurses, doctors, and other children with asthma. An adolescent in an HIV-prevention program is in an environment with friends, sexual partners, parents, teachers, and community leaders. Work-site employees participating in a smoking-cessation program are in an environment with colleagues, health professionals, supervisors, and work-site policies. In a later section of this chapter, we present methods for change at environmental levels. It is important for health promotion planners to realize that individual behavior change is almost always embedded in one or more environmental levels and that methods for individual change need to be complemented with methods for change at those environmental levels.

We combine comparable determinants when they appear in more than one theory, for example, attitudes, beliefs, and outcome expectations. The various determinants are not independent of each other; we will start with knowledge as the basis for many other determinants, such as risk perception, attitude, and skills. Risk perception in turn is a specific part of attitude. Methods described for one determinant may sometimes be used for other determinants as well. The theoretical background for all methods is provided in Chapters Three and Four.

Basic Methods for Behavior Change. Some methods for change at the individual level turn out to be useful for all determinants and also at all levels at which that method is applied. The members of the intervention group, for example, must pay attention to the intervention message, understand the content, and process the information centrally. Table 7.3 lists these basic requirements of health education and promotion at the individual level: attention and comprehension,

TABLE 7.3. BASIC METHODS AT THE INDIVIDUAL LEVEL.

Methods (Related Theory)	Parameters for Use
Participation (Diffusion of Innovations)	Willingness to accept the target population as having an equal status
Persuasive communication (Persuasion Communication Matrix, Elaboration Likelihood Model)	Message is relevant and not too discrepant from target group's experience; can be further stimulated by surprise and repetition
Active learning (Persuasion Communication Model, Elaboration Likelihood Model)	Time, information, and skills
Tailoring (Transtheoretical Model, Precaution Adoption Process Model)	Tailoring variables or factors related to behavior change (such as stage) or to relevance (such as culture or socioeconomic status)
Individualization (Transtheoretical Model)	Personal communication that responds to a learner's needs
Feedback (theories of learning, goal-related theories)	Feedback that is individual, follows the desired behavior closely in time, and is specific
Reinforcement (theories of learning, Social Cognitive Theory)	Reinforcement that is individual and follows the desired behavior closely in time
Facilitation (Social Cognitive Theory)	Changes in the environment

active learning, tailoring, individualization, feedback, reinforcement, and facilitation. We discuss the theoretical and empirical background for these basic methods in Chapter Three. Intervention planners should always consider these methods when identifying promising methods for change.

Methods to Influence Knowledge. Knowledge is a necessary (though not sufficient) prerequisite for most other determinants, such as risk perceptions, behavioral beliefs, perceived norms, and skills. Many methods for other determinants will also change knowledge. Conventional wisdom long held that giving people information could change their behavior and thereby solve health and social problems. However, knowledge does not generally lead directly to behavior change; nor is assuring that the target population attains knowledge necessarily an easy task. Theories of information processing (Kools, Ruiter, van de Wiel, & Kok, 2004) provide several concepts that suggest methods for successfully conveying information. Table 7.4 gives an overview of the methods and parameters for influencing knowledge.

TABLE 7.4. METHODS TO INCREASE KNOWLEDGE.

Methods (Related Theory)	Parameters for Use
Basic methods	See Table 7.3
Chunking (theories of information processing)	Labels or acronyms are assigned to material to aid memory.
Advance organizers (theories of information processing)	Schematic representations of the content or guides to what is to be learned
Images (theories of information processing)	Familiar physical or verbal images as analogies to a less familiar process
Tailoring (Transtheoretical Model, Precaution Adoption Model)	Information tailored to concepts that the learner already has
Discussion (theories of information processing)	Listening to the learner to ensure that the correct schemas are activated
Active learning (Persuasion Communication Matrix, Elaboration Likelihood, Social Cognitive Theory)	Stimulation of elaboration by encouraging the learner to add something to the information to be remembered
Cues (theories of information processing)	The same cues are present at the time of learning and the time of retrieval.
Rehearsal (theories of information processing)	More effective when elaborative: adding helpful information

Methods to Change Risk Perception, Awareness, and Health Beliefs. Before we can motivate people for a health-promoting change, they first need to be aware of a risk for themselves. Table 7.5 presents the methods from various theories that may help people perceive their risk. Most of these methods are derived from theories on risk perception and risk communication; others come from stages of behavioral change theories that start with an awareness stage.

Methods to Change Habits, Automatic Behavior, and Action Control. Health promotion planners often assume that an individual decides on a behavior in a planned and reasoned manner. However, many behaviors are automatic and habitual. Even when people make behavioral intentions, they may fail to follow up on those intentions. Table 7.6 summarizes methods for changing habitual and automatic behaviors, as well as methods to promote action control. The attention of the scientific community to this type of behavior has increased in recent years; however, the evidence for effective methods is still limited.

TABLE 7.5. METHODS TO CHANGE AWARENESS AND RISK PERCEPTION.

Methods (Related Theory)	Parameters for Use
Basic methods	See Table 7.3
Information about personal risk (Transtheoretical Model, Precaution Adoption Process Model)	Messages presented as individual, undeniable, on same dimension, congruent with actual risk, and cumulative rather than for one occasion; messages presented with qualitative and quantitative examples
Scenario-based risk information (Precaution Adoption Process Model)	Plausible scenario with a cause and an outcome; imagery
Loss frame or gain frame (Health Belief Model and Protection Motivation Theory)	More effective to use loss frame for detection behaviors and gain frame for prevention behaviors
Reevaluation, self-evaluation, and consciousness raising (Transtheoretical Model)	Can use feedback and confrontation; however, raising awareness must be quickly followed by increase in problem-solving ability and self-efficacy
Dramatic relief (Transtheoretical Model)	Probably should be done in counseling context so that emotions can be aroused and subsequently relieved
Fear arousal (Health Belief Model, Protection Motivation Theory)	Requires high self-efficacy expectations rather than high outcome expectations alone

TABLE 7.6. METHODS TO CHANGE HABITS, AUTOMATIC BEHAVIOR, AND ACTION CONTROL.

Methods (Related Theory)	Parameters for Use
Basic methods	See Table 7.3
Dissociation of conditioning (theories of learning)	Slow process, especially when reinforcement schedule was intermittent
Counter conditioning (Transtheoretical Model)	Availability of substitute behaviors
Implementation intentions (goal-related theories)	Existing positive intention
Cues (goal-related theories, Health Belief Model, Protection Motivation Theory)	Existing positive intention

Methods to Change Attitudes, Beliefs, and Outcome Expectations. Table 7.7 lists some of the methods that may be used to change people's health-related attitudes. Attitudes are a positive or negative reaction to something; but they can include more specific constructs of beliefs, outcome expectations, assessment of advantages and disadvantages, perceived benefits and barriers, self-evaluation,

TABLE 7.7. METHODS TO CHANGE ATTITUDES.

Methods (Related Theory)	Parameters for Use
Basic methods	See Table 7.3
Belief selection (Theory of Planned Behavior)	Requires investigation of the current beliefs of the individual before choosing the belief on which to intervene
Self-reevaluation (Transtheoretical Model, Social Cognitive Theory)	Stimulation of both cognitive and affective appraisal of self-image
Environmental reevaluation (Transtheoretical Model, Social Cognitive Theory)	Stimulation of both cognitive and affective appraisal and to improve appraisal and empathy skills
Shifting perspective (Health Belief Model, Protection Motivation Theory)	Initiation from the perspective of the learner
Arguments (Persuasion Communication Matrix, Elaboration Likelihood Model)	Arguments new to the individual
Direct experience (theories of learning)	Rewarding outcomes from the individual's experience with the behavior or assurance that the individual can cope with and reframe negative outcomes
Modeling (Social Cognitive Theory)	Reinforcement of the model
Persuasive communication (Persuasion Communication Matrix, Elaboration Likelihood Model, Social Cognitive Theory)	Consideration of the source, message, channel, and receiver
Active processing of information (Persuasion Communication Matrix, Elaboration Likelihood Model)	Individuals with high motivation and high cognitive ability; messages that are personally relevant, surprising, repeated, self-pacing, not distracting, easily understandable, and include direct instructions; messages that are not too discrepant and cause anticipation of interaction
Anticipated regret (Theory of Planned Behavior, Transtheoretical Model)	Stimulation of imagery
Repeated exposure (theories of learning)	Neutrality of original attitude

and motivation to act. Social psychology has devoted much attention to attitude change, and we present a very brief summary of this work here (for a more in-depth review, see Eagly & Chaiken, 1993; McGuire, 1985; Petty, Barden, & Wheeler, 2002).

Methods for Changing Social Influences. The influence of the social environment is an important determinant of many behaviors and as such will be found in many change objectives. One theory that tries to explain social influence is Ajzen's Theory of Planned Behavior (TPB) (1991). This theory states that behavior is determined by intention and that intention is determined by attitudes, subjective social norms, and self-efficacy. Social influence in this theory is seen as social expectations, a cognitive construct, and the theory does not cover social influence in the form of modeling, an environmental construct. Social influence through modeling is a central construct in SCT, which explicates intervention methods that change the social environment as well as perceived social influence (Bandura, 1986). Table 7.8 presents methods for changing both cognitive and environmental social influences.

Methods to Influence Skills, Capability, and Self-Efficacy. Constructs addressed in this section are self-efficacy, perceived behavioral control, perceived barriers, skills and perceived skills, collective self-efficacy, behavioral capability, and com-

TABLE 7.8. METHODS TO CHANGE SOCIAL INFLUENCE.

Methods (Related Theory)	Parameters for Use
Basic methods	See Table 7.3
Visible expectations (Theory of Planned Behavior)	Positive expectations are available in the environment.
Building skills for resistance to social pressure (Theory of Planned Behavior, Social Cognitive Theory)	Skill building for refusal skills; commitment to earlier intention; relating intended behavior to values; psychological inoculation against pressure
Shifting focus (Theory of Planned Behavior)	Must shift focus to a new reason for performing the behavior
Modeling and vicarious reinforcement (Social Cognitive Theory, Diffusion of Innovations Theory)	Attention, remembrance, and skills
Stimulate communication and mobilizing social support (Transtheoretical Model, theories of social networks and social support)	Combines caring, trust, openness, and acceptance with support for behavioral change

munity capability. Self-efficacy is often a crucial determinant in changing health behavior. When people are motivated, the remaining question is whether they are able and feel confident to change their behavior. Self-efficacy is a determinant for the precursors of behavior—intention, preparation to act, and decision to act. But it also directly influences behavior, implementation, and maintenance of behavior change. Self-efficacy and related concepts are all personal determinants, but there is a distinction between perceptions (for example, perceived skills) and reality (for example, real skills). Even with sufficient real skills, people may not try the new behavior when their perceived skills are low. And people with high perceived skills may fail because they have insufficient real skills. Methods to improve self-efficacy are therefore often methods that also improve real skills. Table 7.9 presents methods and parameters to enhance skill and self-efficacy.

Methods for Changing Environmental Conditions

The next section describes methods for changing determinants of environmental conditions, including the behavior of environmental agents. First, we list basic methods for change that can be applied at all environmental levels and then methods

TABLE 7.9. METHODS FOR SKILLS, CAPABILITY, AND SELF-EFFICACY.

Methods (Related Theory)	Parameters for Use
Basic methods	See Table 7.3
Modeling (Social Cognitive Theory)	Attention, remembrance, skills, reinforcement; Credible source, method, and channel
Guided practice (Social Cognitive Theory)	Subskill demonstration, instruction, and enactment with feedback
Enactment (Social Cognitive Theory)	Depends on skills and feedback; should result in mastery experience
Verbal persuasion (Social Cognitive Theory)	Credible source, method, and channel
Physiological and affective change (Social Cognitive Theory)	Must carefully interpret and manage emotional states
Reattribution training (Attribution Theory, Relapse Prevention Theory)	Requires counseling unstable and external attributions for failure
Goal setting (goal-related theories)	Commitment to the goal; goals that are difficult but available within the individual's skill level
Planning coping responses (Attribution Theory, Relapse Prevention Theory)	Identification of high-risk situations and practice of coping response

related to specific environmental conditions at each ecological level. In many of these tables, we refer the reader back to earlier tables of methods for both individual and general determinants, indicating that these methods can be used to change the environmental condition or that the methods are embedded in the environmental change methods.

Basic Methods for Change of Environmental Conditions. Some methods for change turn out to be useful at most environmental levels. Skills training, for example, will be applied in almost any method directed at changing an environmental agent's behavior, even when the form of the training may be different than when this method is applied at the strictly individual level. Table 7.10 lists these

TABLE 7.10. BASIC METHODS AT HIGHER ENVIRONMENTAL LEVELS.

Methods (Related Theory)	Parameters for Use
Basic methods	See Table 7.3
Participatory problem solving (theories of social networks and social support, Organizational Development Theory, coalitions, models of community organization)	Series of steps: diagnosis, feedback, goal setting, action, ownership; training in leadership and consultation; requires culture that accepts change
Advocacy, such as information, persuasion, and negotiation (Stage Theory of Organizational Change, models of community organization, Agenda-Building Theory, Policy Window Theory)	Form of advocacy varies by environmental level, nature of the issue being addressed, and nature of power relationships; must match style and tactics of the collective.
Modeling (Organizational Development Theory, Diffusion of Innovations Theory, Social Cognitive Theory)	Appropriate models will vary by level.
Skills training (Theories of social networks and social support, Organizational Development Theory, Diffusion of Innovations Theory, coalitions)	Nature of skills will vary by environmental level; must include decisions about the type of support needed and must intensively train social skills such as empathy and information giving; individuals and collectives might have goals other than skills training.
Technical assistance (Organizational Development Theory, Diffusion of Innovations Theory, coalitions, models of community organization)	Nature of technical assistance will vary by environmental level.
Facilitating conditions such as cues, reinforcement, and resource availability (Social Cognitive Theory, models of community organization, Diffusion of Innovations Theory)	Facilitating conditions on one environmental level are usually dealt with by intervening on a higher environmental level.

basic tools for the health promoter: participatory problem solving, advocacy, modeling, skills training, and technical assistance. We discussed the theoretical and empirical background for these basic methods in Chapter Four. Intervention planners should always consider these methods when identifying promising methods for change at all environmental levels.

Methods to Change Social Norms. In Chapter Four we presented social norms theory as a community-level theory. However, social norms are influential at all levels. In Table 7.8 we summarized the methods to change social influence, of which social norms are a relevant form. There, the focus was on the individual's perception of, and coping with, social norms. In Table 7.11 the focus is on changing the social norms themselves with methods derived from sociological and social-psychological theories.

Interpersonal Level Methods: Social Support and Social Networks. As discussed in Chapter Four, social networks are the basis for social support. In Table 7.12 we describe methods to change social networks so that they offer support more effectively to their members, help members mobilize support from their networks, and link members with other networks. Networks can engage in participatory problem-solving processes aimed at finding ways to solve specific problems of individuals, families, or communities. We highlight the use of lay health workers specifically. These are natural helpers (community members to whom other persons turn for advice, emotional support, and tangible aid; see Chapter Four) from networks who receive special training to support others, including linking them to the formal service delivery system.

TABLE 7.11. METHODS TO CHANGE SOCIAL NORMS.

Methods (Related Theory)	Parameters for Use
Basic methods	See Table 7.3 and Table 7.10
Mass media role-modeling (Diffusion of Innovations Theory, Social Cognitive Theory)	Conditions for modeling; conditions for persuasive communication
Entertainment-education (Diffusion of Innovations Theory)	Consideration of source and channel; balance of media professional's and health promoter's needs
Behavioral journalism (Diffusion of Innovations Theory, Social Cognitive Theory)	Adequate role models from the community and elicitation interviews to describe the behavior and the positive outcome
Mobilizing social networks (theories of social networks and social support [See Table 7.13])	Presence of a network that can potentially support health behavior

TABLE 7.12. METHODS TO IMPROVE SOCIAL SUPPORT AND SOCIAL NETWORKS.

Methods (Related Theory)	Parameters for Use
Basic methods	See Table 7.3 and Table 7.10
Linking members to new networks by mentor programs, buddy systems, and self-help groups (theories of social networks and social support)	Willingness of networks to reach out; availability of networks that can provide appropriate support and linkage agents
Use of lay health workers (theories of social networks and social support)	Natural helpers in community with opinion leader status and availability to volunteer for training

Methods to Create Health-Promoting Organizations. In Table 7.13 we present methods from organizational development, the Stage Theory of Organizational Change, and Diffusion of Innovations Theory (DIT). These include organizational processes, such as participatory problem solving and team building, that can create changes in organizational norms and practices. DIT and the Stage Theory of Organizational Change provide methods that can be used to direct the adoption of an innovation, such as a nonsmoking policy, as well as the adoption, implementation, and continuation of a full health promotion program. These methods are often led by a consultant, hence the use of technical assistance as a method.

TABLE 7.13. METHODS TO CREATE HEALTH-PROMOTING ORGANIZATIONS.

Methods (Related Theory)	Parameters for Use
Basic methods	See Table 7.3 and Table 7.10
Model availability (Organizational Development Theory)	Models should be organizational rather than individual; identification with model organization.
Team building and human relations training (Organizational Development Theory)	Compatible with the culture
Technical assistance (Organizational Development Theory, Diffusion of Innovations Theory)	Compatible with the culture and with skills of the consultant
Organizational advocacy through information, persuasion and negotiation (Diffusion of Innovations Theory, Stage Theory of Organizational Change)	Must be matched to stage: information and motivation in the earlier stages; skills training and reinforcement in the later stages

' *Methods to Create Health-Promoting Communities.* In Table 7.14 we summarize methods that reflect various types of community change. These include coalition development, conscientization, and community organization (for example, locality development, social planning, social action) that we discussed extensively in Chapter Four. The skillful community organizer uses these models to select processes that fit the context of the community and the key issues to be addressed. These often shift over time. The community methods relate to two separate interventions: (1) that of the health promoter with the community directed to empowerment and community capacity and (2) that of the community toward the environmental agent (see Figure 4.3). For example, the health promoters carry out

TABLE 7.14. METHODS TO CREATE HEALTH-PROMOTING COMMUNITIES.

Methods (Related Theory)	Parameters for Use
Basic methods	See Table 7.3 and Table 7.10
Reflection-action-reflection (conscientization)	Being with the people in the community
Nonjudgmental small group discussion (conscientization)	A safe environment, participation
Question posing (conscientization)	A safe environment; a critical stance
Self-disclosure (conscientization)	A safe environment; participatory and caring dialogue
Grass-roots organizing (models of community organization)	Starting where the community is
Professional organizing (models of community organization)	Starting where the community is
Forming coalitions (models of community organization)	Requires collaboration across various agendas
	Requires attention to stages of partnership development
Lay health workers (models of community organization)	Existence of natural helpers in a social network; lay health workers have opinion leader status in the community and volunteer for training
Framing to shift perspectives (models of community organization)	Match with culture, alter the meaning of concepts, and point to action
Media advocacy to promote community identity, policy and legislative actions, and culturally relevant practice (models of community organization)	Requires both getting media to accept a story and shifting how responsibility for the problem is handled in the story

a facilitated community intervention designed to assist the community in understanding the issues it must face, setting priorities, and developing and implementing action plans to address the key issues. Then the community implements the action plan, using methods of change appropriate to the targeted environmental agent and change. This may involve individuals, organizations, and government. We discuss specific methods for political change in the next section.

Methods to Create Health-Promoting Policy. Political change takes place using many of the methods for individual, organizational, and community change we presented earlier. However, these are in service to theories that explain how policy is formulated, implemented, and modified. In Chapter Four we discussed the Agenda-Building Theory, the Policy Window Theory, and the Advocacy Coalition Framework (Cobb & Elder, 1983; John, 2003; Kingdon, 2003; Sabatier, 2003). These theories provide insight into when to use various individual and community influence methods, such as information giving, negotiation, and advocacy, including media advocacy, and which groups are best suited for involvement (see Table 7.15).

From Methods to Strategies

⟩ *The fourth task in Step 3 is select or design practical strategies for applying the methods to the intervention program.*

As we discussed earlier in this chapter, one method may be accomplished by many strategies, and the planner must decide which strategies best fit the situa-

TABLE 7.15. METHODS TO CREATE HEALTHFUL PUBLIC POLICY.

Methods (Related Theory)	Parameters for Use
Basic methods	See Table 7.3 and Table 7.10
Policy advocacy (Agenda-Building Theory, Policy Window Theory)	Characteristics of effective policy advocates; timing and resources; advocacy coalitions
Media advocacy (models of community organization)	Both getting media to accept a story and shifting how responsibility for the problem is handled in the story
Tailoring to issue initiation (Agenda-Building Theory, Policy Window Theory)	Matching the model by which the issue is getting on the agendas: outside initiative, inside initiative, or mobilization models
Timing to coincide with policy windows (Policy Window Theory)	Consideration of politics, problems, and policies

tion's context. The case studies in Chapters Eleven through Fourteen give examples of the links between objectives, methods, strategies, and programs.

The challenge that this task presents for most health educators is how to think of creative strategies. Many people find themselves stymied by having looked at boxes and arrows for too long. We suggest that health educators step back from the details of the program planning at this point and discuss all the ideas that have been bubbling up for intervention strategies. After that, they must return to the work the planners have done on methods and objectives at each intervention level to evaluate the theoretical and empirical support for their ideas. The determinants in the matrices will help guide the planning toward theoretical methods, and the change objectives, which provide more specification and detail, will help the planning team in selecting or designing strategies for applying the methods. The case study chapters provide detailed examples of strategies linked to methods.

It is important at this time for health educators to revisit the intervention population and the proposed program setting, because strategies will depend greatly on to whom and where the program is being delivered. For example, the Cystic Fibrosis Family Education Program (CF FEP) (Bartholomew et al., 1991) included many SCT constructs, so the planning team might logically have thought of strategies that included a lot of interaction, such as group sessions and role-playing for modeling. However, the team knew from having met with parents and adolescents during the needs assessment that they could reach only about 25 percent of the parent intervention group and almost none of the adolescents in a group setting. They therefore used strategies such as role-model stories in newsletters, and they integrated delivery into the clinical encounter. These types of strategy decisions, based on formative work, are very important. In Chapter Eleven, for example, the authors describe trying to operationalize modeling with role-playing as part of an HIV-prevention program in vocational schools. The teachers, however, had a different idea. They were so uncomfortable with organizing and moderating role-playing that the planners knew they had to resort to another strategy.

The following section provides examples of program elements that illustrate the translation of methods to strategies with careful attention to theoretical parameters.

Stick to the Theoretical Parameters

In the methods tables presented earlier, we provided a consideration of use for each method. These considerations included theoretical parameters and, particularly at the environmental levels, characteristics of the context that program planners must take into account. In the following section, we provide examples of the translation of methods into strategies, focusing on the parameters, the conditions under which the method will work. The challenge for health promotion program planners is to design creative intervention strategies that fit the context and characteristics of the program participants while ensuring that the strategies also address the parameters for the selected methods.

First, we give an example of an intervention that failed to use theory correctly. One strategy that is frequently proposed for school-based programs aimed at the prevention of drug abuse is to have former drug users warn the students about the dangers of drugs. This strategy is very popular among students, teachers, parents, school boards, and politicians. However, evaluation studies have shown clearly that this strategy may lead to a significant *increase* in drug use among students (de Haes, 1987). The program planners made two mistakes in translating the method of modeling into a practical strategy. First, the former drug users provide an incorrect model for the students by showing that even people who start using drugs may end up in a very respectable position—in this case, lecturing in schools. The second mistake is that the focus of the model's message is on the dangers of drug use, whereas the most important determinants of drug use initiation are decision-making skills, skills to resist social pressure, and self-efficacy for those skills. In this case, program planners did not adequately use evidence in the form of theory and empirical data.

When translating theoretical methods into practical strategies, planners have to consider the theoretical parameters very carefully. The following are examples of adequate theory use in this translation process. These examples are from programs that have been empirically shown to be effective (Brug, Glanz, Van Assema, Kok, & van Breukelen, 1998; Schaalma et al., 1996).

Modeling. One of the change objectives of the Dutch HIV-prevention program (Chapter Eleven) was this: "Adolescents express their confidence in successfully negotiating condom use with a sex partner" (Schaalma, Kok, Poelman, & Reinders, 1994). As we reviewed in Chapter Four, in SCT, modeling is a method with the potential to increase self-efficacy (Bandura, 1997). The determinant here is self-efficacy. To find methods for improving self-efficacy, we first turn to SCT (Bandura, 1997). Modeling is effective under specific conditions or parameters:

- The learner identifies with the model.
- The model demonstrates feasible subskills.
- The model receives reinforcement.
- The observer perceives a coping model, not a mastery model.

Using modeling in the final program would be effective only when the parameters for this method are kept in place during the development of the practical materials. Schaalma and colleagues (Chapter Eleven) developed video scenes as part of their program, in which models demonstrate skills for negotiating condom use with unwilling partners. These skills, which were taught earlier in the program, include rejection, repeated rejection with arguments, postponement, making excuses, avoiding the issue, and counterposing (R. I. Evans, Getz, & Raines, 1991). The models were carefully selected to serve as identifiable models for the target population. In all scenes the modeled behavior was identifiable, and the models were rewarded for the behavior with a positive ending. The models were coping models; they were clearly struggling a bit with their task of persuading their partners to use a condom. Keep in mind that these scenes were only a part of the program, in which various methods for many objectives were translated into practical strategies within an integrated program.

Active Learning. Schaalma and colleagues (Chapter Eleven) presented their models in a context of active learning: video scenes presenting high-risk situations were stopped after the situation had developed, and the students were asked to elaborate on what they would do in the situation or to give advice to the role model actor, first individually, then in a group. After the break the video was started again, and the students observed the scene's further development and ending. Again, the group discussed the scene's development. Active learning may be effective in almost any change method, as long as the situation provides sufficient motivation, information, time for elaboration, and skills-related advice. Table 7.16 presents one example from the video, a dating situation in which an adolescent girl stands up to social pressure from her date about going home on time. Note that the role model uses techniques about how to resist social pressure that were taught earlier in the program: rejection, repeated rejection with arguments, counterpose.

In this example we see modeling in combination with active learning, while all parameters of these methods are taken into account: identification, skills demonstration, reinforcement (happy ending), coping model, information (on negotiation skills), and time for elaboration. The parameter of motivation may have been underrepresented. Skills training often needs to be combined with methods to enhance motivation. In this case, the health promoters might have used several methods for increasing HIV-risk awareness and creating an attitude favoring reduction of sexual risk: risk-scenario information, anticipated regret, and fear arousal, among others.

Risk Perception Information. Another change objective in the HIV-prevention school program was this: "Adolescents recognize the possibility of ending up in situations in which contracting HIV/STI [sexually transmitted infection] cannot be ruled out." Here the determinant is risk perception. We turn to theories on risk

TABLE 7.16. SCENE FROM HIV-PREVENTION ACTIVE LEARNING VIDEO.

Video scene: In the discothèque

Boy: Would you like another drink?

Girl: No, I have to go home.

Boy: Come on, don't be lame.

Girl: No, I've got to be home at twelve.

Boy: This is a great tune, let's dance.

On screen: Assignment. Sasja really likes Mike. How can she make clear that she still wants to be home at midnight? How will Mike react? (Video stops, students discuss possible effective reactions. Video starts again.)

Boy: Don't you care about me anymore?

Girl: Yes, but that's not the point. They'll get on my case again if I don't get in before midnight.

Boy: Come on, it can't be that bad.

Girl: How do you know? I just want to go home. Besides, you'll ruin the whole evening if you're going to sulk.

(Boy sinks to his knees in feigned apology.)

Girl: *(Laughs)* Come on, if I'm late, you'll be kneeling for my dad on Saturday.

Boy: So, you'll come on Saturday?

Girl: That's the plan.

Boy: Let's go then.

---

perception and risk communication for methods to improve personal risk perception. These theories suggest the provision of risk information and risk feedback, message framing, self-reevaluation, and fear arousal. For instance, Hendrickx, Vlek, and Oppewal (1989) state that people may base their risk judgments on information that aids the construction of an image of the ways in which a particular outcome may occur. An essential parameter for this method is that the information includes a plausible scenario with a cause and an outcome, instead of only an outcome. Therefore, the peer models in the HIV-prevention program presented scenarios in which they described how they found themselves in risky situations (for example, a sexual relationship over the summer holidays). These scenarios clearly presented a cause and an effect to make these contingencies more likely.

Anticipated Regret. Anticipated regret is a method for attitude change (Schaalma, Kok, Poelman, & Reinders, 1994; Schaalma, Kok, et al., 1996). The TPB suggests an insight in relevant beliefs as the basis of attitude change methods (Conner & Sparks, 1996). Schaalma and colleagues used various methods for attitude change, for example: anticipated regret, active processing of information, linkage of beliefs with enduring values, and association of the attitude object with positive stimuli. The risk-scenario information we discussed earlier may be combined with the method of anticipated regret: asking people to imagine how they would feel after risky behavior such as having had unsafe sex (Richard, Van der Pligt, & de Vries, 1995). The parameter for anticipated regret is that the regret question should stimulate imagery.

Fear Arousal. Many health promotion interventions use some kind of fear-arousing message to promote safer behavior. Theories of fear-arousing communication (Eagly & Chaiken, 1993) and recent meta-analyses (Floyd, Prentice-Dunn, & Rogers, 2000; Milne, Orbell, & Sheeran, 2002) suggest that although fear arousal may enhance the motivation to avert the threat, acceptance of health recommendations is mainly dependent on people's outcome expectations regarding the recommendations (What will happen if I follow the recommendations?) and their self-efficacy (How confident am I that I can do the recommendations?). In addition, high levels of fear may easily inhibit persuasion through processes of denial and defensive avoidance (Ruiter, Abraham, & Kok, 2001), especially when response efficacy or self-efficacy is low (Witte, Meyer, & Martell, 2001). Thus, when using fear arousal, program developers should always provide coping methods for reducing the perceived threat and teach the skills for applying these coping methods.

The use of fear arousal seems to be especially popular in mass media campaigns that aim to reduce preventable causes of death, such as lung cancer due to smoking. A limitation of mass media vehicles such as television commercials or posters is the lack of time and space to present persuasive messages. Thirty seconds for a television commercial may be enough to present the threat by vividly stressing its severity and the person's susceptibility to it, but it is hardly enough to provide sufficient information about the effectiveness and feasibility of the recommended action. For example, in a recent initiative from the Canadian government, cigarette packages vividly displayed the negative consequences of smoking. However, specific recommendations about how to act were not given, or they were implicitly given but at too general a level (that is, stop smoking). This general message could easily trigger a defensive response such as denial (for example, I eat more healthfully than most other smokers, so my risk will not be too serious). Claims that this intervention successfully helps people stop smoking (Hammond, Fong, McDonald, Brown, & Cameron, 2004) are based on inadequate designs and misunderstanding of defensive reactions: people will say that they are impressed, but that is not enough for behavior change (Ruiter et al., 2001).

One way that fear appeals may be better able to motivate people into precautionary action is to include recommendations that can be easily performed, such as calling a help line. First, motivate people by presenting threatening information, and second, provide specific instructions about what to do. The current state of the art with respect to fear arousal in health promotion suggests that health promoters should be rather reserved in scaring their participants. Typically, of the four information components composing a fear appeal, severity information has been found the weakest predictor of protection motivation as compared to susceptibility information and information about the effectiveness and feasibility of recommended action. The optimal strategy might be a combination of creating personal risk awareness without arousing too much fear and developing skills for the desired behavior change. In this respect the current interest in implementation intentions, developing specific action plans about how to perform the desired behavior in practice, may lead to new ideas on effective interventions (Sheeran, 2002).

Combinations of risk-scenario information, anticipated regret, and fear arousal may promote risk awareness and attitude change. In the example in Table 7.17, these three methods are combined in one video scene, again using modeling. This part of the video shows a series of scenes in which students interview fellow students about safe sex. The example interview is introduced as a story of a girl who had contracted a chlamydia infection. Her boyfriend is with her.

In this example, risk-scenario information is combined with anticipated regret and fear arousal. The source of the information is a peer, representing another example of modeling. All the parameters have been taken into account: scenario imagery, cause and outcome, regret imagery, personal susceptibility, outcome expectations, and self-efficacy. Moreover, the parameters for modeling are met, such as reinforcement of the desired behavior. A careful analysis of the parameters makes clear that methods for risk awareness and attitude change have to be combined with methods for self-efficacy improvement and skills training. People need to be motivated for active learning and skills training, but they also need to be self-efficacious for opening up to unpleasant information (Bandura, 1997).

Behavioral Journalism. Many methods may be covered by the strategy of behavioral journalism. *Behavioral journalism* is an approach of media-delivered behavioral modeling that makes use of role-model stories that are based on authentic interviews with the target population (McAlister, 1995). Within every priority population, some people perform the desired behaviors or are at the desired stage of behavioral change. These models give their reasons for adopting the new behavior and state the perceived reinforcing outcomes they received. The use of authentic interviews with actual community members ensures that the content of

TABLE 7.17. COMBINATION OF ANTICIPATED REGRET, RISK SCENARIO, AND FEAR AROUSAL.

Girl: I wasn't with him [current boyfriend] last year. It was a boy I fell in love with on my holiday. So we ended up in bed. I was prepared and had brought some condoms, but he refused to use them. He kept on saying, 'Trust me, no AIDS.' He was very persistent. 'It's okay to do it without, just once.' It was so stupid. But he was such a hunk. I wouldn't pass him up. I've got a much bigger hunk now *(looks at current boyfriend)*. What's more, the boy looked very clean. But I was so stupid. I slept with him without using a condom. I was on the pill at the time.

Interviewer: But why did you do it? It's risky as hell.

Girl: I didn't know what to think anymore. I thought, Maybe it won't come to that. I thought, As long as I'm careful. And I was afraid I'd turn him down. I was doing it for him, basically. It was brought home to me later how stupid it was. I was pretty scared afterward. And sure enough I got a discharge. I went to a doctor, who said I had Chlamydia. I was petrified. It can make you infertile.

Interviewer: That would mean that you could never have children!

Girl: I acted quickly, so it wasn't that bad. I was so angry with him afterward for saying that he cared but refusing to use a condom. Of course, I was angry at myself as well. I was stupid.

Interviewer: So, now you always use a condom?

Girl and Boy: Yes!

Interviewer (to boyfriend): I guess you don't agree with the holiday guy?

Boyfriend: No, I was glad she brought it up.

Interviewer: What do you mean?

Boyfriend: She mentioned it first. I don't talk about it very easy. I was afraid she'd think I jump into bed with any girl.

Girl: Nonsense, I think it's great if a boy brings it up. It means that he really cares about you. I like boys who can talk about it. And sex is more fun if you know you are safe. No worries the next day.

Boyfriend: You bet. She takes care of the pill, and I take care of the condoms. We've got a nice condom joke *(both start laughing)*.

Interviewer: Are you going to let me in on it?

Boyfriend: Before we make love . . . I say I've got to put on a CD!

Interviewer: That's a good one. I've got to remember that.

the message is appropriate to the culture and level of understanding of the at-risk population and gives a realistic and credible picture of the group's lifestyle. Of course, the challenge of behavioral journalism is to find the real-life stories that represent the theoretically correct message, without having to compromise the authenticity of the original interview. This is done by asking interview questions designed to elicit answers comparable with theory and sometimes by combining interviews.

Behavioral journalism is effective in covering various other methods, such as risk scenarios, anticipated regret, and fear arousal. Van Empelen, Kok, Schaalma, and Bartholomew (2003) applied behavioral journalism to a program for HIV-risk reduction for Dutch drug users. Based on interviews with drug users, printed role-model stories were developed and distributed within the network of the drug-using community. For example, comparable with the earlier example of the holiday love, in one of the authentic role-model stories, a risk scenario in combination with anticipated regret and fear arousal was presented in Table 7.17.

Table 7.18 presents an example of a combination of behavioral journalism, modeling, risk-scenario information, anticipated regret, and fear arousal methods. The application takes into account the parameters: identification, skills demonstration, reinforcement, a coping model, cause and effect, stimulation of imagery, regret, personal susceptibility, outcome expectations, and self-efficacy. In contrast to the earlier summer holiday sexual relationship text, this text is almost verbatim from an interview with a drug user. Therefore, the chances that the message is appropriate for the at-risk group are much higher.

Computer Tailoring. Personal risk feedback, provided in reaction to information obtained from a program participant, has been identified as a potentially strong method in motivating people to adopt healthier habits (C. C. DiClemente,

---

TABLE 7.18. COMBINATION OF METHODS IN BEHAVIORAL JOURNALISM.

Etienne (34): I never had condoms on me because I don't want to have sex just for the sex. First, I want to get to know someone. I met my second girlfriend at a rehabilitation centre. She told me she had been on the streets in the past. There wasn't anything going on yet. One evening we had a drink together. We ended up in bed and then it happened. Totally unexpected, so we had sex without a condom. Afterward I thought about it, and I was full of regret. To reassure me she told me she had hepatitis C but not HIV. But I didn't trust her completely, so I took an HIV test, three months after the sexual event. Fortunately, the result was good. But from now on, I want to be well prepared. I will take into account that I might end up having sex with someone without really having planned it. So if I have a date again I will buy condoms in advance, to play it safe.

Marinilli, Singh, & Bellino, 2001; Velicer et al., 1993). Individual counseling used to be the only practical strategy for delivering personal risk information, but now computer tailoring or expert systems can deliver personalized risk feedback to large groups of people at relatively low costs (M. Kreuter, Farrell, Olevitch, & Brennan, 2000; Brug et al., 1998). The personalized messages can be delivered through such communication vehicles as a report, a letter, or computer-assisted instruction. We discuss computer tailoring also in Chapter Eight.

It is essential that health promoters keep the theoretical parameters in place in this process. For example, in studies on determinants of dietary behaviors, researchers have found that lack of awareness is a major barrier for dietary change (Lechner, Brug, de Vries, Van Assema, & Mudde, 1998). According to the Precaution-Adoption Process Model (PAPM) (Weinstein, 1988), risk feedback has been identified as a promising method to raise awareness. However, in order for risk feedback to be effective in raising awareness of personal intake levels, it should include personal risk feedback, comparison with a standard, and normative risk feedback (comparison with a reference group).

For example, computer-tailored feedback could be used to promote a reduction in dietary fat intake. First, the individual receives personal risk feedback on their fat intake, indicating whether it is higher than their self-rated level, to increase awareness. The person then receives feedback on whether it is higher than the recommended intake level (the standard). Last, the individual receives normative feedback in which a person who had a fat intake higher than the peer-average level of intake (the reference group) would receive feedback specifically stating this fact. Later, individuals can also receive feedback on their progress. Normative feedback is only given to people who are doing worse than the mean of the reference group. Normative feedback is especially effective in preventing people from rationalizing away the results of the factual feedback. The personal risk feedback is followed by practical and personalized suggestions for behavioral change (see the earlier discussion on fear arousal).

Examples of Methods and Strategies at Different Levels

We conclude this section with more complete examples of the translation of methods to strategies at the individual, organization, and community levels. Translating methods into strategies for interventions to change environmental conditions, such as those directed toward social networks, organizations, communities, and policymakers, brings in some special considerations. At each of these levels, the environmental agent targeted is influenced by methods addressing change objectives derived from the person's role. For example, outcome expectations for a legislator related to her voting to support funding to provide low-cost mammograms to low-income women might relate to constituent response or to expectations of improved constituent health.

The application of methods and strategies that are used to change determinants vary with ecological level as well. Although the individual methods that we discussed earlier for increasing knowledge, awareness, attitudes, skills, and social influence are used for environmental agents, these methods are often packaged into broader methods or processes that take into account the level and context of the situation. These include participatory problem solving, advocacy, or organizational development.

HIV Prevention for Incarcerated Women.
El-Bassel, Ivanoff, Schilling, Borne, and Gilbert (1997) carefully described an HIV-prevention program for incarcerated women prior to release. Their behavioral outcomes were the reduction of unsafe sex through condom use and abstinence and the reduction of needle sharing. The researchers' program focused on the following determinants: knowledge about HIV and STI risks, perceived vulnerability to HIV and STIs, cognitive behavioral and technical skills tailored to cultural and social factors, motivation to use condoms (that is, attitudes, barriers, pros and cons, and access), social support, and formal and informal help-seeking skills. Theoretical methods were derived from various theories, particularly social cognitive and relapse prevention theories. The methods and strategies are presented in Table 7.19. In addition to the specific methods listed in the table, the researchers used three general methods: relevance (that is, adaptation of the program to knowledge, beliefs, circumstances, and prior experiences of the intervention population based on focus groups and surveys), active learning facilitated by professional group workers, and repetition by trained peer educators (booster sessions).

The program methods were applied in an organized group intervention that consisted of eight weekly sessions of ninety minutes each. A facilitator and a cofacilitator used a standardized protocol to lead the groups of ten women. Group members received a workbook of exercises that could be completed by persons with minimal literacy. Group facilitators were experienced in working with drug users, were credible and comfortable with the group, and valued group work and skills-training approaches.

Within this program various strategies were used to apply the methods. For instance, skills training and guided practice were delivered through discussions and homework exercises. Facilitators reviewed common triggers (that is, places, people, moods, and substance use), and group members learned to identify high-risk situations that served as personal triggers for engaging in risky behaviors. Participants discussed how these triggers influenced their decisions to have unsafe sex

TABLE 7.19. HIV-PREVENTION PROGRAM FOR WOMEN IN JAIL: METHODS AND STRATEGIES.

Determinants	Methods	Strategies
Knowledge	Information	Demonstrations
		Workbook
		Group sessions
Confrontations with risks	Modeling	Personal risk appraisal
Risk perception Skills for identifying high-risk situations	Confrontations with risks Modeling Personal risk appraisal Skill training, with guided practice and feedback	Discussions and homework, including practice identifying triggers from participants' examples Facilitator presentation of examples Awareness exercises
Skills for coping, problem solving, help seeking, and negotiation	Modeling Skill training with guided practice and feedback	Group teaching of skills by facilitators Practice by group members Identification by group members of possible negative outcomes and how to handle them Videotaped stimulus vignettes with evaluation by participants Skill practice in role plays with feedback Booster sessions in the community
Attitudes	Decisional balance Identification of barriers for condom use	Discussion in groups Videotaped stimulus vignettes
Social support	Modeling Guided practice Social comparison	Mobilization through network and contact identification

Source: El-Bassel, Ivanoff, Schilling, Borne, and Gilbert, 1997.

and to use drugs. Using members' examples, facilitators emphasized the powerful, multilayered connections between using drugs (particularly crack) and having unsafe sex. Through awareness exercises in and outside the group, each member identified her own list of triggers. As participants shared their lists of triggers, facilitators and other members helped identify potential steps to minimize, avoid, or counteract the triggers' influence.

Negotiation and assertiveness skills were taught within the context of risk appraisal. The women assessed the possible adverse outcomes of being assertive and identified avenues of escape from partners who might respond abusively. They learned four steps to negotiate safer sex when partners are not interested in using condoms:

1. State what you want.
2. Explain, without blame or accusation, why you want it.
3. Indicate understanding of the other's position.
4. Attain a solution to the problem without compromising your needs.

Members then practiced refusing unsafe sex in situations in which negotiation fails. Facilitators encouraged direct refusal of unsafe sex in situations in which the women are confident that partners will cooperate, and they encouraged indirect refusal when partners are unresponsive or threatening. The program relied on videotaped stimulus vignettes for teaching these and other skills. Participants evaluated the effectiveness of the assertions, negotiations, and refusals used in the stimulus vignettes and generated alternative responses. They then practiced these skills in multiple role-plays. Facilitators provided constructive feedback and support throughout the training.

Prior to the participants' release from prison, counselors met with participants individually to review their triggers for risk behavior, their plans for reducing risk behaviors, the resources they had on the outside, and the steps they would take during the first few days after release to carry out their plans. Individual booster sessions delivered by counselors in the community took place during the first two months after release. During booster sessions counselors and participants linked problem-solving goals and objectives with concrete action plans, and they role-played to access skills and practice plans.

Participatory Problem Solving. Participatory problem solving as an environmental change method includes basic individual methods and those specific to knowledge change, attitude change, skills building, self-efficacy and collective efficacy, and other individual-level determinants. It includes diagnosing the problem, generating potential solutions, developing priorities, making an action plan, and obtaining feedback after implementing the plan. At the social network level, the strategy might take the form of calling together the family, friends, and helpers of an older person living alone for a meeting to discuss what the situation is and how they can come together to handle increasing needs for activities of daily living. At the organizational level, an intervention to improve employee morale might include conducting a survey of employee attitudes, giving feedback on the findings to employees and managers, holding small group discussions of what the findings mean and how to address them, discussing the importance and changeability of the proposed activities, setting priorities, putting the changes into place, and getting feedback concerning their effectiveness through focus groups and surveys. At the community level, the strategy might be a visioning workshop to develop a strategic plan for a community problem, such as obesity. Persons representing government and other organizations in the community meet with residents with a stake in the issue to discuss data concerning the problem, possible solutions, and available community resources. They brainstorm and evaluate strategies for solutions, prioritize them, and develop action plans using committees for different community sectors.

The approach used for adoption and implementation of the Put Prevention into Practice program by Texas primary care clinics provides an example of an organizational intervention using participatory problem solving (Murphy-Smith, Meyer, Hitt, Taylor-Seehafer, & Tyler, 2004; Tyler, Taylor-Seehafer, & Murphy-Smith, 2004). The program is an initiative that consists of a kit of office-based tools, including a guide to preventive services, a health-risk profile, a flow sheet of dates of services and counseling with findings, and patient education materials, all intended to support the provision of clinical preventive services (N. H. Gottlieb, Huang, Blozis, Guo, & Murphy, 2001). Strategies to increase risk assessment and counseling by providers include a process to assess organizational readiness to adopt the program, using a checklist and facilitated discussion and reflection based on an adaptation of the total transformation management process (Mink, Downes, Owen, & Mink, 1994). At that point an advisory committee (strategy) is established to guide the rest of the process and to plan and carry out needed changes in policies, space, continuing education, systems for prescreening charts, clinic flow, referral protocols, and quality measures.

Community Participation. The Healthy Cities movement illustrates strategies for the broad method of community participation, which we discussed in Chapter Four. The World Health Organization (WHO) has developed a tool kit of strategies to facilitate the community participation process (WHO, 2002a). Many of the strategies use group-work techniques, including icebreakers, brainstorming, mind mapping, and research tools such as focus groups. The tool kit is organized around five stages of action planning: assessing needs and assets, agreeing on a vision, generating ideas and plans for action, enabling action, and monitoring and evaluating. Healthy Cities staff choose strategies based on the level of participation required for the task and the community context. Most of the techniques require technical assistance from a planner, trainer, arts worker, community organizer, or evaluator.

Four tools are provided for developing and agreeing on a vision: futures workshops, guided visualization, European awareness scenario workshops, and future search. These tools each describe strategies for community members to work together to create a shared vision. In the guided visualization, for example, participants imagine traveling twenty years and going through a typical day; they are encouraged to build up pictures and images of the future as they would like it to be. Each individual then records the images in words or pictures on movable paper stickers, sharing these first with another participant and then with small groups. The small groups each share their visions, and the entire group develops a collective vision, moving the stickers around. The next step is discussion of the vision in the context of the current condition, barriers, and facilitators to move into action planning.

Three techniques are suggested for assessing needs and interests: community profiles and appraisals, neighborhood and parish maps, and rapid participatory appraisal. Although the nature of these needs assessment processes varies, the important point for participation is that community residents are involved in design, data collection, and interpretation of the data. For example, the neighborhood maps technique has been used in the United Kingdom with groups of local people who, often with a facilitating community arts worker, create a map of their community, often of distinctive landmarks, cultural features, and concern about developments. The mapping process has been done in various media, including painting, collage photography, embroidery, video, and poetry. The maps are then displayed publicly and used to stimulate reflection and discussion.

Three strategies are suggested to facilitate community participation in generating ideas and plans for action: simulation, workbooks, and citizens' juries. In a Planning for Real simulation, over the course of seven to ten days, participants build a small scale model of their neighborhood using a pack of ready-made materials showing land use, including buildings, streets, and conditions. The model is constructed so that components can be moved around. The model is displayed in publicly accessible places, and open meetings are held to discuss ideas for community action and for people to create cards with suggestions concerning such concerns as traffic, local facilities, health, and environment. These are compiled into a report. The workbook process is an interactive technique in which community residents are engaged in identifying ideas and selecting priorities for their area. Citizens' juries are a simulation using witnesses representing different aspects of the issue and a jury (sixteen people who are representative of the community's demographic characteristics). The jury hears the witnesses present both sides of the case, questions them, and then uses a consensus-building approach to agree on recommendations. The recommendations are then disseminated and provided to appropriate groups for implementation.

The tools for enabling action highlight several umbrella strategies for different types of community-based action. For community networks a small planning group develops a network regarding an issue of concern across a number of communities. Through a process of development, the network facilitates and supports community action. Community participation advisory groups and community councils assure widespread community involvement, advise key agencies, and provide a liaison between communities and authorities. Formation of these bodies include the community and key agencies agreeing on a need, deciding on the charge of the group and its membership, providing information and training to members as needed, and supporting the group's function. Theater of the oppressed is an arts-based method based on Freire's conscientization method (1973a, 1973b) (see Chapter Four). Image theater, in which participants use wordless exercises to demonstrate their feelings and experiences and recognize in each other's expressions common experiences and oppression, is another method. Interactive exercises explore how the current situation could be changed and what it would feel like. In forum theater the learning from image theater is used to create a short plan based on the common experiences and oppressions that participants have performed. The audience is asked to consider how things could be changed and are invited to freeze the action and step into the protagonist's role to offer alternative approaches. This allows for empowerment and rehearsal of action that can lead to real-life action (WHO, 2002a).

Community participation in monitoring and evaluation builds on the earlier steps. For example, the story-dialogue strategy involves writing a generative theme (often a controversial issue), writing the "case story" (WHO, 2002a, p. 71) told in the first person to provide deep analysis and understanding, sharing the case story with listeners who reflect on what they have heard, and engaging them in structured dialogue (using question posing as discussed in Chapter Four). Participants create insight cards to record responses to these questions: What do you see happening? Why do you think it happens? So what have we learned? Now what can we do? These cards provide data for evaluation. Case studies can be created by linking individual case stories with information drawn from other sources.

Where Have All the Objectives Gone?

> *The final task in Step 3 is to assure that the final strategies (still) match the change objectives.*

At the end of Intervention Mapping step 3, the planner has moved from objectives to methods, parameters, and strategies. During that process, the planner has made many decisions, from theoretical as well as practical perspectives. The planner has estimated the relevance and changeability of methods and the feasibility of strategies. The planner has anticipated issues in implementation by program users. At this point it is necessary to ensure that all the relevant and changeable objectives that were selected for the program are still matched in the current list of strategies. If that is the case, the planner may continue to the next step; if not, the planner has to decide to leave some objectives out or go back and develop methods and strategies to cover the neglected objectives.

In previous tasks in Step 3, we suggested that the planner make a list of change objectives for each determinant in each of the matrices. In this final task for Step 3, the planning group should return to this list to check that the selected methods or designated strategies address each objective. This is done to make sure that the planning group has not overlooked any of the change objectives. If any of the objectives have been missed, the planning team should either address the objectives by linking them to methods and strategies for other change objectives associated with the determinant or go back through the preceding tasks to select additional methods or strategies for the missing objectives.

Implications for Evaluation

The choice of appropriate methods and strategies for a program will have a lot to do with whether the program is effective or not. However, the direct implications for evaluation of the methods and strategy choices are in the process evaluation. The process evaluation includes whether the theoretical methods that have been chosen are based on evidence and theory to support that they can produce changes in the determinants and change objectives from the matrices. Another question is whether the methods have been operationalized in ways that adhere to the parameters or assumptions inherent in the use of the proposed theoretical change methods. For example, parameters for modeling would include whether a role model is attractive to the participants, credible, and reinforced for the behavior that is performed. Finally, a process evaluation question that relates to this step is whether the correct methods and parameters are apparent in the strategies that are ultimately delivered to participants.

Box 7.2. Stroke Project

↻ *The first task in Step 3 is to review program ideas with the intended participants and use their perspectives when identifying methods and strategies.*

↻ *The second task is to use core processes to identify theoretical methods that can influence change in determinants and identify the conditions under which a given method is most likely to be effective.*

↻ *In the third task the planner chooses program theoretical methods.*

The methods and strategies for the T.L.L. Temple Foundation Stroke Project are shown in Tables 7.20 and 7.21, matched to the categories of determinants from the matrices for the community and the hospital emergency departments (EDs). Methods and strategies for the emergency medical services (EMS) and primary care physicians are not shown. EMS and primary care physician methods and strategies were very similar to those for the EDs. As the tables indicate, the methods are quite similar for the community and professional components of the program with the exception of the addition of organizational development for the hospital EDs. Even though the matrices are different, the determinants are similar, which accounts for the similarity of methods.

Strategies for the two sets of methods are fairly different because even though the determinants are similar, the performance objectives are quite different. The EDs required more skill development and more systems intervention such as the development of protocols for stroke workup and recombinant tissue plasminogen activator (rtPA) administration. Other strategies were equally important to the changes on both matrices. For example, newspaper articles delivered role-model stories that influenced both the lay public and physicians.

The advisory committee that we described in Chapter Five's Stroke Box helped to generate ideas for methods and strategies and also to provide the local role models. We wanted locally recognizable role models who had had strokes and recovered. Three committee members were stroke survivors including the mayor of Lufkin. This multiethnic group of three agreed to be models on billboards, posters, and brochures.

↻ *The fourth task in Step 3 is to select or design practical strategies for applying the methods to the intervention program.*

↻ *Finally, the planner assures that the final strategies (still) match the change objectives.*

To assure that we had methods and strategies to cover all change objectives on all matrices and to assure that all strategies contained well-translated methods, we organized design documents for each strategy that covered intended methods and the

TABLE 7.20. METHODS AND STRATEGIES FOR COMMUNITY MATRICES.

Determinants and Change Objectives	Methods	Strategies
Knowledge of stroke symptoms	Modeling Information	Community members telling their stories in newspaper articles
Knowledge of stroke as emergency— to call 911	Modeling Information Cues to action	Community members telling their stories in newspaper articles Public service announcements (PSAs) showing stroke as emergency Billboards with local role models—stroke is an emergency, call 911 Posters
Skills and self-efficacy for symptom recognition	Modeling Skills training Information	One-to-one instruction at worksites accompanied by a brochure Community members telling their stories in newspaper articles
Perceived social norms to intervene and call 911	Cues to action Modeling Social comparison Reinforcement	Newspaper articles of bystander or significant other recognizing symptoms and intervening—intervention is socially reinforced PSAs showing intervention and reinforcement
Perceived social norms to intervene and ask for priority transport and fast ED care	Cues to action Modeling Social comparison Reinforcement	Newspaper articles of bystander or significant other recognizing symptoms and intervening—intervention is socially reinforced PSAs showing intervention and reinforcement billboards with local role models
Outcome expectations	Modeling	Billboards with local role models—showing good recovery
Barriers	Modeling	PSAs with doctor saying go straight to ED, don't call primary care

TABLE 7.21. METHODS AND STRATEGIES FOR EMERGENCY DEPARTMENT MATRICES.

Determinants and Change Objectives	Methods	Strategies
Knowledge of rtPA study results	Modeling Information	Presentations at medical staff meetings, committee meetings Newsletters delivered to emergency departments (EDs) with science articles and news
Skills and self-efficacy for stroke workup	Modeling Skills training Information	Training in EDs Community mock stroke code
Perceived social norms and standard of care to lower stroke workup times	Cues to action Modeling Social comparison Reinforcement	Newspaper articles of treatment of stroke patients by hospitals in the community Provision of national association guidelines
Perceived social norms and standard of care to treat stroke	Cues to action Modeling Social comparison Reinforcement	Newspaper articles of treatment of stroke patients by hospitals in the community Provision of national association guidelines
Outcome expectations	Modeling Feedback	Newsletters delivered to EDs with role-model stories of physicians treating patients who had good recovery, and reports on treated patients
Reinforcement	Modeling Vicarious reinforcement Feedback	Newsletters delivered to EDs with role-model stories of physicians treating patients who had good recovery, and reports on treated patients
System barriers	Organizational development	Meetings with hospital teams including administration, ED medical and nursing directors, physicians to plan rtPA use, discuss barriers, and develop protocols

change objectives that were to be influenced by that method. Even after all the planning, it is quite easy for a team to become distracted and leave methods out of strategies. For example, the newsletters that went to EDs were each to contain a model of a physician who was reinforced by good patient outcomes for treating with rtPA. As the health educator on the team was reviewing the fourth newsletter, she realized that the role-model story had been deleted and found that the physicians had decided "physicians don't like this sort of thing. We thought we would include just the science." Armed with the design documents and matrices, she lobbied to reinsert the method.

The other important issue when designing strategies is to ensure that as the methods are translated, the parameters under which a particular method could be expected to be effective are present. For example, in order to be effective, the role-model stories had to garner the audience's attention; the role models had to be credible so that people could identify with them; the behaviors that were desired needed to be clearly discernable; and the role model had to be reinforced. We had to keep these parameters in mind for every strategy that included a role model, for example, public service announcements and newspaper articles.

CHAPTER EIGHT

INTERVENTION MAPPING STEP 4: PRODUCING PROGRAM COMPONENTS AND MATERIALS

Reader Objectives

- Consult with the intended program participants to determine preference for program design
- Create program scope and sequence including delivery channels, themes, and list of needed program materials
- Prepare design documents for the production of materials that meet the program objectives and parameters for the methods and strategies
- Review available program materials and select materials that match change objectives, methods, and strategies
- Develop program materials
- Pretest program materials and oversee the final production

The purpose of this chapter is to enable the planner to produce creative program components and materials in support of health education and promotion programs. We speak of materials "in support of" to circumvent the temptation of referring to support materials or products such as newsletters, billboards, and videotapes as the program. The program will usually be a multicomponent, complex entity supported by certain products or materials. The goal is that these products are creative, effective pieces of the planned behavior- and environmental-change program. A challenge in this step is one of translation: getting the support pieces right so that the methods and strategies are adequately (and sometimes brilliantly) operationalized and the change objectives accomplished.

Planning to this point should enable production of creative products that emerge from the thinking captured in the matrix development and the selection of methods and strategies. In particular, the products should do an excellent job of representing the parameters that pertain to the methods that have been chosen. For example, if a planning team decides to use modeling (method), they must ensure that their program's role-model stories (strategies) have models that participants can identify with (parameter). The end product of this step should be a plan for a coherent program that remains true to the planning that has been accomplished in Steps 1, 2, and 3.

Another challenge in this step is to ensure that the final program fits with both the populations to whom it will be delivered and the contexts in which it will be delivered. This step provides an opportunity to revisit the potential program participants to ensure that the program materials result in attention, comprehension, and central processing. Only then will there be a chance that the change objectives will be accomplished and behavior and environment affected. Health educators can use this juncture in the planning process to check not only the depth of their understanding of the intended participants and contexts but also the status of their linkage system with the people who will adopt and implement the program.

In Chapter Nine we present the development of interventions to influence program adoption and implementation. These interventions are directed to the gatekeepers of organizations who will adopt the new program and to the program deliverers who will implement it. In this chapter we focus on program design and materials development. Although our discussion is centered on the health education program that is directed to the client population, the same creative and technical process needs to be applied to the intervention for program adoption and implementation.

Box 8.1. Mayor's Project

The health educator from the mayor's office thought that the task group had jumped the last major planning hurdles. The task group had decided on intervention levels, written performance objectives at all those levels, and then created matrices. Group members even put the matrices aside for a bit and planned theoretical methods and practical strategies with a lot of energy and creativity. They had found ways to listen to everyone's ideas. What a team! At the end of the year, they had enough energy and goodwill to plan a celebratory dinner to commemorate six months of hard work and productive (and sometimes loud) discussions. That dinner was just before the city hit low gear at winter break and everyone took a breather.

Now it was January, and the first meeting of the new year was in full swing. The health educator couldn't believe what was happening. What was all of this regression? Didn't the group members remember the prewinter break ideas about what the program should include? Why was the group talking about what the billboards should look like and what celebrity should narrate the videotape? What billboards? What videotape? The group hadn't decided to have products such as billboards and videotapes as part of the program, and the health educator thought that some members had learned a thing or two about the characteristics of effective role models, but that was the least of the problems. This meeting was beginning to look like a pitched battle. Before members could become entrenched in these resurfaced old ideas, the health educator had to take action. She wanted to make sure that the program components incorporated methods and strategies to accomplish the change objectives.

The mayor's health educator capitalized on the natural energy of the planning group and encouraged group members to dream about what their program could look like—without any of their matrices or previous planning materials in front of them. They worked to keep in mind the objectives and methods they would be trying to deliver.

Participant A: Well, since we want to reach parents and city government, we probably need a coalition of community organizations and agencies. Churches, social service agencies, professional organizations, youth organizations, that sort of thing. The coalition could oversee the program implementation, especially the change directed at the parents and the government approach to the neighborhoods.

Participant B: Since I represent the organization of pastors in the areas of the city that have the biggest violence problem, I think that coalition is a good idea. My congregation would like to be very involved, and I know that my colleagues are interested too.

Participant C: Yeah, and from our point of view at the schools, we need the support of the school district to reach the age groups of youth we are addressing. I think the youth component should have a school focus. Of course, we need a way to reach dropouts as well.
The theme could be . . .

Participant D: OK, let's get down to basics. What would a school program look like? How would we use our methods of modeling, skill building for problem solving, negotiation, resistance skills, planning and studying, goal setting, self-monitoring? Do you think we could use community organization methods in the schools?

Participant C: What about even having the youth from the school program recruit the community agencies for the coalition?

Perspectives

Our perspectives in this chapter are about encouraging full use of the program plan to this point and at the same time encouraging creativity in the development of program components and materials.

Using Steps 1,2, and 3

Planning groups will often shy away when confronted with the perceived complexity of converting all their planning into a program. Members may tend to revert to overly simplistic thinking, such as *We need a videotape.* This was what the mayor's health educator faced, and one thing that helped was staying focused on the thorough work the team had done on Intervention Mapping Steps 1, 2, and 3. In Step 2 the team developed matrices for the at-risk group (the middle school and high school youth) and matrices for various segments of the environment (parents through churches and neighborhood groups and the city government through the mayor and city council). In Step 3 the team developed lists of theoretical methods and practical strategies for each matrix. Further, the planning group had adopted the W. J. McGuire system (1986) of checking all the communications they would develop in Step 4. With these foundations they could use Step 4 to ensure good communications that incorporated the methods and strategies to accomplish the change objectives. Just as Step 3 has two styles of accomplishing the tasks, Step 4 has at least two contrasting styles, but neither of the styles means abandoning the previous work. One style is to take each method and strategy, consider it, and develop a program component to deliver it. Another style is to put away all lists, matrices, and other planning papers and allow the group to bring forth all the ideas that group members have had to this point about what the program should look like. After all, the planning to this point is at its best if it has stimulated many creative thoughts about the program's nature. If the work group chooses this style, then members must check back periodically to their methods, strategies, and change objectives to make sure the program components are actually delivering what they are supposed to deliver.

Allowing Creativity to Flourish

Planning should allow creativity to flourish. In this step program planners liberate all those ideas that have been put on hold during the work of the previous steps. Sometimes they close the books, turn the matrices over, and even close their eyes to dream what a program could look like. The planning group should be cohesive by this point, so it should be all right to come forth with some crazy ideas and to get carried away with some ridiculous themes. Out of this creative mess can emerge a great program. The foundation is laid; the design task should be fun. A related point is making use of the real talents of any production contractors the team may have. In this chapter we build on the planning documents developed to this point to create design documents that can guide contractors without hamstringing them.

Designing Culturally Relevant Program Materials

> The first task in Step 4 is to consult with the intended program participants to determine preference for program design.

Aiming at Cultural Relevance

We believe that if a program is not culturally grounded at this point in the planning process, the project is in trouble. From the program's very inception and through each step, community members will have been involved if the health promoter knows his or her business. However, the issues of cultural relevance resurface when the planning team begins to think of materials. Resnicow, Baranowski, Ahluwalia, and Braithwaite (1999) define what we mean by cultural relevance (although they label it cultural sensitivity). They describe this characteristic to exist to "the extent to which ethnic/cultural, characteristics, experience, norms, values, behavioral patterns and beliefs of a target population as well as relevant historical, environmental, and social forces are incorporated in the design, delivery, and evaluation of targeted health promotion materials and programs" (p. 13). Even though there is sparse evidence about the impact of cultural relevance on the effectiveness of health promotion interventions or materials, there is considerable expert agreement that cultural relevance is closely related to the principle of participation in program development and is a good thing (M. W. Kreuter, Lukwago, Bucholtz, Clark, & Sanders-Thompson, 2003; Resnicow et al., 1999).

Resnicow and colleagues (1999) define two primary dimensions of culture that are relevant to public health and to program development in particular: deep structure and surface structure. Deep structure refers to the factors that influence the health behavior in the intervention's proposed recipients. We have dealt with this aspect of creating a culturally relevant program repeatedly in the Intervention Mapping steps to this point. We hope that it is clear that if the planner has not understood the behaviors or the determinants of those behaviors correctly to this point, attention to cultural relevance of materials is unlikely to be effective because the program will not have salience to the intended cultural group.

Assuming that the planner has worked with the cultural group to adequately bring to bear the group's insights into the behaviors and determinants, he or she can turn attention to surface structure and the creation of materials. According to Resnicow and colleagues (1999), surface structure comprises the superficial but still important characteristics of a cultural group such as familiar people, language, music, clothing, and so on.

M. W. Kreuter and colleagues (2002) propose five categories of mechanisms by which health promoters can work to achieve attention to both surface and deep aspects of culture in their program planning.

- *Peripheral processes* match materials' characteristics to the culture's surface characteristics. This attempt to make materials familiar and comfortable to the intended audience relies heavily on visual aspects of production (Kostelnick, 1996; Moriarty, 1995; Schiffman, 1995).
- *Evidential strategies* remind the cultural group of the significance of the health problem to them, for example: "African American children suffer twice the hospitalizations for asthma as white children."
- *Linguistic strategies* provide programs and materials in the language of the cultural group.
- *Constituent-involving* approaches cover several strategies for involving the intended program group, including hiring staff from the cultural group, using lay health workers from the group, and continuing to work with the group as members of the planning team.

Sociocultural strategies embed health education in the context of broader cultural values and issues.

Preproduction Research

Atkin and Freimuth (1989) describe two types of formative research: preproduction and production. Preproduction research discovers characteristics of the intended participants that relate to message, medium, and situation; whereas production testing (pretesting) is a process in which prototypes of program materials are tested for audience reaction. We develop a description of the processes of pretesting and further pilot testing later in the chapter. However, working with the people who will use and those who will benefit from the program begins as soon as the work group begins to have program ideas, and it continues throughout the process of developing materials.

In the preproduction research phase, health educators explore interpersonal as well as media channels. Freimuth (1985) also suggests ascertaining the credibility of vehicles and sources and the recall of previous messages on a topic. Preproduction testing can include both informal feedback and ratings of sources, messages, themes, persuasive arguments, and stylistic devices. Focus groups are a good mechanism for preproduction testing. Work at this point can be very important in determining program messages. For example, in the development of the Cystic Fibrosis Family Education Program (CF FEP) (Bartholomew, Seilheimer, Parcel, Spinelli, & Pumariega, 1989) we held focus groups with children, adolescents, and parents who would be using the program. One issue that stood out was the adolescents' discussion of being different from their peers. The program developers had thought that they should deal explicitly with the young people's worry about being different in the program. However, the adolescents with cystic fibrosis said in no uncertain terms that they are not different and would object to program materials that addressed their "differentness." With this and other feedback, it was back to the drawing board for the developers.

Culture-Oriented Preproduction

Resnicow and colleagues (1999) describe a process of explicitly culturally oriented preproduction activity. They use focus groups, for example, "to explore the thoughts, feelings, experience, associations, language, assumptions, etc. regarding the target health behavior" (p. 15). They suggest exploratory research with both the population of interest and with a comparison group to clarify ethnic differences. They work primarily in African American communities, and with these groups they suggest asking specific questions about how the group members see the health behavior. They find that the perceptions of African Americans about the health behavior often differ relative to European American communities. In a smoking-cessation project, for example, the African American participants saw cigarette smoking as a significant stress relief whereas the "white folk . . . can just take a vacation" (Resnicow et al., 1997, p. 15). They also use an approach they call ethnic mapping, in which aspects of the health behavior can be rated by the cultural group as compared to another group. In the work of Resnicow and colleagues, aspects of behavior are rated as one of these three options: mostly a black thing, equally a black and white thing, or mostly a white thing. They used this technique to classify foods for a nutrition project but also suggest its usefulness to gain culturally centered information about other behaviors such as brand preferences, quitting techniques, and perceptions about smokers; physical activity; HIV-prevention practices; and substance use (Resnicow et al., 1999).

Reciprocity in Teaching and Learning

In coming up with program ideas, successful teams keep in mind the reciprocity between the teacher and the learner. A powerful way to strive for culturally competent health education programs is to be in constant interaction with program participants so that the creation of meaning is both shared and fluid. This inter-action does not require that the health educator be of the same ethnic group as the community, and health educators may become complacent if they have a team member who can be the designated cultural match to the community. This un-fortunate tokenism does not guarantee any real cultural similarity between the re-source group and the community. We are not saying that recruiting ethnic diversity to program development teams is not essential; it is! But it is not enough to en-sure culturally competent practice. Culturally competent practice is based on rec-iprocity in teaching and learning as described by Ladson-Billings (1992, 1995). She describes three broad categories of characteristics of culturally competent teachers. In their conceptions of self and others, culturally competent teachers seem to see themselves as members of the community, and they see community members as capable of changing and learning. They believe in the Freirian no-tion of "teaching as mining," in other words, as facilitating the emergence of ex-isting capabilities and competencies (Freire 1973a, p. 76). They see social relations as fluid within a community of learners, and they encourage program participants to learn collaboratively and be responsible for one another. Finally, they see knowl-edge as needing to be created jointly between teachers and learners and viewed critically. If the information flows both ways, then health educators have some op-portunity to be congruent with the learner's culture. Program components based on reciprocity make the creation of meaning a mutual task between teacher and learner. To put it another way, with reciprocal activities every participant is both a teacher and a learner. Such methods should be used in every complex health education situation. For example, Majumdar and Roberts (1998) describe a method of AIDS awareness in which women were organized into like-culture groups with a facilitator from that cultural group. They then planned the way the program would be delivered in their group.

Checking in with Potential Implementers

Planners at this stage should pay particular attention to the characteristics of their program's setting. What is the school, hospital, or community really like? Who will be involved in implementing the program? Is there any group involved in im-plementation that has not been involved in development? What additional facts about the setting does the planner need to consider in program design? Step 5, which requires the development of an adoption and implementation plan, really begins at the beginning of program development with consideration of a linkage system (see Chapter Five) and resurfaces here. As planners conceptualize program components, they need to consider how to implement them and what implemen-tation will require of the implementers. Planners must also consider the impact of perceived program characteristics on the gatekeepers, those responsible for adoption decisions (see Chapter Nine).

Creating the Initial Program Plan and Structure

⊃ *The second task in Step 4 is to create the program scope and sequence, delivery channels, themes, and a list of needed program materials.*

The product of the first part of this step is a plan that outlines the scope and sequence of the program, all the program vehicles and materials that must be produced, and the budget and resources for the program materials. The program plan should account for every intended contact of the program participants with some element of the program. The health educator should specify both the amount of the program that is expected to be delivered and the way the program should look at each interface with participants. The summary plan's format will vary from program to program, but it should include at least three elements: the program scope and sequence; a description of each population group and program interface with a list of the program materials and staff required for that interface; and a program budget for materials production.

Program Ideas

Gedney and Fultz (1988) address the problem that plagues communicators, that is, how to have a good idea. They suggest having more than one idea and even having hundreds of possibilities. Planners often use brainstorming to generate ideas that encompass the entire program (We could go to schools and do X) or to address specific methods and strategies (The role-model stories could contain Y). This step is a good time to throw away all preconceived notions and program constraints. Planners should ask themselves, What would we do if we could do anything that comes to mind? What would be the most powerful things we could do? Brainstorming allows no evaluative comments and is therefore a good mechanism to generate, generate, generate! When the group gets stuck, planners can try a paradoxical approach: If we wanted to have the opposite effect, what would we do? One of us often uses a more visual brainstorming at this point and has the group draw what the program would look like.

The core processes (Chapter Two) also will be useful here. A literature review can elucidate to some extent the types of strategies and programs others have used. Using theory can help with generating thoughts about methods and ways to use them. Finally, going to the potential participants and continuing to fuel the process with their ideas is imperative. Focus groups can be used for this purpose and are particularly suited because stimulus materials in the form of learning and change objectives are available. You can phrase questions in this way: If you were trying to figure out how to [change objective X], what would you do? For example, If you were going to increase the confidence of teenage girls in negotiating condom use, what would you do? Bartholomew and colleagues (2005) are working on messages to encourage older persons to be vaccinated for influenza. When they conducted their formative research in community grocery stores, they also asked participants if they would be willing to return to work with the team on communications about influenza. The team then met with African American, Hispanic, and white groups and asked for ideas about how to influence the factors related to influenza vaccination found for that group (Bartholomew, Selwyn, Sablotne, Chronister, & Livoti-Debellis, 2005).

Scope and Sequence

Health education and promotion programs have components (units or modules) with an identifiable scope and sequence. However, unlike targets of typical curriculum planning, which are cognitive or academic skills, these program components have more diverse change objectives. Therefore, the modules or units might be, for example, combinations of methods, strategies, and delivery mechanisms aimed at various objectives. A program might comprise messages that neighborhood volunteers deliver one-to-one and mass media messages delivered in public service announcements (PSAs) and billboards, all loosely tied together across time with a theme.

Scope is the breadth and amount of a program, whereas *sequence* is the order in which programs are delivered across time. For example, the Safer Choices 2 program has been delivered in alternative high schools intensively over a period of two to two and a half months because the attrition from school is high and the planning team wanted to reach as many adolescents in as short a period as possible (Tortolero, Markham et al., 2005) (see Table 8.1).

Themes

A *program theme* is a general organizing construct for a program. A program often has a theme as well as several recurring visual and linguistic subthemes or ideas. Both themes and recurring subthemes can be based on the health topic, such as the themes for the stroke project (see Chapter Five). Themes may be based on the behavioral or community change objectives. For example, the Watch, Discover,

TABLE 8.1. SAFER CHOICES 2 PROGRAM SCOPE AND SEQUENCE.

Timing	Lesson	Activities
Week 1	1. What This Means to Me	An introductory activity helps students understand some of the pressures that young people face related to sexual relationships. Students and the facilitator generate agreements for classroom discussion. This lesson introduces "My Choices," the journaling component of the curriculum.
	2. Understanding Sexually Transmitted Infections (STIs) and Human Immunodeficiency Virus (HIV)	Using visual materials, the facilitator provides an overview of six common STIs including how they are spread, symptoms, treatment, and prevention. Students play a game to learn about the ways in which HIV is transmitted. They brainstorm reasons that teens might not get tested for STIs or HIV and identify ways to address these barriers.
Week 2	3. Making Choices (Video)	Students view the video "Choices." The video shows three teenage couples facing decisions about sex. It also depicts some of the consequences of unprotected sex.
	4. Setting Personal Limits	Students discuss the need for setting personal limits regarding sexual behavior and discuss three steps to avoid making unsafe choices. In a journaling activity, students address their personal limits regarding sex.
Week 3	5. Talking with a Person Infected with HIV	A guest speaker shares his or her experience living with HIV infection or AIDS. A question-and-answer period follows the speaker's presentation. In a journaling activity, students personalize how being infected with HIV would affect their lives.
Week 4	6. Ways To Say "No!"	Verbal and nonverbal refusal skills are introduced and demonstrated through scripted role plays. Discussion and practice using a half-scripted role play help students distinguish between ineffective and effective statements and actions.
	7. More Ways To Say "No"	After reviewing characteristics of clear "no" statements, two new refusal skills are modeled: alternative actions and delay tactics. Students practice refusal skills in small groups using half-scripted role plays.
Week 5	8. Healthy Relationships	Students identify the characteristics of healthy and unhealthy relationships. Students rank the qualities that are personally important to them in a boyfriend or girlfriend and assess their values and expectations in dating situations.

TABLE 8.1. SAFER CHOICES 2 PROGRAM SCOPE AND SEQUENCE, Cont'd.

Timing	Lesson	Activities
	9. Healthy and Un-healthy Relationships	This lesson reinforces what the students learned in Lesson 8. Through the use of case studies, students identify the characteristics that make a relationship healthy or unhealthy. Students brainstorm tips to avoid and end an unhealthy relationship.
Week 6	10. Using Protection: Condoms	This lesson focuses on the use of condoms to protect against HIV, STIs, and unintended pregnancy. Students discuss barriers to planning, getting, and using condoms along with solutions. After the facilitator demonstrates the proper use of condoms, students examine condom packages to identify characteristics and practice correct steps for condom use.
	11. Using Protection: Not Having Sex Without a Condom	Students practice responding to typical pressure lines in role-play situations in which young people are being pressured to have unprotected sex.
Week 7	12. High-Risk Situations	Through role plays, students review and practice methods to avoid high-risk situations that might promote sexual behavior. Students discuss how drugs and alcohol affect an individual's decision to avoid unwanted or unprotected sexual activity.
	13. Personalizing the Risk for Pregnancy and Methods of Protection	Students participate in an activity to personalize their risk for unintended pregnancy. HIV, STIs, and pregnancy prevention methods commonly used by teens are presented and discussed. Students differentiate between methods that offer little or no protection, those that reduce the risk of pregnancy only, and those that reduce the risk of HIV, STIs, and pregnancy.
Week 8	14. Playing It Safe	Students brainstorm common barriers to using condoms and contraception and ways to overcome these barriers. Students practice communication skills for talking with a partner about using protection in half-scripted role plays.
	15. What You Can Do	Students reflect on what they have learned from the program and complete the final journaling activity, making a personal commitment regarding responsible sexual activity.

Think, and Act program's theme of an intervention for asthma is based on the self-regulatory processes taught in the computer program. It became the program title and a structure for recurring visuals (Figure 8.1) (Shegog, Bartholomew, Gold, et al., 1999; Shegog, Bartholomew, Gold, Pierrel, et al., 1999). Themes may be unrelated to the program content. The third-grade component of the CATCH program (Perry et al., 1997) used a theme of space creatures that had come to earth to teach earth children about diet and physical activity (Figure 8.2). Themes may also derive from characteristics of the at-risk groups, cultures, or preferred learning styles. In the CF FEP (Bartholomew et al., 1991), the theme of the adolescent modules was "taking charge" of one's health and one's life and was based on an adolescent developmental task (Figure 8.3), whereas the modules for the school-age children emphasized exploration and mastery, a developmental task of children this age.

FIGURE 8.1. WATCH, DISCOVER, THINK, AND ACT SCREEN WITH SELF-REGULATORY ICONS.

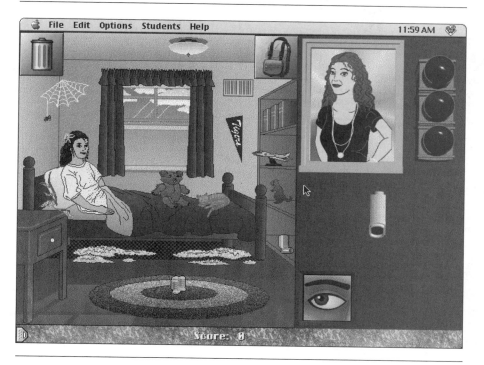

FIGURE 8.2. CATCH THEME.

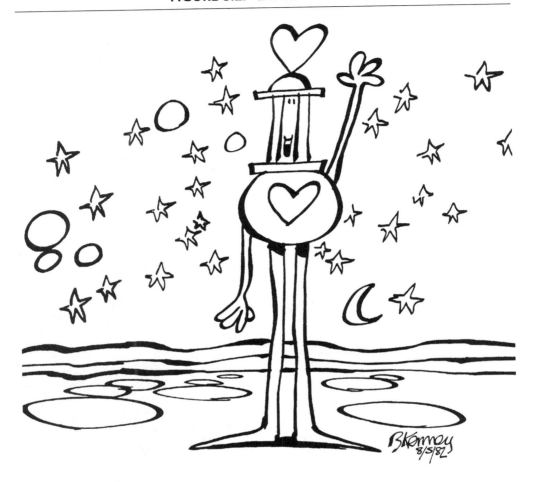

Hi there, Earthlings! I'm Hearty Heart,
With a heart health story I'm about to start.
My planet's called "Strongheart," right next to that star;
When I travel by spaceship, it doesn't seem far.

FIGURE 8.3. CYSTIC FIBROSIS FAMILY EDUCATION PROGRAM THEME.

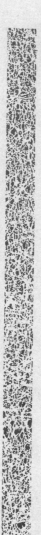

feature story

Finding Your Inner Voice

Finding a personal problem-solving style takes a while. Getting in tune with your own way of solving problems goes hand in hand with gaining more independence.

As Nicole, 23, says, "I was out on my own for a while before I started to listen to my own voice and know what was right and wrong for me. I started to get gut feelings about things: Is this going to work for me? Has it worked in the past?"

Some people like to think over problems for a long time and then try a solution. Others like talking to friends, family, or the medical team before trying out a solution. It all depends on what works for each person.

Stopping Problems Before They Happen

No matter what we do, problems happen. But some problems you can almost see coming. What can you do to prevent some of these?

"First of all, you really learn from your mistakes," says Kelly, 16. "I remember going on a trip with my friends. Because nobody wanted to eat as often as I needed to eat, I wasn't getting enough calories. On the next trip with my friends I brought some snacks I could eat between meals. That worked for me."

Thinking through problems ahead of time seems to be a way of avoiding some of them.

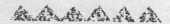

A Step at a Time

Laurel, 22, thinks about problem-solving this way: "I compare it to cleaning the house. If your whole house is a mess and you think, 'I gotta clean this whole place up right away,' you get overwhelmed. So, I divide it up into small tasks. I start by cleaning out a drawer, a closet, or a sink. Then I clean a little bit each day. Pretty soon the whole house is clean. A step at a time."

"I compare problem-solving with cleaning a house. You take it a step at a time."

The most important factor in choosing themes and organizing subthemes or ideas for a program is whether the chosen idea will aid participants' attention, awareness, and comprehension (Petty & Cacioppo, 1986a; Petty & Wegener, 1998). As a second tier of effectiveness, it is possible that themes can also affect determinants and change objectives directly. For example, in the stroke program materials, the theme of urgency paired with the theme that treatment is available was meant to directly affect certain change objectives.

A good example of the development of a comprehensive program theme designed to appeal to the intended participants is Project Parents and Newborns Developing and Adjusting (PANDA) (Mullen, DiClemente, Carbonari, Nicol, Richardson, Sockrider, et al., 1999) (Chapter Thirteen). When Mullen and her colleagues first characterized a program to help women who had quit smoking during pregnancy not to return to smoking, they thought of the theme "tender loving care for the mother." As they worked on program development and talked to the women, they became even more convinced that a theme that enabled the mother to focus on herself and get ready for the baby would garner the prospective mother's attention, whereas a theme more closely related to cigarette smoking would not.

Channels and Vehicles for Program Methods, Strategies, and Messages

Program design demands decisions not only about themes but also about messages and how to deliver them. A communication channel can be interpersonal or mediated; a vehicle is more specifically how a message is actually packaged and delivered. Before the planners can choose channels and vehicles for delivery of program components, they must ascertain the preferred media use by intended audiences:

- Do they watch television, listen to the radio, and read newspapers and magazines?
- Do they attend mostly to certain ethnic media?
- Who are credible sources?
- What amount of time do they spend with each medium?
- What content do they attend to (for example, news, talk shows, PSAs, entertainment)?
- What channels are used to get information about the program topic?

Various communication vehicles are described in Table 8.2, with examples of the methods and strategies the vehicles often carry. Choosing vehicles is a matter of balancing the needs and preferences of the intended program participants with logistics and budget. With children, for example, planners look to school-based education using teachers and peer leaders; to health care providers; to magazines, radio, and television targeted to children; and to computer and video

TABLE 8.2. COMMUNICATION CHANNELS AND VEHICLES.

Channels and Vehicles	Typical Uses, Methods, and Strategies	Advantages	Disadvantages
Interpersonal Community volunteers Peer leaders	Skill training Social reinforcement Modeling Tutoring Small-group discussion	Powerful source of influence and persuasion Inexpensive Involve community and enhance capacity	Difficult to train and motivate multipliers
Interpersonal Teachers	Mastery learning Tutoring Small-group discussion Lecture Modeling	Expert in teaching techniques Fit organizational context of school	Can be resistant to truly interactive techniques Can be crippled by curriculum time constraints
Interpersonal Health care providers	Skill training Social reinforcement Modeling Counseling	Powerful source of influence and persuasion Expert in patient assessment and counseling Captive audiences interested in personal health issues	Difficult to train and motivate Lack of time Have difficulty integrating counseling techniques if they are used to a more directive "medical model" Can be perceived as too dissimilar from the patient
Circulating Print Newspapers	Letters to the editor Editorial commentary Role-model stories Information Persuasion Vicarious reinforcement	Inexpensive Wide audience Extends expertise Detailed Very flexible Positive consumer attitudes about vehicle Can be niche based	Depend on literacy Reach only certain segments Short life span Clutter (many vehicles on the market compete for attention) Not for demonstration Poor visual quality Require health educator cultivation of relationship with gatekeepers such as health reporters at the newspaper

TABLE 8.2. COMMUNICATION CHANNELS AND VEHICLES, Cont'd.

Channels and Vehicles	Typical Uses, Methods, and Strategies	Advantages	Disadvantages
Circulating Print Newspapers, (Cont'd)			Require health educator to capitalize on short media attention span for issues
Circulating Print Magazines	Editorial commentary Role-model stories Information Persuasion Vicarious reinforcement	Good audience segmentation High audience receptivity Credibility and prestige Long life span Visual quality	Lack of flexibility Lack of control of distribution
Circulating Print Newsletters	Letters to the editor and editorial commentary Role-model stories Information Persuasion Vicarious reinforcement	Good audience segmentation High audience receptivity Strong possibility for tailoring Control of distribution	Require high degree of novelty
Display Print Billboards Posters	Attention Awareness Cue to action	Can be very effective in calling attention to a campaign	Can only effect limited learning and change objectives (such as knowledge and awareness) Expense can be significant
Display Print Brochures Flip-charts	Skill training Modeling Information with extensive detail Persuasion Vicarious reinforcement	Can effect a variety of learning and change objectives	No standard distribution routes exist as they do for circulating print.
Radio News items Interviews	Information Awareness Role-model stories	Good audience segmentation High audience receptivity	Require cultivation of relationship with station gatekeepers

TABLE 8.2. COMMUNICATION CHANNELS AND VEHICLES, Cont'd.

Channels and Vehicles	Typical Uses, Methods, and Strategies	Advantages	Disadvantages
Radio, (Cont'd) Public Service Announcements (PSAs)	Persuasion		Require ability to capitalize on short media attention span for issues; also short life span
			Require high degree of novelty
			Role-model stories not supported by visuals
Television News stories Talk shows Interviews	Skill training Modeling Information with extensive detail Persuasion Vicarious reinforcement	Wide distribution Possibility for segmentation	Lack of control over content
			Require cultivation of relationship with station gatekeepers
			Require ability to capitalize on short media attention span for issues; also short life span
			Require high degree of novelty
			Competition with broadcast clutter
Television Entertainment TV	Intense role-model stories	Wide distribution Natural segmentation Norm changing capabilities	Require relationships with producers Can be very long
Television PSAs	To stimulate awareness	Wide distribution Natural segmentation	Channel surfing cuts down on audience. Must have excellent production qualities Often used at off-peak or not used
Television Infomercials	Product awareness and persuasion	Can provide large amounts of detail	Channel surfing is problematic.
Computer-assisted instruction	Skill training	Has a very wide and quickly expanding repertoire of vehicles such as CD-ROM,	Can be costly to develop Programming skills are rare and in high demand.

TABLE 8.2. COMMUNICATION CHANNELS AND VEHICLES, Cont'd.

Channels and Vehicles	Typical Uses, Methods, and Strategies	Advantages	Disadvantages
Computer-assisted instruction (Cont'd)		Decision-support, simulations, games, learner-controlled instruction	
Videotape	Just about anything	Control over content	Can be costly
Training Documentary			Distribution systems must be planned.

Source: Adapted from Elder, Geller, Hovell, and Mayer, 1994; Wells, Burnett, and Moriarty, 1998.

games and instruction. Techniques from social-marketing market segmentation can help define the communication vehicles that will reach certain population groups (Andreasen, 1995; Lefebvre & Flora, 1988; Maibach, Ladin, Maxfield, & Slater, 1996; Slater, 1995).

One program can use both interpersonal and mediated channels as well as many different vehicles. The A Su Salud program used both media (circulating print, radio, and television) and interpersonal communication through community volunteers to promote smoking cessation among Mexican Americans in south Texas (A. L. McAlister et al., 1995; A. G. Ramirez et al., 1995). Program implementers, using the strategy of behavioral journalism, worked with mass media journalists to produce news and features with information regarding cessation and with stories of real-life people from the population at risk who were in various stages of change regarding the behavior. Trained volunteers then handed out calendars containing the times of the news and talk show broadcasts, tips for quitting, and information of public interest (for example, the high school basketball game schedule); encouraged their friends and acquaintances to consider quitting smoking; and reinforced any efforts those friends made.

This approach was also used in the AIDS demonstration projects funded by the Centers for Disease Control (CDC), (CDC, AIDS Community Demonstration Projects Research Group, 1999; Corby, Enguídanos, & Kay, 1996; A. L. McAlister et al., 1995; Pulley, McAlister, Kay, & O'Reilly, 1996). In one city the AIDS project chose runaway youth as the focus, and it targeted condom use and either not shooting up or using clean needles and used micromedia in the form of small cards that contained role-model stories. Although the role-model stories were true ones obtained through interviews with members of the at-risk groups, the pictures and names were fictitious. In this case because the chosen at-risk group was small and the behaviors were private, using a mass-media channel would not be possible or effective. A major advantage of using role-model stories from the population is that they are culturally appropriate when ascertained properly. The role models speak, think, look, and act like members of the at-risk group because, in fact, they are. Making these early adopters of a healthy behavior more visible to others in the population increases the rate of diffusion of the behaviors in the population (A. G. Ramirez et al., 1995).

In addition to community volunteers, interpersonal channels include teachers and health care providers (who also likely use print and video media). Teachers may use tutorials (one-on-one instruction), group discussions, and lectures, depending on the context and on the content and objectives of the instruction. Tutorials and small group learning have the advantage over lectures in that learner performance can be elicited and feedback provided with greater individualization.

More abstract and interactive vehicles for change, such as community coalitions, are also frequently used in health promotion programs. For example, the stroke project (L. B. Morgenstern et al., 2002) included a community committee of people with a stake in stroke treatment, such as health care providers, community groups, and stroke victims. The Walk Texas! program (Texas Diabetes Program/Council & Texas Department of State Health Services, 1998), a community program aimed at getting Texans to exercise, is conducted by local health departments and other community-based organizations. An early task was to identify and connect to partners who could establish local walking groups. Advocacy is a central part of many programs, such as those directed to reducing exposure of youth to tobacco, to increasing support of coordinated school health, and to preventing various chronic diseases (Altman, 1995a, 1995b). Blueprints for accomplishing these performance objectives are comparable to the program design documents we discuss later in this chapter for the development of media and small group communications. These blueprints include guidelines for selecting coalition members, guidelines for meeting agendas, protocols for legislative visits, and sample letters for advocacy. These channels for delivering methods and strategies to accomplish program objectives should be considered as a possible part of every program.

Computer-Assisted Intervention. The current computer environment in health education is one of great promise. Street and Rimal (1997) define interactive technology as that which includes both user control, the extent to which the user can modify the form and content of the computer environment and can determine what topics and services are selected, and responsiveness. *Responsiveness* is the extent to which the program takes into account the user's previous activities. A highly responsive program gives feedback on health choices made within a program and provides opportunities to practice new skills (Funk & Buchman, 1995). Another aspect of interactive media is that they comprise modular units that are linked together to enable the program to employ an array of databases such as animation, narration, graphics, and services and to enable the user to move from one part to another (Dede & Fontana, 1995). These characteristics are attractive for program development in health education because they provide a powerful medium for delivering methods and strategies that influence a wide range of determinants.

Interactivity promotes active information processing and satisfaction (Dede & Fontana, 1995; Rafaeli, 1988; Schaffer & Hannafin, 1986) and may contribute to central processing as discussed by Chaffe and Roser (1986), Petty and Cacioppo (1986a, 1986b), and Webber (1990)(see Chapter Three).

Another advantage of interactive multimedia is that a single application can support a wide variety of learner needs (Rimal & Flora, 1997). For example, users who lack sufficient background (including language skills) can supplement text learning with other modalities, such as pictures, and can be presented significant redundancy across modalities. Redundancy is needed because a novice learner has to construct cognitive schema and then attach new information. On the other hand, users who already have the schema can reduce redundancy and cut to the chase. The computer environment also is an excellent mechanism for balancing novelty (to acquire and maintain attention) and redundancy (to facilitate processing). Rimal and Flora cite Singer and Singer (1979) who compare the public television programs *Sesame Street* (high novelty) with *Mister Rogers' Neighborhood* (high redundancy). With computer-assisted instruction, both environments are available simultaneously. A further advantage is temporal flexibility. The user can control not only when to get the message but when and how to manipulate the message. All these types of user control—the ability to control when the program is used and the aspects of novelty and redundancy—can facilitate learning and the development of self-directed learning skills (Lieberman & Linn, 1991).

Despite the potential of computers in health education, Hawkins and colleagues (1997) warn against a "If you build it, they will come" attitude (p. 79). They suggest that the program developer build tools, start small, and not be afraid of being captivating. They applied these principles to the Comprehensive Health Enhancement Support System (CHESS), an example of the explicit use of theoretical methods such as problem solving, decision support, self-monitoring, social support, and action planning in a multimedia environment. CHESS also is a good example of developing a carefully limited design and adhering to it across content domains. The program is intended for people who have health crises; and the first problem areas to be developed were breast cancer, HIV, sexual assault, adult children of alcoholics, academic crisis, and stress management (Gustafson, Bosworth, Chewning, & Hawkins, 1987; Gustafson et al., 1993). The program shell consisted of three components:

- Information delivered through an instant library, questions and answers, "ask an expert," and help and support
- Decision and planning support delivered through decision analysis, action planning, and risk assessment
- Social support delivered through personal stories and a discussion group

The HIV component has been evaluated and found to result in better quality of life for the program users as compared to a control group (P. Brennan, Ripich, & Moore, 1991). Quality of life included better cognitive functioning, less degeneration over time in activities of daily living and social activities, more effectively managed medical care visits, and less hospitalization. Other programs, such as one linking caregivers of persons with Alzheimer's disease patients and one providing social support to persons with advanced AIDS (P. Brennan et al., 1991), have also demonstrated the ability to incorporate sound theoretical methods such as social support into computer-assisted health promotion. Furthermore, the programs seem to be used equally across demographic segments, including men and women and both disadvantaged and more advantaged individuals. One study indicated differential use between older and younger participants, however, with older individuals using the program less often (F. A. Brennan & Fink, 1997).

Other program developers have demonstrated that the computer-assisted instructional environment is a good way to teach self-management skills and to enhance self-efficacy (Brown et al., 1997; Lieberman, 2001). Lieberman (1997) describes a series of Health Hero video games that provide simulated self-management environments for diabetes and asthma and that solidify negative attitudes regarding smoking. She notes that children will continue playing games until they can easily complete them. Bartholomew and colleagues had the same experience with the Watch, Discover, Think, and Act program (Chapter Twelve) (Bartholomew, Gold, et al., 2000; Bartholomew, Shegog, et al., 2000). Children would often encourage entire families to wait for them in the clinic so that they could just get one more scene done in the asthma management program. All these programs have design elements geared toward promoting attention and active processing, motivation, knowledge and skills of disease management, self-efficacy, communication, and social support. Watch, Discover, Think, and Act makes use of the computer's capabilities by enabling children to enter their personal asthma characteristics, which the computer then uses to modify the simulations to be more lifelike for the individual child.

Telephone-Assisted Interventions. Soet and Basch (1997) point out that the telephone has been used as an instrument of health care since its debut. They cite a large literature on the use of the telephone as an instrument of health education and promotion, ranging from simple information hotlines, through a midrange of standardized messages aimed at health behavior, to more complex computerized counseling for behavior change (Ramelson, Friedman, & Ockene, 1999). There are now protocol-supported telephone interventions that support tailoring of messages (Zhu et al., 1996). The telephone as a delivery mechanism has many advantages. It is interactive, and messages can be not only tailored but also individualized. Visual privacy can make intervention less stressful and more productive for individuals who are reluctant to discuss a particular issue. The telephone also can reach dispersed or homebound populations and can accommodate low literacy and language differences. There is some risk of loss of meaning in this medium (as there is for print vehicles) because 65 percent to 95 percent of social meaning comes from visual cues in face-to-face interaction. However, it is possible that the novelty and different set of expectations for electronic media may liberate the delivery from the burden of interpersonal empathy as long as the messages are developed with appropriate counseling sophistication.

Perhaps the most exciting development in telephone delivery is the combination of expert system technology and interactive (digitized voice) telephone counseling. This technology enables a real-time assessment and contingent delivery of messages and feedback regarding attempts to perform a health behavior. Automated systems are being used more and more in managed care situations and other health care settings. For example, Ramelson and colleagues (1999) describe the *Telephone Linked Communication* (TLC) system, which can function as an at-home monitor, educator, and counselor for patients and consumers (Friedman, Stollerman, Mahoney, & Rozenblyum, 1997). The TLC has been used to counsel smoking cessation (Ramelson et al.), improve medication compliance for hypertension (Friedman et al., 1996), promote physical activity (Cullinane, Hyppolite, Zastawney, & Friedman, 1994; Jarvis, Friedman, Heeren, & Cullinane, 1997; King et al., 2002), promote dietary changes (Delichatsios et al., 2001; Dutton, Posner, Smigelski, & Friedman, 1995), and promote screening (Friedman, 2000). A sample conversation from the smoking intervention is included in Figure 8.4.

Computerized Tailoring of Interventions.

Computerized Tailoring of Interventions. For the past fifteen years, health education researchers have been testing computerized expert systems that enable tailoring of communications to certain participant characteristics (Bental, Cawsey, & Jones, 1999; Brug, Campbell, & Van Assema, 1999; M. W. Kreuter, Caburnay, Chen, & Donlin, 2004; M. Kreuter, Farrell, Olevitch, & Brennan, 2000; Revere & Dunbar, 2001; V. J. Strecher, 1999). Although there is need for further research to determine exactly on what characteristics tailoring should be based (that is, what characteristics influence the intervention's effectiveness), there is enough evidence of effectiveness to continue to work in this area and to import these strategies into common practice, with the caveat that the characteristics on which to

FIGURE 8.4. COMPUTERIZED TELEPHONE SYSTEM FOR SMOKING COUNSELING.

Figure A: Example of contemplation dialogue

The callers' responses to the questions posed by the system are underlined. The dashed lines represent a jump to another part of the conversation.

Hello Mr. [Name]. I'm glad that you called in today. About how many cigarettes are you now smoking a day?   25

You are smoking more cigarettes than the last time we spoke. I hope you will be able to cut down when we speak next. In the conversation, we will identify reasons that you smoke and reasons why you want to quit. This will help me to give you specific suggestions to help you quit.

- -

If you haven't smoked for a while, do you get a strong craving or desire to smoke? Press 1 for yes and 2 for no.   1

Write down on your list the words, "I smoke to satisfy my craving for a cigarette." Press 1 when you are done.   1

Do you smoke to give yourself a lift or to keep yourself from slowing down? Press 1 for yes and 2 for no.   2

Do you smoke when you are under stress or feeling depressed? Press 1 for yes and 2 for no.   1

Write down on your list the words, "I smoke to reduce stress." Press 1 when you are done.   1

- -

Now I would like to identify reasons why you want to quit. This will help me to give you specific suggestions to help you to quit. Do you want to quit for your health? Press 1 for yes and 2 for no.   2

Dr. [Name] recommends that you quit for your health. Passive smoking occurs when you smoke around other people. They inhale your cigarette smoke and the cancer-causing substances in it. Do you want to quit for the health of those close to you? Press 1 for yes and 2 for no.   1

Write down on your list the names of the people who you are thinking about. Press 1 when you are done.   1

- -

The money that you spend on cigarettes adds up to a lot. Since you started smoking, approximately how many cigarettes on an average day would you say that you have smoked?   30

Approximately how many years have you been smoking?   25

Do you realize that over the time that you have smoked, you have spent $27,375 on cigarettes? I'll bet that you wish you had that money now. Well, it's not too late to quit smoking and save money now. If you continue to smoke for the next ten years, you will spend another $16,425 on your habit. Do you want to quit to save money? Press 1 for yes and 2 for no.   1

We have finished making our lists. I would like you to put these lists in a place where you will see them every day—like near your telephone or on your fridge. Try to look at them at least once a day. You might think of more reasons why you want to smoke and why you want to quit. Add them to the lists as you think of them.

FIGURE 8.4. COMPUTERIZED TELEPHONE SYSTEM FOR SMOKING COUNSELING, Cont'd.

Figure B: Example of preparation dialogue

Did you try to quit on [your quit date]? Press 1 for yes and 2 for no.	1
Don't be discouraged. Most smokers need several tries before they quit. Did something unexpected come up that made it hard for you to quit? Press 1 for yes and 2 for no.	1
I understand. I hope that you will try again. Are the suggestions that we discussed helping you? Press 1 for yes and 2 for no.	2
We will review the suggestions, and if you want, I will give you some other ones to help you out. After we do this, I will ask you to choose another goal for quitting.	
You told me that you smoke to satisfy a craving. You wanted to satisfy your craving by taking ten deep breaths. Did you try this suggestion? Press 1 for yes and 2 for no.	1
Did this suggestion help you with your cravings? Press 1 for yes and 2 for no.	2
Don't be discouraged. I will give you some other ideas to help you to quit. If you get a strong urge for a smoke, try putting something in your mouth instead of a cigarette. You can carry around with you a carrot, celery, cinnamon sticks, chewing gum, or toothpicks. Do you think you will do this? Press 1 for yes and 2 for no.	1
Write down on your list the thing that you will put in your mouth when you get a craving. Examples are carrot, celery, and cinnamon sticks. Press 1 when you are done.	1

Source: Reprinted from *Patient Education and Counseling, 36*(2), Ramelson, H. Z., Friedman, R. H., & Ockene, J. K., "An Automated Telephone-based Smoking Cessation Education and Counseling System," copyright 1999, with permission of Elsevier.

tailor in a particular program must be well justified empirically and theoretically (Brug, Glanz, Van Assema, Kok, & van Breukelen, 1998; Brug, Steenhuis, Van Assema, & De Vries, 1996; Dijkstra, De Vries, Roijackers, & van Breukelen, 1998a, 1998b; Kreuter & Strecher, 1996; Kreuter & Wray, 2003; Rimer et al., 1994; C. S. Skinner, Strecher, & Hospers, 1994; V. J. Strecher et al., 1994; Vandelanotte, de Bourdeaubhuij & Brug, 2004). The literature is somewhat unclear about exactly what aspects of tailored messages have been the effective components. Table 8.3 provides a summary of the variables that have been used in studies of tailored communications.

Velicer and colleagues (1993) define an *expert system* as a collection of facts and rules about something and a way of making inferences from the facts and rules. The most common type of expert system in health education is a computer program that generates behavior-change messages tailored to the receiver's specific characteristics. In other words, the expert system contains one or more databases of messages based on theoretical constructs that vary as they apply to different characteristics of individuals and algorithms for matching the messages to the individual. The message channel could be anything that facilitates delivery of the

TABLE 8.3. TAILORED ON WHAT?

Study	Characteristics Used in Intervention
Curry, Wagner, & Grothaus, 1991; Curry, McBride, Grothaus, Louie, & Wagner, 1995	Intrinsic motives for quitting, self-efficacy, self-control
Prochaska, DiClemente, Velicer, & Rossi, 1993; Velicer & Prochaska, 1999	Stages and processes of change from the Transtheoretical Model
Strecher, Kreuter, Den Boer, Korbin, Hospers, & Skinner, 1994	Smoking behavior, stage of change, perceived benefits, and barriers
Rimer, Orleans, Fleisher, Cristinzio, Resch, Telepack, et al., 1994	Stage of change, quitting needs, and smoking habits
Skinner, Strecher, & Hospers, 1994	Mammography beliefs, stage of change, risk factors, and barriers
Brug, Steenhuis, van Assema, & de Vries, 1996; Brug, Glanz, van Assema, Kok, & van Breukelen, 1998	Fat, fruit and vegetable intake, attitudes, perceived social influences, self-efficacy expectations, and awareness levels
Dijkstra, De Vries, & Roijackers, 1998	Consequences of smoking, benefits of quitting, barriers to quitting, high-risk situations
Bull, Kreuter, & Scharff, 1999	Stage of readiness to change, exercise goal, motives for and perceived barriers to reaching the goal, and preferred type of physical activity
Kreuter, Caburnay, Chen, & Donlin, 2004	Presence of smoke detector, smoker living in the home, living above the first floor, stairway in the home, car and car-seat ownership, baby's vaccination history, mother's breastfeeding history, participation in Special Supplemental Nutrition Program for Women, Infants, and Children (WIC), and next scheduled appointment
Kreuter, Lukwago, Bucholtz, Clark, & Sanders-Thompson, 2003	African American cultural characteristics: religiosity, collectivism, racial pride, and perception of time
Lusk, Ronis, Kazanis, Eakin, Hong, & Raymond, 2003	Use of hearing protection devices, type of device used most often, perceived hearing ability, and predictors of use of devices

message. In the expert system by Velicer and colleagues, for example, the vehicle is a report; but the message could also be delivered by newsletter, video, or computer-assisted instruction. In the Velicer work, messages were based on the Transtheoretical Model (TTM) and included processes of change tailored to the stage of the individual in regard to quitting smoking. Feedback included current smoking status and stage of change, current use of change processes, suggested quitting strategies, and high-risk situations. Feedback was compared against a normative database as well as against the participant's own progress. All the systems described in the literature are based on similar configurations (Figure 8.5), with a theoretical framework and specification of relevant hypothesized determinants of the health behavior; use of the determinant model to create a data collection tool and a series of messages; several databases, including at least a data file and a feedback message file; decision rules and a tailoring program; communications; and delivery vehicles (Dijkstra & De Vries, 1999; Rhodes, Fishbein, & Reis, 1997).

FIGURE 8.5. DEVELOPING TAILORED FEEDBACK.

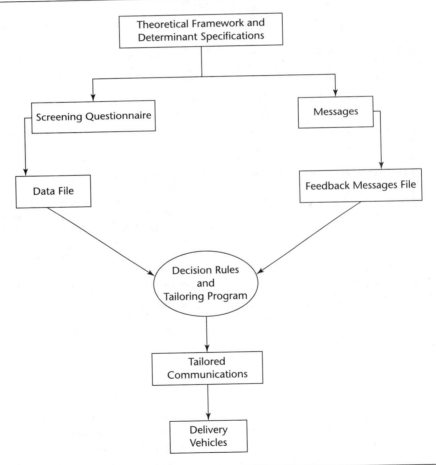

Source: Adapted from Brug, Steenhuis, Van Assema, and De Vries, 1996.

Preparing Design Documents

⤸ *The next task in Step 4 is to prepare design documents for the production of materials that meet the program objectives and parameters for the methods and strategies.*

The next task in Step 4 is to develop design documents to guide the process of program creation. Sometimes members of the planning group will develop the support materials for health education programs. In other cases the budget will allow hiring of a variety of creative consultants. Either way, planners must prepare documents to guide the producers to produce what the planners intend for the program.

Hiring and Working with Creative Consultants

In an ideal budgetary world, health educators should take the advice of Balderman (1995), who says that if you weren't trained to do something, don't do it. A creative consultant should be hired when the health educator does not have the specific skill needed to create a component of the program. Commonly used creative resources include graphic design studios, copywriters, instructional designers, video and film writers, and video and film directors. In addition, production resources can include photographers, illustrators, talent (models and actors), location search companies, printers, videographers, and computer programmers.

In order to find the creative or production resources they need, experienced health educators talk to people. Good sources of referrals are printers or other people who have produced work and can introduce a designer, photographer, or illustrator. Branching out from the health field can often help. Balderman (1995) suggests the following ways to recruit talent to a project:

- Put together a synopsis of the job including approximate budget, length, purpose, concept, and producing agency
- Send the synopsis with a request for statements of interest. Schedule meetings with the persons who respond. Interviewing talent is a good way not only to look for help on the current job but also to build a file of possible resources for future work.
- Look at the portfolio of work. Is there any evidence that this person has conveyed the type of message needed and gotten the desired response? Does the planning team like the work? Does the range of previous work of the creative person include the type of work needed for the project?

- Ask about several of the projects in the portfolio. Is a range of budgets represented? Ask the person to talk about each project. If the type of product the team wants is not represented in the portfolio (which is the best of the best), then it is probably not available from this vendor.

Remember that members of the team will not be designing the piece; the creative consultant will. Health educators should at no point have to take over for the creative person. That person should understand the project's intent well enough that he or she brings to the team something that is even better than what the team imagined. This scenario implies that the person should not only be creative but also willing to thoroughly understand the team's intent. How does this creative person present herself? Is this purely a salesperson, or does he or she ask questions to understand the project? Is the person too quick to assume that it is just like other projects he or she has done? Does the person seem insensitive to the team's needs, making statements such as, "But I'm the producer" or "We never do it like that"? If so, proceed cautiously.

A word about second-guessing the creative resources: don't. Health educators should give their creative people the most understandable background possible and then try not to interfere with their creativity. The opportunity to allow a creative resource to create something independently is one of the reasons for all the planning up to this point. The creative people hired for the project will produce their best effort, and fiddling with it will decrease the quality in some way. It is possible that the person you hire for a project just cannot deliver acceptable work, and health educators must know when to end the relationship with the vendor. If the initial ideas, preliminary sketches, or other proposed work are not acceptable, the health educator may want to look for other talent. The health educator might ask for one more attempt after reviewing the project background and the matrices. But after a couple of unsuccessful tries, the health educator should go back to the hiring process.

Design Documents: Conveying the Project Intent

The first step in working with a creative resource is conveying initial project parameters. The first design document includes answers to the following questions:

- What pieces will be produced?
- What creative and production elements will be necessary to produce the project, and who will provide them?
- How and when will each piece be produced?

- What is the deadline?
- What is the budget?
- What preexisting pieces can the production resource of the planning team provide (for example, videotape, photos, illustrations, logos, copy)?
- Does the piece need to follow a particular format?
- Does the group have a corporate or agency manual of style?
- Whom does the piece need to acknowledge?
- What will the approval process be?
- Who will be involved in approval?

The planning team members who are working with creative resources want them to understand the project as well as possible and to wholeheartedly adopt the planning group's intent. The team members want the creative person to understand their plan for the program materials and then to bring his or her talent to producing it. The person's creative additions should bring to life rather than override or misinterpret the team's understanding of the problem and its solution. Some creative people are unable to stay within the project parameters. Planners may encounter the video producer who, no matter what, will try to turn the team's role-model story into her documentary or the graphic designer who wants the team's newsletter to be his award winner. The key to working with the creative production team is to create design documents so that the producers come to fully understand what the planning team intends.

To get started with a creative person, health educators usually invite him or her to a team meeting to talk about the project once the team can give a fairly consistent message. If possible, the health educator takes the creative person to visit with members of the community. Sometimes the creative person can go to focus groups or interviews. The persons that he or she encounters at these meetings may end up in the final materials. For example, the women consulted in focus groups for formative research for Project PANDA (Chapter Thirteen) were interviewed for the resulting videotape as well.

In an ideal situation, the designer (or writer or producer) can work with the team almost from the beginning of planning, offering ideas as to format and serving as an expert witness on what is (and is not) doable. The next best approach is to bring the designer in when the matrices, strategies, and methods have been hammered out but before the team has decided on the formats of the support materials. This approach allows the designer to bring his or her creativity to the table as the planning team figures out what precise form the product will take. The earlier the designer can enter the process, the more his or her skills will enrich the it. Designers and other creative consultants need to be compensated for their time in participating in the planning process.

Writing Design Documents

Planners must communicate in words what someone else will return in various forms of pictures, stories, movement, color, sound, and so forth. We have already talked about including the creative people in meetings with the team and the intended audience, but doing so does not alleviate the need for documents to convey the team's intent in detail. We suggest two types of design documents:

- A series of design documents from the health educator to the creative people
- A series of production design documents from the creative people to the health educator

The first design documents from the planning team to the creative team are the matrices, with all the change objectives that are pertinent to a given product highlighted. A second document from the planning team is a project prospectus that gives the length of the product, a brief description of the audience, the way that the user will interact with the product, the purpose of the piece (the intended impact), the central messages, and the target budget.

The design documents then become more specific to the desired product. For example, Table 8.4 illustrates the initial design documents used for Project PANDA. This project delivered methods through a series of newsletters directed to pregnant women and another series directed to their partners. It also included a videotape for each partner, delivered to their home; the man received his just prior to the baby's arrival and the woman just after. This design document gives an overview of the women's intervention across time and across the weeks of pregnancy.

A second design document (Table 8.5) for project PANDA is included to show the progression from the overview to a more detailed description of the content to be developed for one specific newsletter. The PANDA development team decided to write the first draft of the newsletter copy themselves, so the development team members used the design document in-house to convey intent to all the team members who were writing copy.

Preparing design documents for a computer-assisted program requires a particularly intensive process, usually entailing creation of an initial description of the program, various flowcharts, and one or more storyboards (a sequential depiction with words and pictures of the product). Table 8.6 is an initial design description from the Health Heroes video-game series (Lieberman, 1997).

Figure 8.6 presents the overview flowchart that the team for Project Promoting Colon Cancer Screening in People 50 and Over (Project PCCaSO) (Vernon, 2004) developed to guide themselves, the video writer-producer, and the computer programmer through developing the message, writing video scripts for role-model stories and narration, and programming the computer-assisted instruction. The

TABLE 8.4. PROJECT PANDA PRELIMINARY DESIGN DOCUMENT—NEWSLETTER.

Women's Intervention: Smoking Over Time

	29–30 Weeks	32–34 Weeks	34–36 Weeks	Immediate Postpartum	2 Weeks Postpartum	4–6 Weeks Postpartum
Target	Smoking: Precontemplator Contemplator	Smoking: Contemplator	Smoking: Contemplator	Smoking: Action	Smoking: Action	Smoking: Action
	Action (model all 3; have them find selves)					
	Passive Smoking: Contemplator	Passive Smoking: Contemplator	Passive Smoking: Contemplator	Passive Smoking: Action	Passive Smoking: Action	Passive Smoking: Action
			Action			
Outcome	See self as nonsmoker Attribute success to self Reassess benefits of nonsmoking	Be a healthier you	Acquisition of further skills for not smoking Preparing for delivery and return home as nonsmoker	Relapse prevention: Stress reduction Modeling Emotional support	Relapse prevention: Specific smoking, cognitive, and behavioral strategies for healthy lifestyle	Relapse prevention: Specific strategies for coping with resurfacing of environmental cues
Primary Messages	Where are you now?	Personal health and recovery	Aids for creating a nonsmoking environment Cognitive and behavioral strategies for staying off cigarettes post-delivery	Having that new baby at home is like nothing before. We've been there. Here's what to do for you.	Baby and you: A healthier lifestyle; order out of chaos	As you settle in: preparing for return to work or settling into new schedule
Medium	Print	Print	Print	Video	Print	Print

Consistent contexts: (1) from your health care provider; (2) health of new family (not just smoking)

TABLE 8.5. PANDA NEWSLETTER DESIGN DOCUMENT.

Women's Intervention Number 3: 34–36 Weeks: Newsletter

Description	Content	Impact
Element 1: Bulletin board Working title: "Let the Preparation Begin!" Assignment: Sarah	Preparing bags for the hospital: what to bring and what not to bring Preparing the house: freeze food for use after delivery; hang no-smoking signs; have some of your favorite things around for when you return from the hospital See home and hospital as places not to smoke (don't pack cigarettes in hospital bag)	Use strategies to enhance environment and control stimuli
Element 2: Feature story Working title: "Using Your Senses" Assignment: Sarah and Kay	Using senses to experience newborn baby: new baby smell, feel of new skin, and so on A quasi-research report that talks about the role of senses in mother and includes those senses that are enhanced after quitting smoking	Focus on benefits of not smoking
Element 3: "No Smoking" signs (these are separate from newsletter so mother can post) Messages on back of signs Assignment: Marianna	For the home and car Slogans: "Please don't smoke—tiny lungs at work." Cigarette with circle and slash through middle "I'm a new mom, and I cared enough to quit." Effects of passive smoke: "Thanks, Mom, you've saved me from [number] of colds and doctor visits." Reasons not to smoke: list from baby's point of view	Stimulus control: cues Decide not to smoke and to not let others smoke for the baby's sake Protect the baby

TABLE 8.5. PANDA NEWSLETTER DESIGN DOCUMENT, Cont'd.

Women's Intervention Number 3: 34–36 Weeks: Newsletter

Description	Content	Impact
Element 4: Tip sheet (detachable) Working title: "Baby's Message to Relatives and Friends" Assignment: Maryann and Angie	Yes, the baby's cute, but Mom needs the most attention and help right now. Suggestions for helping Mom: cooking, grocery shopping, cleaning, laundry	Use tip sheet to structure help after delivery Lessen environmental stress
Element 5: Special feature Working title: "Creating Your Own Smoke-Free Zone" Assignment: Pat	"Because you know the effects of passive smoke and others might not, you'll need strategies for helping other people not to smoke around you or your baby." Validate woman's effort to remain smoke-free Provide concrete tips on how to be assertive with others about where they can and cannot smoke—modeling Phrases to use in certain situations Encourage assertive control over amount of smoke that reaches their babies Focus on husband's smoking and how to deal with it	Recognize they have the skills to assertively deal with problematic smoking situations Remember passive smoke issues
Element 6: Cartoon Assignment: Sarah	Mom in a tank protecting her baby's "smoke-free zone"	Feel empathy for difficulty of controlling passive smoke
Element 7: Small box Working title: "Baby Status Report" or "Baby Facts" Assignment: Marianna	What's happening with your baby right now (describe development at 34–36 weeks)	Stay interested and feel informed

TABLE 8.6. DESIGN DOCUMENT FOR HEALTH HERO VIDEO GAMES.

Goals	Design Features
Attention and Active Processing	
To reduce psychological distance, increase attention to the content, and make the content seem personally relevant to young people	Present content on the popular video game medium in a format young people perceive to be targeted to them
To boost players' self-esteem, increase attention, optimize credibility, and increase likelihood that young people will emulate characters' behaviors	Use attractive, competent role-model characters who have the same health condition as the target user group and are about two to three years older
To increase attention, involvement, learning, and retention	Provide cognitive challenges, compelling characters and relationships, experiential learning, user control over the action, and individualized feedback
Motivation	
To make games motivating, engaging, and appealing	Present clear, intriguing, and challenging goals; provide continual updates on progress toward the goals; provide individualized interaction and feedback
To enhance enjoyment and individualize the learning experience	Allow game players to customize the content according to preferences and to match their own health status (for example, player can select the frequency and dose of a diabetic character's daily insulin)
Knowledge	
To teach explicit content	Use direct instruction; include game strategies that require the player to learn information in order to succeed in the game; use very graphic and memorable illustrations such as disgusting tar, plaque, and debris shown in a smoker's body
To teach skills	Present animated demonstrations such as how to use an inhaler for asthma medication; provide opportunities to rehearse skills and solve problems in simulations that show realistic outcomes based on the player's actions
To ensure that players will retain the information and skills they have learned in the game	Repeat information and animated demonstrations for review when players give a wrong answer; make the game difficult enough that players will repeat game levels dozens of times and therefore will be exposed repeatedly to the same content
Attention and Active Processing	
To correct mistakes and improve performance	Provide constructive feedback about the player's actions and choices, and offer remediation as needed

TABLE 8.6. DESIGN DOCUMENT FOR HEALTH HERO VIDEO GAMES, Cont'd.

Goals	Design Features
To provide background information on demand	Enable easy access to dynamic databases such as a food chart showing the food exchanges in a serving of each food that players may select in the game
To provide a cumulative record of performance in the game, increase the player's understanding, and encourage the use of personal logbooks	Use on-screen, automatically updated logbooks that record, for instance, medications the character has taken and blood glucose or peak flow measurements attained in each game level
Perceived Self-Efficacy	
To increase player's perceived self-efficacy for prevention and self-care	Create opportunities for players to rehearse new skills and to apply new knowledge in the game until they are successful
To help players feel more confident and willing to discuss their health concerns with peers, parents, and caregivers	Present issues and questions that players must address in the game, thereby allowing them to rehearse the answers while playing alone or to discuss the answers when others are present
To encourage social interaction that can increase peer tutoring, learning, and retention	Offer a two-player option in the game
To provide a springboard for discussion about prevention or self-management	Create an appealing game that young people will want to talk about and will be proud to play

Source: Lieberman, 1997.

theoretical framework for Project PCCaSO is the TTM (C. C. DiClemente & Prochaska, 1985; C. C. DiClemente et al., 1991). The planning team worked from the matrices to develop a flowchart to show the components of the intervention addressed to each stage of change. The team then worked from each part of the flowchart to develop a more detailed flowchart, one arm of which appears in Figure 8.6. The storyboards depict both the visuals and the messages for the five types of content: assessment and feedback on stage of change, instructions for navigating the program, information about colorectal cancer and screening, role-model stories about screening, and a fictitious role-model story depicting stages of change to match the learner and provide a guide for stage movement (one part of which is shown in Figure 8.7).

The production design documents that flow from the creative person to the health educator are usually more than written words. They might be written, as in a concept for a videotape, or they might be a combination of words and pictures,

FIGURE 8.6. PCCaSO FLOWCHART DESIGN DOCUMENT.

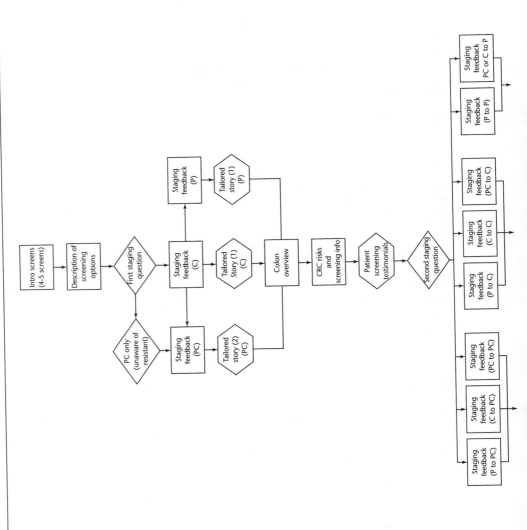

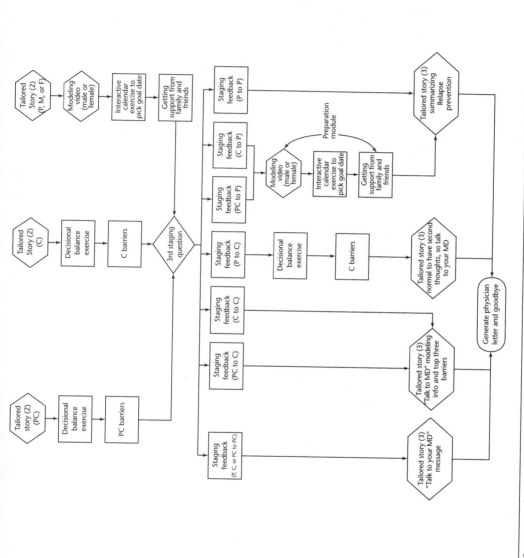

Key: PC = Precontemplators; C = Contemplators; P = Preparation; A = Action; CRC = Colorectal cancer; Tailored story = Serial role-model story tailored to stage of change and gender

FIGURE 8.7. DETAIL FROM PCCaSO FLOW DIAGRAM.

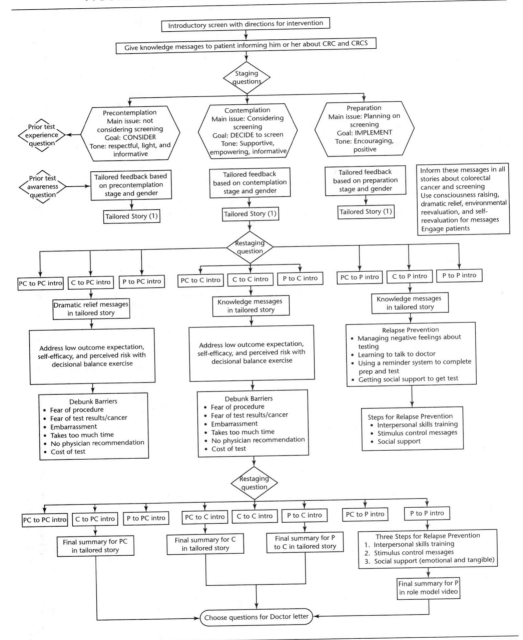

Key: PC = Precontemplators; C = Contemplators; P = Preparation; A = Action; CRC = Colorectal cancer; CRCS = Colorectal cancer screening; Tailored story = Serial role-model story tailored to stage of change and gender as in a storyboard or a rough sketch of a layout. They also might be illustrations or photographs in a layout or rough-cut videotape. These documents are all elements of conveying the creative person's image of the final product as it is developed first in the mind of that person and then in some medium. The number of these intermediate production design documents the health educator requires will affect the budget.

Creating Design Documents for Community Processes

At this point readers who are planning an intervention that includes only such methods and strategies as policy development, coalition building, and media advocacy may be thinking: "All this discussion about design documents doesn't refer to me! I won't be developing traditional materials." However, design documents can be very helpful to guide program components that are not products such as videotapes, public service announcements (PSAs), and the like. Products can be processes such as advisory board and committee meeting structure and function, coalition development and maintenance, and lobbying. Each of these products needs a design document and sometimes more than one. Coalitions, for example, need a design document that specifies how coalition members will be recruited, how meetings will be run, how minutes or meeting summaries will be constructed and delivered, and so on. A coalition might also need training for membership, and the training session will need a design document. Not only can these documents prevent breakdowns in communication, such as occurred in the mayor's group, but they can also make the processes smooth, productive, and reinforcing to the participants.

Box 8.2. Mayor's Project

The mayor's task force was well on its way to the production of support materials for the multicomponent program. The health educator, while busily looking at portfolios, choosing designers, and trying to understand what the video writer–producer would require in terms of design documents, received a panicky call from the chair of the group working on the community coalition strategy. She and her cochair were in the neighborhood, so the health educator decided on a spur-of-the-moment, face-to-face discussion of whatever was engendering the panic.

Group chair: Oh my gosh! We had our first coalition organizational meeting, and it was a free-for-all. I couldn't get hold of the agenda. I know it is supposed to be a participatory agenda. I've read the books.

This was participatory, all right—participatory by one small group! They took over at the beginning, and none of the rest of us could say a thing!

Cochair: Yeah, and one woman felt her ideas were so criticized that she walked out right in the middle of the meeting.

Group chair: Several of our most dedicated supporters stopped me afterward and said they didn't know if they could stand to come back. And on top of all that, we are not sure whether we can develop cohesion with this new group after all the groundwork the planning group has already laid.

The health educator helped the two plan a strategy. Before their next meeting, the cochairs put together a couple of meeting design documents. One was on how a participatory agenda would be created; the other was a format for meeting summaries that used the meeting that had just occurred. Finally, they put together the coalition overview and task document that would serve as a beginning for group development and task orientation in the coalition.

Figure 8.8 is a coalition design document showing the steps used in recruiting community partners for the Walk Texas! program (Texas Diabetes Program/ Council & Texas Department of State Health Services, 1998). Local health departments followed the steps in the design document to establish community walking groups. Coalitions must not only recruit members, they must do so in a manner that ensures inclusiveness and a broad representation of appropriate stakeholders. K. Johnson, Grossman, and Cassidy (1996) suggest a three-columned worksheet as a design document. The first column is a listing of appropriate community sectors (for example, local government, media, and parents). The second column is for the name of a recruitment contact within each sector, and the third column is for listing the level of participation that each has agreed to. Similar worksheets and other design documents can be deceptively simple but keep the group pointed in the right direction.

In another illustration of design documents for the common tasks of advocacy by coalition members, examples of advocacy design materials include a guide for three-person teams to interview legislators (Figure 8.9). A less elaborate guide can be used for preparing coalition members to make telephone calls to state or national legislators. A typical guide might outline how an advocate should identify him- or herself as well as provide talking points or brief summaries of relevant data, the conclusion the advocate wishes the legislator to make from this data,

FIGURE 8.8. WALK TEXAS! DESIGN DOCUMENT.

Recruiting community partners can be an exciting challenge when you proceed in an organized, well-planned manner.

Step 1: Determine the characteristics of your ideal partner and list them. Here are some attributes of an ideal community partner:

- One who reaches the community (that is, a gatekeeper to audiences such as nutrition centers, senior centers, and churches)
- One whose goals and priorities are in line with your organization
- One who is willing to join a partnership
- One who has credibility (people respect them; they do what they say they will)
- One with resources (time, money, expertise, facilities, and so on)
- One who is enthusiastic and willing to work
- One who is a leader in the community
- One who can serve as a positive role model
- One who will champion the cause

Step 2: Find potential partners

- Satisfied past partners are easy to sell
- Ask everyone you talk to for more names of potential partners
- Talk to people who have influence in the community
- Participate in promotional activities (advertising, booths, and so on)
- Use lists and directories; don't forget the library

Step 3: Do your homework; gather information about the individual and the organization

Step 4: Make an appointment

Step 5: Prepare your presentation

- Know what you want to accomplish at the meeting
- Make it clear what's in it for them, but let them express and work through reservations

a straightforward statement of support (or opposition) to a specific piece of legislation, and an appropriate close (Center for Pediatric Research, 1997). A legislative contact report allows simple but structured record keeping of such telephone calls and can be used to plan follow-up. A contact report might, for example, provide room to record the caller's name, the name of the person called, the topic of the discussion, check boxes for indicating the legislator's overall reaction, space for significant comments or suggestions from the legislator, and the caller's comments

FIGURE 8.9. ADVOCACY DESIGN DOCUMENT: ORGANIZING THE INTERVIEW TEAM.

The interview team should consist of three members, each of whom has a specific function. The functions should be thoroughly delineated, and there should be no overlapping of function.

1. *The leader or team captain:* This is the person who sets the tone of the interview. He establishes rapport with the candidate. He is a "nice guy" type. He must be friendly and courteous and never show any hostility. He asks the question—objectively—and supplies whatever background information is needed.

2. *The listener or reporter:* After this person says, "How do you do?," he doesn't say anything at all. He bends all his efforts toward being perceptive and committing as much of the interview to memory as possible. *He does not take notes.* Nothing inhibits free discussion more than a pencil and notepad in someone's hands. He not only listens to what is said but also listens for attitudes, for signs of strain. (Example: Every time salary is mentioned, the candidate pulls his earlobe. What could this mean?) He tries to spot the candidate's "hidden agenda." Why is he seeking office?

3. *The track man:* This man has either a big job or a small one depending on how the conversation goes. If the interview seems off on a tangent, he can courteously interrupt with phrases such as, "You said a moment ago that . . ." "Did you mean . . ." or " I think Mr. Leader meant to ask if . . ." The track man keeps the interview moving and could signal its change of pace or termination. *But* he should not attempt to stifle a discussion that is giving some insights, ever though it is off track. He keeps the conversation from meandering fruitlessly.

DO	DON'T
1. Be prepared to state your views clearly	1. Don't prolong the interview
2. Have appropriate materials to leave	2. Don't tip off the best answer
3. Be on time	3. Don't do all the talking; sometimes silence will bring out interesting information
4. Be friendly, positive, and constructive	
5. Be specific about your position	4. Don't let the candidate interview you
6. Be brief! Be brief! Be brief!	5. Don't attempt to exact rash promises; obtain reasons for opposition and ask what you can do to help support efforts

or recommendations for follow-up (Virginia Department of Health, Division of HIV/AIDS, Regional Consortia, 2005). Such materials provide how-to information for members and could be used as part of an advocacy training session; as with legislative contacts, letter and telephone scripts can in themselves serve as micromedia messages.

Reviewing Existing Materials

⟳ *The next task in this step is to review available program materials for possible match with change objectives, methods, and strategies.*

After working from the matrices to prepare initial design documents, planners should consider using existing materials when available. However, if existing materials are considered to be acceptable after the review described here, they must be pretested with the intended participants, just as one would test materials that have been newly developed (National Cancer Institute, Office of Cancer Communications, 2002).

Planners should ask the following questions:

- Do the program materials enable the change objectives to be met?
- Do they deliver the intended theoretical methods and practical strategies?
- Do the materials fit with the intended audience?
- Are the materials attractive, appealing, and culturally relevant?

To determine the answers to these questions, the planning team reviews existing materials against matrices and lists of methods and strategies. The match should be almost perfect. Questions to ask include the following:

- Are all the messages that are needed to influence change objectives included?
- Are the required methods executed appropriately? For example, do role-model stories use coping models, and are they derived from a group that matches the community on important characteristics?

It is difficult to make all these matches, but sometimes parts of existing programs work well.

Determining Production Quality and Suitability

Existing materials that match objectives, methods, and strategies can be reviewed for production quality and suitability (Doak, Doak, & Root, 1996; Glynn & Britton, 1984; R. C. Parker, 1988; Rudd, 2002; Strong, 1990; Wells, Burnett, & Moriarty, 1998; White, 1988; R. Williams, 1994). Doak and colleagues (1996) describe factors that can contribute to reading difficulty. In addition to attributes measured by readability formulas, these are the print size and type style, color contrast between ink and paper, the difficulty of reading the text, the number of concepts in each paragraph, and the unfamiliar context that may be represented by health or medical topics. The Suitability Assessment of Materials (SAM) is a useful guide to reviewing the appropriateness of materials (Doak, Doak, & Root, 1996). SAM guides the scoring of materials in six categories: content, literacy demand, graphics, layout and typography, learning stimulation, and cultural appropriateness. This yields a final score and indicates whether the materials are superior, adequate, or not suitable. The SAM scoring rationale is presented in Table 8.7. One factor that is often missed in assessment of materials is their appropriateness in terms of showing nonstereotypical power and social relations. Check to see whether there is anything stereotypical about the materials. (For example, are only mothers portrayed giving certain kinds of care to children? Do the materials display stereotypical power relations, with only males or only females in certain occupations or with only whites as physicians and people of color as patients? Does the text make inappropriate assumptions as to the reader's socio-economic status or environmental resources?)

Determining Availability. Before engaging in a thorough evaluation, however, the planner should determine whether the materials are available in the needed quantity and time frame. Some agencies may allow reproduction. Some materials may be available in electronic form, for instance, as a PDF file over the Internet. In some cases copyright holders allow materials to be adapted, but any changes must usually be made with the express permission of the copyright owner (Fishman, 1997). Materials produced by the U.S. government are free for use by U.S. citizens, and more and more such materials are available on the World Wide Web. The National Institutes of Health (NIH), for instance, are making a concerted effort to upload their patient education material onto the Web. For example, the Cancer Control Planet Web portal is a collaborative effort aimed at providing access to data and resources that can help cancer control planners, health educators, program staff, and researchers design, implement, and evaluate evidence-based cancer control programs (National Cancer Institute, 2005). If a piece is adapted or reproduced, all copyrights, adaptations, and permissions must be acknowledged on every piece; and it is appropriate to provide courtesy copies to the people who created the original material.

Determining Reading Level. Reading levels indicate a grade level beyond which the message is likely to be difficult to decipher. Reading levels are almost always an issue for written materials—actually two issues: What should the reading level be for a program's intended audience? What is the actual reading level of the material? Pertaining to the first question is the persistent finding that a significant proportion of adults in the United States have limited reading skills. The National

TABLE 8.7. SUITABILITY ASSESSMENT OF MATERIALS (SAM) RATIONALE.

Factor to be Rated	Considerations for Rating
Content	
Purpose	Readers should be able to discern the purpose readily.
Content	The content is about what the reader is expected to do without superfluous information.
Scope	The scope is limited to the objectives.
Summary or review	Reviews are included that help the reader process the main points.
Literacy Demand	
Reading grade level	Ninth grade or more is usually not suitable; grade should match the intended readers' competence.
Writing style	Text should be active voice and conversational with simple sentences.
Vocabulary	Common, explicit words should be used. Imagery words are good. Concept and category words are avoided, or examples are used.
Context	Tell the purpose first
Learning aids	Headers, topic captions, and statements of what will be presented (advance organizers) help orient the reader and aid encoding to memory.
Graphics	
Cover graphic	The first thing the reader sees can determine attitude. It should portray the purpose, be friendly, and get attention.
Type of graphic	Illustrations should be familiar, age-appropriate, and without symbols and distracting details.
Relevance of illustrations	Illustrations should tell the key messages visually with no distractions.
Lists, tables, figures	Graphics must include step-by-step directions for interpretation.
Captions	Captions should tell the reader what the graphic is and where to focus.
Layout and Typography	
Layout factors	Most of the following should be present: low-gloss paper, high contrast of paper and ink, consistent information flow, visual cues such as shading or arrows to guide the reader, illustrations next to text, adequate white space, appropriate and focused use of color.
Typography	Text is uppercase and lowercase; type is serif and at least 12 points;, typographic cues such as size and color emphasize key points. Avoid all caps.
Subheads and "chunking" of information	Lists should be grouped so that people do not have to remember more than a few points.

TABLE 8.7. SUITABILITY ASSESSMENT OF MATERIALS (SAM) RATIONALE, Cont'd.

Factor to be Rated	Considerations for Rating
Learning Stimulation, Motivation	
Interaction used	Enhances central processing to solve problems, respond to open ended questions, make choices
Behaviors	Behaviors are modeled, specific, and reinforced. Learner must be able to distinguish and practice the exact behaviors to be learned.
Self-efficacy	People are more able to engage in the task and persist when they are confident about their task-related ability.
Cultural Appropriateness	
Matching	Matching in logic, language, and experience will facilitate engagement, reading, and learning.
Images and examples	All learning materials should present positive, culturally relevant images.

Source: Adapted from Doak, Doak, and Root, 1996.

Adult Literacy Survey was a survey of 24,944 adults that assessed functional literacy (Kirsch, Jungeblut, Jenkins, & Kolstad, 1993). Prose literacy was based on newspaper stories, quantitative literacy on bus schedules, and document literacy on job applications. Findings indicated that 46 to 51 percent of the adults in the United States have limited or extremely limited reading and quantitative skills and that approximately 21 to 23 percent would have difficulty using these skills for everyday tasks. The organization also reported that many adults with these low skill levels did not see themselves as limited and do not seek help with reading tasks (Kirsch, Jungeblut, Jenkins, & Kolstad, 1993). Poor readers share certain characteristics. They often read (decode) one word at a time; they skip over common words and do not classify or categorize information; they often miss the context of the information; and they fail to make inferences from data (Doak, Doak, & Root, 1996).

Low literacy, including the ability to use formal oral language, has well-documented implications for health status including disease outcomes (National Institutes of Health, 1994, 2003; Schillinger et al., 2002). The mechanisms of the link between literacy and health status may include the impact on diagnostic assessment of patients (Parikh, Parker, Nurss, Baker, & Williams, 1996; B. D. Weiss & Coyne, 1997); the inability to understand and follow a care plan for chronic illness (D. W. Baker, Parker, Williams, & Clark, 1998; Kalichman & Rompa, 2000;

M. V. Williams, Baker, Honig, Lee, & Nowlan, 1998; M. V. Williams, Baker, Parker, & Nurss, 1998) and acute care (Chew, Bradley, Flum, Cornia, & Koepsell, 2004; Estrada, Martin-Hryniewicz, Peek, Collins, & Byrd, 2004); communication between patient and physician (Schillinger, Bindman, Wang, Stewart, & Piette, 2004; M. V. Williams, Davis, Parker, & Weiss, 2002) and the influence on use and access to health care (D. W. Baker, Parker, Williams, & Clark, 1998; D. W. Baker et al., 2002; D. W. Baker, Parker, Williams, Clark, & Nurss, 1997).

Studies have addressed whether materials are written at levels that patients can be expected to read and have found that many health and health care topics are presented at levels beyond patient skills: for example, patient medication inserts (Basara & Juergens, 1994), medication instruction (Estrada, Hryniewicz, Higgs, Collins, & Byrd, 2000; Estrada et al., 2004), emergency department discharge instructions (D. M. Williams, Counselman, & Caggiano, 1996), nutrition education (Dollahite, Thompson, & McNew, 1996), cancer information (Cancer Research Center and Centers for Disease Control, 2005; Glazer, Kirk, & Bosler, 1996), and patient education for chronic diseases such as diabetes, arthritis, and epilepsy (Foster & Rhoney, 2002). Recently, L. S. Wallace and Lennon (2004) tested the readability of a random sample of 171 patient education materials from the American Academy of Family Practice and found that over 70 percent of materials were at a ninth-grade or higher reading level.

A large number of studies has measured patient reading skills and compared them to the materials that patients were expected to comprehend. For example, many studies have noted the gap between the reading ability of cancer patients and cancer education materials (Beaver & Luker, 1997; Cooley et al. 1995; Foltz & Sullivan, 1996; Michielutte, Bahnson, Dignan, & Schroeder, 1992). Materials for other illnesses may also represent a mismatch. For example, materials for patients with diabetes (Hosey, Freeman, Stracqualursi, & Gohdes, 1990), arthritis (Hill, 1997), and lupus (Hearth-Holmes et al., 1997) fell between a seventh- and thirteenth-grade reading level, whereas the patients were able to read between a sixth- and tenth-grade level.

The most reliable way to determine what the reading level of any print materials should be is to assess the health literacy of the intended program participants. This is commonly done in patient education settings and less commonly practiced in community settings, although short assessments based on instruments such as the Rapid Estimate of Adult Literacy in Medicine (REALM) or the Test of Functional Health Literacy in Adults (TOFHLA) (Parker, Baker, Williams, & Nurss, 1995) may be feasible. The REALM is a three- to five-minute test in which the participant is asked to read a list of health-related words arranged from very simple one syllable words to multisyllable words (Davis et al., 1991). The test, as well as a shortened version, correlates well with the Wide Range Achievement Test-Revised

(WRAT-R) (Bass, Wilson, & Griffith, 2003), although there appears to be some discrepancy between scores of African Americans and Caucasians (Shea et al., 2004). Another option is the shortened version of the TOFHLA (s-TOFHLA), which uses a modified Cloze procedure (W. L. Taylor, 1953) on two passages of health-related material. The passages lack every fifth to seventh word, and the respondent chooses the correct word from multiple-choice passages (Baker, Williams, Parker, Gazmararian, & Nurss, 1999).

The second issue is how to assess the reading level of a document. Many techniques are available; most include an assessment of the average number of words in a sentence and the average number of syllables in a word. The former is used as a measure of complexity and the latter as a measure of vocabulary level. There is more to complexity than the length of a sentence and more to vocabulary level than the number of syllables, but in precomputer days the pioneers developed these methods as workable substitutes. Many word-processing and grammar-checking programs will now do the math, but the programs are still using algorithms set up in the precomputer era. Common protocols include the SMOG formula, the Fry Readability Graph, the Flesch Reading Ease score, and the Flesch-Kincaid grade level (Flesch, 1974; Fry, 1977; McLaughlin, 1969). These various protocols will not necessarily give comparable results: a first draft of five paragraphs from this chapter had a Flesch Reading Ease score of 47.7 (grade level required: 13.3, that is, three months into the first year of college; U.S. adults who understand: 54 percent). The same five paragraphs had a Flesch-Kincaid grade level of 10.5 and a Gunning Fog grade level of 13.4. We suggest picking one protocol to use consistently (Trapini & Walmsley, 1981). By using one protocol, the health educator learns over time to write very close to a target grade level and to edit passages to achieve the target.

Many health educators find it simplest to use the protocols included with Microsoft Word: Tools→Options→Spelling and Grammar→Show Readability Statistics. To fine-tune their assessment, writers can use a graded vocabulary list (for example, Mogilner, 1992). Such a list gets past the assumption that a longer word is necessarily a harder word (*grandfather* is a first-grade word in the United States, despite its three syllables). Using words at a third-grade level and below ensures capturing an audience with fifth-grade reading skills. Health educators may find such restrictions difficult, but they can inspire genius; it was such an assignment that launched the career of Theodore Geisel as Dr. Seuss.

Several other approaches have been applied to reading levels (Holcomb & Ellis, 1978; Irwin & Davis, 1980; Mosenthal & Kirsch, 1998). A different approach to assessing document complexity is the PMOST/KIRSCH document readability formula, which looks at both the organizational pattern (simple list, combined list, intersected list, nested list) and density (number of labels and number of items) (Mosenthal & Kirsch, 1998). This formula is an attempt to evaluate the readability of charts, graphs, tables, forms, and other nonlinear presentations of written words. In conjunction with Tufte's works on visual display (1983, 1990, 1997), it may prove a useful adjunct to standard reading-level formulas.

Developing Program Materials

⮑ *The next task in Step 4 is to develop program materials.*

It is beyond the scope of this book to provide specific instruction on every task for the production of the wide variety of possible program materials. We attempt to give some insight into the number and types of tasks for print materials and videotapes or DVDs as models and briefly discuss the added tasks when the product is more complex, such as a multimedia program. We also provide some instruction on writing messages.

Once the planner has created initial design documents and the team has added creative resources to its membership when needed, the original group and the new participants will work together to produce program materials. We present Figures 8.10 and 8.11 to give a sense of the steps involved in the production process for two types of materials (a print piece and a video or DVD) and also of the back-and-forth movement between the health promotion development team and the creative consultants who will produce the materials. These figures give an idea of how important the communication of ideas is in this process. A large part of that communication burden falls on the health educator.

Producing Printed Material

Figure 8.10 gives an example of the process involved in producing print material. Whoever is doing the design and managing the production must have read several design documents and must understand the team's intent for the piece by this phase of the process. Designers may benefit from contact with the intended audience for the piece as well. The design document should have already given a clear description of the audience, its special needs, and the contexts in which the material will be used. Material that is to be published in a three-ring binder, for instance, normally calls for larger type than does a brochure, because readers will set it on a table for reading. An item that a parent will be consulting while bathing a baby had best be waterproof. All the facts must be clear before the design process

FIGURE 8.10. TASKS FOR PRODUCING A PRINT PIECE.

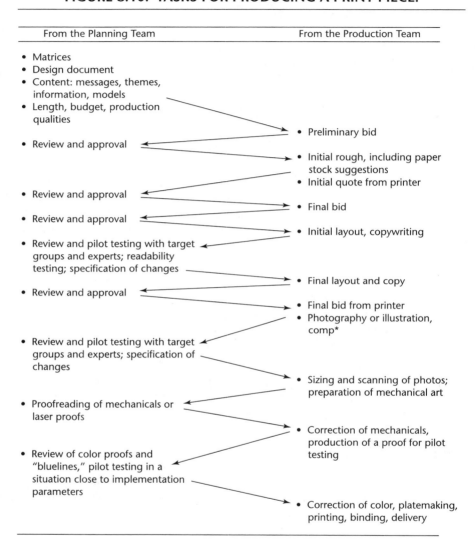

From the Planning Team	From the Production Team
• Matrices	
• Design document	
• Content: messages, themes, information, models	
• Length, budget, production qualities	
	• Preliminary bid
• Review and approval	
	• Initial rough, including paper stock suggestions
	• Initial quote from printer
• Review and approval	
	• Final bid
• Review and approval	
	• Initial layout, copywriting
• Review and pilot testing with target groups and experts; readability testing; specification of changes	
	• Final layout and copy
• Review and approval	
	• Final bid from printer
	• Photography or illustration, comp*
• Review and pilot testing with target groups and experts; specification of changes	
	• Sizing and scanning of photos; preparation of mechanical art
• Proofreading of mechanicals or laser proofs	
	• Correction of mechanicals, production of a proof for pilot testing
• Review of color proofs and "bluelines," pilot testing in a situation close to implementation parameters	
	• Correction of color, platemaking, printing, binding, delivery

*A comprehensive or "comp" represents the finished product in a more accurate form and detail than a rough. It shows as closely as possible how the final product will look. These are for presentation and pretesting only. They can be required but will add to the budget.

FIGURE 8.11. TASKS FOR PRODUCING A VIDEOTAPE.

From the Planning Team	From the Production Team

- Matrices
- Design document
- Content: messages, themes, information, models
- Length, budget, production qualities

- Attendance at team meetings, interviews and/or focus groups, preliminary bid

- Approval
- Initial concept from the producer/writer

- Approval
- Final bid and contract

- Approval
- Script treatment or storyboard

- Review with target group and experts specify changes
- Final script treatment or script

- Review and approval
- Preproduction scheduling of subject or actors, locations and videography for messages and background scenes

- Review and approval
- Videography

- Requirements vary with working relationship
- Offline editing, first rough cut

- Review of first rough cut
- Pilot of rough cut with target groups and experts
- Specifications of revisions
- Correction of first rough cut

- Review (and approval) of second rough cut
- Pilot of rough cut
- On-line editing and delivery

- Approval of final
- Mass duplication

starts. In the production phase, the designer will work with the team to consider the following:

- What design elements or types of copy will the piece have? Examples to consider are levels of subheads, lists, tables, graphs, charts, illustrations, captions, pull quotes, footnotes or references, interviews, and step-by-step instructions. The more elements there are, the more complicated the design process, though the best result is usually something with a simple design.
- When and how will the project need updating?
- What are the costs and constraints?
- What are the graphics standards of the organization producing the piece?
- What process will be used to review the piece?
- What aspects of the production process is the team responsible for?
- Who will produce the camera-ready copy?
- Will the piece be photocopied or printed?

Next, the designer lists the elements of the design that will be needed to carry the important messages. Will the piece have line illustrations, photos, or frequent bulleted lists? This list includes all the elements the design will have to accommodate. Should there be places for people to enter personal information? Does the piece serve as a reference tool in which people have to find a particular section quickly? It is also important to consider how the finished piece will be put together. For example, if a piece is lengthy and requires frequent additions or changes, a three-ring binder is a good choice.

Once a designer offers an acceptable design, the content will have to be edited to conform to it. Asking for changes to a completed design is counterproductive; changing the design will cost more money and decrease the resulting quality. Also, a good adage to remember is: "You can get it good, you can get it fast, and you can get it cheap; but you can't have all three." Health educators aim for two out of three by talking with suppliers about how long it will take to get the quality of product they desire. We also refer the reader to works on basic design principles. Understanding a little about the designer's process can help health educators work with rather than against the designer (Doak, Doak, & Root, 1996; R. C. Parker, 1988; White, 1988; R. Williams, 1994).

Writing and Organizing to Help the Reader. The greatest design in the world can't make up for poor writing or confusing organization. Refer to SAM (Table 8.7) to consider the elements of good writing for health promotion materials. Here are a few pointers for writing copy:

- Match the reading level of the intended audience
- Write in active voice
- Make lists understandable without introductory sentences (For example, in a list of things people should not do, every item should begin with "Do not.")
- Write as clearly as possible (For example, if the meaning is "do not," copywriters should not use the term *avoid*. Readers often interpret the word to mean "try not to do this, but do it when you have to.")
- Present the material in the order the reader will need it
- Include only messages in support of the change objectives; remove superfluous material unless it provides an appropriate context
- Use subheads to break up or chunk the test
- Use a careful hierarchy to support comprehension
- Use advance organizers (see Chapter Three) (Glynn & Britton, 1984)
- Use sentences and designs that encourage interaction, such as checklists with boxes that readers can check
- Use one- and two-syllable words and short, simple sentences with definitions of more difficult words in appositional phrases and parenthetical statements
- Provide visual cues
- Use strong topic sentences for paragraphs

It seems self-evident, but an intervention program should not use print media if the intended participants can't read (Torrence & Torrence, 1987). Sometimes technical material is difficult to write below a fifth-grade level without losing meaning and becoming patronizing. Such technical material is perhaps better presented through another medium. Copywriters should avoid the trap of replacing commonly heard words with less commonly heard (but shorter) words (for example, replacing medicine with meds); doing so may lower the computed reading level but will interfere with comprehension. When possible, health educators can prepare the group for the material by determining what the group members need to know before they read (for example, vocabulary) and teaching it and by discussing the point of the material (that is, what readers are supposed to get from it).

Producing a Video

Videotapes or DVDs can be a good solution to some problems. Many people do not read well enough to learn skills from print materials, for example. The production costs for videotapes are in producing the master; the individual copies are very inexpensive. The more copies you purchase, therefore, the more cost-effective the medium of videotape is. VCRs, DVD players, and televisions are ubiquitous in many countries; and the equipment to make a videotape is also commonplace. Unfortunately, this easy access can lead to the fallacious assumption that making a useful videotape consists of pointing, shooting, and running off copies.

Contracts and Budgets. Figure 8.11 presents processes in the production of a videotape. Early in the process, the producer must develop an understanding of what the development team has planned, and optimally the producer has participated in some contacts with the intended audience. An early step in working with a video producer is agreeing on the contract. The contract and the budget should include a rough-cut review and approval. A rough cut is usually an off-line edit of the production prior to final online editing, which is when all the bells and whistles, such as music, are added to a tape. In our experience, the rough cut is the moment to perform pretesting with the development team, the intended participants, and the gatekeepers or program implementers. The budget must contain money for production at this intermediate stage and for revisions. It helps greatly if the health educator has been at the video shoots so that the material included in the rough cut does not come as a surprise. Other examples of contract considerations are casting approval, credits, and copyright. The program development team (not the video producers) should have the assigned copyright so that the organization can recycle the video images from one medium to another. Any artwork bought for the videotape will also have a contract with it that specifies who owns the material. It is important to have legal title and custody of the master tape. Health educators should obtain from the production company copies of all releases and should make sure that everyone signs a release before filming begins.

Scripts and Script Treatments. A vital component of video and DVD production and a centerpiece of work between a development team and a video producer is the script or script treatment. A script works from the design document that the development team has written to detail the audio and visuals for every scene, whereas a script treatment—a scene-by-scene message, a look-and-feel description, or a storyboard with the same information plus visuals—is used when stories will be obtained directly from members of the community and edited together. A script is very different from material that is meant to be read; it is meant to be seen and heard. In addition, a video has about fifteen seconds to grab the audience's attention, and it has to recapture that attention every few seconds after that. To use the video medium to best advantage, it is important that the picture tells the story and that words complete the messages. A producer should first offer a preliminary script treatment. After receiving approval at this stage, the producer can move to creating the final script treatment or script.

Script approval is a formal process and a key point in the creative cycle. The planning team will want to list the number of people who should approve the video, because it is easy to underestimate the number of stakeholders. These same people also should review the script. Reshooting can break the budget and in some situations may not even be possible, so incorporating changes at the script stage often makes more sense. If the same video is needed in more than one language, the script should be translated as soon as the stakeholders have approved the original. For live-action shots, it can be cost-efficient to shoot all language versions at the same time. For voice-over footage, producers need to allow for the difference in length of the narration and shoot the footage to allow for the longer narration time.

The final script should be compared against the budget, because, the more complex the script is or the more difficult it is to shoot, the greater the shooting and editing costs will be. Health educators should consult an experienced videographer before approving the final script. Script approval is also the time for everyone to approve the credits and the copy for the labels and packaging. Although the credits can seem a simple task, if left to the last minute, they will invariably contain errors; and revising credits can be quite time-consuming for the production house.

Script approval is followed by preproduction. Preproduction includes such tasks as finding locations, actors, and props and scheduling the film crew. Although some preproduction can be done in tandem with script development, some items are contingent on the final script.

Postproduction. The first task of postproduction is the creation of a rough cut that can be checked for appropriate execution of methods and strategies and then pretested. Checking the rough cut is a crucial point in program development. For example, in Project PANDA (Mullen et al., 1999), the videotape for women who had stopped smoking during pregnancy was to be delivered to their homes immediately postpartum, when stress and sleep deprivation are at their height. Even though the program planners had been present during shooting and had seen the raw tapes, the rough cut came as a surprise. The development team was looking for role models for the immediate postpartum period, and the video producer (who had not yet had children) had included only the most "together" women. These mastery models seemed to have handled the transition to nonsmoking parenthood flawlessly, and they might have caused the self-efficacy of the target women to decrease in comparison. Before pretesting the tape, the development team asked for a second rough cut that would include more models who were moving toward success rather than models who were already there. Following approval of the rough cut, the music soundtrack, graphics, and credits are finalized; and a final master tape is produced.

Creating a Multimedia Program

Producing a computer-assisted multimedia program contains many of the same production steps as producing a videotape except that it is more complex and involves a computer programmer as a part of the production team. With computer-assisted instruction, the program is able to deliver tailored messages in real time. Depending on the amount of user control, the program can also deliver an individualized learning experience. Because the vehicle has branching pathways for the learner and may contain many different methods and strategies, the design documents are more complex, as illustrated by the flowcharts (Figures 8.10 and 8.11).

For example, in Project PCCaSO, a learner might interact with the following program components, depending on their current moment-to-moment intentions regarding colorectal cancer screening: role-model video vignettes with professional actors, computer graphics, interactive decisional balance exercise, video interviews with laypeople, and a personalized letter for their doctor regarding their plans for colorectal cancer screening. Following the initial charting of the program flow, the planning team worked with the production team to create storyboards to serve as the main source of communication between the planning team and the computer-programming design team. The storyboard presented each proposed screen in the computer program (Figure 8.12), with a visual layout of the screen and the following elements: module and screen number, screen title, screen objective, screen description, video description (if applicable), graphic description, dialogue

FIGURE 8.12. STORYBOARD: PROJECT PCCaSO.

Module/Screen Number: 3.2 (C, Female)

Title: First role model duo conversation

Objective: Engage patients in conversation between two friends, to generate interest in continuing program

Description: Thirty- to sixty-second video between two friends (AA-F/W-F)

Video Description: Opening shot appears in the frame we saw in the open. Two women in their fifties are talking as they walk in the park for exercise. They're dressed in sports clothes—T-shirts and workout pants. Corrine, an African American woman, is walking a little faster than Anna, a Caucasian woman, as they come toward the camera.

FIGURE 8.12. STORYBOARD: PROJECT PCCaSO, Cont'd.

Dialogue:

Anna and Corrine: Missing Jen

(Anna is in the contemplation stage, and Corrine is in preparation.)

Scene 1: Bring music in and under as we hear dialogue.

Anna (wincing): Corrine, can we stop and stretch some? I've got a cramp in my leg.

Corrine: Sure.

(Women pause by a bench or other area where they can stretch and take a breather. Anna rubs her calf and tries moving her leg up and down. Corrine looks over at Anna as they stretch.)

Anna: I sure wish Jen were here. . . . It's just, you know, I can't believe she has colon cancer.

Corrine (looking down and nodding): I'm still in shock, too. It seems strange to be exercising without her, since we always do this together. She is usually the first one down the trail. . . . I miss her.

Anna: I hadn't thought about colon cancer much before. I mean, you just don't think someone you know will actually have it. It makes me feel so helpless.

Corrine: I know—just hearing the word *cancer* is scary. But I found out that there are things we can do. I think the key is getting that test.

Anna: Have you been tested before?

Corrine: Yeah, I have. A few years ago I had a colon test, and I found out I had polyps, you know, these little abnormal growths on my colon. But I had them removed before they grew into cancer. I didn't know I would ever need to have it repeated though, but Jen says that her doctor told her everyone over fifty is supposed to get tested every so often. It makes me realize that I do need to go in again to get checked out. It's been too long.

Anna: So colon cancer testing is that important?

Corrine: Yeah, I'm starting to think that it is! The earlier you find cancer, the easier the treatment, and the better chance you have of a cure. If Jen had gone in before she had symptoms, her doctor might have been able to find her cancer even earlier. . . . Should we keep walking?

(Anna nods, and they start down the trail.)

Navigation buttons: repeat and back

Data to capture: Time spent on screen, navigation buttons used

Processes: Dramatic relief and consciousness raising

Notes: Role-model "guide duo" will be matched to gender. The "guide duo" will reflect the same stage as the participant as they move through the intervention, moving forward and back as the participant's ideas about CRCS change.

(narration and video vignettes), navigation buttons, data to be captured, and project team notes. There were practical elements specifically for the programmers (that is, data to capture, navigation buttons needed); organizational elements for the project team (that is, module number, screen title); and theoretical elements (that is, screen descriptions, dialogue) that were included so that both teams could have the performance and learning or change objectives from the matrices at their fingertips at all times. The high level of detail in the storyboards was instrumental in communicating with the computer programmers; it allowed them to truly understand the processes that were at work behind the program's components.

Writing Program Messages

Many health promotion program materials contain two types of messages. One is a focused attempt to accomplish a change objective. For example, in Project PCCaSO, the team provided some information in order to influence the change objective regarding risk perception and provided feedback occasionally to remind the participant of his or her stage of change. The other type of message is contextual. These messages might tell the reason for the first type of message, for example: "To help you understand your likelihood of getting colon cancer, we are going to give you some facts and figures." Or contextual messages might flesh out the vehicle for the presentation of the change-oriented messages. In Project PCCaSO the team embedded many change messages in a story about two friends who were worried about a third friend with colon cancer (Vernon, 2004) (see Figure 8.12). A contextual message might also be related to the health and well-being of the intended audience, though not specifically to the targeted health behavior. In Project PANDA, Mullen and colleagues (Chapter Thirteen) realized that women who had quit smoking during their first pregnancy probably would be more interested in contextual pregnancy messages than in messages about not returning to smoking. For both the women and their partners, the program change messages were a part of a wider pregnancy and entry into parenthood context.

Writing messages to create change requires working from the change objectives in the matrices and from the design documents. For example, one of the design documents in the T.L.L. Temple Foundation Stroke Project (L. B. Morgenstern et al., 2002) showed a newsletter for emergency department staff. Each newsletter had three types of stories:

- A role-model story of physician experience with providing medication for stroke
- Local news about the stroke program
- Scientific updates about stroke treatment

The program team created specific messages for each type of story.

Messages, a part of all health promotion materials, are focused attempts to accomplish a change objective. The following processes can get a health educator started on message development:

- Think about the methods and strategies that the team has decided on for a particular set of objectives and that will fit together in a particular vehicle, such as a newspaper story
- Decide what vehicle would be appropriate to deliver the methods and strategies
- Note the change objectives organized by determinants
- Draft messages matched to each change objective
- Draft contextual messages that will be incorporated into the vehicle

In illustration of both change messages and contextual messages, Figure 8.12 presents a storyboard for one scene in the multimedia program in Project PCCaSO. The following types of messages can be found in this document:

- Contextual: the visual of the two women on the track and the words, "Corrine, can we stop and stretch some? I've got a cramp in my leg." Other messages pertain specifically to change objectives from the project matrix.
- Dramatic relief: Anna says: "I sure wish Jen were here . . . It's just, you know, I can't believe she has colon cancer." Corrine looks down and nods. "I'm still in shock too. It seems strange to be exercising without her since we always do this together. She is usually the first one down the trail . . . I miss her."
- Positive outcome expectations for screening: Anna says: "So, have you been tested before?" Corrine replies: Yeah, I have. A few years ago I had a colon test, and I found out I had polyps, you know, these little abnormal growths on my colon. But I had them removed before they grew into cancer."

A Cultural Perspective on Writing Messages. Many cultural characteristics directly influence both how people communicate and how they understand and respond to the messages they receive. Message writers will want to know a lot about the preferred communication styles of the intended program recipients and will also want to pretest the messages with them. Many aspects of cultural preferences can affect message writing. For example, communication is very different between collectivist (high-context) cultures and individualist (low-context) cultures (see Table 8.8). In collectivist cultures communicators are more likely to focus on the perceiver of information than on themselves, and they may communicate to please the receiver. In a more individualist culture, one presents the best arguments first in order to gain attention. As Table 8.8 shows, other aspects of communication may differ, including the structure of the argument, the use of words, and the

TABLE 8.8. COMMUNICATION PREFERENCES IN
COLLECTIVIST AND INDIVIDUALISTIC CULTURES.

Individualistic	Collectivist
• Important characteristics are expert knowledge, credibility, and intelligence.	• Important characteristics are family, age, gender, and status in the group.
• Anticlimactic argument style presents best arguments first to get attention.	• Climactic argument style builds up from peripheral arguments in order not to offend the perceiver.
• Emphasis is on content, specificity, and precision in word usage.	• Prefers intuition, ambiguity, generality, vagueness, and bland expressions
• Silence is negative indicating hostility, rejection, disagreement, weakness, unwillingness, shyness, anxiety, and lack of skill.	• Emphasis is on the unspoken; too many words spoils their value. Silence is okay.
• Inductive argument: fact, fact, fact: conclusion	• Need face-to-face contact because of the importance of paralinguistic communication
• The opinion of the in-group hierarchy is less important.	• Deductive argument: conclusion: supportive evidence
	• The opinion of the in-group hierarchy is very important.

standards used to judge credibility. For instance, in high-context cultures the individual presents the argument climactically, starting with peripheral arguments and ending with the main argument in order not to offend and in order to gauge the listener's response. Most often health educators will create messages that match a cultural group's communication expectations. Interestingly, Triandis (1994) points out that message construction can help people respond more or less in a collectivist or individualistic fashion.

Health promoters must be particularly careful to clearly understand a cultural communication method before using it. Airhihenbuwa (1994) gives the example of the pitfalls of superficial use of oral culture (ear to mouth) versus visual culture (eye to object) storytelling methods. He points out that stories are a reciprocal vehicle that depend on the listeners' interaction with the teller to create the learning. Any adaptation that makes this vehicle a one-way street loses the method's power. On the other hand, he points out that imposing a delivery vehicle from outside the culture has different pitfalls. For example, if posters are used to convey information in an oral culture, learners will face problems with attention, comprehension, and memory because the learner will first have to learn to attend to this novel source of information.

Translation. Translation of health education and promotion materials into another language is usually aimed at symmetry: a translation that is loyal to the meaning of the source language while ensuring equal familiarity and colloquiality in both languages. Another term for this symmetry is decentering (from the source language). Decentering implies a deemphasis of the developer's language in such a way that the system of symbols supersedes a single culture. At best, decentering eliminates the distinction between source and target language. Decentering requires a multistage translation that allows for paraphrasing the meaning of the source materials and of the translation before deciding on a translated version. The translation is then translated back to the original language, and the versions are compared. The process of translation and back translation are continued until the two versions are acceptable. The goal is a dynamic equivalence in which a cultural symbol in the source language is translated into a cultural symbol in the target language that evokes the same functional response from the reader or listener. For example, Werner and Campbell (1973) relate the problem of finding a Navajo word for measles; presenting a list of symptoms might have evoked a more meaningful response than trying to find one word that did not originally exist in a language. They relate an even more significant problem of meaning when they explain that the literal translation of the word *meningitis* into Navajo would be "the covering of the brain is getting red." Translation is at best approximate, and program development is better done using methods and strategies that are built from within the intended participants' language and culture. When that is not possible, the health educator should use a decentering approach to translation, introduce redundancy into the text, and use a rich context (Werner & Campbell, 1973).

The translation period is another good time to work with focus groups to understand the words used to describe certain phenomena. In creating the Spanish version of the Watch, Discover, Think, and Act program, Bartholomew, Shegog, and colleagues (2000) used focus groups to discover the ways people described asthma and related concepts such as wheezing and inhaler. Many of these words related to asthma had no equivalents in Spanish.

Creating and Choosing Program Visuals

Kreuter and colleagues (2002) suggest that visuals, unlike text, can be perceived and understood almost immediately. Visuals should help the materials developer to gain attention, interest and credibility for the message (Moriarty, 1995; Schiffman, 1995). Furthermore, the visuals can and should capture elements that are familiar and pleasing to the cultural groups that will use the materials. For example, in the Familias program development (Chapter Fourteen), Fernández and colleagues (2000) (Bartholomew, Sockrider, et al., 2000; Fernandez, Bartholomew,

Lopez, et al., 2000) picked fabric and objects with Mexican and Central American designs and worked with the community advisory committee members to choose which of the objects to photograph to provide the visual backgrounds in the multimedia program.

In addition to visuals being pleasing to the audience and stimulating interest, Doak and colleagues (1996) argue strongly that visuals should assist the reader with deciphering and remembering a message. According to these authors, the visuals should have the following characteristics:

- Be realistic rather than symbolic
- Be simple with little distracting background
- Be used to reduce text by showing, for example, steps in a procedure
- Show all important elements of a gestalt, for example, the entire body rather than just the chest so that the reader does not have to struggle with orientation
- Be used to stimulate interaction

Pretesting, Revising, and Producing Program Components

The final task in Step 4 is to pretest and pilot-test program components; oversee production of materials.

Pretesting is the process of trying out the specific messages of the program products with the intended participants before final production. Pilot testing is trying out the program as it will be implemented with both the implementers and intended participants prior to the actual implementation. Both pretesting and pilot testing are crucial to determine whether planning to this point has resulted in appealing, understandable messages and whether the program can be implemented. Program materials must be culturally relevant and the implementers culturally competent as well. In other words, not only must the program and its delivery be understandable in a particular culture and not offensive, it must also make use of particular cultural concepts related to the health, behavior, and community changes inherent in the program and leave the community with greater capacity than before the program.

Sometimes program planners do not conduct pretesting and pilot testing because the planners are experiencing a time crunch at this point in production. No matter how big the hurry, planners must make time for pilot testing. One of us has had the experience of consulting with an AIDS-prevention agency that had an advertising firm develop a series of messages. The agency refused to pretest and produced and implemented messages that had the reverse of the intended effect: the messages made people feel that they were safe from AIDS under certain circumstances that were actually irrelevant to risk. The ad campaign might actually have increased risky behavior among the intended audience.

Sometimes the planning team may object to pilot testing by pointing out that the planning group already contains representatives of the potential program participants. Representatives, however, have probably come to value the program they have developed in a way that colors their objectivity. This step requires going back out into the communities you are serving, talking to community members, and getting their responses to ideas and to all the various aspects of support materials: graphics, illustration, photography, messages, and delivery.

Methods for Pretesting

Table 8.9 presents various pretesting and pilot-testing methods. This is a brief overview, and we refer readers to other sources of information on pretesting (NCI, 2002). The first pretesting that health educators conduct is to test initial program concepts, including key phrases and visuals proposed to portray the main ideas. Focus groups and interviews are good for this purpose. A very important reason for this process is to discover the words, phrases, and vernacular that members of the at-risk group use when discussing the topic.

In addition to the methods of focus groups and in-depth interviews, the techniques of central location–intercept interviewing and theater testing are good for pretesting. In central location intercept, interviewers armed with questionnaires ask for responses from people in high-traffic areas such as malls and grocery stores. In theater testing for television spots, groups of watchers are asked to respond to programs or other television components amid simulated television clutter. For example, spots are aired between two thirty-minute television shows. After the first show, spots appear between irrelevant material; and after the next thirty-minute show, viewers are tested for recall. Viewers are then shown the messages again and asked about specific characteristics. Day-after recall can also be used to assess what participants remember from various program materials a day later.

Program developers must also conduct gatekeeper reviews and use testing so that the people who will implement and maintain the program review the components; the materials must also be tested in real life or a simulation of real life. This review is to ascertain how participants perceive the materials in terms of characteristics that have been shown to influence adoption and implementation. Such testing can also uncover potential problems with implementation plans. (See Chapter Nine for more on adoption and implementation.) For this pretesting it is important to find potential implementers and gatekeepers who have not been a part of program development.

For final pretesting the various program components are executed in preliminary formats and are tested to determine attention, comprehension, strong and weak

TABLE 8.9. PRETESTING AND PILOT-TESTING METHODS.

	Concept Testing	Readability Testing	Executing the Message	Impact on Determinants	Adoption/Implementation Characteristics
Purpose	To test the key phrases and visuals that portray the main ideas; to discover vernacular	To estimate school-grade reading level required to read text	To determine whether program material messages are attended to, comprehended, appealing, and culturally relevant	To get a sense of possible impact or to actually measure impact	To see how the materials are perceived in terms of complexity, trialability, observability, and relative advantage To determine problems with implementation
Participants	Program participants	Program participants	Program participants and implementers	Program participants and implementers	Program adopters and implementers
Materials and Strategies	Interviews and focus groups	Text and readability formula or computer program	Interviews, focus groups, questionnaires after exposure, theater testing	Interviews, focus groups after exposure Measurement via instruments designed from the determinants columns of the matrices	Interviews, focus groups after review by potential adopters and implementers Observation of trial implementation
Instructions	Use concept ideas as stimulus materials; ask people how they would convey an idea	Apply the program or formula to each component	Ask people to explain what they "got" from the product; separate components Assess identification with questions such as, "How much did these people seem similar to you? What thoughts and feelings did they express that you might have?"	See Chapter Ten	Ask for review by naïve potential implementers, not those who have worked on development Make the pilot as realistic as possible.
Can't Be Used For	Nothing at this stage attributable to the executed materials	Determining whether intended readers will understand text	Estimating total impact	This is only a formative evaluation. Without a comparison group, change is not attributable to the program.	

points, and personal relevance. At this point program planners can gauge potential objection to sensitive or controversial issues. A major question at this stage is how to get materials in final-enough form to be good stimulus material without spending too much extra money. For example, videotapes can be presented in storyboard format, as can PSAs. Radio PSAs can be read aloud, and newsletters can be produced with a word-processing program. However, as much of the final product as possible should be included: illustrations, photographs, and graphics for newsletters rather than just the words, for example. It is also important to evaluate individual aspects of materials rather than just the whole. For example, two panels of consultants, one of women and one of partners, reviewed the Project PANDA newsletters. Response boxes were included for each newsletter article (see Figure 8.15).

Checking for Parameters of Theoretical Methods

As we discussed in Chapters Three, Four, and Seven, theoretical methods can produce changes only if they are used as intended. The pretesting period is a good time to review and check how well methods were operationalized. In Intervention Mapping Step 3, program planners made decisions about theoretical methods and practical strategies. For instance, in the development of the HIV-prevention program (Chapter Eleven), the developers selected modeling, active learning, and feedback as methods for improving self-efficacy. For the strategies the developers chose to create an interactive video presentation: peer models present scenarios on video; the students stop the video and have a group discussion about solutions; the peer models on video present a solution; and the teacher gives the students feedback on their solutions. Although this video presentation is only a part of the program, it requires that the methods be well operationalized.

For instance, an assumption for the use of peer models is that students will find these models attractive (Bandura, 1986). Pretesting of the program should provide assurance that this assumption was correct. The developers of the HIV program tested their video segments with members of the potential audience and found all but one role model to be attractive and believable to the youth. Another assumption for the educational program was that students will pay attention because they think that the program is personally relevant (McGuire, 1986). Again, pretesting should address this assumption, and the developers assessed this variable again in the process evaluation (Chapter Ten).

Making Sense of Pretest Data

At every step of pretesting, there is the likelihood of obtaining conflicting data. Table 8.10 presents one method for organizing data from the participant review. This method does not include the opinions of gatekeepers and implementers. The

TABLE 8.10. MAKING SENSE OF PRETEST DATA.

Material Title: Managing HIV in Your Child

Pretest Methods: Waiting Room Use (N = 6) and Parent Focus Groups (N = 10)

Category → Component ↓	Role Modeling	Skill Training	Technical Content	Other
Module 1: Observing Signs and Symptoms	Comments: The stories are just a waste of space.(1) The stories are great. I felt exactly like that.(1) In response to specific question about stories: Leave them in. They're okay. Not bad, not good.(8) Implications: Leave in. There will be damage to methods if role modeling deleted.	Comments: Steps are not broken down enough.(2) Implications: Observe teaching; break steps down further	Comments: This is not what I was taught by the nurse.(3) Implications: Check with nurses; observe teaching again	Comments: I always thought this was the doctor's job. No one ever told me I had a role.(3) Doctors do not ask me what I have observed.(6) Implications: Work with physicians to help them ask about and use parent observations
Module 2: Treating Infections	Comments: Same as above Implications:	Comments: Steps are not broken down enough.(6) Cards with medications are too easy to lose. Implications: Combining drug information will give some families names of drugs they are not using.	Comments: Implications:	Comments: Implications:
Module 3: Maintaining Good Nutrition	Comments: Same as above Implications:	Comments: Impractical(1) Can't do this(3) My child won't eat these things.(4) Implications: Work with parents to devise more practical nutrition advice	Comments: Implications:	Comments: Implications:

point is to use some mechanism to make clear what program participants are saying about the program and how strongly they hold their opinions. The note labeled implications reminds the planner to consider what would be left out of the intervention in terms of methods, strategies, and messages if the material was changed on the basis of reviewers' comments. For example, according to Table 8.10, some reviewers did not particularly like the role-model stories. The developer then has to decide whether to leave the stories as they are, change them, or delete them. If the developer deletes the stories, then he or she deletes the method of role modeling (and the strategy of role-model stories) and should replace them by an equally powerful method or reexecute them in a different strategy with different messages. Making appropriate use of pretest data requires working back through messages, strategies, and methods to matrices to ensure that changes in the program materials do not leave gaps in the intervention chain of causation.

Implications for Evaluation

This chapter has two categories of evaluation implications. The first is formative evaluation. We have given an overview of pretesting and pilot testing, evaluation that is done while program materials are being developed and that seek to incorporate the opinions of both intended recipients and intended adopters and implementers into the final materials. The second category is part of summative evaluation, and it includes a later assessment of how the audience received the materials during implementation and whether the methods and strategies were well enough operationalized to have an impact on the change objectives (Chapter Ten).

Box 8.3. Stroke Project

The first task in Step 4 is to consult with the intended program participants to determine preference for program design.

As we mentioned in Step 1, the planning team included university faculty along with community members. The community members included persons who had had a stroke, significant others of those who had suffered stroke, media representatives, health care providers, and members of various organizations. Working with these community members, we decided that the program should have two major components, one for the health care providers (emergency departments (EDs), emergency medical services (EMS), and primary care providers (PCPs)) and one for lay members of the community. The group was involved in all of the decisions related to these two components.

⊃ *The second task in Step 4 is to create the program scope and sequence, delivery channels, themes, and a list of needed program materials.*

The program's two major components, community and professional, each had multiple channels and vehicles to deliver the major messages (Table 8.11). Each intervention module had more detailed sequences of its own. As Table 8.11 indicates, the professional module activities began ahead of the lay activities to assure that community services were in place as the demand for emergency care for stroke increased. The scope and sequence of the stroke project needed to accommodate the methods and strategies chosen in Step 3. For the community these methods and strategies were role models for treating stroke as an emergency, delivered by radio and television PSAs in English and Spanish and by billboards and posters; and skill training in recognizing stroke symptoms by one-to-one training, role modeling, and information transfer through brochures and newspapers.

Changes in the behavior of health care providers were created and reinforced in three ways:

- Organizational change consultation to assess awareness, increase perceptions of need, and diagnose needed support for change in EDs and EMS. (Most hospitals and emergency medical services needed support for getting revised stroke care guidelines in place, including individualized guideline development and staff training.)
- Skill training individualized to the provider and the setting
- Reinforcement for using new treatment protocols through newsletters and newspaper stories of successes

Of course, all these activities could not happen at once, and many of them depended for their success on prior requisite activities, thus the need for a well-defined program sequence.

The program had two themes:

- Every minute counts—call 911
- Is there life after stroke? (with positive outcome expectation messages)

⊃ *The next task in Step 4 is to prepare design documents for the production of materials that meet the program objectives and parameters for the methods and strategies.*

⊃ *The fourth task in this step is to review available program materials for possible match with change objectives, methods, and strategies.*

⊃ *The fifth task in this step is to develop program materials.*

Table 8.12 shows the materials for the stroke project's community component and highlights from the design documents. The team decided that materials available from

TABLE 8.11. SCOPE AND SEQUENCE OF THE T.L.L. TEMPLE FOUNDATION STROKE PROJECT.

Weeks 1–2	Weeks 2–8	Weeks 8–16	Weeks 16–32	Weeks 32+
Professional Module 1: Meetings to plan change with hospital emergency departments (EDs)	Professional Module 2: Orientation meetings with hospital medical staff	Professional Module 3: Training meetings with ED and EMS teams	Professional Module 4: Review training meetings for ED and EMS teams	Professional Module 5: Reinforcement for protocol use via newsletters
Professional Module 1: Meetings to plan change with local emergency medical services (EMS)	Professional Module 2: Guideline and protocol development meetings with medical staff and critical care committees	Community Module 1: One-to-one train the trainer and brochure	Community Module 1: One-to-one train the trainer and brochure	Community Module 1: One-to-one train the trainer and brochure
	Guideline and protocol development with EMS directors and medical directors	Community Module 2: Placement of billboards and public service announcements (PSAs)		Community Module 2A: Change out billboards and PSAs to use real stories
		Community Module 3A: Newspaper stories and news releases introducing the program and objectives; coverage of the mock stroke code	Community Module 3B: Newspaper stories regarding stroke symptoms, new treatment, and steps to take	Community Module 3C: Newspaper stories about stroke treatment successes

TABLE 8.12. MATERIALS AND DESIGN DOCUMENT HIGHLIGHTS.

Material	Design Document Highlights
Community Module	
Billboard	Recognizable community role models participating fully in life after stroke
	Is there life after stroke?
	Every minute counts: call 911
Public Service Announcements (PSAs) time one–bystander response—TV	Use actors to depict response to stroke
	Show rapid treatment
	Show recovery
	Reinforce bystander for acting
PSAs time one–physician response—TV	Show physician saying that his patients should call 911
	Stroke is an emergency.
	Review symptoms
PSAs time one–radio	Same as above for TV
Brochure	Review symptoms
	Call 911
	Treatment results in better outcomes
One-to-one training	Review symptoms
	Call 911
	Treatment results in better outcomes
PSAs time two–TV	Same as above with actual local cases
Newspaper story–intro type	What is the T.L.L. Temple Stroke Project?
	What the community can expect
	Stroke is an emergency.
	Call 911
Newsletter story–stroke code	Coverage of local hospitals and EMS practicing stroke response

TABLE 8.12. MATERIALS AND DESIGN DOCUMENT HIGHLIGHTS, Cont'd.

Material	Design Document Highlights
Newsletter story–symptom recognition and response	Review stroke symptoms
	Call 911
	New medication
	Better outcomes
Newsletter story–success story	Local individual experienced stroke
	Bystander or significant other called 911
	Good outcome
	Reiteration of symptoms

various voluntary health organizations and government agencies did not present messages well-matched to the change objectives. Table 8.13 shows a full design document for four items from the stroke project. For each product the planners thought about what methods and strategies they had decided to use to influence the change objectives. They decided on vehicles to convey those methods and strategies, and partial planning for four of the vehicles is shown in the table. Finally, the planners composed first drafts of the messages to be contained in the newspaper stories, newsletter, and billboard they were planning.

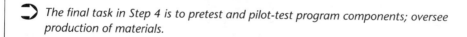 *The final task in Step 4 is to pretest and pilot-test program components; oversee production of materials.*

All stroke materials were drafted by the project health educator, reviewed by the neurologist for stroke content, and then reviewed by the project advisory committee. Because much of the project material was newspaper stories or television and radio PSAs, the media gatekeepers on the advisory committee were particularly helpful as reviewers and potential implementers of the public education part of the program.

TABLE 8.13. MESSAGE DEVELOPMENT GUIDE FOR THE STROKE PROJECT.

Proposed Vehicle	Change Objectives Grouped by Determinant	Methods and Strategies	Message Content
Emergency Departments (EDs) and Community Physicians			
Newspaper Article	Social norms: Recognize that other physicians in the community respond rapidly to symptoms of stroke	Modeling through role-model stories	"I had a stroke patient who got to the hospital on time; the hospital emergency department treated my patient."
	Believe that other EDs are lowering their workup times for stroke		
	Outcome expectations: Expect that stroke patients (especially those presenting with moderate disability) can recover function with acute treatment of stroke	Testimonials	"I wasn't sure about this new treatment before, but I am really pleased with the improvement I saw in my patient."
	Reinforcement: Prepare and share patient success stories because there can be a lack of feedback to emergency department staff	Vicarious reinforcement	From the patient or family's point of view: "I am back (or my family member is back) to full functioning. The doctor saved our quality of life by acting quickly."
Newsletter	Knowledge: Describe the results of the rtPA clinical trial	Information transfer–science article	Stroke clinical trial article and references
	Social norms: Recognize that other EDs are lowering workup times and treating patients	Modeling through physician testimonials	Article from physician's view point of actual treated case
	Reinforcement: Recognize that patient did well after treatment	Reinforcement	Article about patient treated in ED
	Outcome expectation: Recognize that when workup times are lowered patients can get function-saving treatment	Modeling through actual hospital role-model stories	Article about patient treated in ED

Community Members

Billboard	Knowledge: Describe importance of calling 911 for stroke symptoms	Modeling through familiarity of community member	Call 911
			Every minute counts
	Outcome expectations: Expect that getting to the ED fast will allow treatment to minimize effects of stroke	Modeling through familiarity of community member	"Is there treatment for stroke?" (Ask Annon Card, stroke victim who is playing golf.)
Newspaper Story	Knowledge: List symptoms; describe to call 911	Information transfer	Symptom list
	Skills: Recognize symptoms	Information transfer, modeling	Symptom list and someone responding to symptoms
	Outcome expectations: Describe that treatment can prevent disability	Modeling through role model story with vicarious reinforcement	Some bystander or significant other does the right thing; the patient is treated; the outcome is good.

FIGURE 8.13. STROKE PROJECT BILLBOARD.

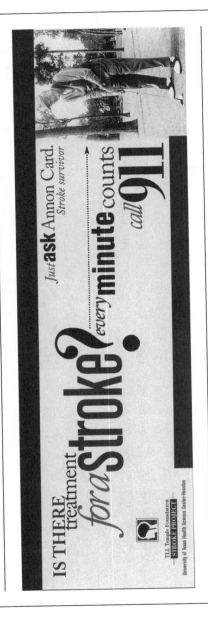

FIGURE 8.14. NEWSLETTER.

September – October 1999
2nd Issue

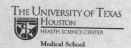

THE UNIVERSITY OF TEXAS
HOUSTON
HEALTH SCIENCE CENTER
Medical School

*code*stroke

a publication of the University of Texas Health Science Center at Houston and the Temple Foundation Stroke Project

MARY KING
Health Educator
409/637-3771

LEWIS MORGENSTERN, MD
Newsletter Editor
Assistant Professor of Neurology
University of Texas Health Science Center–
Houston
713/500-7099

TREAT STROKE → PREVENT DISABILITY AND SAVE A LIFE!

Local Doctor's view on rt-PA

An interview with Gavin McGown, MD, Director of Emergency Medicine, Nacogdoches Medical Center

Dr. Gavin McGown, MD, Emergency Medical Director of Nacogdoches Medical Center for the past 17 years, is pleased with the changes he has seen in stroke care. Dr. McGown had the opportunity to recently treat one of Dr. Randall Vinther's patients, Mrs. Lois Moss. Mrs. Moss, a very active 73-year old, was rushed to the Nacogdoches Medical Center after suffering from aphasia and experiencing left-sided paresis. "As soon as Mrs. Moss came through the door we began the protocol. We felt very comfortable with it", stated McGown. "Mrs. Moss met the criteria and we administered rt-PA. She showed almost immediate improvement."

"Saving time with stroke is the most important thing," stated Dr. McGown. "We know we only have 3 hours. If the EMS can call ahead, we can clear the CT scanner, and help streamline things once the patient arrives." Dr. McGown says that if he or a family member suffered a stroke, he would want rt-PA.

Local Medical Staff "Make the Grade"

Are the tri-counties prepared for treating an acute stroke with rt-PA therapy? The answer is an overwhelming "yes!"

On July 20-21, 1999, mock stroke codes were held in Lufkin, Nacogdoches, and Center. Volunteers were coached on stroke symptoms and then suffered a "stroke" at a predetermined time and location. Emergency Medical Services were alerted.

Dr. Robert Felberg, who was in attendance from the Temple Foundation Stroke Project was impressed by the professionalism and efficiency of the hospital staff and ambulance crews. The ambulance crews remembered the 3 tenets of EMS stroke care:

1. Load and Go
2. Determine last time seen normal
3. Call ahead to the Emergency Department

The crews did not treat hypertension en route and a witness was asked to ride along.

The emergency departments also showed the professionalism and competence that has made the tri-county region the envy of many Texas counties. All patients were appropriately screened and CT scans performed quickly. Blood samples were drawn by the EMS crews and handed off to the triage nurses who personally ensured delivery to the lab. The hand-off of labs cut about 20 minutes off work-up time. Overall, participation and knowledge were outstanding. CONGRATULATIONS from The T.L.L. Temple Project for a job well done.

FIGURE 8.15. NEWSPAPER ARTICLE (*THE DAILY SENTINEL*).

The Daily Sentinel
Sunday, June 18, 1999

Son's Quick Action, New Therapy
Help Woman Recover From Stroke

Her son Jeremy discovered Ms. Moss could not get up, was totally paralyzed on her left side, had facial droop and garbled speech. He immediately called 911.

By ROBBIE GOODRICH
Sentinel Staff

It began as a normal day.

Lois Moss, 73, had been to Henderson to get her hair done and had returned to her home off FM 343 at around 2:30 p.m. that day.

Her son, Jeremy, had given her a plant that she wanted to plant outside. She grabbed a set of post hole diggers and headed for the yard.

"I had my post hole diggers in my hand, and suddenly, I fell to the ground," Ms. Moss said. "That's all I remember."

She estimates that she was on the ground for as long as 30 minutes before someone saw her. That "someone" happened to be Jeremy.

"I had tried to get up, but I couldn't," Ms. Moss said, adding that it didn't occur to her at the time she had suffered a stroke. "I didn't have any symptoms of a stroke. I just fell, and I don't remember much after that."

Jeremy hadn't planned on stopping by his mother's house that day. But he found himself in that part of the county and decided to check on her. He guessed she would have gotten home from taking care of errands in Henderson.

As he pulled into the driveway, he saw her and thought at first she was just kneeling down.

But when he spoke to her, and she didn't respond, he knew something was wrong.

He discovered Ms. Moss could not get up, was totally paralyzed on her left side, had facial droop and garbled speech. He immediately called 911.

Paramedics from the local volunteer fire department arrived within 15 minutes, and an ambulance arrived within another 15 minutes. Ms. Moss was taken to Nacogdoches Medical Center.

At the hospital, doctors asked Jeremy about the time of onset, and he was told his mother likely suffered a stroke. It was then that Jeremy was told of a clot-busting agent—tissue plasminogen activator, or TPA—that had proven effective in stroke victims if it is administered within a three-hour time window.

"It's very new," Dr. Randal Vinther, internal medicine physician, said. "There's been a lot of research in the past two or three years, but it's been only within the past six months that it's becoming common to use as state-of-the-art therapy for stroke treatment. And you have to get to the patient within three hours of developing symptoms, so it's very important to be evaluated immediately."

Almost immediately after receiving TPA, Ms. Moss' symptoms began to disappear. Prior to receiving TPA, she had been completely unresponsive, had significant neurological deficits and a facial droop. By the time Vinther got to the hospital and saw her, she was beginning to move her left side. By the next day, the facial droop was gone, and she was moving her left side.

Vinther said he was convinced that had Ms. Moss not received TPA, she would be totally paralyzed on one side.

"But now, she's able to resume a fairly normal quality of life," he said.

Ms. Moss said that she's been extremely weak since suffering her stroke, but she's been getting better. She also said being administered TPA so quickly in the hospital "made all the difference" in her quality of life.

But Vinther said the public needs to understand that TPA may not be the answer in every circumstance.

"There is a potential for complication," he said.

One such complication is bleeding, Vinther said. TPA restores blood flow into me brain, as a result, a person can bleed into the stroke, such as in the case of Ms. Moss. However, that problem was countered with blood pressure control, he said.

There is risk in using TPA on anyone who has undergone recent surgery or had recent CPR chest compression. It's also risky in using on anyone with high blood pressure that can't be brought under control quickly.

But given the right circumstances, the potential for benefit outweighs the risk, Vinther said.

"It's been my experience, given the right circumstances without these complications, the drug whould be very seriously considered and administered in the majority of cases," he said.

Mary King, health educator with T.L.L. Temple Foundation Stroke Project, contributed to this story.

CHAPTER NINE

INTERVENTION MAPPING STEP 5: PLANNING PROGRAM ADOPTION, IMPLEMENTATION, AND SUSTAINABILITY

Reader Objectives

- Identify potential uses of the health promotion program and reevaluate the planning group and linkage system to assure representation of potential program users
- Specify performance objectives for program adoption, implementation, and sustainability
- Specify determinants of adoption, implementation, and sustainability
- Create program use matrices
- Select methods and strategies to address the determinants
- Design interventions and organize programs to affect change objectives related to program use

Effective health education and promotion programs will have little impact if they are never used or if they are discontinued while still needed to create the desired health impact (Oldenburg, Hardcastle, & Kok, 1997; Parcel, Perry, & Taylor, 1990). Without a planned intervention, the health promotion program may stay on the developers' shelf if the program is not adopted or on the organization's shelf if the program is adopted but not implemented. If the program is not sustained, it returns to the shelf after initial implementation. Systematic planning for each stage of program use is essential if the program is to optimally affect the population for whom the developers designed it (Caburnay, Kreuter, & Donlin, 2001; Heath & Coleman, 2003). For new programs, demonstration projects, and research projects, the focus of Step 5 is on planning for program use for initial testing of the program's efficacy or effectiveness. If the program proves effective, then its greater impact on public health will depend on a greater exposure of populations to the program, and developers can use Step 5 to plan a larger program diffusion.

In Step 5 of Intervention Mapping, the focus is on planning an intervention component to ensure that the program developed in the previous steps will be used and maintained over time as long as it is needed. The purpose of this chapter is to enable health educators to consider how programs will be initially adopted and implemented and how they will be continued. The chapter also guides the application of the Intervention Mapping process in the development of program components that affect the program's successful use.

Perspectives

In this section, we discuss the importance of planning for program use and the effectiveness of planned dissemination programs.

Planning for Program Use Is Essential

The impact of a health education program will be determined not only by the effectiveness of the interventions but also by the quality of program implementation and the proportion of intended participants exposed to the program (Parcel, 1995). In this chapter we take the perspective that preparing for program use is an essential component of an effective health education or health promotion program. Program failure can often be traced to problems with program adoption and use (L. W. Green & Kreuter, 1999). Therefore, program planning must include this step.

The type of objectives needed for program use will depend on how involved the people who will use the program have been in its development. Also, some health education programs may be self-selected and self-directed by the audience; however, most programs require someone to deliver the program. Often the person or persons who deliver the program will be different from the program developers; therefore, the developers cannot assume that the implementers will know the what and how of program implementation. Under these circumstances, especially, planning is needed for interventions to increase the likelihood that the program will be used and continued over time.

Most programs have people who deliver the program and who are actively involved in the program activities. Some examples of program users are teachers who present health education programs to students and nurses who present programs to patients. In contrast, some programs are delivered without a person implementing intervention activities. However, these mediated programs still need to get to the intended participants through a delivery system. Gatekeepers for delivery systems, even though they are not program users like the teacher and nurse, may still be program adopters because they are necessary to get the program to the end users. For example, the principal in a school may not be the user of a health education curriculum, but his or her support for the program may be critical for adoption. A program manager at a radio station may not be directly involved in conducting a mass media campaign, but his or her support in getting the program on the air is essential.

Planned Interventions Can Make a Difference

We have experience with programs whose implementation was characterized by the echoing lament, "We should have thought about that." Bartholomew and colleagues' computer-assisted instructional program for self-management of asthma was one of these. In the first implementation, we relied on research assistants for implementation and underestimated the roles of clinic nurses and physicians. Without having specified in advance what these individuals would need to do to implement the program and without having delineated determinants (and methods and strategies to change them), we received little cooperation from the health care providers (Bartholomew, Gold, et al., 2000).

On the other hand, we have experience with very well-conceptualized diffusion interventions that have supported program adoption and implementation. For example, Heart Partners was a program to enable schools to adopt and implement programs for prevention of heart disease. The American Heart Association developed a network of school heart partners (usually on-site school staff) who acted as program champions to acquire and enable heart-health program adoption and implementation (Roberts-Gray, Solomon, Gottlieb, & Kelsey, 1998). The average number of American Heart Association curriculum kits used in Heart Partner schools was 3.6, as opposed to 1.9 in schools without the program. The number of Texas schools with the Heart Partners program increased from 637 the first year of the program to 2,734 the fourth year of the program, and its success in Texas led to the institutionalization of the program nationally (Roberts-Gray et al., 1998).

Dissemination activities to promote full use of programs as depicted in the Heart Partners program can be planned with Intervention Mapping steps and core processes. However, even if the program is to be implemented in a single community, school, or work site, the tasks in Step 5 will help to ensure that the program is adopted, implemented, and sustained over time.

Program Users and Linkage System

Intervention Mapping can be used to promote the use of programs first on a small scale for demonstration and evaluation and subsequently on a wider scale after effectiveness has been demonstrated for diffusion into broader use. Planning for program use involves two aspects. The first is to design the health education program in ways that enhance its potential for being adopted, implemented, and sustained. The second is to design interventions to influence adoption, implementation, and continuation.

⊃ *The first task in Step 5 is to identify potential uses of the health promotion program and reevaluate the planning group and linkage system to assure representation of potential program users.*

Who Will Adopt and Use the Program?

Figuring out who will decide to use a program and who will implement its components begins in the earlier steps of Intervention Mapping and continues here. Planners will work with the potential program users and seek to incorporate their concerns during all steps of the planning process. It is especially critical in Step 3, program design, to know as much as possible about the program users to ensure a good fit. As we discussed in Chapter Eight, planners need to involve potential program users as part of the planning process, know the context in which the program will be implemented, know how the potential program users typically practice, and conduct pilot tests of program components with potential users (Renaud & Paradis, 2001).

At this step, the planner will formalize answers to the following questions:

- Who will decide to use the program?
- Who will the decision makers need to consult?
- Who will implement the program?
- Will the program require different people to implement different components?
- Who will assure that the program continues as long as it is needed?

Box 9.1. Mayor's Project

The mayor's task force is chugging along with program development. Group members are planning support materials and considering implementation networks. The team is really a team now—a model of a cohesive working group. Its members have a commitment to inclusivity, and along the way they have added members. Anyone who wanted to work hard on preventing violence was welcome. For a while it seemed that every new meeting generated a new member, and every planning success attracted another contingent of community members. The health educator handled this by creating an orientation packet for new members, with information designed to quickly bring a new member up-to-date on the planning milestones the group had accomplished and alternate paths it had considered. So far, so good.

The planning committee members were pleased with their efforts to keep an intact linkage with the community. Members who joined the task force along the way included representatives of churches, community centers, and advocacy groups. However, as the subgroup on implementation began to enumerate the types of people and agencies that might be involved with the program, they were astounded by who was not at the table. Neighborhood social groups, parent organizations, and (interestingly enough) other arms of the mayor's city government were absent. Where were the police, juvenile justice, child protective services, alternative schools, and city job programs?

The task force went back to the streets. The members were assigned to recruitment efforts, and the mayor personally invited her colleagues from other city departments to meet and discuss the history of the violence prevention task force with her and the health educator. She encouraged department heads to assign both management and neighborhood specialists to the task force. Fortunately, the group members prided themselves on inclusivity, and the health educator had been facilitating integration of new individuals all along. The group understood the need to encourage a certain amount of covering old ground and even reinventing programs to integrate these new members, who were so crucial to the linkage system. Soon the group returned to making progress toward planning the adoption, implementation, and sustainability of program objectives.

Revisiting the Linkage System

In Chapter One we presented the notion of participation in the planning group including a linkage system that involves potential adopters and implementers of the program. The linkage system should provide a means to exchange information and ideas between planners and users, to ensure access to the planning process for program users, and to facilitate the development of user-friendly programs (Ammerman et al., 2002; Havelock, 1971; Kocken, 2001; Kolbe & Iverson, 1981; Orlandi, 1986; Orlandi, Landers, Weston, & Haley, 1990). The linkage system serves a dual purpose: to enable collaboratively developed user-relevant health education programs and to accomplish program adoption and implementation. Health promoters should establish the linkage system at the beginning of program planning because it aids the program planners at each stage of the Intervention Mapping process and aids the user system in expressing needs, expectations, and limitations for the health education program. Glasgow, Marcus, Bull, and Wilson (2004) suggest that the developing organization assure potential diffusion of a program by forming a partnership with an organization that has a ready-made network for implementation. They give the example of the Cancer Information Service, a network of health education offices funded by the National Cancer Institute at cancer centers that are well positioned to develop programs in partnership and then implement them broadly.

The *resource system* is the agency or organization supporting and developing the health education program. The resource system could be a university group, a community group, a governmental office, a hospital department, an educational agency, a service group, or a coalition of groups. The resource system includes the personnel, funding, materials, and services available to support the development of the health education program. The user system includes the individuals or groups that will implement the health education program and might be located in schools, work sites, hospitals, clinics, service agencies, mass media outlets, neighborhoods, or communities. The linkage system comprises representatives of both the resource system and the user system with the addition of any change agents who facilitate collaboration or who may be in positions to influence changes necessary to support the adoption, implementation, and continuation of the health education program. Advisory groups, training workshops, and consultation are examples of activities facilitating linkage systems. Schwartz and colleagues (1993) have described a linkage system for translating the findings of research and demonstration programs for cardiovascular disease risk reduction supported by federal public health agencies through the linkage system of state health agencies to communities. The researchers listed technical assistance, quality assurance, training, funding, and on-site coordination as activities bringing together the state health agencies and community program implementers.

Chapter Eleven describes a linkage system for the Dutch AIDS prevention program for vocational schools (H. Schaalma, Kok, Poelman, & Reinders, 1994). To anticipate problems with future adoption and implementation of the program, the program developers formed a linkage board to bridge the gap between the research and development team and the school system. This board was made up of representatives from the research and development team, the school advisory services, the organizations that provide sex and AIDS education to secondary schools, and an association of biology teachers. The role of the board was to provide feedback on the program's performance and change objectives and to give advice on implementation issues. The linkage board gave careful consideration to the secondary school context for the program and to the teachers who would use it.

The Heart Partners program created a linkage system of school-based volunteers specifically to mediate between the teachers and the American Heart Association. The role of each heart partner was to promote awareness and use of the school-site programs, to conduct training sessions, and to reinforce teachers who conducted the programs. The Heart Partners program also used a linkage system composed of American Heart Association staff, teachers who were knowledgeable about the association and its resources, and university program developers (Roberts-Gray et al., 1998).

The linkage system can be organized with varying degrees of formality. In the system's simplest form, health promoters can invite potential users of the program to be members of the program-planning group and participate fully in each step of the Intervention Mapping process. This simple form can be extended by having the user system select members to represent it and by having these representatives report and obtain feedback on the program development's progress. The size or complexity of the project will influence ways of creating and structuring the linkage system. Another influence will be the goal for sustaining the program. A program that will depend on the hospitality and resources of many agencies should have these community partners present throughout its development in order to foster as much commitment and ownership as possible as well as to foresee barriers and facilitators to implementation.

For a very large project, either in scope of the program to be developed or in the number of organizations to be involved in planning and implementation, the linkage system may need to be more formal; health promoters may need to create a new entity to carry out the linkage function. The structure of a linkage system and the makeup of individuals participating in it will be unique to each program and situation. An important consideration in selecting individuals to participate in the linkage system is to ensure representation of different views and receptivity toward the innovative program. Often program planners rely entirely on volunteers who are already committed to the implementation of a new program. If individuals who are reluctant or opposed to using the program are not included in the planning process, the program may fail to be adopted and implemented because the planning process has not taken into consideration the divergent views. Representation of potential decision makers for adoption and institutionalization, in addition to those who will implement the program, will ensure that program developers consider the larger organizational perspectives. The following examples from two health promotion projects illustrate this more formal approach.

The Partners in School Asthma Program (see Chapter Twelve) is a research and demonstration project to develop and evaluate a multicomponent school-based program to improve the management of childhood asthma (Bartholomew, Czyzewski, Swank, McCormick, & Parcel, 2000; Bartholomew, Gold, et al., 2000). To help develop the interventions and achieve program adoption and implementation, health promoters created a linkage system with two components. The first was an advisory committee that included the director of school health services, a school nurse, an elementary school principal, the director of risk management, the director of building maintenance and services, and a parent of a child with asthma. This group's primary role was to engage in planning to develop and carry out interventions to ensure program adoption and implementation. The second component was a small group of selected pilot schools to serve as sources of information on needs, expectations, and limitations of program users and to test intervention components. This group's major role was to ensure that the health promotion program was compatible with program users and was a good fit for the schools' structure and context. Both of these formal groups functioned as partners in the program-planning process.

Another example of a linkage system is from a project designed to promote the diffusion of an effective program to prevent tobacco use, Smart Choices (Brink et al., 1995; Parcel, 1995; Parcel et al., 1995). The project goal was to influence as many school districts as possible within two educational service regions of the state of Texas to adopt and implement a program to prevent adolescent smoking (Parcel, Eriksen, et al., 1989). The linkage system used for this project also had two components. One pilot school served as a model for program adoption and implementation and then shared its experiences with other school districts through video and print communications. The second component of the linkage system comprised the regions' two educational service centers. Each center employed a health educator responsible for working with schools to help them identify and adopt health education programs. These health educators served as links between the research group and the school districts. They enabled the planners to have more direct contact with potential adopters and implementers and help them gain a better understanding of how to design the diffusion interventions. The two also assisted with implementing the diffusion intervention.

Performance Objectives for Adoption, Implementation, and Sustainability

⊃ *The second task in this step is to specify performance objectives for program adoption, implementation, and sustainability.*

The point of this task is to figure out who has to do what in order for the program to be used across the phases of program diffusion. The work of E. M. Rogers (1983, 1995, 2003) and others over several decades has laid the groundwork for how to get programs adopted, implemented, and continued over time. Often this process is referred to as diffusion and focuses on program adoption and initial use (see Chapters Three and Four for a discussion of Diffusion of Innovations Theory). However, since the 1980s, researchers have given increasing attention to the processes involved with both program implementation (J. L. Monahan & Scheirer, 1988; Roberts-Gray, Solomon, Gottlieb, & Kelsey, 1985; M. A. Scheirer, 1981, 1990, 1994) and program continuation (R. M. Goodman, McLeroy, Steckler, & Hoyle, 1993; R. M. Goodman & Steckler, 1989; R. M. Goodman, Steckler, & Kegler, 1997; M. A. Scheirer, Shediac, & Cassady, 1995; Shediac-Rizkallah & Bone, 1998).

Diffusion is a process of moving from awareness of a need or of an innovation, through decisions to adopt the innovation, to initial use and program continuation. Program use has three stages (R. M. Goodman & Steckler, 1989; Oldenburg et al., 1997; Parcel, Eriksen, et al., 1989; Paulussen, Kok, & Schaalma, 1994; Paulussen, Kok, Schaalma, & Parcel, 1995):

1. Adoption, a decision to use a program, which depends on knowledge of an innovation, awareness of an unmet need, and the decision that a certain innovation may meet the perceived need and will be given a trial (adoption can depend on active dissemination of a program)
2. Implementation, the use of the program to a fair trial point
3. Sustainability, the maintenance and institutionalization of a program or its outcomes

The program planner will need to write performance objectives for each of these phases.

Adoption

An *innovation* is an idea, practice, or product that is new to the adopter, which may be an individual or an organization. Healthy behavior, such as being physically active, stopping smoking, and using contraceptives, may be innovations for individuals, as may interventions to promote these behaviors in organizations. Further, new programs demand change in individuals and organizations (Mullen & Mullen, 1983). The program that health promoters plan with Intervention Mapping Steps 1 to 4 can be thought of as an innovation because the program will be new to its users and will require changes in what they do and how they do it. Therefore, in order for the health promotion program to be put into use, someone or a group of people must decide to adopt the program.

Program adoption by organizations is a more complex event than is adoption by individuals, and it often involves key agents. For example, a teacher team leader may hear about a program at a professional meeting and discuss it with other teachers and staff. The team leader may then request the curriculum coordinator or superintendent (depending on the school district's size and personnel structure) to adopt the program.

Implementation

Program adoption does not guarantee program implementation. Program users are often asked to implement a program without having a clear understanding of what program implementation means, especially of what a well-implemented program should be (M. A. Scheirer, 1981, 1994). Program developers and evaluators are often concerned about three dimensions of implementation: fidelity, completeness, and dose (Baranowski & Stables, 2000; Linnan & Steckler, 2002; Rossi, Lipsey, & Freeman, 2004; M. A. Scheirer, 1981). *Fidelity* is the degree to which the program is implemented with its methods and strategies intact; *completeness* indicates the proportion of program activities and components that are delivered; and *dose* indicates the number of units or amount of the program that participants receive. For example, in the Cystic Fibrosis Family Education Program CF FEP, some cystic fibrosis centers taught all the program modules (good completeness) but neglected to perform goal setting with the families (inadequate fidelity) (Bartholomew, Czyzewski, et al., 2000). An important process in developing performance objectives for implementation is to answer these questions: What exactly is the program? What would constitute a level of fidelity and a level of completeness consistent with program effectiveness?

Program developers must know what constitutes a well-implemented program. On the other hand, a defining characteristic of program implementation is mutual adaptation (Hall & Loucks, 1978; Ringwalt et al., 2004). Both the innovation and the organization must adapt to each other's objectives, processes, and structures. Mutual adaptation is so ubiquitous that E. M. Rogers (1995) described it as a stage in organizational innovation, calling it reinvention. Quite a bit of reinvention takes place; various studies have found that more than 50 percent of adopting institutions reinvent the programs they adopt, making anything from small insignificant changes to major revisions. From the perspective of the adopting institution, reinvention is a positive process that fosters program owner-ship and commitment. In the diffusion of the CF FEP, we encouraged cystic fi-brosis centers to reinvent the program to fit their ways of practicing (Bartholomew, Czyzewski, et al., 2000). From an intervention perspective, it may be best to an-ticipate this process and facilitate it within the boundaries of program effective-ness. The resulting ownership is important not just for program implementation but for sustainability, which we discuss next in this chapter.

Sustainability

A final stage of program use has been described as institutionalization, that is, in-corporating a program into organizational routines so that it survives beyond the presence of the original program funding, adopters, or program champion (R. M. Goodman et al., 1997; R. M. Goodman & Steckler, 1989; Kegler & McLeroy, 2003). However, a broader construct, sustainability, can stimulate the health pro-moter to choose among several possible program continuation goals. Shediac-Rizkallah and Bone (1998) theorize that sustainability includes three possible goals: maintenance of health benefits from a program, institutionalization of a program within an organization's routines, or capacity building in the recipient community.

E. M. Rogers (1983) describes institutionalization as routinization, the pro-gression of an innovation to an indistinguishable part of the individual or organi-zational host's practices. However, R. M. Goodman and Steckler (1989) pointed out that health education and promotion interventions can be fragile and expend-able innovations unless health promoters plan for and nurture institutionalization. These authors built on the work of R. K. Yin (1979) to define dimensions of in-stitutionalization as the extensiveness of a program's integration into the subsys-tems of a host organization and intensiveness, or the depth of program integration into each organization subsystem. Yin identified three degrees of intensiveness:

1. Passages: anniversaries of the intervention, such as the number of fiscal year beginnings that the intervention has survived
2. Routines: operating structures and functions into which program protocols are embedded
3. Niche saturation: complete integration into a subsystem's structures and functions

Once a program has achieved a certain level of health effects, the program con-tinuation goal may be to continue the program's effects rather than the program itself. Some programs are needed in their original form to continue the effects (Hoelscher et al., 2004). Shediac-Rizkallah and Bone (1998) give the example of a measles disease-prevention program that was effective in controlling measles outbreaks only while it was functioning. Two years later the rates were at the preprogram level; other types of programs were needed to maintain the effects of the initial program. In the World Health Organization efforts to eradicate smallpox (Fenner, Henderson, Arita, Jezek, & Ladnyi, 1988), an initial program of mass vaccination was followed by one of surveillance and aggressive follow-up of suspected cases. Both these programs were in service of the same health objective and represent program sustainability. As another example, Lichtenstein, Thompson, Nettekoven, and Corbett (1996) describe efforts to continue tobacco control activities, rather than the initial program, after the COMMIT trial.

Sometimes the best way to diffuse and sustain a program is to go beyond organizational boundaries. Both intact programs and program components intended to guard health effects may need multiple community agencies to sustain them. Bracht and colleagues (1994) describe how community agencies made efforts to sustain components of the Minnesota Heart Health Program, a program begun by university-based researchers. Agencies and their networks may need training and technical assistance and developmental support to expand their capacity to house new programs. The specific areas of capacity enhancement that may need to be included in diffusion interventions to continue programs are skills, structures, and functions to encourage participation, leadership, group process, conflict resolution, leverage of resources, and network maintenance.

Performance Objectives

Looking at the phases of program use, the planning group can think about the potential decision makers and users and write performance objectives. The performance objectives for Step 5 are similar to the those in Step 2 for health-related behavior and environmental change except that the behaviors in Step 5 are adoption, implementation, and (depending on goals selected for sustainability) either maintenance, institutionalization, or capacity building for sustaining health effects. The performance objectives make clear what performance will constitute use with acceptable fidelity and completeness.

Adoption Objectives. The adoption of a health education program by an organization or practitioner means that someone decides to use the program. The someone could be an individual, such as a practitioner or an administrator, making an independent decision; or it could be a group, such as a committee or governing board, making a collective decision. Program adoption can also be decided sequentially or concurrently at multiple levels of responsibility within an organization. For example, the school board and superintendent may decide to adopt an innovative health promotion program for a district; a principal may make the decision for a school; and a teacher may decide for a classroom. Knowing ahead of time who will make the adoption decision and how will greatly assist the program planners in specifying the performance objectives for adoption.

Program adoption behavior can be specified in this way: [someone] adopts the [innovative program] as indicated by [the evidence or document to indicate adoption]. For example: the curriculum committee of the Star Independent School District decides to adopt the Smart Choices smoking prevention program as indicated by the superintendent signing the program adoption form. The answer to the following question specifies the performance objectives for adoption: What do the potential program adopters need to do to constitute adoption of the health education program?

The example just given can be used to state the general question more specifically: What does the curriculum committee of the Star Independent School District need to do to perform an adoption of the Smart Choices program? Answers to this question are possible performance objectives. For example, the curriculum committee will do the following:

- Review the Smart Choices program materials
- Note the program's objectives, methods, and relative advantages
- Obtain parent, administrator, and teacher reaction to the program
- Obtain information on the experiences of other school districts using the Smart Choices program
- Identify barriers for implementation as perceived by potential program users
- Seek information and consultation from the linkage system or resource system for addressing barriers and concerns
- Gain support for program adoption from teachers (implementers) and key administrators (principals, director of curriculum, and superintendent)
- Prepare a statement of recommendation for adoption of the Smart Choices program
- Complete the adoption form for the Smart Choices program, have it signed by the superintendent, and return it to the resource system for processing

Implementation Performance Objectives. Implementation of a health education program can also be stated in behavioral terms. However, to a greater extent than for adoption, implementation is often multiple tasks performed by a variety of individual roles. For the CATCH program, for example, implementation is performed by classroom academic teachers, physical education teachers, food service staff, and administrators (C. L. Perry et al., 1997). Parallel to the statement of adoption behaviors, implementation behaviors can be stated in this way: the [role of implementer] will [perform specific implementation task] with fidelity and completeness as indicated by [quality standards for fidelity and completeness]. The statement must answer the question: What do the program implementers need to do to implement the program with acceptable fidelity and completeness?

The planners of Smart Choices asked what teachers and principals need to do to implement the program, and they developed this set of implementation objectives:

- Health teachers will participate in training to prepare for implementing the *Smart Choices* curriculum.
- Health teachers will schedule and incorporate the Smart Choices curriculum into the lesson plans for all health classes for each semester.
- Health teachers will teach all six lessons in the Smart Choices curriculum using the teaching methods specified in the lesson plans.
- The principal at each middle school will form a policy committee that includes teacher, student, staff, and parent representation to establish policies for tobacco control at the school.
- The policy committee will follow the Smart Choices Tobacco-Free Policy Guidelines to review current tobacco control policies and will revise or form new policies to establish a tobacco-free school.

Sustainability Performance Objectives. Before specifying performance objectives for sustaining a program, the planner will decide on a goal: institutionalization, continuation of health effects, capacity building, or some combination of these. The example we give here is for institutionalization. Institutionalization objectives answer the question: What do the organizational decision makers need to do to incorporate the program into the organization's routines for the long term? Here are the performance objectives for institutionalization of the Smart Choices program within a school district:

- District coordinators will include training of new health teachers to implement the Smart Choices curriculum in their yearly plans.
- Book and curriculum warehouse managers will order and maintain inventory of the curriculum.
- Principals will include implementation of the Smart Choices curriculum in teacher job descriptions and evaluations.
- The principal at each middle school will include the Smart Choices program as a line item in the budget.

- The school district curriculum committee will write Smart Choices into the district curriculum guide for middle school science.
- The policy committee will report the results of the program to the parent teacher association each year.

If multiple organizations in the community are interested in the continuation of the program after the initial cycle of funding, the objectives should be written to include those organization decision makers would do to continue the program in their organizations. For example, at the conclusion of the Stanford Five-City project, the project group first attempted institutionalization through a nonprofit community health promotion center. When this approach encountered barriers related to continued funding and program development, the focus shifted to capacity building among health educators employed by local organizations, with leadership provided by the local health department (Jackson et al., 1994).

Determinants of Program Use

⊃ *The third task in this step is to specify determinants of adoption, implementation, and sustainability.*

As with the performance objectives of health-related behaviors and environmental conditions, the performance objectives for program use will have a set of determinants, that is, factors that are likely to influence their performance. The determinants may be personal (located within the individuals responsible for adoption and implementation) or external (social or structural factors that might serve as barriers or facilitators).

The processes for selecting determinants are the same as the ones recommended for selecting determinants of health-related behavior and environmental conditions. The team should begin by brainstorming a list of factors that will facilitate or serve as barriers to accomplishing the performance objectives for adoption, implementation, and sustainability (Elliott et al., 2004). To refine or add to this list, the group should review the literature and the information from potential program users. A review of the literature starts with studies that report findings of determinants of use of similar programs in similar settings. If there is not a large body of literature on comparable program use in health education and health promotion programs, the team may need to search in other fields (Oldenburg, Sallis, French, & Owen, 1999).

Next, the team can review the literature on theories that have been used to explain the adoption, implementation, and continuation of innovations and the literature from general theories that includes some of the identified determinants. For example, if the preceding review of the literature identified relative advantage as a possible determinant of the adoption of an innovation, it would be useful to go to the literature on Diffusion of Innovations Theory (DIT), for which relative advantage is a central construct. A review of DIT may suggest other constructs that the team might consider as important determinants of the program adoption and implementation. A review of theory should not be limited to theories of diffusion. For example, in the Smart Choices diffusion project, the planning team used Social Cognitive Theory (SCT) (Bandura, 1986) to hypothesize determinants of adoption and implementation such as outcome expectations, expectancies, reinforcement for adoption, and behavioral capability and self-efficacy for implementation (Parcel, Eriksen, et al., 1989; Parcel, Taylor, et al., 1989). Best and colleagues (2003) suggest the use of systems theory to conceptualize determinants and methods to enhance health promotion program adoption and implementation.

E. M. Rogers (1995, 2003) describes three types of knowledge of an innovation that can be important to a decision to adopt. *Awareness* is knowing that the innovation exists. The adopter must also have procedural knowledge (knowledge about how to use the innovation) and principles knowledge (the underlying mechanism of the innovation or how it works). SCT provides explanations of the psychological mechanisms by which adoption decisions are made (Bandura, 1986).

Before program users can adopt an innovation, they must be aware of the innovation, hold positive outcome expectations and expectancies for it, and have sufficient self-efficacy and behavioral capability for both adoption and implementation. For example, positive outcome expectations by the potential adopters of self-management programs might include beliefs that the program will lead to better self-care and increased health and quality-of-life outcomes among patients and to increased job satisfaction and career enhancement for health care providers. Negative outcome expectations could include beliefs that the program will disrupt patient-provider relationships, lead to inappropriate or detrimental self-care based on faulty self-management decisions, and result in a decline in health status. Expectancies are how much each of the outcomes is valued. Intervention messages would seek to increase positive outcome expectations and values and decrease negative ones. Self-efficacy, or confidence in implementing the innovation, is also important for adoption. However, it increases in importance as a person or organization tries to implement the new program.

Another important set of factors often related to the decision to adopt a program are the characteristics of the innovation (Oldenburg et al., 1997; E. M. Rogers, 1995; Berwick, 2003). These characteristics are the potential adopters' perceptions of what the program is like. They include the relative advantage of the innovation compared to what is being used, compatibility with the intended users' current practice, complexity, observability of the results, impact on social relations, reversibility or ease of discontinuation, communicability, required time, risk and uncertainty, required commitment, and ability to be modified. The planning team must consider each of these characteristics of an innovation as either a predictor of or a barrier to adoption, both in program design and in the creation of an intervention to influence program adoption.

The social interaction among stakeholders who seek to maximize their own goals and interests during adoption and implementation is complex. Organizational decision makers may adopt the program to accomplish the organization's goals or to reduce pressure from interest groups. Implementers may wish to conduct the program as they would like rather than as the developers designed it. The decision to retain the program may compete with other organizational activities. The program may be a source of career advancement for some but an undesired added workload for others. In any event, there are multiple competing views of whether to adopt the program, how to implement it, and whether to retain it.

As attention shifts from adoption to the implementation of a health promotion program, the determinants shift to an emphasis on behavioral capability, skills, self-efficacy, and reinforcement. A challenge in planning interventions to promote implementation is to correctly estimate the level of skills and related self-efficacy necessary to implement the program. For example, the CF FEP required many different types of skills for putting this complex program into clinical practice. The clinic coordinators who had to direct its use perceived skills as important determinants of implementation, and the diffusion intervention emphasized skill building. In comparison, necessary skills were sometimes underestimated in the program diffusion in spite of careful planning. The planners seriously underestimated the training intensity required to develop skills in communication domains such as mutual goal setting. Skill requirements are also often neglected or taken for granted in community interventions based on activities such as coalitions. Some researchers have suggested that coalition members receive training on how to be part of an effective coalition as a part of the implementation of a coalition-based health promotion program (Holmes, Neville, Donovan, & MacDonald, 2001).

Another important determinant of program implementation can be reinforcement. Usually, the innovation will eventually be intrinsically reinforcing because the implementers will see its effects. In the CATCH program, the food service workers liked seeing the children choose low-fat foods and were reinforced by the good feelings from their role in creating a healthier environment for the children. However, at the beginning of an implementation, positive reinforcement is delayed and change can be punishing (with the implementers seeing the change as a hassle or a disruption). Therefore, extrinsic reinforcements may have to be built into an implementation intervention. Extrinsic reinforcements can sometimes simply highlight program outcomes that may be difficult for implementers to see.

The application of the Theory of Planned Behavior (TPB) (Ajzen, 1991) to the identification of determinants for program adoption and implementation is illustrated in Figure 11.1 and in Chapter Eleven, which describes a Dutch AIDS-prevention program in the schools. Paulussen and colleagues (1994, 1995) hypothesized both endogenous and background variables to influence teacher adoption of an AIDS curriculum. The background variables are thought to influence adoption and implementation through their effects on the TPB variables in the top half of Figure 11.1. Instrumentality refers to the teachers' perceptions of whether the curriculum meets their planning concerns and includes clarity of instructions, anticipated student reactions, time required, and ease of teaching. The authors found that subjective norms, instrumentality, and descriptive norms (perceived colleague behavior) explained a considerable amount of the variability in teachers' adoption of AIDS curricula.

Because program adoption and implementation often involve organizations and community groups making decisions and changing practices to make use of an innovation, the application of organizational change and community development models is critical to identifying the external determinants of program adoption and implementation (J. A. Hogan et al., 2003). The brainstorming and the literature review provide informed but nevertheless hypothesized relationships of determinants to the adoption and implementation objectives. If there is a long list of determinants at this stage, the planner may need to test the hypothesized relationships of determinants in order to select the most important determinants to guide intervention development. If the list of determinants is small, the planner may need to collect data from the potential program users to identify additional determinants. In either case, the planner can use both qualitative and quantitative methods.

Qualitative methods, such as focus groups or interviews, can be helpful in generating new ideas for determinants or in verifying some of the findings from the research literature. Quantitative data collection using questionnaires that measure the determinants and interest or intentions to adopt and implement a program can be especially helpful in judging the strength of the association between determinants and potential adoption and implementation. With both types of data collection, planners can obtain some estimate of the presence or absence of the determinant in the user system.

In the Smart Choices diffusion project, for example, the program developers had assumed that teachers and school administrators would need to be convinced that it is important for the schools to conduct programs to prevent student tobacco use. Therefore, modeling and messages were created in the adoption intervention to influence teachers to place a higher value on the schools' conducting smoking prevention programs. However, the baseline data collected for program evaluation showed that the teachers and administrators already placed high value on smoking prevention; because this possible determinant was high, it could be reinforced rather than introduced in the intervention (Parcel, Eriksen, et al., 1989; Parcel, Taylor, et al., 1989).

Eventually, the planning team must refine the list of determinants. A long list of determinants is not practical for program development. To assess the list of determinants, planners should begin by rating each determinant in terms of importance (that is, strength of association with program adoption and implementation) and changeability (that is, how likely it is that a diffusion intervention influences a change in the determinant). The planners should give priority to those determinants that have high importance and high changeability. However, planners may want to retain some determinants with high importance and low changeability because the determinant is likely to be a critical factor in program adoption or implementation. For example, the cost of adopting a health promotion program may be a strong determinant, but there may be little that planners can do to lower the cost. Because cost may be a major barrier to adoption, it needs to be addressed in the intervention so that the planner can find ways to compensate (that is, find additional funding sources) or demonstrate that the program's costs are worth the benefit.

Matrices and Plans for Promoting Program Use

⮐ *The fourth task in Step 5 is to create program use matrices.*

This task links performance objectives and determinants for adoption, implementation, and sustainability to create change objectives. Essentially, the planner is now repeating the task from Step 2, but instead of focusing on behavioral and environmental outcomes, the focus is on outcomes for adoption, implementation, and sustainability of the health promotion program.

We present a matrix for the diffusion of the CF FEP in Table 9.1. This planning was conducted in order to effectively disseminate the program to the approximately 120 cystic fibrosis comprehensive care centers in the United States, Canada, and Australia (Bartholomew, Czyzewski, et al., 2000). The matrix in Table 9.1 was created, like the matrices that were developed for planning the intervention, by entering performance objectives on the left side of the matrix and determinants across the top of the matrix. Then the program planners assessed each cell to decide whether the determinant was likely to be important to the

TABLE 9.1. CYSTIC FIBROSIS FAMILY EDUCATION PROGRAM (CF FEP) MATRIX.

Performance Objectives	Personal Determinants					External Determinants	
	Knowledge	Skills and Self-Efficacy	Outcome Expectations	Attitudes		Team Functioning	Logistics
Adoption							
PO.1. Staff members evaluate patient education needs in CF Center.	K.1.a. Describe ways to evaluate patient education needs K.1.b. Summarize needs K.1.c. Prioritize needs	SSE.1. Express confidence in performing a needs assessment	OE.1. Expect that by becoming more aware of patient education needs will be able to choose programs to better meet needs				
PO.2. Center directors and staff members decide whether CF FEP will meet needs.	K.2.a. Increase awareness of CF FEP K.2.b. Explain the advantages of the CF FEP to meet patient education needs		OE.2. Expect that using the CF FEP will improve patient health outcomes and quality of life	A.2. Review characteristics of CF FEP and react favorably (relative advantage and so on)			
PO.3. Center directors and staff members decide to adopt CF FEP.	K.3. Describe how CF FEP compares to other available programs		OE.3. Expect that using the CF FEP will be accepted by center staff	A.3. Review characteristics of CF FEP and react favorably (relative advantage and so on)		TF.3. Center directors discuss pros and cons of the program with staff.	
PO.4. Center directors and staff members identify program champion.	K.4. List characteristics of a good program champion					TF.4. Center directors discuss need for program champion with staff.	

Implementation

Performance Objectives	Knowledge	Skills/Self-Efficacy	Outcome Expectations	Attitude	TF	L
PO.5. Staff members work with families using the CF FEP with completeness and fidelity.	K.5.a. Describe the units of the CF FEP by developmental stage. K.5.b. Describe how the CF FEP is supposed to be used	SSE.5.a. Demonstrate working on various models with families depending on staff role. SSE.5.b. Express confidence at being able to work with families on the models in a goal-setting and counseling mode	OE.5.a. Expect to be successful in working with families. OE.5.b. Expect that when families and children work on the program, they will learn to perform better self-care. OE.5.c. Expect that better self-care as a result of the program will result in better health and quality of life.	A.5. Describe the added work of doing the program as being "worth it"	TF.5.a. Center directors and program champions create a CF FEP implementation team. TF.5.b. Team members participate in decision making about CF FEP.	L.5. Time and space are set aside for the use of the program.
PO.6. Program champions work with staff to develop implementation plan.	K.6. Describe components of implementation plan, such as who will teach which modules	SSE.6. Express confidence in being able to organize a plan with staff				
PO.7. Staff members document program use.	K.7. Describe documentation form and where to find it		OE.7. Expect that by documenting progress, team members will be able to reinforce families' increases in self-management.	A.7. Judge documentation forms to be useful, not too complex	TF.7.a. Center directors authorize documentation forms. TF.7.b. Center staff members revise forms to suit needs.	L.7. Center administrators make documentation forms available in medical record or special file.
PO.8. Staff members review patient CF FEP progress in rounds.			OE.8. Expect that discussion of patient education progress during rounds will elevate importance of the self-management process.		TF.8. Center directors and staff members plan to add patient education progress to team discussions.	

TABLE 9.1. CYSTIC FIBROSIS FAMILY EDUCATION PROGRAM (CF FEP) MATRIX, Cont'd.

Performance Objectives	Personal Determinants				External Determinants	
	Knowledge	Skills and Self-Efficacy	Outcome Expectations	Attitudes	Team Functioning	Logistics
Maintenance and Institutionalization						
PO.9. Program champions and supervisors use CF FEP in orientation of new staff.	K.9. Recognize the importance of finding ways to integrate the CF FEP into center routines		OE.9. Describe how integrating the CF FEP into training will contribute to its continued use		TF.9. Program champion and supervisors integrate CF FEP content into training protocol.	
PO.10. Program champions work with supervisors to write CF FEP into care paths or continuous quality improvement plans.	K.10. Recognize the importance of finding ways to integrate the CF FEP into center routines		OE.10. Describe how integrating the CF FEP into continuous quality improvement (CQI) will contribute to its continued use		TF10. Center directors approve integration of the CF FEP into CQI activities.	

achievement of the performance objective. Next, the planner wrote change objectives for the appropriate cells. The process for writing change objectives is the same for adoption and implementation matrices as for the health education matrices (see Chapter Six).

The program was tested over a period of two years in one cystic fibrosis center using a quasi-experimental evaluation design and was shown to be effective in improving self-management skills and clinical outcomes (Bartholomew et al., 1997). More than one hundred multidisciplinary cystic fibrosis centers care for approximately twenty thousand cystic fibrosis patients in the United States (Cystic Fibrosis Foundation, 1995). For the program to have a meaningful impact on helping patients and families self-manage cystic fibrosis, the next phase of program development had to address the program's adoption, implementation, and institutionalization in the cystic fibrosis centers throughout the three participating countries. To accomplish the outcomes of program adoption, implementation, and institutionalization, the planning team designed a diffusion intervention to address both personal and external determinants.

Methods and Strategies for Dissemination

Program use within organizations is complex and requires consideration of a variety of organizational-level factors (Beyer & Trice, 1978; R. M. Goodman et al., 1997; Riley, Taylor, & Elliott, 2003). Planning interventions to promote use of a health promotion program should consider the organization's goals, authority structure, roles, rules and regulations, and informal norms and relationships (E. M. Rogers, 1983). The decision to adopt an innovation within an organization can be made by an individual independent of others, collectively by consensus among the members of the organization or a subsystem within it, or by a person or persons with authority for the organization. An intervention to influence an adoption decision must be clearly oriented to how that decision is being made. Implementation success will depend on the degree of ownership that those who must carry out the tasks feel and the support they give. These attributes may depend in part on how the adoption decision is made.

A powerful influence toward the adoption of new programs in organizations can be program champions (Riley, 2003). Program champions are likely to be sophisticated, analytical individuals with strategic linking locations in organizations. They often have intuitive skills in discovering the program adopters' and users' goals, and they have interpersonal and negotiating skills in order to troubleshoot both adoption and implementation (R. M. Goodman & Steckler, 1989). A champion can be a force to facilitate adoption of programs and to prevent discontinuation (J. L. Monahan & Scheirer, 1988). Compared to their colleagues, program champions have been described as taking more risks, being more innovative, and initiating more attempts to influence others (Howell & Higgins, 1990). Program champions must be credible to their colleagues, and when an innovation is costly or represents a radical new direction for the organization, the champion must be in a powerful organizational role.

> **⊃** *The fifth task in Intervention Mapping Step 5 is to select methods and strategies to address the determinants.*

The same core processes used in other Intervention Mapping steps can be applied here. The program planners start with the list of change objectives for determinants and performance objectives and brainstorm methods that they think can influence a change. Next, they review the relevant research and practice literature to confirm, refute, or modify the provisional list of methods. The best approach is for planners to start with the literature on the diffusion of health promotion programs and then review diffusion literature related to other innovations that may have some common elements with the adoption and implementation of health promotion programs. Planners also need to explore the literature on theories of change related to specific theoretical constructs on the final list of determinants. For example, self-efficacy may be considered an important determinant of program implementation, but it may not be specifically addressed in the literature on diffusion. However, a review of the theoretical literature on self-efficacy would lead to SCT, which discusses methods shown to be effective in changing self-efficacy (Bandura, 1986). Finally, it may be useful and necessary to collect additional data from potential adopters and program users to test out some items on the provisional list of methods to determine acceptability and appropriateness for use in an intervention.

The planning team then uses the revised list of methods to design practical strategies to influence program adoption and implementation. As we discussed in Chapter Seven, the selection of methods and strategies may be a back-and-forth process. In reviewing the adoption and implementation objectives, planners may find that ideas for strategies occur to them before ideas for methods do. They can then assess the strategy in order to link it to a theoretical method. For example, planners are brainstorming methods and strategies to influence families to adopt a program to survey and correct household hazards for childhood injuries. One of the strategies they think would be effective is to communicate through mass media the stories of parents who have successfully adopted the program and discovered hazards that might have been very harmful to their children. This strategy of role-model stories (Pulley, McAlister, Kay, & O'Reilly, 1996; A. G. Ramirez et al., 1995; Suarez, Nichols, Pulley, Brady, & McAlister, 1993) can be linked to the theoretical method of modeling from SCT (Bandura, 1986). The planners can then review the theoretical principles that guide the use of modeling in order to influence possible determinants of program adoption such as perceived norms, outcome expectations, and self-efficacy. They can then design interventions that take advantage of what others have learned about the method of modeling and how it can be applied to their idea for using role-model stories as a strategy.

The methods discussed in Chapters Three, Four, and Seven can be applied to interventions to accomplish program adoption, implementation, and continuation. Planners can address personal determinants such as knowledge of program compatibility and relative advantage, attitudes toward the program, outcome expectations for the program, self-efficacy, and behavioral capability for doing the program activities with methods based in social psychology, such as persuasive communication, modeling, skills training, incentives, reinforcement, and social comparison (Bandura, 1986; McGuire, 1985). Methods to address external determinants for program adoption, implementation, and continuation, such as social support, program advocacy, resources, organizational structures and practices, and policies, can also be found in Chapters Three and Four. Table 9.2 presents methods and strategies for the CF FEB; Table 9.3 presents them for Smart Choices.

Adoption, Implementation, and Sustainability Plan

⊃ *The last task in this step is to design interventions and organize programs to affect change objectives related to program use.*

The final task in Step 5 is to design a plan for an intervention to influence program adoption, implementation, and sustainability outcomes. The plan for getting a program adopted and implemented is as important as the intervention plans discussed in Chapter Eight. It should include a scope and sequence of activities, staffing, and budget. Any materials that are needed for the adoption or implementation such as training manuals or newsletters should be described in the design documents and produced with the same care described in Chapter Eight for the program materials. As an example, the scope and sequence for the CF FEP diffusion is included in Table 9.4.

Implications for Program Evaluation

The tasks completed in Step 5 will be useful for completing the tasks in Step 6, whose products are plans for both process and effectiveness or efficacy evaluations. The development and evaluation studies of health promotion programs have tended to focus on efficacy and effectiveness without addressing the other

TABLE 9.2. CYSTIC FIBROSIS FAMILY EDUCATION PROGRAM (CF FEP) DIFFUSION INTERVENTION PLAN.

Diffusion Stage	Change Objectives (See Matrix Table 9.1)	Theoretical Methods	Intervention Strategies
Adoption performance objectives: PO.1. Staff members evaluate patient education needs in CF Center. PO.2. Center directors and staff members decide whether the CF FEP will meet needs. PO.3. Center directors and staff members decide to adopt the CF FEP. PO.4. Center directors and staff members identify program champion.	Knowledge Skills and self-efficacy Outcome expectations Attitude Team functioning	Persuasion Modeling Cues to participate in training Information	*Pharmaceutical-style product detailing of program to CF centers:* Contact person recruitment of workshop registrants Distribution of color program guide charts Workshop invitation and confirmation Scientific presentations and exhibits at CF medical meeting
Implementation with families in CF centers performance objectives: PO.5. Staff members work with families using the CF FEP with completeness and fidelity. PO.6. Program champions work with staff to develop implementation plan. PO.7. Staff members document program use. PO.8. Staff members review patient CF FEP progress in rounds.	Knowledge Skills and self-efficacy Outcome expectations Attitude Team functioning Logistics	Modeling Skill training Reinforcement Persuasion Skill building with guided practice Information	*Regional workshops:* Discussion Problem analysis Role playing Lecture Videotape modeling and information to use in center Team meeting to plan implementation Print implementation guides *Newsletters:* Role-model stories Resources Information *Regional coordinators:* Technical and social support Social reinforcement Role modeling
Institutionalization performance objectives: PO.9. Program champions and supervisors use the CF FEP in new staff orientation and write CF FEP into job descriptions. PO.10. Program champions and supervisors write the CF FEP into care paths or continuous quality improvement plans.	Knowledge Skills and self-efficacy Outcome expectations Attitude Team functioning	Problem solving Reinforcement Social support Skill training	*Regional coordinators:* Technical support Social support Social reinforcement Role modeling *Newsletters:* Role-model stories Resources Information

TABLE 9.3. SMART CHOICES DIFFUSION.

Diffusion	Target Outcome	Variables to Be Addressed	Social Cognitive Theory Methods	Practical Strategies
Dissemination	Teachers and administrators indicate awareness of the Smart Choices program.	Preconditions—knowledge and awareness	Symbolic modeling Direct modeling	Dissemination videotape Workshop for school personnel Diffusion network
	Teachers and administrators view the Smart Choices program favorably.	Outcome expectations Attitudes Expectancies	Dual-channel communication	Newsletter
	Teachers and administrators discuss the Smart Choices program.			
Adoption	School districts adopt the Smart Choices program.	Outcome expectations Expectancies Vicarious reinforcement	Symbolic modeling Incentives Contracting	Newsletter Adoption form
Implementation	Teachers use the Smart Choices program with acceptable completeness, fidelity, and proficiency.	Behavioral capability Self-efficacy	Direct modeling Symbolic modeling Guided enactment Self-directed application of acquired skills	Training workshop Training videotape
Maintenance	After one year, teachers continue to use the Smart Choices program with acceptable completeness, fidelity, and proficiency.	Self-efficacy Outcome expectations Expectancies Reinforcement	Feedback and reinforcement	Recognition Material rewards Special status for school district Feedback on performance

Source: Parcel, Taylor, and others, 1989.

TABLE 9.4. SCOPE AND SEQUENCE OF THE CYSTIC FIBROSIS FAMILY EDUCATION PROGRAM DIFFUSION INTERVENTION.

Months 1–2	Months 2–4	Months 4–6	Months 6+
Pharmaceutical style detailing:	*Regional training meetings:*	*Newsletters:*	*Newsletters:*
Contact person recruitment of workshop registrants	Discussion	Information on the program	Role-model stories on successful adoption and implementation
Distribution of color program guide charts	Problem analysis	Information on how to do implementation	
Workshop invitation and confirmation	Role playing		
	Lecture		
	Team meeting to plan implementation		
	Print implementation guides		
	Problem solving		
Scientific presentation CF conference	*Use of videotape orientations in centers:*	*Regional coordinator contact:*	*Regional coordinator contact:*
	Orientation to the materials	Calls to encourage implementation	Sharing role model success stories
	How to get the program adopted in the CF Center	Technical support	Technical and social support, social reinforcement
	How to organize implementation	Social support	Role modeling
	How to work with families	Social reinforcement	
		Role modeling	
	Newsletters:		
	Information on the program		
	Information on how to do implementation		

dimensions needed to more fully evaluate a program and determine its potential for affecting population health (S. S. Bull, Gillette, Glasgow, & Estabrooks, 2003). Glasgow and colleagues (R. E. Glasgow, Lichtenstein, & Marcus, 2003; R. E. Glasgow, Klesges, Dzewaltowski, Bull, & Estabrooks, 2004) have developed the Reach, Efficacy or Effectiveness, Adoption, Implementation and Maintenance (RE-AIM) model, in which they emphasize expanding program evaluation to five dimensions that should be planned for and evaluated in the process of translating health promotion research into practice.

These processes are the focus of process evaluation, which we discuss further in Chapter Ten. A logical starting point for process evaluation is to determine whether the program was adopted for use. The performance and change objectives for adoption stated as part of Step 5 can be used to guide the formation of questions to evaluate the evidence for program adoption. *Reach* refers to the extent to which the intended target population for the program is exposed to the program. Knowing who was exposed to the various components of the program can help to interpret the findings related to the impact of the program. Program implementation is concerned with completeness, how much of the program was delivered, and with fidelity, whether the program was delivered as designed. The performance and change objectives stated for program implementation can help guide the formation of questions to measure implementation completeness and fidelity. Finally, questions to evaluate the sustainability of the program can be based on the performance and change objectives to address maintenance, institutionalization, adaptation, and capacity building (Lytle, Ward, Nader, Pedersen, & Williston, 2003). As we discussed in Chapter Six, the matrices prepared in Step 2 are used to develop measures for impact evaluation; similarly, the matrices prepared in Step 5 are used to form questions and measures for process evaluation.

Box 9.2. Stroke Project

Identify potential uses of the health promotion program. Revisit the planning group and linkage system to assure representation of potential program users.

The T.L.L. Temple Foundation Stroke Project was a demonstration project in East Texas. Most of the program components were designed to be implemented by the project health educator. Nevertheless, our development advisory committee was important to assure good placement of our community media. The other members of the committee also contributed to setting the context for cooperation of work sites for the one-to-one messages and to hospitals and emergency medical services for the training and organizational development components.

CHAPTER TEN

INTERVENTION MAPPING STEP 6: PLANNING FOR EVALUATION

Reader Objectives

- Describe program outcomes for quality of life, health, behavior, and environment and write objectives and evaluation questions
- Write evaluation questions concerning performance objectives and determinants as expressed in the matrix of change objectives
- Write process evaluation questions based on the descriptions of methods, conditions, strategies, program, and implementation
- Develop indicators and measures
- Specify evaluation design and write an evaluation plan

The product of Intervention Mapping Step 5 is a plan for an evaluation of the process and outcomes of a health education program based on the products from the previous Intervention Mapping steps. In this chapter we do not describe in detail the general techniques of evaluation. A wealth of literature is available for that purpose (Patton, 1997; Rossi, Lipsey, & Freeman, 2004; Shadish, Cook, & Campbell, 2002; Wholey, Hatry, & Newcomer, 1994; Windsor, Clark, Boyd, & Goodman, 2003). The purpose of this chapter is to help planners (also called evaluators in this chapter) use the previous steps of Intervention Mapping to facilitate program evaluation. Therefore, the chapter is organized following the steps of intervention development.

Perspectives

We attempt in this section to clarify evaluation terms, underscore the importance of conducting program evaluations, and remind planners to involve stakeholders.

Evaluation Terms

The development of an evaluation plan is the final step of Intervention Mapping. However, thinking about the evaluation is a parallel process with program planning and begins with the needs assessment. As a matter of fact, most evaluation texts (see Rossi et al., 2004) include program planning or understanding the program as the first part of evaluation. In the evaluation, planners determine whether the intervention was successful in meeting program goals and objectives and why the intervention was or was not successful. Process evaluation is necessary to understand the results from an evaluation of program outcomes.

Outcome evaluation (sometimes referred to as effect or impact) describes the differences in outcomes with and without the program. Possible outcomes of interest include quality of life, health indicators, behaviors, environmental conditions, and program objectives (determinants, performance objectives, and change objectives). Outcome evaluation involves determining whether these factors change as a result of the intervention, which usually means comparing the group that had the opportunity to participate in the program to one that did not. An evaluator does not usually propose to measure all intended program outcomes in an evaluation plan. Proposed measurement will depend on the logic model for the intervention as well as on evaluation resources, stakeholders' interests, and purposes. Outcome evaluation can be described as efficacy, meaning a program evaluated under optimal conditions, for instance, with motivated volunteers who will take part in the program no matter how much time and effort is required, and effectiveness, meaning a program evaluated under real-world circumstances, for instance with representatives of the at-risk group some of whom will not take part or will drop out (Cochrane, 1971; Williamson, 1978; Sackett, 1980; Flay, 1986; Windsor et al., 2003).

Process evaluation seeks to describe program implementation and explanations for implementation status (M. A. Scheirer, 1994; Steckler & Linnan, 2002). Program implementation questions include the following: Is the program being delivered to the persons for whom it was intended? Is the program being delivered in a form that maintains fidelity to its original design? Further, this aspect of process evaluation includes whether theoretical methods have been appropriately operationalized in the program strategies. Process evaluation also attempts to describe the program, organizational, and implementation factors related to why an intervention is being implemented in a certain way. For example, an intervention can be well designed but not well implemented because the planners misjudged the needs of the at-risk group (R. E. Glasgow, Lando, Hollis, McRae, & La Chance, 1993). Alternatively, it can be poorly implemented because the implementers lack certain skills or because there is no one to champion the program in an organization (Bartholomew, Czyzewski, Swank, McCormick, & Parcel, 2000). A program can be poorly implemented at a more basic level if the program designers have not adhered to assumptions inherent in the use of the proposed theoretical change methods, a problem Rossi and colleagues (2005) consider part of the evaluation of the program logic model. In contrast to effect evaluation, which often makes comparisons between groups, process evaluation is concerned with the group that received the intervention. Some process indicators, for example, judgments by the participants about the intervention, can be elicited only from the intervention group. Researchers may also collect process data in the control group, but they do this mostly to find out whether any unplanned intervention may have contaminated the evaluation.

Planners evaluate a program's efficiency in terms of its costs and effects. A cost-benefit analysis monetizes both the inputs and the outputs of a program, whereas cost-effectiveness describes only program inputs in terms of money. Cost-effectiveness avoids controversy that may arise from computing a monetary value for a program's health or social effect by describing the program outputs in programmatic units rather than money. For example, a cost-effectiveness evaluation of a health program that seeks to prevent cases of measles might report the cost of a case of measles averted rather than determining the monetary value (possibly by determining the productivity loss averted). Knowing how program outcomes compare in terms of their cost is important to deciding whether to expand, continue, or terminate an innovative program. The program plan includes a budget and a description of all other program inputs that should provide a basis for an efficiency analysis. This chapter does not present the methodology for efficiency analyses; for these, we refer the reader to other works (M. F. Drummond, O'Brien, Stoddart, & Torrance, 1997; Gold, Siegel, Russell, & Weinstein, 1996; Green and Kreuter, 2005; Rossi et al., 2004; Windsor et al., 2003; Yates, 1997).

Formative and *summative* are terms used to describe the purpose of an evaluation rather than to refer to specific evaluation questions. A formative evaluation is done to obtain information to guide program development or improvement, whereas the primary purpose of a summative evaluation is to make a judgment on whether a program met its goals and objectives.

Reasons for an Evaluation

Evaluation may commonly be thought of within the context of determining efficacy and effectiveness, or it may be thought of as formative pretesting of programs and support materials. However, it is equally important to conduct evaluation as part of program management to provide feedback to improve programs and enable the greatest benefit from scarce program resources (Preskill, 1994). One key to establishing accountability and improving the health promotion program is first to frame the performance and change objectives for both behavioral and environmental outcomes and for program implementation and then to assess whether the program has met these objectives. Our experience is that successful health promotion practitioners tightly monitor the implementation and outome of their programs in order to improve them as they are being conducted, to ensure their ongoing quality, and to justify them for continued allocation of resources.

Perhaps the most exciting reason to perform program evaluation is to generate knowledge. Knowledge about effective programs, good implementation, and useful evaluation methods enriches the field of health education and promotion. A program planner who has used a systematic planning framework, such as Intervention Mapping, should be able to express in the scientific literature the theory of the intervention, its operationalization, and its implementation. If so, a contribution to knowledge will be possible and should depend on the quality of the evaluation, because a poorly conceptualized or described intervention (the downfall of some evaluations) should not be an issue.

Involving Evaluation Stakeholders

An important goal of an evaluation should be that someone uses the results (Torres, Preskill, & Piontek, 1996). To ensure that evaluation results are used, the evaluator must engage the attention of the evaluation stakeholders, including the program consumers, funders, planners, and implementers. Table 10.1 describes possible evaluation stakeholders. Getting an evaluation used requires identifying stakeholders and gaining their participation. Not all types of stakeholders will be relevant for every evaluation, but most programs have multiple stakeholders. The steps in ensuring stakeholder participation (Reineke, 1991) are the following:

- Identify stakeholders and involve them early
- Plan structures for involving stakeholders in the ongoing evaluation process
- Help stakeholders plan how to use evaluation data
- Present evaluation results in multiple forms

Some evaluators would argue that the most important stakeholders from an ethical point of view are a program's intended beneficiaries. These persons stand to be most affected by both formative and summative evaluations. Even when program planners have sought their opinions regarding the program, they often leave program beneficiaries out of the evaluation process. Participatory evaluation

TABLE 10.1. EVALUATION STAKEHOLDERS.

Policymakers and decisionmakers	Persons responsible for deciding the fate of a program including funding, startup, continuation, expansion, and change
Program sponsors and funders	Organizations that initiate and fund a program (can overlap with policymakers and decisionmakers)
Evaluation sponsors and funders	Organizations that initiate and fund the evaluation (health education program and evaluation sponsors often are the same)
Beneficiaries	Persons, households, communities, or other units who are intended to receive the intervention and its benefits
Program adopters	Persons in an organization, community, and linkage system who are responsible for deciding to bring the program in and use it
Program developers	Persons in the resource system and the linkage system who create, choose, or modify the program
Program managers	The personnel responsible for overseeing the intervention
Program staff and implementers	Personnel responsible for delivering the program components or for supporting those who deliver the program
Program competitors	Organizations or groups that offer competing programs and compete for available resources
Contextual stakeholders	Organizations, groups, and individuals who form the immediate environment of a program
Health education community	Health education professionals who read the health education literature and learn from the successes and failures of their peers
Evaluation community	Evaluation professionals who read evaluations and learn from their technical contributions

Source: Rossi, Freeman, and Lipsey, 1999, p. 55.

should include the program's stakeholders, including the at-risk group, and many evaluators are beginning to consider an empowerment approach that includes enhancing the capacity of program stakeholders to perform and use evaluations (Fetterman, Kaftarian, & Wandersman, 1996; Greene, 1988; Mark & Shotland, 1985; Papineau & Kiely, 1996; Torres et al., 1996).

Reviewing the Program Logic Model

Throughout the Intervention Mapping process, a planning group will have developed logic models in order to understand how a program is supposed to work to produce change. We reintroduced the logic model in Step 2 (Chapter Six) and review it here with types of evaluation added (Figure 10.1). Reviewing the

FIGURE 10.1. INTERVENTION LOGIC MODEL.

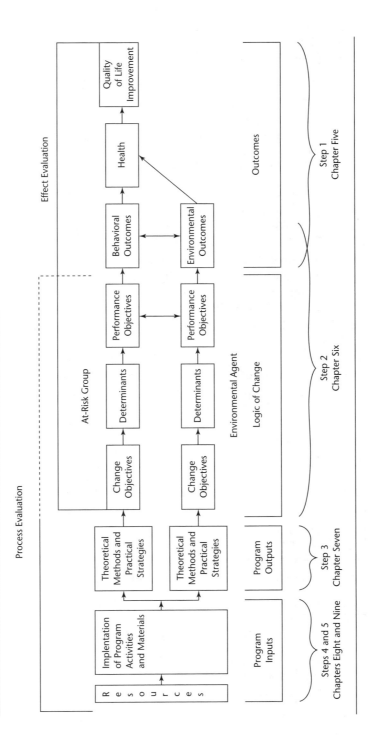

program logic model will enable evaluators to perform the first three tasks of evaluation planning:

1. Describe program outcomes for quality of life, health, behavior, and environment and write objectives and evaluation questions
2. Write evaluation questions based on the matrix; address performance objectives and determinants as expressed in the change objectives
3. Write process evaluation questions based on the descriptions of methods, conditions, strategies, program, and implementation

Program evaluators first need to understand the program they are evaluating and what types of program effects they can expect within the time frame of the program implementation and evaluation. They need to be guided by the theory of the program (Rossi et al., 2004).

If the evaluators are part of the program development team and if the team has used a systematic framework to plan the program, then understanding the program is a fairly simple descriptive step, as explained in this section. However, evaluators are sometimes asked to evaluate a program after it has been developed. In this case the evaluator must backtrack and reconstruct the steps in the planning process. Rossi and Freeman (1993) state, "Clearly, it would be a waste of time, effort, and resources to estimate the impact of a program that lacks measurable goals or that has not been properly implemented" (p. 218). Wholey (1994) suggests an evaluability assessment that includes a description of the program model, assessment of how well defined the model is, and identification of stakeholders' ability to use the evaluation results. An important first finding of an evaluation may be that the needs assessment, formulation of objectives, choice of methods, and translation of methods and strategies into a program or implementation were not appropriately executed.

Rossi and colleagues (2004) describe the evaluation model as the theory of the program and refer to the logic of the pathways for accomplishing program outcomes. Other evaluation experts refer to a theory of action (Patton, 1997) and to causal models (M. A. Scheirer, 1994). Program pathways comprise two parts: the impact pathway, how the program is expected to cause change, and the process pathway, how the program is implemented. In addition, the description of the program pathways includes careful specification of the intended participants.

Box 10.1. Mayor's Project

Our health educator is hard at work finishing up the program plan to present to the city council the next week. She has spread matrices and audiovisuals all across the floor of her office. Just the finishing touches have to be put on the chart that explains the scope and sequence of program activities and the graphic that outlines all of the program partners. Then she can tackle the evaluation plan.

The department head drops in to make sure that everything is progressing for the next week's meeting.

Department head: How is everything coming?

Health educator: Oh, just great. Sixteen members of the task force will be at the meeting. Here's the agenda for the flow of the presentation. You can see that you are giving the introduction. Then later on I have you slated to hand out certificates of appreciation.

Department head: Sounds good. Looks like you are just finishing up here.

Health educator: Yes, I just have to write the evaluation plan.

Department head: (barely under control) What do you mean, write the evaluation plan? Why did you wait until the last moment?

Health educator: (pointing out the folder for the evaluation part of her presentation to the mayor) Look, here's the evaluation model. Of course, I didn't wait until the last minute! You know me better than that!

The whole intervention planning process is, in a way, developing the evaluation plan as you go along. See, here are our health and quality-of-life objectives, behavior and environment changes, change objectives, methods and strategies, program and resources. Here are the pages that show how we are going to measure each outcome, and here is our plan to monitor the process. I just have to wrap some words around it. The plan has been formulating itself for a long time.

The program logic model contains the two program pathways. All the information needed to complete the model should be available from the work done throughout Intervention Mapping. Evaluating the logic of the program pathways is a first step in both determining program evaluability and in evaluating a program (Wholey, 1994). To evaluate program pathways, the planner judges the logic in the causation as well as the evidence and theory used to develop the logic. If planners have carefully used Intervention Mapping core processes to access evidence and theory at each step, then the model should be sound. However, when the evaluator determines that the logic is flawed, the evaluation may stop at that point and the evaluator may recommend that the planners correct the program logic. If the intended intervention has little likelihood of creating the desired impact, then using resources to create and execute an evaluation plan to measure the intended impact would be a waste. The evaluator can help program planners and administrators correct the theory of the program, the program's intent.

Another aspect of evaluating the program pathways is to make sure that the processes being implemented are the ones intended. The program logic model should include enough details to analyze whether the program is being implemented with fidelity to the proposed methods and with the quality and quantity of activities intended.

Impact on Health, Quality of Life, Behavior, and Environment

⊃ *The first task in Step 6 is to describe program outcomes for quality of life, health, behavior, and environment and write objectives and evaluation questions.*

Working from the right side of the model (Figure 10.1), the evaluator looks at the intended impact of the program on health, quality of life, and on the behavioral and environmental causes of the health problem. The planning team will have written program objectives about expected changes in these factors in the needs assessment (see Table 5.4). These objectives form the basis for evaluation questions:

- How much was the health problem changed in the designated time frame?
- How much was the quality-of-life problem changed in the designated time frame?
- What changes in behavior and environmental conditions were achieved?

Determining an Evaluation Time Frame

Determining the evaluation questions, especially about outcomes, requires thinking about the time frame for expected effects. For instance, health and quality-of-life outcomes for the school program to prevent HIV infection (Chapter Eleven; see Table 10.2) could not be evaluated because of the logic and the timing of expected effects from the program (H. P. Schaalma, Kok, et al., 1996). Because the program was designed to reach students before they began having sexual intercourse, changes in behavior were outside the time frame for an initial program evaluation. The behavior of interest was expected to occur a year or more from the time of the program. Therefore, behavior change was not an appropriate short-term evaluation goal, even though it certainly belonged in the program logic model. The short-term impacts that the program developers expected were

TABLE 10.2. EVALUATION OF
A SCHOOL HIV-PREVENTION PROGRAM.

Intervention Mapping Step	Question Focus	Process Evaluation Variable	Effect Evaluation Variable
Step 1: Needs Assessment	*Quality of Life	n/a	Quality of life related to worry about AIDS Quality of life related to AIDS
Step 1: Needs Assessment	*Health	n/a	HIV-Infections AIDS cases Mortality
Step 1: Needs Assessment	Behavior	n/a	Condom use
Step 1: Needs Assessment	Environment	n/a	Condom availability
Step 2: Matrices of Change Objectives	Components of behavior	Correctness of objective specification	Condom use performance objectives
Step 2: Matrices of Change Objectives	Components of environmental change	Correctness of objective specification	Environmental agent objectives
Step 2: Matrices of Change Objectives	Determinants	That chosen determinants are the correct ones That all important behavioral domains are covered	Knowledge Skills Self-efficacy
Steps 3 and 4: Methods and Strategies	Choice of methods Use of methods according to parameters Acceptability of program and materials	Evidence that methods can effect expected change (For example, modeling is effective in stimulating steps of condom use; skill training results in students' ability to make counterarguments against taking risk and demonstrate refusal and condom use.) That strategies convey methods appropriately (For example, students attend to and remember modeled material.)	n/a

TABLE 10.2. EVALUATION OF
A SCHOOL HIV-PREVENTION PROGRAM, Cont'd.

Intervention Mapping Step	Question Focus	Process Evaluation Variable	Effect Evaluation Variable
		That materials and program are culturally relevant— students and teachers find the program salient	
		That materials and program are acceptable to intended users and implementers (both students and teachers like the program)	
Step 5: Program Adoption, Implementation, and Sustainability	Interaction of intended intervention group with intervention	That program is delivered to intended recipients	n/a
		That program is adopted	
		That program is implemented with fidelity and completeness—teachers do all lessons as designed; students read magazine and do homework	
		That program is sustained, routinized, and institutionalized	

*Not included in the final evaluation model because of time frame

changes in knowledge, self-efficacy, and skills. They expected the program to have a longer-term impact that would be observable when the students reached an age at which they were beginning to have intercourse (within a year or two).

Having a clear understanding of the time frame for being able to create certain program outcomes is important to making sure that the expectations for measuring program effects in an evaluation are realistic. Some program funders, planners, and other stakeholders are satisfied with positive outcomes in the process evaluation, such as participation of the at-risk group; others will not be satisfied until they see evidence of a relevant reduction in the health problem and improvement in quality of life (Fishbein, 1996). Our position is that the evaluation should be realistic and take into account the complexity in influencing a health problem. First, intervention outcomes require time to develop. Second, health education is often directed at people's future behavior at a time when a risk behavior has not yet emerged. In this case the desired changes may become observable only years after the intervention. An example of this situation is the promotion of condom use in adolescents who have not yet become sexually active. Third, the intervention itself needs time, especially when the intervention is targeted for long-term change, such as empowerment and community development.

Determining the feasibility of achieving evaluation goals may be a challenge. On the one hand, the planner wants to show outcomes that are meaningful in relation to the health problem. On the other hand, the planner may not reasonably expect certain changes in health outcomes or risk factors to occur shortly after an intervention. An essential part of the evaluation plan is to decide in advance on the level of effects that can be expected within a given time frame. In the example of the HIV-prevention program for schools, the final evaluation goals after two years are for behavior change, in this case for consistent condom use, and changes in determinants, that is, knowledge, self-efficacy, and skills. H. P. Schaalma, Kok, and colleagues (1996) did not include any health or quality-of-life outcomes in the evaluation plan because they did not expect health changes in that respect from the program within the given time frame.

When health changes are not expected or measured in the evaluation plan, the planner must have strong evidence and logical arguments to justify any assumption of causation that is beyond the evaluation's scope. For instance, the planner must document the relation between skills improvement now and the use of condoms and a reduction in HIV infections later. The epidemiologic or experimental evidence and arguments could include:

- The relation between behavior or environment change and change in the health problem
- The relation between change in determinants and change in behavior or environment
- The relation between methods and change in determinants

That last type of evidence is often difficult to document, but it may be based on earlier intervention studies. For instance, there is now some evidence that smoking prevention programs that influence adolescents' perceptions of norms and self-efficacy and that refusal skills can lead to a reduction in the onset of smoking (Centers for Disease Control and Prevention [CDC], 1994a).

Impact on Change Objectives

⟲ *The second task in this step is to write evaluation questions concerning performance objectives and determinants as expressed in the matrix of change objectives.*

Next, moving to the left in Figure 10.1, the planner specifies expected changes in objectives from the matrices, that is, performance objectives and change objectives (see Chapter Six). The first questions concern behavior and are derived from the performance objectives. For example, questions regarding the behavior of the emergency department physicians in the stroke example included the following: Did the physicians perform workups for stroke more quickly after the intervention than they had before? Did physicians order and read CT scans within the time by which treatment must start more often than they had before the intervention? In the HIV-prevention example, questions about behaviors included the following: Did the teens who received the program follow the preparatory steps for condom use more often than the teens who did not receive the program? Did the teens who received the program follow more of the preparatory steps than other teens?

Change objectives combine hypothesized determinants with expected performance, and both should be well specified and documented from Intervention Mapping Step 2. Planners can write evaluation questions looking at the change objectives by determinants (the columns of the matrices). In the HIV-prevention evaluation, the following evaluation questions were derived from the Intervention Mapping work on change objectives: Did the teens who participated in the program increase their knowledge of condom use as compared to teens who did not receive the program? Did teens who participated in the program increase their skills and self-efficacy as compared to teens who did not participate? The importance of the exploration of mediator and moderator variables to explain intervention effects is being widely discussed and demonstrated in the literature (Baranowski, Anderson, & Carmack, 1998; Holmbeck, 1997; MacKinnon, Lockwood, Hoffman, West, & Sheets, 2002; Baranowski, Klesges, Cullen, & Himes, 2004; Baranowski, Lin, Wetter, Resnicow, & Hearn, 1997; Baron & Kenny, 1986; MacKinnon, 1994). Intervention Mapping guides planners to make an explicit model of these variables throughout planning so that evaluators can analyze their relations to the outcomes in the presence of and without the intervention.

Program Process

⟲ *The third task in Step 6 is to write process evaluation questions based on the descriptions of methods, conditions, strategies, program, and implementation.*

The next part of describing the program pathways is to look at the process components, specifically with a description of the intended interactions of the participants with the program. Measuring and attributing outcomes to a program, without insight into whether a program was delivered, what program was delivered, and how it was delivered, is a black box evaluation (Harachi, Abbott, Catalano, Haggerty, & Fleming, 1999; Patton, 1997). A black box evaluation contributes little to any field because the evaluator does not know why a program succeeded or failed. If a program was not successful, the cause could be in the program's impact pathways (that is, the program's theoretical methods and practical strategies cannot cause the intended effects). Or it can be a problem with the process pathways. Patton (1997) offers one extreme example in which the effect of a parenting program was measured before and after the program and compared with a group that did not receive the program. When the results were presented to policymakers, they ended the program because of its ineffectiveness. Several years later the evaluators found that the program had never been implemented at all because of political sensitivities. This situation is an extreme, but not impossible, example of a black box evaluation.

Rossi and colleagues (2004) call these intended interactions with the delivery system of the program the program's utilization plan, which are depicted in Figure 10.2. These interactions are the practical program strategies in operation.

FIGURE 10.2. OVERVIEW OF PROGRAM PATHWAYS.

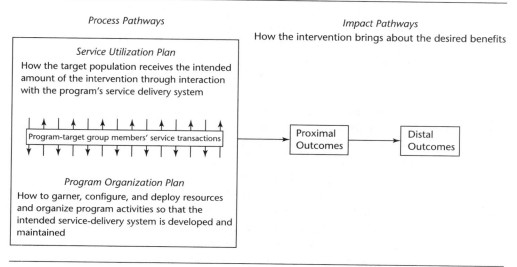

Source: Rossi, Freeman, and Lipsey, 1999, pp. 99–100.

They are the acting out of the methods that the program is intended to deliver to effect change, that is, actualization of the impact pathway. No matter how good the program's utilization plan is, if the interactions with the intended participants do not happen or do not happen according to the parameters necessary to make a method effective, the impact pathway breaks down.

The planner has a description of the intended interactions of the target group members with the program components and should also be able to describe the implementation plan for the program and the program inputs in terms of costs and other resources. Planners should know what theoretical methods they intend to deliver and how those methods were operationalized into deliverable strategies with consideration of the important parameters for the methods. A word of caution: evaluators must remember to verify how the program is actually working in addition to knowing how it should be. Rossi, Lipsey, and Freeman (2004) suggest using both interviews and observations to ascertain what is actually happening in a program. For example, in the Cystic Fibrosis Family Education Program (CF FEP), the developers considered goal setting to be an important theoretical method in the program. However, implementers often delivered the program without setting goals with the patients and families (Bartholomew, Czyzewski, et al., 2000).

The process evaluation will carefully check all the decisions and assumptions that the program developers have made within Intervention Mapping Steps 2, 3, and 4. That information is essential for the interpretation of the findings of the outcome evaluation. If the program fails to show an intervention effect, the process evaluation data can help determine why the program failed. A better understanding of why the program does not work can improve decision making about program modifications. It is very important to the field of health education and promotion that planners critically analyze programs that are not effective to learn from these programs and share the learning with other program planners.

Process evaluation has a place in both formative and summative evaluations and a place in both onetime evaluations and ongoing program monitoring. Process questions generally focus on two points: the amount of the program that is going to the intended participants and the fidelity of the program that is being delivered. Process evaluation can also include exploration of why programs are being delivered the way they are (that is, with or without sufficient quantity and fidelity). Because the focus of Intervention Mapping is on program development, health educators are also very concerned in process evaluation with determining if and to what degree the decisions they have made about program methods and strategies were appropriate. Further, they want to ensure that the necessary parameters have been met as the methods and strategies are translated into a program.

Looking at the process components of the program logic model in this way, first the planner needs a correctly implemented intervention (as stated in the adoption and implementation objectives in Chapter Eight), in which all the assumptions that were made in the methods and strategies steps are realized (Chapters Six and Seven). Then the planner may expect changes first in the determinants and change objectives and then in behavior and environmental conditions. Finally, changes are expected in health outcomes and quality of life (as stated in the measurable objectives related to the health problem and the quality-of-life indicators in Chapter Five).

Linnan and Steckler (2002) describe the following key process evaluation components:

- Context: aspects of the larger social environment that may affect implementation
- Reach: the proportion of the intended audience to whom the program is actually delivered
- Dose delivered: the amount of intended units of each program component that is delivered
- Dose received: the extent to which participants engage with the program
- Fidelity: the extent to which the intervention was delivered as intended
- Implementation: an overall score that shows the extent to which the program was implemented and received
- Recruitment: a description of the approach used to attract program participants

Table 10.3 shows the plan for a process evaluation based on these dimensions. This is the initial plan for evaluating the process of a program intended to deliver a computerized telephone intervention to increase uptake of colorectal cancer screening in veterans.

In the HIV-prevention program for schools, the first evaluation issue was to determine whether the program was implemented completely and correctly. After that the evaluators could explore whether execution of the program met assumptions made in program design, including selection of theoretical methods and practical strategies. If the program was well implemented and the design assumptions were met, the health educators could expect changes in determinants. In other words, they could expect to observe changes in knowledge, negotiating skills, and self-efficacy as those factors pertain to the performance objectives, and they could expect changes in the performance objectives as well, for example, buying and using condoms.

Fidelity and Reach

To formulate process questions, the planner must first fully describe the program that should be delivered. What is each program component? What are the program support materials? What is entailed in complete and acceptable delivery of

TABLE 10.3. PROCESS EVALUATION INDICATORS AND PROPOSED MEASUREMENT.

Components	Indicators	Method
1. Context	Changes in Veterans Administration (VA) colorectal cancer screening (CRCS) guidelines or veterans' access to health care VA's organizational capacity Participant exposure to non-VA CRCS health promotion efforts	Communication with VA staff Tracking CRCS guidelines and reimbursement policies, CRCS demand and VA's ability to meet demand, VA CRCS programs, materials, and policies
2. Reach	Percentage of the intended participants who used the program	Project records during the delivery period
3. Dose delivered	Tailored phone number and length of completed calls and booster sessions	Project records during the delivery period, including phone counselor checklists and telephone counseling system–generated reports
4. Dose received	Percentage calling to request educational materials Attention, remembrance, understanding, and credibility Time and effort spent thinking about the messages	Toll-free phone records Participant recall and reaction to intervention Interviews with random sample of those getting CRCS and those not getting CRCS
5. Fidelity	Degree to which the message is linked to a theoretical methods and strategies and to determinants Match of message to stage of change	Narrative analysis of message concept booklets against Intervention Mapping (IM) matrices, intervention scripts and flowcharts, checklists, and transcripts of conversations

the program? How should the program methods be translated in order to ensure that they produce change? For example, a program might include four meetings with individual families whose children with diabetes were experiencing frequent high blood sugar. A description of the program would include the specifications that the meetings would follow a defined schedule of a meeting every two weeks for two months. Each of the meetings would follow a format in which a self-management problem is delineated and problem-solving steps are used to address the problem.

Process evaluation questions related to the program reach would include the following (R. E. Glasgow, Vogt, & Boles, 1999):

- What proportions of the intended groups are participating in the program? Which groups are underrepresented?
- Are any persons who are not members of the intended groups participating in the program? How many? Do any of them suggest new groups that should be included?
- How much of the program are intended participants receiving? What are the patterns of incomplete doses? What are the main causes?

Process evaluation questions related to fidelity could include questions related to both the program utilization plan and the program organization plan. Questions related to the program organization include the following: Are the type of staff delivering the program those specified in the plan? Do the staff have available program materials? Is time scheduled for the program? Questions related to utilization include these: Is the protocol followed in program delivery? How often is the protocol or parts of the protocol omitted? Which parts are omitted?

Inherent in any process evaluation are performance standards, the minimum level of performance described by experts in a special area (Windsor, Baranowski, Clark, & Cutter, 1994). In the diabetes example just discussed, the program manager could express performance standards or acceptable levels of adherence to both the visit schedules and the protocol elements within the visits. Windsor and colleagues suggest creating an implementation index that combines the reach of the program with the performance standard. Table 10.4 presents a calculation of implementation indices from the hypothetical diabetes program. In the program staff selected seventy-five children with poor blood glucose control for the program. Their parents were notified of the new program and encouraged to enroll. Those who enrolled were invited to counseling sessions every two weeks for two months. The performance standards were that 80 percent of those invited enrolled and that the proportion completing each session showed no more that a 5 percent loss from the session before. The implementation index for program reach was calculated by dividing the proportion reached by the performance standard. In addition, the manager set the standard that 80 percent of the program's intended characteristics should be met in each counseling session. Table 10.5 shows the observation sheet for implementation characteristics that the manager used to judge the implementation. The implementation index for fidelity was calculated by dividing the proportion of implementation guidelines adhered to by the performance standard.

Further, the manager, concerned that the program implementation might change over time, extended the process evaluation table to include implementation beyond the first 75 children (the bottom half of Table 10.4). In the continuing implementation not as many children were eligible because most of the

TABLE 10.4. HYPOTHETICAL PROCESS EVALUATION OF DIABETES COUNSELING PROGRAM.

Procedures	Eligible (A)	Exposed (B)	Percent Reached (B/A) = C	Performance Standard for Reach (D)	Implementation Reach Index (C/D) = E	Percent of Protocol Followed* (C^f)	Performance Standard for Fidelity (D^f)	Implementation Fidelity Index (C^f/D^f) = E^f
Initial Implementation								
Screening for poor control	200	200	100	80	1.20	n/a	n/a	n/a
Enrollment contact	75	75	100	100	1	63	80	.79
Counseling session 1	75	70	93	95	.98	72	80	.90
Counseling session 2	75	67	89	90	.99	80	80	1
Counseling session 3	75	60	80	85	.94	62	80	.78
Counseling session 4	75	59	79	80	.99	64	80	.80
Counseling session 5	75	58	77	75	1.03	70	80	.88
Counseling session 6	75	55	73	70	1.04	62	80	.78
Program Maintenance								
Screening for poor control	125	125	100	100	1.20	n/a	n/a	n/a
Enrollment contact	25	25	100	100	1	72	80	.90
Counseling session 1	25	18	72	95	.76	72	80	.90
Counseling session 2	25	16	64	90	.71	80	80	1
Counseling session 3	25	15	60	85	.71	79	80	.99
Counseling session 4	25	14	56	85	.66	70	80	.88
Counseling session 5	25	14	56	85	.66	70	80	.88
Counseling session 6	25	14	56	85	.66	71	80	.89

*Average percent across all family sessions initial implementation

Source: Adapted from Windsor, Baranowski, Clark, and Cutter, 1994.

TABLE 10.5. IMPLEMENTATION CHECKLIST FOR COUNSELING SESSIONS.

	Present	Absent
The counselor:		
1. Asks how the family has been since last session or from intake	☐	☐
2. Establishes or reviews goal statement	☐	☐
3. Reviews progress on each step of the problem-solving framework, or if first session teaches framework	☐	☐
4. Reviews data collected or presents forms for self-monitoring	☐	☐
5. Reinforces approximations to the problem-solving steps	☐	☐
6. Shows video sequence with role-model story	☐	☐
7. Has the family practice appraisal	☐	☐
8. Has the family practice generation of alternative solution strategies	☐	☐
9. Has the family practice evaluation of alternative strategies	☐	☐
10. Elicits the family's thoughts and feelings about the process	☐	☐

Percent of protocol followed equals number from the "Present" column divided by 10.

children who had less than adequate control were recruited and participated initially. However, there were some newly eligible children and also some children whose parents had dropped out of the program in the first phase. As can be seen in Table 10.4, that group was somewhat more difficult to involve, and reach was not as good. On the other hand, the manager had tightened the training requirements for the staff who implemented the protocol, and the fidelity index improved. The performance standard column of Table 10.4 is the average across all families of the proportion of implementation criteria met in each session. Table 10.5 indicates clearly that the checklist was devised from the Intervention Mapping steps because it represents both implementation guidelines and attention to the detail of how the health educator planned that methods such as role modeling would be operationalized.

In the HIV-prevention program evaluation, Paulussen, Kok, Schaalma, and Parcel (1995) asked teachers about program adoption and use (Table 10.2). For instance, they asked about familiarity with the program and whether the teachers used the program in the previous year. Fidelity was assessed with the question, How did you use the program? Teachers could answer with the following choices: "took some ideas," "took many ideas," "as a guiding principle," "followed most of the instructions," "followed the instructions completely." The teachers were also asked, Have you used other materials along with the program materials?

Reasons for Fidelity and Reach

In the next part of the process evaluation, the evaluator will want explanatory data for the extent and fidelity of implementation. What barriers were there for implementation? For example, in the CF FEP evaluation of program diffusion and implementation, the evaluators found that the program was implemented with only moderate fidelity. A major reason for the lowered fidelity was the lack of skills of program implementers to engage in the goal-setting process (Bartholomew, Czyzewski, et al., 2000). In the HIV-prevention program evaluation (H. P. Schaalma, Kok, et al., 1996; H. Schaalma, Kok, Poelman, & Reinders, 1994), teachers were also asked questions or presented with statements that could explain implementation failure, such as this: "Is AIDS prevention a structural part of your curriculum?" (The answer choices were "yes" or "no.") "The program is sufficiently flexible to be used in classes with substantially different subgroups (ethnicity, sexual experience)." (The answer choices were "agree" or "disagree.") Schaalma and colleagues interviewed teachers a second time, based on their responses on the questionnaire, to better understand implementation barriers.

Methods and Strategies

Questions related to the decisions made in program planning, that is, questions about program methods and strategies and their operationalization, have been addressed to some extent in the pretesting and formative evaluation of the program (see Chapter Eight). The only difference is that now the planner can test the intervention in its final form and its final setting instead of in a provisional form and in a simulated setting. Again, evaluators do not deal with effects here but with judgments, such as satisfaction, positive emotional reaction to the materials, an understanding of the message, a determination of whether the program was of help, or conversations with peers about the program.

Selecting and Developing Measures

⟩ *The fourth task in Step 6 is to develop indicators and measures.*

The development of measures will be guided by the matrices developed in Step 2 (Chapter Six). A planner usually sets program objectives that are stated in terms of health status, functional status, behavior, environment, and determinants. These objectives may specify an amount of change and a time frame, but they usually do not specify an indicator of the change. The first task in determining an indicator is to define the construct being measured. For example, a program objective may be to increase the functional status of elementary school children with asthma by 25 percent in two years. An evaluation question may be: How much did the functional status of elementary school children with asthma change? Now the problem is, What is an indicator of functional status in children that can be measured in a program evaluation? The construct of functional status can be defined as the ability to conduct normal activities of daily living unlimited by disease. Children are usually not limited by disease if they can attend school, can have achievement congruent with aptitude, and can engage in playtime and physical activity with other children. So indicators of functional status in children with asthma could be number of school days attended, grades, achievement, participation in physical education, and time spent playing after school.

A *measure* is a device for quantifying or categorizing an indicator. A measure usually entails applying numbers to indicators. For example, an evaluator interested in grades achieved could measure this construct in many different ways. A measure could be a year-end achievement test, an average of numerical grades achieved in all subjects, an average of numerical grades achieved in math and language arts (core subjects), and so forth. Likewise, the other indicators of functional status can be measured in numerous ways. Using the asthma program objective from the previous paragraph, the indicator of participation in physical education could include the number of days the child attended school, the number of days without a doctor- or parent-excused absence, time spent in moderate to vigorous movement, and so forth.

This section presents some guidelines for defining constructs from Intervention Mapping and for developing the measures of the constructs. However, advice on measurement theory and on the ways that other evaluators have measured similar constructs must come from the measurement literature (DeVellis, 1991) and from the literature on a specific construct.

Reliability and Validity

Validity in measurement basically means that the evaluators are measuring the construct they think they are measuring. Rossi and colleagues (2004) describe demonstrations of validity as depending on a comparison that shows that the measure "yields the results that would be expected if it were, indeed, valid" (p. 220). Examples of these comparisons are the following:

- When the measure is used with other measures of the same variable, results should be the same.
- When the measure is applied in situations thought to be different on the variable, the results should be different.

- Results on the measure are correlated with other characteristics expected to be related to the outcome.

If planners have used Intervention Mapping carefully, they have clearly specified the health, quality-of-life, behavioral, environmental, and determinant constructs that will eventually be measured and have provided a good basis for beginning to establish validity. Intervention Mapping Steps 3, 4, and 5 also provide the basis for clarity about what the program is and how it is to be implemented, constructs that will be important in process evaluation.

Reliability, on the other hand, is stability in measurement. If evaluators measure the same construct at two points in time, or if two different observers record the same event, will they get the same answer? Reliability concepts include consideration of sources of error. For example, a child may understand questions about asthma symptoms or self-efficacy or any other construct differently at two points in time based on the question's complexity, a distraction in the environment, or help received. Reliability can also be diminished through procedural problems, such as asking the question in different ways or transcribing data inaccurately.

Intervention Mapping contributes much less to the consideration of reliability of measurement than to validity questions, and again we refer the reader to the evaluation and measurement literature.

Selecting Versus Creating Measures

Often researchers receive requests to use measures from their program evaluations from health educators who are looking for valid and reliable measures with which to evaluate their interventions. These requests always bring forth the question of how close a match is the instrument under consideration to the specification of the construct they are trying to evaluate. Certainly, considerable effort goes into the development and pilot testing of measures, but even a highly reliable measure will do an evaluator no good if it is not valid for the intended measurement purpose. In a hypothetical example, an evaluation team wanted to assess whether a program has met its goal of increasing asthma knowledge among school-age children; it must decide whether to use an existing measure or to create one. The team looked at a recently published report of a measure of asthma knowledge for children. It has good reported internal consistency and test-retest reliability. It also was found to be sensitive to pretest and posttest program change. Should the team use that measure? Well, that depends. What does it measure? It is possible that an instrument could measure a very broad construct asthma knowledge without the specification of the construct matching what the asthma team needed. What were the items on the measurement blueprint from which the items for the measure were sampled? What domains of asthma knowledge do they represent? How well do the domains and items match the knowledge that was taught in the program the team is assigned to evaluate? Table 10.6 represents the domains of asthma knowledge in which the evaluators were interested compared to the domains reported in the published article. There is not a good match; therefore, the published measure is not appropriate for the new purpose. This point about validity to the purpose will become even clearer as we describe measurement development from Intervention Mapping in the next section.

Outcome Measures

In the planning for the effect evaluation, evaluators will have stated questions related to program impact on quality-of-life and health problems from the measurable objectives the planners defined in the needs assessment. They also will have stated questions related to change in behavior and environmental conditions that are thought to have an impact on quality-of-life and health problems, and they will have identified questions related to the hypothetical determinants that must be changed in order to have an impact on behavior and environment. The evaluators' next task is to develop indicators and measures that will enable them to generate answers to each of the questions.

Determinants

Change objectives are the most specific objectives for program development and for effect evaluation. Using the same principle as for intervention development, the evaluator organizes the change objectives by determinant to create a blueprint for each measure related to evaluation questions concerning change in determinants.

TABLE 10.6. COMPARISON OF DOMAINS OF ASTHMA KNOWLEDGE.

Published Measure Domains	Domains Underlying the Program to Be Evaluated
Anatomy of the respiratory system	Monitoring asthma symptoms
Physiology of asthma	Figuring out personal triggers
Causes of asthma exacerbations	Using an asthma action plan
Rescue and control medicines for asthma	Managing an episode
	Staying in control

For example, if there is an evaluation question about change in knowledge, then the change objectives for knowledge (the knowledge column in a matrix) can be used as a blueprint for measuring knowledge. Looking at the columns of a matrix as blueprints for measuring a construct in the specific way it was used for program development is a good way to begin developing construct validity for the specific evaluation purpose. Thus, the indicators for program evaluation are the determinants specified in Step 2, and the change objectives linked to each of the determinants serve as the basis for items in a scale to measure the determinants. The program evaluator then constructs scales for each of the determinants following the measurement methodologies typically applied to the specific type of determinant. For example, if change objectives for adolescents in a program to prevent sexually transmitted infection (STI) included self-efficacy for performance objectives related to condom acquisition, use, negotiation, disposal, refusal, and so on, then the blueprint includes self-efficacy change objectives for all these behaviors. However, the evaluator must go to the literature on self-efficacy to determine how the construct is typically measured and use this literature as a guide for developing the actual instrument (Basen-Engquist et al., 1999; Forsyth & Carey, 1998; E. Maibach & Murphy, 1995; Maurer & Pierce, 1998). The evaluator should also consult an original source regarding the construct and its measures, in this case Bandura (1997).

The *Familias* matrices presented in Chapter Six can be used as an example. To devise measures of determinants of asthma management, the evaluator can look down the columns on the matrix (Table 6.6) for change objectives related to determinants such as knowledge ("Describe possible symptoms of asthma"; "Identify patterns of asthma symptoms over time") and self-efficacy ("Express confidence in identifying symptoms and environmental conditions"; "Express confidence in being able to notice symptoms"; "Express confidence in being able to link symptoms to exposures"). For every change objective in a column, the evaluator may formulate one or more questions. To measure knowledge, for example, the evaluator may ask directly, "What are the symptoms of asthma?" and provide people with a list of alternatives or ask an open-ended question.

Behavior and Environmental Conditions

Most health problems have a combination of behavioral and environmental causes. Sometimes it is easy to choose a behavioral evaluation objective, for instance, the consistent use of a child restraint device to prevent serious damage to the child in case of an accident. Often the decision is more complex; for example, there are many components to a healthy diet to prevent cardiovascular diseases. One behavior evaluation objective could be a reduction of fat intake by consumers; an environmental condition evaluation objective could be the industry's reduction of the percentage of fat in some popular foods. The best indicator for behavior is the list of performance objectives for behavior changes in Intervention Mapping Step 2, and the best indicator for environmental conditions is the list of performance objectives for environmental changes, also in Step 2.

From the list of performance objectives, measurement items can be selected based on the objective's importance, pilot testing of the measure, statistical analyses such as factor analysis, and feasibility of administration. The evaluator should make sure to select items that represent all domains of objectives and that domains are not underrepresented after the planners have tested the measure and deleted poorly performing items.

For example, based on Project SPF's needs assessment of sun exposure in young children, a number of behaviors for parents and teachers (the child's interpersonal environment) were identified to reduce sun exposure for the child (Tripp, Herrmann, Parcel, Chamberlain, & Gritz, 2000). The following behaviors were chosen for parents and teachers in the children's interpersonal environment:

- Apply SPF 15+ to children before their exposure to the sun
- Reapply SPF 15+ sunscreen to children when no longer effective (every 1.5 to 2 hours, or after swimming or profuse sweating)
- Dress children in protective clothing, such as hats, sleeved shirts, long shorts, and sunglasses
- Direct children to play in shaded areas

Measurement of these behaviors might best be conducted by observation. However, they could also be measured by self-report of behavior or intentions, for instance, "I (plan to) apply sunscreen (SPF 15 or higher) to my child at least thirty minutes before going outside" (with answer categories of "always," "frequently," "sometimes," "rarely," and "never"), and "I (plan to) reapply sunscreen to my child every 1.5 to 2 hours after the child has been swimming or sweating profusely" (with the same answer categories).

These five behaviors related to sun exposure can be described in more detail that identifies performance objectives. For example, the performance objectives for the first behavior, "Apply sunscreen (SPF 15 or higher) to child at least 30 minutes before child goes outside" are the following:

- Purchase or obtain sunscreen (SPF 15 or higher)
- Spread sunscreen evenly
- Cover all exposed areas from head to toe

In order to measure the behaviors (or intentions) in more detail, questions about these performance objectives could include, "I (plan to) purchase or obtain sunscreen (SPF 15 or higher)" (with answer categories of "always," "frequently," "sometimes,' " rarely," and "never"), and "I (plan to) spread sunscreen evenly over my child" (with the same answer categories).

These questions are examples of a self-report approach to measuring behavior. When evaluators use self-report measures they should, when feasible, validate them against observation. In the sunscreen example, parents may think that they apply the sunscreen correctly, but they do not; or parents may answer the questions in a socially desirable way so that they make a good impression on the researchers, when in fact their behavior is different from what they report. Observing the actual behavior—for example, of the parents in the sunscreen program—may be a necessary additional measure of behavior.

Observation may be necessary for testing the validity of self-report questions in a pilot test. Then, if there is a large discrepancy either observation should be used or if that is not feasible the evaluators can test methods of improving self-report (Aday, 1996). Such methods include the "bogus pipeline" in which those providing self-report are informed that they may be observed or some other source of verification may be used (Roese & Jamieson, 1993). Another option is to include response options that are socially more desirable than the target behavior (Mullen, Carbonari, Tabak, & Glenday, 1991; Mullen, Cabonari, & Glenday, 1991).

For some behaviors the measurement issues and methods are very complex and will require the program evaluator to become knowledgeable about the scientific basis for their measurement. For example, behaviors such as smoking (Prokhorov, Murray, & Whitbeck, 1993), nutrition (De Moor, Baranowski, Cullen, & Nicklas, 2003; McPherson, Hoelscher, Alexander, Scanlon, & Serdula, 2000; F. E. Thompson & Byers, 1994; Warneke, Davis, De Moor, & Baranowski, 2001), and physical activity (Masse et al., 1998; Pereira et al., 1997; Sidney et al., 1991; Treuth et al., 2004) have established and tested standardized instruments or methods for measurement. Many government agencies and institutes have developed compendia of measures on their health and behavior issues. The National Institute on Alcohol Abuse and Alcoholism (NIAAA) and the National Institute on Drug Abuse (NIDA) both have good examples (U.S. Department of Health and Human Services, NIAAA, 1995; U.S. Department of Health and Human Services, NIDA, 1997). For each of these behaviors, there is extensive scientific literature on measurement. The program evaluators will need to review this literature and decide whether existing measurement tools match well with the stated performance objectives. If several options are available, then the decision will be to choose the one that best fits the performance objectives and program participants.

If there is not a good fit with the performance objectives, then the evaluators may find it necessary to develop new questions or instruments to measure the behaviors. The design of reliable and valid instruments to measure the evaluation objectives is beyond the scope of this chapter; however, readers can use several texts to help guide them (Devellis, 1991; Mahoney, Thombs, & Howe, 1995; National Cancer Institute, 1989; Osterlind, 1989; Tryon, 1985; Windsor et al., 2003).

Health and Quality of Life

The primary source for deciding what to measure to determine whether the health promotion program had an effect on health is the needs assessment (Chapter Six). In the needs assessment, the program planners identified the health conditions that contributed to poor quality-of-life outcomes and were caused by behavior and environmental conditions. The needs assessment led to the statement of measurable objectives for health and quality-of-life outcomes. Choosing measurable evaluation indicators that are related to the health problem, as was done in the needs assessment, can be simple or difficult. In an example of fireworks injuries on New Year's Eve, a reasonable health outcome indicator is injuries caused by fireworks. In an example of patient education for chronic diseases, a health outcome indicator could be a reduction in emergency visits to the hospital, which also can be accomplished in a fairly short time frame (Mesters, van Nunen, Crebolder, & Meertens, 1995). However, in cancer prevention establishing a health outcome indicator is more difficult. A reduction in cancer morbidity and mortality could only be described over an extended time period (ten to twenty-five years or more). Therefore, the best short-term indicators for cancer morbidity and mortality are probably to be found in behavior changes, such as smoking and diet, and not in health outcomes.

Sometimes evaluators can identify indicators for the health problem that are measurable at an earlier stage. AIDS diagnoses, for example, follow the infection after about ten years, but a measurable short-term indicator would be a reduction of cases of HIV infection after a limited number of years, depending on the intervention. An alternative would be to use STI cases as a proxy indicator. For cardiovascular diseases, indicators could be serum cholesterol levels, blood pressure, and weight. However, the consensus on these indicators is not always strong. Moreover, many health education programs are directed at younger people, anticipating effects on future behavior, which means that the health outcome evaluation objectives are all long-term objectives. Once the indicators are selected, the evaluator develops a protocol for measurement. For example, a typical protocol for the measurement of lung function would include the daily calibration of the spirometer, the performance of three measures, and the use of the best score.

The selection of indicators for the measurement of quality of life is also based on the needs assessment. In the needs assessment, program planners identified specific outcomes that they considered to be the consequences of the health problem or the behavioral factors and environmental conditions (see Chapter Five) (Green & Kreuter, 2005). The indicators may be stated at the individual level, such as days lost from work, happiness, self-esteem, and alienation; or at a societal level, such as crime, crowding, discrimination, and unemployment. Thus, measurement can be made by collecting data from the population to evaluate the program outcomes for individuals as well as by collecting data from organizations or governmental agencies that track potential social indicators of quality of life. The field of quality-of-life measurement is developing at a fast pace, concurrent with the incorporation of this type of measurement into many clinical trials. In the public health field, quality of life is increasingly being considered as an important outcome for health promotion and disease prevention programs (R. E. Glasgow et al., 1999; Hennessy, Moriarty, Zack, Scherr, & Brackbill, 1994). Recently, extensive efforts have been directed at developing measures of quality of life that are especially relevant to and sensitive to health-related factors. The CDC has developed indices for health-related quality of life (HRQOL) based on a series of survey questions that are used in the Behavioral Risk Factor Surveillance System (CDC, 1994; Hennessy et al., 1994; Hough, 1999). The advantage of using a standard measure of quality of life, such as the HRQOL measure, is that results from one study or program evaluation can be compared with data from the Behavioral Risk Factor Surveillance System or to findings from other studies. Such a comparison allows the program evaluators to know how quality-of-life indices for their population compare to those of other populations and allows evaluators to determine whether quality of life improves as a result of the program. The disadvantage of a standardized measure of quality of life is that it may not be specific to the health problem that the program addresses and therefore not sensitive to change even if the health outcomes do improve.

The measurement of quality of life has important time-related factors that need to be considered when developing a program evaluation model. The time needed to detect an improvement in quality-of-life outcomes, as in health outcomes, may be long after the health promotion program takes place, especially for broad societal measures that may require decades of intervention to make a difference. Some of the individual-level indicators, such as happiness or days lost from work, may be more sensitive and therefore measurable within the time frame for evaluating the health promotion program. The point is to select those measures of quality of life that are sensitive to change within the time period allocated to evaluate the program's effectiveness.

Design Issues

⟳ *The final task in this step is to specify evaluation design and write the evaluation plan.*

Qualitative Methods for Process Evaluation

Qualitative research paradigms range from an inductive method (Lincoln & Guba, 1985; A. Strauss & Corbin, 1990) that uses grounded theory, in which theoretical propositions emerge from the empirical research, to a deductive approach (Miles & Huberman, 1994; R. Yin, 1994), which uses conceptual models of the objective world and pattern matching. Qualitative methods include the case study, focus groups, interviews, observations, document review, and open-ended questions on surveys.

The data obtained using qualitative methods must stand up to scrutiny in terms of reliability and validity. Qualitative study designs must enable the accumulation of valid and reliable observations. Reliability has been defined as the extent to which the same observational procedure in the same context yields the same answer however and whenever it is carried out (Kirk & Miller, 1986). Other approaches to reliability emphasize dependability or auditability, meaning that other researchers can follow the decision trail of the original investigator (Lincoln & Guba, 1985). Validity is viewed as the truth value or credibility of the findings. Credibility is increased through prolonged engagement; through the investment of sufficient time to understand the phenomenon being studied; through persistent observation to understand what aspects of the situation are most relevant; and through triangulation of sources, methods, investigators, and theories. Other techniques include peer debriefing and member checks (Lincoln & Guba). Construct validity can also be viewed as the relationship between the conceptual model being studied and the evidence collected in the field (R. Yin, 1994). A study of a human experience is credible when people who have had the experience can recognize the description as their own or if those who have not had the experience can recognize it even though they have only read the study (Sandelowski, 1986). Internal validity, which relates to causal relationships in quantitative methods, is closely related to truth value and credibility. R. Yin suggests the techniques of pattern matching and explanation building to enhance internal validity.

N. H. Gottlieb, Lovato, Weinstein, Green, and Eriksen (1992) used focus groups, structured interviews, and written comments of surveys to identify factors associated with the implementation of a restrictive work-site smoking policy. They used a conceptual model in which the smoking policy concept and organizational context produced an implementation process, including communication, administrative procedures, and management support, which resulted in intended and unintended outcomes. A quantitative survey assessed exposure of communication regarding policy, beliefs, policy-related behaviors, and tobacco use among employees. The triangulation of these methods enabled the investigators to gain a clearer understanding of the policy implementation and impact.

The Purpose of Designs for Outcome Evaluation

The purposes of designs for process evaluations and for outcome evaluations are different. In an outcome evaluation, the purpose of the design is to enable the evaluator to answer two questions:

- How do indicators of desired program effects compare before and after the program?
- Can changes noted be attributed to the intervention being evaluated?

The first question requires a design in which the evaluators measure program outcomes before the program implementation (usually referred to as baseline or pretest measures) as well as after the program has been conducted (follow-up or posttest measures). Sometimes multiple follow-up measures are made to monitor how long it takes for change to take place or how long change is sustained once it does occur.

However, change in the outcome measures over time may result from influences other than the health promotion program being evaluated; these call for the second question and the need for designs that include a comparison group. For example, if a smoking-cessation program is implemented and evaluated during the same period as a national trend in reduced rates of smoking, the possibility exists that the observed evaluation outcomes are the results of secular trends rather than the program interventions. Therefore, the evaluator also needs to know whether there is a difference between people participating in the program and those not participating. This added feature leads to a design containing pre- and postprogram measures in exposed and nonexposed groups. An important methodological principle in program effect evaluation is ensuring comparability between treatment and control groups on as many factors as possible that may influence the outcomes of interest. This principle is most easily adhered to by using an experimental design with random assignment of participants to the intervention group and a control group. However, it can also be accomplished with a number of quasi-experimental designs in which the treatment group is compared to itself at more than two time points or is compared to another group that is not defined by random assignment (Shadish et al., 2002).

In health education practice, randomly assigning individuals is often impossible. For instance, students from secondary schools cannot randomly be assigned to a school program or a control program, because the program is schoolwide or at least classwide. In that case it is possible to randomly assign units to the program condition or the control condition. When randomization of individuals or units (that is, schools, clinics, work sites, communities) is not possible, quasi-experimental designs allow the evaluator to compare two or more groups that are as similar as possible. Evaluators have to expect that the groups are not completely equivalent, meaning not completely comparable on a number of relevant characteristics, and evaluators cannot even assume that they know all the relevant characteristics. Statistically, evaluators can control for most of these differences, but only when the differences are measured before the program starts (Shadish et al., 2002; see H. P. Schaalma, Kok, et al., 1996, for an example). We encourage the reader to consult texts on program evaluation (Shadish et al.; Rossi et al., 2004; Windsor et al., 2003) for more specific guidance on selecting a design for program evaluation.

Whether evaluators use a random assignment or a quasi-experimental design, they sometimes want to find out whether their intervention is more successful than the standard program or practice. In this situation the control or usual care comparison is not a condition without a program but a condition with the usual program. The evaluators are estimating program effects for the new program compared to usual care or practice. This group is usually called a comparison group rather than a control group. Randomized experimental design using these two groups provides the strongest basis for straightforward answers to the question, Did the program have an effect? However, an experimental design for program evaluation is not always possible and not always the preferred design for all program evaluations.

The Evaluation Plan

An evaluation plan includes the evaluation questions, design, indicators and measures, and timing of the measures. The plan should also include a description of how the evaluator will analyze and present the resulting data to the stakeholders. Finally, the plan should outline the resources required to conduct the evaluation. Table 10.7 provides an outline for the evaluation plan and includes examples from the school HIV-prevention program that was presented in the discussion of evaluation models earlier in this chapter (H. P. Schaalma, Kok, et al., 1996; H. Schaalma et al., 1994). The evaluation plan should contain details about how the evaluation will be carried out: what data will be collected, who will collect it, what resources will be needed, and how the data will be analyzed and reported. For example, the plan in Table 10.7 suggests that a survey instrument will be developed that includes

TABLE 10.7. EVALUATION PLAN SUMMARY: SCHOOL HIV-PREVENTION PROGRAM.

Evaluation, Variables, and Proposed Design	Measures	Sources	Data Collection Timing and Resources	Data Analysis	Reporting
Process Evaluation Plan					
Adoption					
• Awareness	Survey	Teachers	Prior to program, project research assistant (RA)	Frequencies	Report to the linkage system
• Agreement to conduct program	Record review	Project records	Prior to program, RA	Frequencies	Report to the linkage system
• Participation in teacher training	Observation	Teacher training	Prior to program, RA	Summary memos on observations	Report to the linkage system
Implementation					
• Lessons completed	Teacher records	Teachers	During program, RA	Frequencies	To the development team, scientific literature, schools, and funder (each implementation indicator)
• Activities executed	Observation	Research staff	During program, RA	Frequencies	
• Time per lesson	Surveys	Students	During program, RA	Means	
• Scheduling of lessons	Interviews	Teachers	During program, RA	Means and summary memos	
• Use of video	Surveys	Students	After program, RA	Summary memos	
Intervention Assumptions					
• User evaluation	Surveys	Teachers	1 week following program, RA	Frequencies	To the research team, scientific literature, schools, funder, and participants (all intervention assumption indicators)
• User evaluation	Interviews	Students	1 week following program, RA	Comment summaries	
• Participant exposure	Surveys	Students	1 week following program, RA	Means	
• Method and strategy assumptions	Content analysis	Materials and lesson review	Before program, project team leaders	Table of content analysis	

Effect Evaluation Plan

Quality of Life(QOL)					
• QOL Health	Not measured	n/a	n/a	n/a	n/a
• HIV infection	Not measured	n/a	n/a	n/a	n/a
• AIDS cases	Not measured	n/a	n/a	n/a	n/a
• STI cases	Health Department Registry of STIs	Health Department surveillance	Baseline and years 3,4,5	Change in pre- and post-intervention incidence rates compared between groups	To research team, schools, funders, scientific literature, and participants
Behavior					
• Condom use	Survey questions	Intervention and control groups	Baseline, six-month, and one-year follow-ups	Pre- and post-intervention change scores compared between groups	To research team, schools, funders, and scientific literature (behavior and environmental condition)
Environmental Condition					
• Availability of condoms (condom machines)	Observations	Businesses	Baseline and one-year follow-ups	Pre- and post-intervention change scores compared between groups	
Determinants					
• Knowledge and self-efficacy	Knowledge and self-efficacy scales	Intervention and control groups	Baseline, six-month, and one-year follow-ups	Pre- and post-intervention change scores compared between groups	To research team, schools, funders, scientific literature, and participants
• Cues	Observation	Schools	Baseline, six-month, and one-year follow-ups	Pre- and post-intervention change scores compared between groups	
• Skills	Not measured	n/a	n/a	n/a	

scales to measure the personal determinants of knowledge and self-efficacy and questions to measure the performance of using a condom. The survey will be administered to subjects in an intervention group and a control group both at baseline before the intervention and at follow-ups six months and one year after the intervention. An observation instrument will be developed and used to measure an increase of condom machines in locations where adolescents have access and to measure the placement of posters that serve as cues for using condoms. Finally, health department reports on STI cases in adolescents will be used as a proxy measure of HIV infections at three, four, and five years following the intervention's implementation. The plan also includes the decisions not to measure quality of life, because the time period would not allow for HIV prevention to have an impact, and not to measure skills, because developing a reliable and valid measure of skills that could be applied to a large number of people would be difficult.

Box 10.2. Stroke Project

Figure 10.3 is the final logic model for the stroke project. It enabled us to review all of the possibilities for asking evaluation questions. Because this was a pilot project with limited funding, we were unable to complete an evaluation of all aspects of the project. In this part of the stroke example, we indicate the evaluation questions we asked and answered and those that we would have addressed if a more complete evaluation had been possible.

FIGURE 10.3. INTERVENTION LOGIC MODEL FOR EVALUATION.

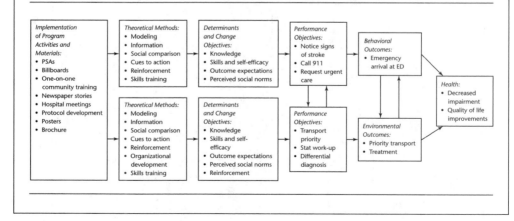

Evaluation Questions

⮫ *The first task in the evaluation step is to describe program outcomes for quality of life, health, behavior, and environment and write objectives and evaluation questions.*

We did not ask evaluation questions about health status and quality of life. These questions had been addressed in the trials of the stroke treatment, recombinant tissue plasminogen activator rtPA. Had we asked this level of evaluation questions, they would have concerned decreases in disability and case fatality rates from stroke. However, we asked both process evaluation questions and questions regarding behavior. We present the tasks related to asking and answering these questions together in this section.

⮫ *The next task in the evaluation step was to write questions based on the matrix.*

⮫ *Another task is to write process evaluation questions based on the descriptions of methods, conditions, strategies, program, and implementation.*

⮫ *A final task covered in this section is to develop indicators and measures.*

We also did not ask evaluation questions based on the change objectives and determinants because the cost was too high. These questions would have concerned change in the determinants of knowledge, skills, self-efficacy, outcome expectations, perceived social norms, and reinforcement.

The major focus of this evaluation was in changes in behavior of community members and the health care environment. See the evaluation plan in Table 10.8. The questions concerned whether the program decreased the time between stroke onset and arrival at the emergency department and whether stroke patients received treatment.

Evaluation Design and Plan

⮫ *The final evaluation task is to specify evaluation design and write a plan.*

The study used a quasi-experimental comparison-group design within two communities. The intervention was located in the community of the sponsoring agency. The comparison community was chosen to provide matched hospitals and similar nonurban demographic characteristics. Both communities were in east Texas, and they did not have overlapping media orbits. Each community was far enough from Houston so that referral to Houston for acute stroke care was prohibitive without an initial stop at a local hospital. The intervention community contained five hospitals in Angelina, Nacogdoches, and Shelby counties, Texas. The comparison community contained five hospitals in Jefferson and Orange counties, Texas.

TABLE 10.8. EVALUATION PLAN.

Variable	Evaluation Question	Indicator	Measure
Effect Evaluation—Behavior of Community			
Time to emergency department (ED)	Did the intervention have an impact on time between stroke onset and arrival at the ED?	Time between last seen normal to ED arrival	Minutes from medical record
Effect Evaluation—Health Care Environment			
Receipt of stroke treatment	Did the intervention increase the proportion of patients receiving rtPA?	Patients receiving rtPA	Medical record indication of receipt (as against all stroke and all eligible by time window)
Process Evaluation			
Reach	How many community members were reached with one-on-one intervention, posters, and brochures?	Persons counted in trainings	Sign-in sheet
Fidelity	Did the strategies and program components contain appropriate role models and role model stories?	Presence or absence of messages from matrix determinants	Analysis of program materials and activities

Findings

The community with the intervention increased the proportion of eligible patients (those who arrived within the three-hour time window) who received treatment to about 70 percent, up from about 12 percent. The comparison community increased from about 5 percent to about 20 percent. Among all stroke patients, the treatment community increased treatment from less than 1 percent to almost 10 percent, and the comparison community increased from no treatments to about 1 percent.

We conducted 488 community train-the-trainer workshops resulting in 634 trainers to deliver personal messages to 49,527 persons. The trainers distributed sixty thousand brochures. We placed five thousand posters in work sites, placed five billboards, and produced and aired two rounds of public service announcements on radio and television.

With health care providers, we were able to conduct the organizational change intervention with all five hospitals and 3 emergency medical services. We held protocol development meetings, trainings, and opportunities to practice called mock stroke codes. We delivered newsletters to emergency departments throughout the implementation and used the community news media to link community and health care environment methods.

PART THREE

CASE STUDIES

CHAPTER ELEVEN

A SCHOOL HIV-PREVENTION PROGRAM IN THE NETHERLANDS

Herman Schaalma and Gerjo Kok

Reader Objectives

- Conceptualize how to perform a study of determinants for program planning
- Use theory to guide the selection of determinants and methods
- Translate methods into practical strategies

HIV infection and AIDS in the Netherlands are mainly limited to men having sex with other men. In 1994, when this program was developed, 337 people in the Netherlands were diagnosed with AIDS; 63.7 percent were men having sex with other men (Nationale Commissie AIDS Bestrijding, 1995). However, at the time we developed this program, there had been a small increase in the AIDS prevalence among the heterosexual population. In 1994 17.5 percent of the diagnosed AIDS cases were attributed to heterosexual contact, 12.4 percent to intravenous drug use.

Despite the low prevalence of AIDS cases among young people, there were several reasons to address HIV prevention programs to this population. A significant spread of HIV among the heterosexual population could not be ruled out. Because of HIV's long incubation period, young adults diagnosed with AIDS might have contracted HIV as teenagers; by November 1994 in the Netherlands, 22.3 percent (527) of the people diagnosed with AIDS were young adults, ages 20 to 29. A considerable proportion of the general population, including young people, did not practice HIV-preventive behaviors (Brugman, Goedhart, Vogels, &

Van Zessen, 1995; Vogels & van der Vliet, 1990), and because of the growing epidemic of HIV infection, young people faced increased risk of exposure. In addition, a health education program targeted prior to the population's formation of the risky behavior patterns could result in primary prevention of infection (Basch, 1989). Finally, it is relatively easy to expose young people to HIV prevention activities through the school system, whereas it is rather difficult to reach them after they have completed their secondary school careers.

This chapter presents the development of an HIV prevention program in Dutch secondary schools. At the time we began this project, one of us (Kok) also was developing Intervention Mapping. We were following Intervention Mapping steps without necessarily naming them so, and this chapter represents in part a post hoc analysis of the program development in Intervention Mapping terms.

Perspectives

Health educators and promoters are often in the position of developing programs without a clear understanding of the determinants of behavior or environment relevant to the health problem. The emphasis in this chapter is the use of a careful study of determinants in program development. Even though health educators are not always able to perform an extensive determinants study, attention to developing a strong (hypothetical) list of facilitators and barriers to behavior is always necessary.

Intervention Mapping Step 1: Needs Assessment

The needs assessment focused on behavioral and environmental risk factors for HIV/AIDS and the determinants for those factors found to be important and changeable.

Behavioral and Environmental Risk Factors

For Dutch young people, the behavioral risk factors related to HIV infection are having vaginal or anal sex without using a condom; performing oral sex so that ejaculate, vaginal fluid, or menstrual blood enters the mouth; injecting drugs with shared hypodermic needles; and receiving a tattoo with infected needles. Of these behaviors unprotected heterosexual intercourse, primarily vaginal intercourse, is the most prevalent mode of HIV transmission (Brugman, et al., 1995; Vogels & van der Vliet, 1990).

In 1986 the Alan Guttmacher Institute presented the results of an international comparative study on teenage pregnancy (E. F. Jones, 1986; E. F. Jones, Forrest, Henshaw, Silverman, & Torres, 1988). The Netherlands was reported to have the lowest rate of unwanted pregnancies among teenagers of all industrialized countries. The researchers of the Guttmacher Institute attributed this low rate of unwanted pregnancies to effective use of contraceptives, especially birth control pills. The Institute report further attributed the effective use of contraceptives to a pragmatic and liberal attitude toward sexuality and sex education, the high quality of information and education on sex and contraception at secondary schools and in the mass media, and the wide availability of confidential and low-cost contraceptive services. In line with this climate regarding sex education, the large majority of schools provide education on HIV prevention (Paulussen, Kok, Schaalma, & Parcel, 1995), and condoms can be purchased in every drugstore and in almost every supermarket. Neither school policy favoring HIV education nor condom availability seem to be major environmental risk factors for HIV infection among young people, but both may be positively related to young people's safer-sex behavior.

Determinants of Safe Sex

When we began program development, there were very few studies of the determinants of safe-sex behaviors among Dutch youth (H. P. Schaalma, Kok, Braeken, Schopman, & Deven, 1991). Therefore, we needed to explore these determinants before undertaking intervention development. We hypothesized major determinants of behavior based on the Theory of Planned Behavior (TPB) (Ajzen, 1991; Montaño & Kasprzyk, 2002) (see Figure 11.1). These determinants were attitudes toward safe sex, beliefs concerning the consequences of practicing safe sex, beliefs about social influences regarding practicing safe sex, perceptions of others' sexual behavior, and beliefs about self-efficacy with regard to practicing safe sex (Bandura, 1986).

We used both qualitative and quantitative methods to explore the determinants (see Figure 11.2). First, we conducted a review of the literature using the topic approach (see Chapter Three) about young people's contraceptive and HIV-preventive sexual behavior to get initial ideas about the determinants of safe sex. To highlight and broaden these ideas, we used focus group interviews with students as well as interviews with youth workers, local health educators, and secondary school teachers. Table 11.1 provides an outline of focus group and interview questions. Subsequently, we administered two surveys to the youth: the first addressed the determinants of condom use and sex without intercourse, HIV and AIDS knowledge, sexual behavior, and risk perceptions; the second addressed condom use.

FIGURE 11.1. THEORY OF PLANNED BEHAVIOR.

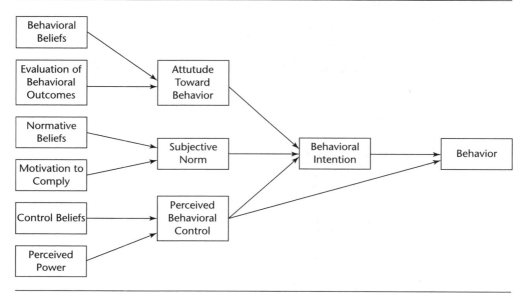

Source: Montaño, Kasprzyk, and Taplin, 1997, p. 92.

TABLE 11.1. EXAMPLES OF FOCUS GROUP AND INTERVIEW QUESTIONS.

Do you think young people should practice safe (or safer) sex when having sexual intercourse? Do you think that the prevention of human immunodeficiency virus (HIV) and other sexually transmitted infections (STIs) is relevant for people your age? Why? Why not?

Do you think that infection with HIV or another STI is relevant for you personally? Why? Why not?

What are, in your view, the most important advantages of condom use when having sexual intercourse? Why?

What are, in your view, the most important disadvantages of condom use when having sexual intercourse? Why?

Do you think that your peers and classmates practice safe sex to prevent HIV and other STIs? Have you ever discussed safe sex with your friends? If so, can you elaborate on that?

In your view, what is the opinion of your parents and brothers and sisters with regard to safe sex and young people? Have you ever discussed safe sex with your family? If so, can you elaborate on that?

Have you ever had sexual intercourse? Did you practice safe sex? Why? Why not?

Suppose you decide to practice safe sex in the future. When or in what situations might this be a difficult thing to do? Do you expect any difficulties with bringing safe sex into practice? Which? When? Why?

FIGURE 11.2. AN ITERATIVE APPROACH TO DETERMINANT STUDY METHODS.

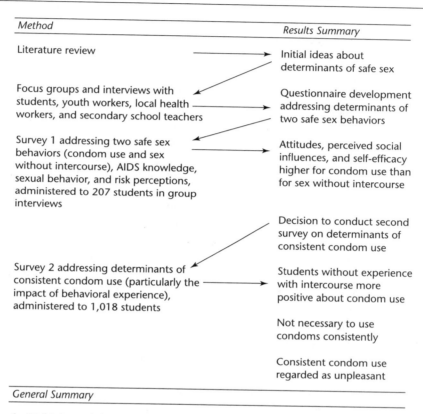

Method

Results Summary

Literature review

Initial ideas about determinants of safe sex

Focus groups and interviews with students, youth workers, local health workers, and secondary school teachers

Questionnaire development addressing determinants of two safe sex behaviors

Survey 1 addressing two safe sex behaviors (condom use and sex without intercourse), AIDS knowledge, sexual behavior, and risk perceptions, administered to 207 students in group interviews

Attitudes, perceived social influences, and self-efficacy higher for condom use than for sex without intercourse

Decision to conduct second survey on determinants of consistent condom use

Survey 2 addressing determinants of consistent condom use (particularly the impact of behavioral experience), administered to 1,018 students

Students without experience with intercourse more positive about condom use

Not necessary to use condoms consistently

Consistent condom use regarded as unpleasant

General Summary

1. Well informed about HIV; some confusion between HIV and AIDS

2. Did not consider personal risk

3. Did not perceive relationships as short

4. Experience with intercourse and condoms related to less positive attitudes

5. Condom use not perceived as practice of peers

6. Trouble resisting pressure to practice unsafe sex

7. Self-efficacy in ability to negotiate use related to intention to use

Table 11.2 provides an outline of the first survey questionnaire. The team pretested the questionnaire using group interviews with students to assess comprehensibility, length, and language. We then administered it to 207 students (mean age 15.8 years). This survey revealed that attitudes, perceived social influences, and self-efficacy expectations concerning condom use were more positive than were attitudes, social influences, and self-efficacy expectations concerning sex without intercourse. Consequently, students' intention to use condoms was significantly higher than their intention to have sex without having intercourse. This finding implies that education should emphasize condom use to prevent HIV because this behavioral option seems to be the most realistic for young people. We therefore decided to focus a second survey on the use of condoms to prevent HIV infection.

The second survey emphasized the impact of behavioral experience on the determinants of consistent condom use (H. Schaalma, Kok, & Peters, 1993). Experience of intercourse may affect beliefs about condom use, perceived social norms, and self-efficacy (Bandura, 1990; Fishbein & Ajzen, 1975). Information about the impact of behavioral experience on the determinants of condom use is sparse, even though it may be particularly relevant for HIV education. We administered a questionnaire to 1,018 students (mean age 15.1 years).

The results confirmed the hypothesis that, in addition to attitudes, perceived social influences and self-efficacy expectations were important determinants of intentions to use condoms. We also learned detailed information about beliefs and expectations that differentiated students with positive condom use intentions from those with negative intentions.

On average, Dutch students seemed to be quite well informed about AIDS and HIV prevention. However, misunderstandings existed with regard to the distinction between having AIDS and being HIV-positive, HIV's incubation period, and HIV transmission. Although students were generally well aware of the risk of HIV transmission, they did not consider it to be their problem, especially not when having a relationship they regarded as being steady. They did not seem to endorse the fact that their relationships are usually short (about three months) and that being monogamous within these relationships is not an effective method of HIV prevention.

Students without experience with intercourse generally had positive attitudes toward consistent condom use, but there was a marked decline in the popularity of condom use after students had begun having sexual intercourse. Although students with experience regarded using condoms consistently as a sensible thing to do, they did not consider it necessary, especially when having intercourse with a partner they knew relatively well. Moreover, they were likely to regard consistent condom use as being unpleasant, creating an annoying interruption, reducing sensitivity, and decreasing pleasure.

TABLE 11.2. OUTLINE OF DETERMINANTS SURVEY QUESTIONNAIRE.

Variables	Questionnaire Items
Demographics	What school do you attend?
	What is your grade level?
	What is your age?
	What is your religious background?
Knowledge (answers range from "yes" to "no" to "don't know")	You can tell from a person's looks whether or not he or she is infected with AIDS.
	You can contract AIDS by sharing toilets or bathrooms with an AIDS patient.
Risk (five-point scale from "very little" to "a very great chance")	Suppose you have unprotected sexual intercourse with a one-night stand. What are, in your view, the odds of contracting AIDS?
Attitude (seven-point scale from "agree" to "disagree")	The use of condoms reduces the pleasure of lovemaking.
	If you want to use condoms because of AIDS, you distrust your sex partner.
Social influence (seven-point scale from "they do" to "they do not")	Do you think your parents want you to use condoms consistently to prevent HIV infection?
	Do you think your best friends use condoms consistently to prevent HIV infection?
Self-efficacy (seven-point scale from "yes" to "no")	Do you think you have the guts to buy condoms in a drugstore?
	Do you think that you are able to use condoms when you are drunk?
	Suppose you are on holiday and you have a date with a nice boy or girl. One night you both want to have sex. You took condoms along and planned to use them.
	Do you think you are able to bring up the subject of condom use?
	Do you think you are able to resist pressure to have sex without a condom?
Behavioral intention (seven-point scale from "yes" to "no")	Suppose you want to have sexual intercourse with a girl whom you have been dating for a couple of months. She is using oral contraceptives. Do you plan to use a condom?

Most students endorsed the health-related advantages of condom use. These advantages, however, did not differentiate students who used condoms from those who did not. Beliefs about the disadvantages of condom use in general (for example, reduced pleasure), disadvantages of condom use because of HIV (for example, distrust), and beliefs about the necessity of condom use in specific situations (for example, when having intercourse with a regular date) did differentiate students with low intentions to use condoms from their counterparts with high intentions.

Although perceived social influences with regard to using condoms consistently were moderately positive, young people did not perceive condom use as current practice among their peers. Generally, students had the idea that their parents, peers, and friends might favor safer sex, although a lot of them had no idea what others think or do with regard to AIDS prevention. The positive social influence of parents was striking and conflicting with the general assumption that young people tend to become more independent of adults and to conform to their peer group. Perceived social influences of young people without experience with intercourse were more positive than were those of their counterparts with experience of intercourse.

Although most students without sexual experience were quite optimistic about practicing safer sex, a considerable proportion of students with sexual experience had trouble resisting social pressures to practice unsafe sex. Generally, students' self-confidence in their ability to negotiate condom use was strongly related to their intentions to use condoms. A considerable proportion of the students expected problems with purchasing condoms, carrying them regularly, maintaining consistent use, and negotiating their use. Students without sexual experience, especially girls, were the most likely to expect difficulties with purchasing and regularly carrying condoms, whereas students with experience of intercourse were the most likely to expect difficulties in maintaining consistent use within a steady relationship.

When age and educational levels were considered, the study showed that young teenagers in vocational schools, and, to a lesser degree, students in schools for general secondary education (both types of schools are high school age in the United States) were potentially at risk for infection with HIV or other sexually transmitted infections (STIs) (H. Schaalma et al., 1993). Among these teenagers we found the lowest levels of HIV and AIDS knowledge and a relatively high prevalence of sexual intercourse without the use of either condoms or oral contraceptives. These findings are similar to those of other studies (Brugman, et al., 1995; Vogels & van der Vliet, 1990).

Step 2: Matrices

In this step, planners selected the intervention population, decided which health promoting behaviors and environmental conditions to focus on, and wrote performance objectives. They then settled on a final set of proposed determinants and developed matrices.

Selection of an Intervention Population

On the basis of the needs assessment and practical considerations, we directed the HIV-prevention program to students in the lower grades of schools for secondary education. The large majority, about 80 percent, of these students does not have experience with sexual intercourse. However, these young teenagers in secondary and vocational schools are potentially at the highest risk for HIV infection (H. Schaalma et al., 1993; Vogels & van der Vliet, 1990). These students begin sexual activity at younger ages than do students in other types of schools, and the prevalence of unprotected sexual intercourse is fairly high. Their level of HIV and AIDS knowledge is fairly low, and their attitudes toward condom use to prevent HIV infection are somewhat negative. Furthermore, this was a relatively underserved group in that most Dutch HIV-prevention programs had been developed for young people in the higher grades of secondary schools.

When demographic variables are considered, this population of teenagers can be characterized as having, on average, a low socioeconomic status and a variety of religious affiliations (nonreligious, Protestant, Catholic, and Islamic). The students are from various ethnic backgrounds, especially in the big cities (native Dutch, Turkish, Moroccan, Surinamese, Antillean).

We considered whether or not to differentiate the intended audience on the following variables: experience with sexual intercourse, age, ethnicity, and gender. The question regarding differentiation is whether either the determinants or the performance objectives differ by group. If they do differ and the effect is large, program planners must develop different matrices for the group; if the effect is small, a single matrix will do (see Chapter Five).

We had already seen from the needs assessment that it might be useful to differentiate between young people with and without experience with sexual intercourse, because these two groups differ to a large extent on the psychosocial determinants related to practicing safe sex (H. Schaalma et al., 1993). Experience with sexual intercourse was related to more negative attitudes and perceived social influences toward using condoms consistently. In addition, young people without experience with sexual intercourse primarily anticipated difficulties with buying condoms and initiating a conversation about condom use, whereas experienced students primarily anticipated difficulties with using condoms consistently within a steady relationship. Because sexual experience is to some extent related to age and grade level, it might have been possible to develop different programs for students in the lower and higher grades. However, from a practical point of view, creating two programs would be more costly and would possibly have impeded widespread diffusion of the program. We differentiated the population on the variable of sexual experiences, and differences were considered within the matrices and during program development, so that different messages could be included for the two groups. We focused on young teens so that the program group did not have to be differentiated by age.

Differentiation also could have been gender-based. The needs assessment demonstrated significant gender differences with regard to buying condoms and taking responsibility for condom use. Again, even though gender-specific education may not be a feasible or practical option for classroom practice, we took the differences into consideration during matrix and program development.

Although the role of parents in HIV education is not very clear, we thought it might be worthwhile to include them in a prevention program. We decided not to do this for several reasons. First, involving parents and increasing parent-teen communication about sexual topics may be very difficult to accomplish (D. Kirby et al., 1994). Moreover, Dutch schools are not familiar with the inclusion of educational activities that go beyond the classroom, and a community-based education approach could impede widespread implementation because these approaches are very time-consuming and require intensive organization.

Another possibility would be differentiation based on religious affiliation or ethnicity. Although the needs assessment did not reveal significant differences between the beliefs and behaviors of nonreligious, Catholic, and Protestant students, it demonstrated differences between students with a Dutch background and those with a Muslim background. We did not want different programs based on ethnicity to interfere with the program's nationwide character. Moreover, Muslim girls strongly stated that they did not like the idea that they would be treated as a special group. Therefore, we considered these differences within the matrices and during program development to ensure appropriate role models and messages.

Health Behaviors and Environmental Conditions

Because the needs assessment clearly indicated that condom use is the most realistic option for young people to prevent HIV infection, we focused the program primarily on condom use. After the program students should use condoms when having sexual intercourse, and they should continue condom use during at least their teenage years. Because the population has a mixed religious affiliation, the program should not only address condom use but also nonpenetrative sex and abstinence. This decision was primarily based on implementation considerations: the inclusion of alternative safe-sex options would facilitate widespread diffusion of the program among religious schools.

Regarding environmental conditions, condom use might be increased by a school policy favoring HIV education and by an easy availability of condoms in schools. Because condoms are relatively easy to access in the community, we decided to address condom availability as an external determinant and to focus on students' self-confidence and skills regarding purchasing condoms instead of focusing on condom availability in schools. Moreover, interviews with teachers revealed that school management would strongly oppose making condoms available in their schools. School policy on HIV education had improved in the last several years: for national schools, it had become compulsory, and this education had to go beyond a mere transfer of information.

Performance Objectives, Determinants, and Matrices

In order to effectively use condoms, students should be able to do the following:

- Make an adequate decision about future condom use to prevent HIV infection
- Buy condoms
- Carry condoms regularly
- Communicate about condom use with potential sex partners within the context of both one-night stands and regular dates
- Use condoms correctly and consistently
- Maintain condom use in their teenage years
- Use condoms in relationships that are perceived as steady

The needs assessment and other studies showed that risk perceptions, attitudes, social influences, and self-efficacy expectations are relevant determinants of young people's intentions to use condoms to prevent HIV infection, as well as determinants of actual condom use. Research also showed that young people's attitudes toward condoms, condom use, and communication about condom use are moderately positive and that they perceive norms that slightly favor safe sex. However, many young people do not seem to regard AIDS and HIV prevention as something that affects them personally. Although they generally regard using condoms as a sensible thing to do, many associate condoms primarily with casual sex. Research also revealed that many young people, especially girls, expect difficulties with buying condoms and with carrying them regularly. Furthermore, a lot of young people seem to expect difficulties with communicating about condom use, because this is an embarrassing thing to do and seems to indicate a lack of trust in the partner, especially in steady relationships.

Although research showed that levels of HIV and AIDS knowledge do not differentiate students who practice safe sex from those who do not, basic knowledge is a prerequisite for risk perceptions and other determinants. Therefore, the program should influence knowledge about AIDS and HIV prevention, and it should establish that young people regard HIV prevention as personally relevant.

Subsequently, it should develop and reinforce attitudes and social norms favoring safe sex, and it should enhance students' self-efficacy beliefs with regard to the various behaviors related to safe sex.

Most of the research information is about determinants of the individual's decision making or planning with regard to condom use to prevent HIV infection. There is little information about the antecedents of the specific behaviors related to safe sex that we formulated as performance objectives: buying condoms, carrying them regularly, communicating about condom use, using condoms, and maintaining condom use. Our needs assessment provided some information about attitudes toward communicating about condom use (for example, it is embarrassing, it implies lack of trust, and it is difficult to counter the notion that condoms reduce pleasure) and toward condom use (for example, condom use is annoying and reduces pleasure). The assessment provided specific self-efficacy information about buying condoms, taking them along, communicating about and negotiating condom use, and maintaining condom use. Self-efficacy expectations of students without experience with sexual intercourse were quite low with regard to interrupting sex to put on a condom and with regard to the use of condoms when drunk or when having sexual intercourse with a sex partner for the first time. Furthermore, the needs assessment showed that these students had low self-efficacy expectations with regard to buying condoms in drugstores or from vending machines, although they generally thought that they could manage to get a condom if they wanted to. Self-efficacy expectations with regard to carrying condoms regularly (for example, on a date or at a party) were generally low. Although young people were generally optimistic about their communication skills, many expected difficulties with resisting social pressure to practice unsafe sex (especially boys) and with maintaining safe sex within a steady relationship. In summary, we designed the HIV education program to address the following determinants of students' condom use:

- HIV knowledge and risk perceptions
- Attitudes, especially attitudes regarding the consistent use of condoms for the purpose of HIV prevention
- Perceived social influences, again especially influences regarding the consistent use of condoms for the purpose of HIV prevention
- Self-efficacy beliefs regarding students' ability to buy condoms, take them along regularly, negotiate their use, and use them adequately

See Table 11.3 for a final determinant delineation.

The last task in this step in Intervention Mapping is the translation of performance objectives and determinants into the most immediate focus for program impact, that is, into change objectives. We developed one matrix for this program (Table 11.4).

TABLE 11.3. FINAL DETERMINANT DELINEATION: PERFORMANCE OBJECTIVES—BEHAVIOR.

Determinants	Importance	Changeability	Evidence
Knowledge	+	+++	Basic knowledge about AIDS and human immunodeficiency virus (HIV) prevention is a precondition for a positive attitude toward safe-sex behavior.
Risk perceptions	+	++	Students should at least endorse the fact that HIV prevention is also their concern, even when having sex with relatively well-known sex partners (serial monogamy).
Attitudes	+++	++	Positive attitudes are a major antecedent of condom use, communicating condom use, and maintaining condom use; buying condoms is seen as a male responsibility.
Social influences	++	+	Attitudes and intentions toward condom use are related to perceived social norms; "it takes two to tango."
Self-efficacy	+++	+	Among students without sexual experience, intentions to use condoms are strongly determined by self-efficacy regarding buying, carrying, and using condoms.
			Among students who have sexual experience, condom use is strongly related to self-efficacy regarding communication, use, and maintenance.

Step 3: Intervention Theory-Informed Methods and Practical Strategies

The next step in Intervention Mapping is to link the desired change objectives to theoretical methods. We selected theoretical methods based on a review of theories about changing behavior in general and changing behavior by means of education in particular (general approach to theory selection; see Chapter Three). In addition, we reviewed school-based programs on sex education and health education that had been shown to be effective (topic or issue-related approach to theory selection; see Chapter Three).

This review suggested that an HIV-prevention program based on social cognitive and social influence approaches can be effective (Flay, 1985; D. Kirby et al.,

TABLE 11.4. PERSONAL CHANGE OBJECTIVES.

Performance Objectives	Knowledge	Risk	Attitude	Perceived Social Norms	Self-Efficacy	Availability
PO.1. Plan condom use	K.1.a. Explain the difference between human immuno-deficiency virus (HIV-positive (HIV-positive) and AIDS (HIV incubation) K.1.b. Describe other sexually transmitted infections (STIs) and their characteristics (such as, which ones are most serious and contagious; how to prevent, recognize, and treat) K.1.c. Discuss basic facts about contracting and preventing HIV infection (how it is contracted, what works for prevention, how it affects the immune system)	R.1.a. Recognize that HIV and STI infection is related to behavior, not to risk groups R.1.b. Describe accurate perceptions of the prevalence and incidence of AIDS and other STIs R.1.c. Recognize that they might land in situations in which contracting HIV and STIs can't be ruled out	A.1.a. Perceive that condom use has advantages that are not related to health (such as, absence of regret, lower chance of early ejaculation, no postcoital discharge of sperm) A.1.b. Describe their strong perception of the health-related advantages of condom use and other safe-sex options A.1.c. Recognize that advantages of safe sex outweigh disadvantages A.1.d. Anticipate disadvantages of condom use	PSN.1.a. Explain that peers plan to use condoms		
PO.2. Buy condoms	K.2.a. Name three places where they can buy condoms			PS.2.a. Explain that both boys and girls buy condoms	SE.2.a. Express confidence in ability to buy condoms SE.2.b. Express confidence in ability to deal with embarrassment when buying a condom	A.2.a. Name three places where they can buy condoms

PO	K	A	R	PSN	SE
PO.3. Carry condoms regularly				PSN.1.a. Describe peers as carrying condoms	SE.3.a. Express confidence in carrying condoms regularly SE.3.b. Describe a plan of where to carry condoms
PO.4. Communicate about condom use	K.4.a. Describe the steps of successful negotiation	A.4.a. Express the belief that negotiation will lead to condom use		PSN.4.a. Discuss accurate perceptions of what young people think, fear, and do with regard to AIDS and STI prevention PSN.4.b. Explain the process of social influence and conformity PSN.4.c. Adduce arguments countering proposals to have unsafe sex	SE.4.a. Demonstrate negotiation of condom use or other safe-sex options with potential sex partners (bringing up the subject; resisting proposal to have unsafe sex)
PO.5. Correctly and consistently use condoms	K.5.a. Describe how to put on, take off, and dispose of a condom				SE.5. Demonstrate effective condom use
PO.6. Maintain condom use		A.6.a. Describe a plan to cope with the disadvantages of condom use			SE.6.a. Express confidence in practicing safe sex in difficult situations
PO.7. Use condoms with regular partners			R.7.a. Describe their sexual behavior as "serial monogamous" (rather than monogamous)		SE.7.a. Express confidence in being able to negotiate condom use with regular partner

1994). These approaches posit that the likelihood of an action such as using condoms is affected by the following:

- An understanding what must be done to avoid infection with HIV or another STI (knowledge)
- A belief in the anticipated benefits of risk-reducing sexual behavior (outcome expectations, beliefs about advantages and disadvantages)
- Perceived and actual social influences
- The belief that one can effectively practice risk-reducing sexual behaviors (self-efficacy)

Social Cognitive Theory (SCT also posits change methods of social modeling and peer modeling; skills training, especially social skills; and guided practice in applying information and skills in difficult situations (Bandura, 1986).

In addition to this general theoretical approach, we looked for other theories to address change in the determinants. For example, authors of theories on risk perception and the construct of unrealistic optimism suggested various methods to communicate risk and to attract young people's attention to the program (Hendrickx, Vlek, & Oppewal, 1989; Van der Pligt, 1994; Weinstein, 1989). Theories of attitude change suggested methods for the presentation of information (Eagly & Chaiken, 1993). Theories of fear-arousing communication suggested methods to motivate young people to action (Eagly & Chaiken, 1993; Hale & Dillard, 1995; Holtgrave, Tinsley, & Kay, 1995). Theories about social comparison (J. Suls & Wills, 1991) and conformity (J. C. Turner, 1991) suggested methods to deal with social influences. We discuss these methods in detail later in this chapter.

The next task in Intervention Mapping includes the translation of theoretical methods into practical strategies, such as classroom exercises and educational materials. An essential feature in this step is that theoretical methods are operationalized into effective communication variables (McGuire, 1985, 1986). Although there is extensive information on teaching methods and activities that are frequently used in school-based primary prevention projects (Sussman, 1991), little is known about the effectiveness and practicability of specific teaching strategies. Program developers can overcome their lack of understanding of appropriate strategies by developing programs in collaboration with teachers, educational experts, and students; diagnosing teachers' wishes, needs, and abilities; and pretesting strategies and materials with both students and teachers (Kok & Green, 1990).

In general, students' attention may be enhanced by a positive message and by attractive and appealing information sources and materials. Messages should be geared to students' levels of sexual experience, and the program should use appealing media formats, such as those used by popular television programs and teen magazines. To enhance attraction and comprehension, the program should match students' language and their priorities and values, taking into account differences between genders, ethnic groups, and educational levels (Bunton, Murphy, & Bennett, 1991). Strategies to enhance comprehension are clear organization of information, repetition, and explicit conclusions (Burgoon, 1989). Print materials added to video and class activities may also enhance comprehension, and peers may be a useful source for translating expert knowledge into comprehensible information. Furthermore, teaching strategies based on active learning and participation, such as inquiry teaching and classroom discussion, can enhance elaboration of the message and comprehension (Petty & Cacioppo, 1986a, 1986b). Tables 11.5 and 11.6 summarize the team's choices of methods and strategies.

Change in Risk Perception

Considering the communication aspects of the process of behavior change, a major problem that had to be dealt with was students' perceptions of invulnerability to HIV. Although adolescents are generally very eager to receive education about HIV and AIDS prevention, most students seem to regard themselves as personally invulnerable (Abrams, Abraham, Spears, & Marks, 1990).

Theories of risk perception suggest that these perceptions of invulnerability may be due to unrealistic optimism (Weinstein, 1989). Students may consider themselves as being invulnerable because they underestimate what others do to protect themselves and because they have a stereotypical image of high-risk groups. With regard to the first, the needs assessment showed that a considerable proportion of students had no knowledge of their peers' protective behavior. With regard to the latter, the needs assessment showed that students' perceptions of AIDS risk were strongly related to their ideas about monogamy and promiscuous sex. In their view HIV prevention is especially relevant for people having many one-night stands, and people who have sex only within steady relationships may not be at risk. To deal with risk perceptions and unrealistic optimism, we provided information about the protective behavior of similar others (peers) and about the risks of certain behaviors (such as serial monogamy), so that the adolescents could come to feel that not being in certain risk groups did not protect them.

Studies on risk perception and decision making suggested that people not only base their risk judgments on frequency-based risk information (probability statistics) but also on "information that may aid the construction of an image of the ways in which a particular outcome may occur" (Hendrickx, 1991, p. 28). Various studies have revealed that the cognitive availability of an explanation for an event (for example, catching a disease) increases the assessment of the likelihood of that event and that events that are rated as easy to imagine are judged as more

TABLE 11.5. METHODS AND STRATEGIES.

Method	Theory (Parameters)	Practical Strategies
For Risk Perception		
Scenario-based risk information	Risk Perception (use controllable, small-scale risks with low prevalence; imagery; should describe cause and effects)	Role-model stories in textbooks; videotaped role modeling
Fear appeals	Protection Motivation Theory (moderate fear; present effective coping strategies—high self-efficacy)	Inquiry teaching role-model stories in textbooks; videotaped role modeling
For Attitude Change		
Active processing of information	Elaboration Likelihood Model (high motivation, cognitive ability; personal relevant, surprising, repetition; self-pacing; no distraction; direct instruction; understandable; moderate discrepancy)	Inquiry teaching; group discussion; questionnaire; quiz; interviews
Arguments and persuasive communication	Persuasion Communication Matrix (consideration of source, message, channel, and receiver; reliable and attractive source; strong, new arguments)	Information in print materials; role-model stories in textbooks; videotaped role modeling
Self-reevaluation, linking beliefs with enduring values	Transtheoretical Model, Congruity Theory (stimulate both cognitive and affective appraisal of self-image, cognitive ability)	Role-model stories in textbooks; group discussion; videotaped role modeling
Anticipation of regret	Economic decision making (cognitive ability; must stimulate imagery)	Role-model stories in textbooks; videotaped role modeling; group discussion
Mere exposure	Theories of learning	Print material; classroom demonstration; video demonstration
Associating attitude object with other positive stimuli	Theories of learning	Instruction about pleasurable sexual activities in print material and video
For Dealing with Social Influences		
Social comparison of fears, beliefs, intentions and behavior	Social Comparison Theory; group polarization (identification; positive expectations available in social environment)	Role-model stories in textbooks; videotaped role modeling; group discussion

TABLE 11.5. METHODS AND STRATEGIES, Cont'd.

Method	Theory (Parameters)	Practical Strategies
Enhancement of refusal skills	Social Inoculation Theory (commitment to intentions; motivation)	Counterarguments in print material; group discussion; role-model stories in textbooks; videotaped role modeling; video-guided role playing
For Skills and Self-Efficacy		
Modeling	Social Cognitive Theory (requires attention, remembrance, skills, reinforcement; needs attractive, positive role modeling; coping model)	Role-model stories in textbooks; videotaped role modeling
Enactment	Social Cognitive Theory (should lead to mastery experience; needs feedback and reinforcement)	Video-guided role playing; small-group discussion

TABLE 11.6. SELECTING METHODS: RELEVANCE AND CHANGEABILITY.

Methods from List *(Selected Methods in Italics)*	Relevance	Changeability
Active learning	++	+++
Personalized feedback on risk behaviors	++	++
Risk-scenario information	+	+
Risk-frequency information	+	+
Fear arousal	+	+
Consciousness raising	++	++
Self-reevaluation	++	++
Persuasive communication	++	++
Dramatic relief, anticipated regret	+	++
Heuristic appeals	+	+
Mere exposure	++	+
Social modeling	++	+++
Guided practice	++	++
Feedback and reinforcement	++	+++
Social comparison	++	++
Mobilizing social support	++	+++
Resistance to social pressure	++	++
Prompting	+	+
Forewarning and pre-exposure	++	++
Goal setting	+	+++
Reattribution	+	+

likely to occur than events that are rated as difficult to imagine (Carroll, 1978; Hendrickx et al., 1989; S. J. Sherman, Cialdini, Schwartzman, & Reynolds, 1985). According to Tversky and Kahneman (1983), "a scenario that includes a cause and an outcome could appear more probable than the outcome on its own" (p. 307). Experiments on risk judgments and decision making concerning personally controllable, small-scale risks revealed that available scenario information was more important than frequency information in making risk judgments (Hendrickx et al., 1989). These studies on risk perception guided us to provide the adolescents with scenarios that include a cause and an outcome to make certain contingencies seem more likely.

We used fear-arousing messages that adolescents are personally vulnerable to AIDS and to the losses that would occur with HIV infection. However, we also provided coping methods for reducing the threat and taught the skills for applying the coping methods. Theories of fear-arousing communication suggest that fear appeals may enhance acceptance of health recommendations but that high levels of fear may elicit persuasive-inhibiting responses such as defensive avoidance (Eagly & Chaiken, 1993). Reactions to fear appeals and fear-reducing recommendations mainly depend on people's outcome expectations regarding the recommendations (What will happen if I follow the recommendations?) and their self-efficacy expectations (How confident am I that I can follow the recommendations?).

To arouse moderate levels of fear, we personalized the risk information by using the strategies of inquiry teaching, peer-led teaching, role-model stories in print, and videotaped role modeling. We used strategies to enhance elaboration of the information, including classroom and small group discussion and exercises in which students have to apply the information that is provided, such as completing a quiz or questionnaire, developing an information brochure, and interviewing classmates. Inquiry teaching is preferable to the didactic approach because it reduces resistance to the message and encourages discussion and consensus among group members, which in turn promotes more central processing (see, for example, Flay et al., 1988). We used various sources to provide information. Teachers or experts may be most useful for providing factual information, but peer models or peer educators seem to be most useful for providing scenario-based information. Peer modeling can be included in videotape or in print material by means of role-model stories.

Attitude Change

To change students' attitudes, we chose persuasion, exposure to condoms associated with positive stimuli, stimulation of anticipatory regret, and the promotion of elaborative processing of persuasive arguments that are not too discrepant from the students' current beliefs. Theories of attitude formation and attitude change (for an overview, see Eagly & Chaiken, 1993) suggest that attitudes may change because of new persuasive arguments, preferably regarding short-term consequences of the behaviors involved, and because of the enhancement of the salience of information already possessed, for instance, by linking beliefs with enduring personal values. Reception of information and its persuasiveness may be enhanced by motivating students to engage in elaborative or systematic processing of the information (Eagly & Chaiken; Petty & Cacioppo, 1986). This implies that the HIV-prevention program should not be based on a one-sided transfer of information but that students should be motivated to actively elaborate the information that is presented. The framing of arguments as rhetorical questions, repetition of arguments, and active learning techniques may enhance message-relevant thinking.

Theories of attitude change do not provide clear suggestions for other factors that may affect the persuasiveness of a message, such as its organizational structure, the ordering of arguments, logic, the number of arguments, and the explicitness of conclusions (Burgoon, 1989). However, a two-sided message acknowledging the advantages and disadvantages of condom use may be most valid and as such most preferable because most students will have been or soon will be exposed to arguments opposing the use of condoms.

Social judgment theory (O'Keefe, 1990) suggests that people's existing attitudes distort their perception of the positions advocated in communicators' messages. The theory posits an inverted U-shaped relation between message discrepancy and attitude change: moderate message discrepancy may cause the highest attitude change; extreme levels of discrepancy might even result in boomerang change, in which the person changes away from the position advocated in the communication. This premise implies that the discrepancy between HIV-preventive recommendations and students' current attitudes should not be too large.

Theories of economic decision making (Bell, 1982; Loomes & Sugden, 1982) suggest that choices between behavioral options are determined by the anticipated regret associated with each of these options. Attitudes may change when the potential affective responses to the behavioral options are aroused. We used this principle by enhancing the link between unsafe sex and negative affective reactions, such as regret and worry, as well as the link between safe sex and positive affective reactions, such as relief.

Classical learning theories suggest that attitudes toward condoms may be modified by means of mere exposure (Bornstein, 1989) and by the association of condom use with other positive stimuli (Zimbardo & Leippe, 1991). The first premise implies that students should be exposed to condoms frequently. The latter can be accomplished by means of erotic instructions (Tanner & Pollack, 1988).

Therefore, we exposed students to condoms and paired the exposure with scenes of positive relationships and pleasant sexual behavior.

Change in Perceptions of Social Influences

Methods to influence the way students deal with social influence are information on group norms and skill training for refusal skills. Social comparison theory (J. Suls & Wills, 1991) assumes that people tend to conform to the attitudes and behavior of similar others, partly because those others provide information about social reality and partly because conformity may be socially rewarding. Young people, however, do not usually communicate about sexuality and AIDS prevention, and most of them have only vague ideas about what their peers think and do. We cleared up perceptions of group norms regarding safe sex by providing information about the way peers respond to sexuality and AIDS prevention and by enhancing communication among young people about sexuality and AIDS prevention.

Research on group polarization has shown that group discussions may strengthen group members' initial position because of an exchange of arguments favoring the prediscussion position and because of a comparison of views (Isenberg, 1986). This finding implies that group discussion may lead to a risky shift when the group's average prediscussion position favors unsafe sex. We helped teachers to be alert for shifts to discussion favoring unsafe sex. Teachers were trained to end group discussions when the majority of their students strongly favored unsafe sex. Teachers learned that they also might break with an undesired shift by supporting arguments and views favoring safe sex and by presenting support from other reference groups.

A useful method for dealing with social pressure to practice unsafe sex is the enhancement of students' refusal skills. Skills training based on psychological inoculation (W. J. McGuire, 1964) and social inoculation (R. I. Evans, Getz, & Raines, 1991, 1992) may improve students' ability to cope with their peers' influence toward unsafe sex. The concept of social inoculation (R. I. Evans et al., 1992) suggests a method to increase young people's resistance to social influences to practice unsafe sex by inoculating them with both knowledge and a repertoire of social skills to help them resist such pressures. R. I. Evans, Smith, and Raines (1984) suggest different coping mechanisms for different levels of perceived peer pressure:

- Low-level peer pressure: simple refusal
- Moderate-level peer pressure: persistent refusal, delay of decision, and making excuses
- High-level peer pressure: avoidance and counterpressure

Our program dealt with the interchange of attitudes and values among peers by the strategies of classroom and small group discussion. We included exercises in which values and attitudes were anonymously communicated, such as exercises in which students responded on paper to statements about safe sex, and used these exercises as the basis of subsequent group discussion. Strategies used to accomplish social modeling were role-model stories in print material and role models on videotape. Psychological inoculation was accomplished by providing counterarguments by teachers, experts, or peers presented by means of print material, videotape, and small group or classroom discussion. Role-playing techniques provided students with opportunities to practice counterarguments. Videotapes showed peer models negotiating safe sex in difficult situations, offering models of negotiating skills. Various subskills, for example, purchasing condoms, were enacted in easy situations followed by group discussion or feedback provided by teachers.

Self-Efficacy Enhancement

Methods for self-efficacy enhancement include skills training, mastery experiences, and modeling—all with feedback and reinforcement. To increase their self-belief regarding condom use and related skills, students need encouragement and successful experiences with purchasing condoms, taking them along on a date, negotiating their use, and using them adequately (Basen-Engquist & Parcel, 1992; H. Schaalma et al., 1993). Bandura (1986, 1990) suggests a teaching process with four distinct phases:

1. Breaking up complex behavior into subskills that are easier to handle
2. Modeling to facilitate comprehension of the behavior
3. Guided enactment of the behavior in easy situations, followed by feedback
4. Guided enactment of the behavior in more difficult situations, followed by feedback

Social modeling and peer modeling seem to be effective methods to enhance skills. Adequate feedback and reinforcement may be essential elements in the acquisition of skills.

In the class situation, we limited skills training regarding safe sex to behaviors that are related to the actual sexual behavior, such as decision making, communicating, and resisting social pressures. To compensate for this limitation, we included materials that explicitly demonstrated condom use and ways to handle lifelike high-risk situations.

Step 4: Creating a Coherent Program

Creating a program involves developing a plan that fits the context of the delivery system, designing the program's scope, sequence, and delivery vehicles, and then pretesting and producing program materials.

Understanding the Program Context

Dutch secondary schools can be categorized by religious affiliation and by educational level. Although most of the HIV-education programs that have been developed for different school types have similar goals and methods, possible differences in norms and values should be taken into account. We encountered these differences when the organization of Protestant schools refused to distribute an AIDS program because of what it saw as a one-sided emphasis on condom use. We therefore decided to embed HIV prevention into the broader context of relationship formation and to pay attention to prevailing norms and values regarding sexuality and related matters.

The analysis of the school system further revealed the following issues:

- Schools generally have limited instruction time for HIV education (total for a school year is about four classroom periods; four to six hours).
- The predominant teaching strategies are the didactic approach and the use of textbooks and videotape.
- Most teachers are not familiar with role-playing techniques and are reluctant to implement role-playing.
- Teachers are not willing to invest a lot of time in program preparation or teacher training for an AIDS program.
- Most teachers perceive problems with initiating classroom discussions about sexuality.
- Teachers perceive that students in the lower grades of secondary schools are not able to concentrate on one topic for long.
- Students in the lower grades of secondary schools may have difficulty putting their attitudes and opinions in writing.

Program Scope, Sequence, and Delivery

On the basis of the review of potentially useful strategies and the practical limitations of the school system, we developed four one-class-period lessons that are embedded in a comprehensive program on sexuality (H. Schaalma, Kok, Poelman, & Reinders, 1994). The sexuality program covers topics such as falling in love, the first intercourse, and homosexuality. The program's four lessons are presented in Table 11.7.

TABLE 11.7. PROGRAM SCOPE AND SEQUENCE.

Lesson Number and Goal	Strategies
Lesson 1: To increase knowledge and to change risk perceptions	Inquiry teaching
	Classroom discussion
	Exercises to apply the information that is provided (such as making an information brochure, completing a quiz, interviewing peers)
	Teachers lecture and experts give information in print
Lesson 2: To change attitudes about condom use and safer sex in general	Classroom discussion on the basis of a homework assignment addressing facts about AIDS and sexually transmitted infection (STI) prevention
	Role-model stories in print material covering attitudes about safe sex and problems with practicing safe sex
	Classroom discussion on the basis of statements about practicing safe sex (students respond to statements orally or in writing)
	"Pencil-and-paper"-subgroup discussion
Lesson 3: To strengthen values, social influences, and communication skills regarding the prevention of AIDS and STIs	Homework assignment requires students to respond to situations addressing social pressures ("What would you do when . . .")
	Classroom discussion subsequent to homework
	Teacher-delivered information about the process of social influence (didactic approach or inquiry teaching)
	Peer models discussing safe sex and telling about their attitudes, values, and experiences by means of dramatized videotape and subsequent classroom discussion about videotape modeling
Lesson 4: To enhance students' self-efficacy regarding negotiating and condom use skills	Homework assignment on buying condoms
	Subsequent classroom discussion about buying experiences
	Demonstration and practice of condom use on fingers
	Video-animation of effective condom use
	Interactive videotape showing peer models negotiating real-life troublesome situations and subsequent classroom discussion

The program consists of the following support materials:

- A teacher's manual providing background information and fully worked-out lessons in terms of objectives, materials, and strategies
- A student magazine, similar to popular teen magazines, that presents information about facts, attitudes, fears, and values regarding sexual behavior and HIV and STI prevention

- A videotape showing the process of social influence and conformity, introducing positive role models, and demonstrating dialogues concerning safer sex in difficult lifelike situations

Both the magazine and the video deal with young people's beliefs and values concerning safe sex, reasons for having risk-taking sex, barriers to the practice of safe sex, communication about safe sex, and ways to stand up to direct and indirect pressures to practice risk-taking sex. Besides facts about HIV and other STIs, the magazine provides information about attitudes and values regarding sexual activity and HIV and STI prevention by means of peer role-model stories about values, attitudes, expectations, problems, and experiences.

In order to introduce skills training in the classroom, we developed a dramatized two-part videotape. The first part presents a group of young people making a television program for a local broadcasting company. The video shows them interviewing peers about safe sex and discussing these interviews during the production of their program. The video also presents a girl demonstrating condom use on her boyfriend's fingers and a computer animation of condom use. The second part of the video presents four scenes concerning standing up to social pressures regarding sex. First, a realistic high-risk situation is introduced, for example, a boy pressing his girlfriend to have intercourse. Halfway through the dialogue, the teacher stops the tape, and students complete the dialogue in subgroups guided by specific questions. After these discussions the video resumes playing and presents a positive outcome to the situation. The dialogues, viewing exercises, and teacher instructions for the discussions are based on a framework for resistance to increasing peer pressure based on social inoculation (R. I. Evans et al., 1991, 1992) and are intended to help students build their resistance to social pressure against safe sex in up to six steps:

1. Say what you want
2. Think about the arguments
3. Stick to your opinion
4. Present alternatives
5. Give counterpressure
6. Walk away (avoidance) if counterpressure does not work

Pretesting and Production

An essential element in program development is pretesting, because it allows program planners to gauge the reactions of experts and members of the population at an early stage in a program's life. We tested the intervention materials for attractiveness, comprehensibility, relevance, credibility, acceptability, undesired side effects, and workability with the adolescents. We also tested the feasibility of the program with teachers and educational experts. Interviews addressed the suitability of teaching methods and examined expectations about how long preparation and instruction would take. Some of our originally proposed strategies, such as strategies to disclose sexual values, were deemed to be too radical a departure from usual teaching. Consequently, we revised the program and slightly narrowed the variety of strategies.

The student magazine was first pretested on 147 students, who completed a questionnaire that addressed the page layout and the illustrations' attractiveness. Generally, they evaluated the magazine positively: 79 percent of the students liked it; 54 percent liked the illustrations; 69 percent found it well organized; and 88 percent liked the balance between text and illustrations. In a second pretest, we tested the comprehensibility and persuasiveness of the magazine on 119 students using a pretest and posttest comparison group design. Respondents completed a questionnaire that assessed students' level of HIV knowledge, and the students evaluated the magazine's quality, clearness, usefulness, newsworthiness, and closeness to real life. Both pretests led us to make content and style changes to the magazine.

A synopsis of the video was pretested by means of two group interviews with students. Respondents evaluated the ideas that the video contained and provided suggestions for translating the synopsis into a scenario. We pretested a model scenario among 44 students, using content response coding (U.S. Department of Health and Human Services, National Cancer Institute, 1984), and the off-line montage was previewed by 83 students, who assessed it for attractiveness, credibility, and closeness to real life. Again, pretesting led to changes. We also frequently consulted a student panel during the later development of the program.

Several people contributed to the program's production. A research and development team, including researchers and school health educators, produced the teacher's manual. The student magazine was developed in cooperation with a professional copywriter, graphic designers, and an illustrator. The videotape was developed in cooperation with a professional scenario writer and a film producer. To guarantee the linkage between materials and theoretical methods and strategies, the research and development team closely supervised all activities.

Step 5: Specifying Adoption and Implementation Plans

In this section, we describe how we supported the program's adoption and implementation using materials and training.

Linkage Board

To anticipate problems with program adoption and implementation, we formed a linkage board to bridge the gap between the development team and the school system (Orlandi, Landers, Weston, & Haley, 1990). This board comprised representatives from the development team, the school advisory services, the organizations that provide sex and HIV education to secondary schools, and an association of biology teachers. A member of the development team acted as change agent. The board's role was to provide feedback on the program's performance and change objectives and to give advice on implementation issues.

Performance Objectives, Determinants, and Change Objectives

The next tasks in developing an adoption and implementation plan begin with a decision about performance objectives based on a description of what would occur if the program were well adopted and implemented. Once performance objectives are determined, developers can hypothesize performance determinants and create a matrix of change objectives by combining the performance objectives with the determinants. In order to do these tasks, we explored the determinants of teachers' intentions to teach HIV education.

In the Dutch educational system, the autonomy of schools and teachers is the prevailing norm. No external authority can interfere in the details of the curriculum in schools. Dutch teachers are not mandated to provide HIV and AIDS education, but they can make individual or small-team decisions to adopt and implement HIV-education programs. Teachers of biology, social studies, religious education, or health education are the usual providers of education on sexuality and HIV-prevention, if they choose to do so. Therefore, teachers should be the ones to adopt and implement a program such as ours. The performance objectives for teachers were the following:

1. Become aware of the availability of the new program
2. Adopt the new program
3. Teach the new program according to the development team's guidelines

A questionnaire survey among a sample of 956 Dutch secondary school teachers provided insight into the determinants of their intentions to provide classroom AIDS education (Paulussen, Kok, & Schaalma, 1994). This study, based on a conceptual model with elements of the TPB (Ajzen, 1991), addressed determinants of awareness and adoption of four nationally disseminated HIV-prevention programs. It revealed that teachers' knowledge about HIV programs largely depended on diffusion networks within schools. Both the perceived behavior of colleagues and the frequency of interaction with colleagues played an important role in teachers' acquiring information about HIV-prevention programs. Adoption of HIV education in general was associated with perceived subjective norms, self-efficacy beliefs, perceptions of responsibility, sexual morality, and formal school policy toward HIV education. Neither teachers' general intentions to provide this type of education nor their intentions to adopt a specific program were associated with beliefs about learning outcomes. This finding suggests that teachers are more motivated by immediate concerns, such as ease of program implementation and student response, than they are by expected health or other beneficial outcomes.

The teacher survey further revealed that most of the teachers who were aware of national AIDS curricula (60 percent) had received information about the curricula by written communication (for example, publishers' overviews or direct mail); 16 percent had received information through personal communication with external experts. A considerable proportion of teachers named colleagues as an information source; 63 percent of them knew about a colleague using one of the curricula, and 34 percent had discussed the materials with a colleague. Teachers' awareness was most strongly related to descriptive norms and frequency of collegial interaction (Paulussen et al., 1995).

One out of two teachers had initially implemented one of the HIV curricula. A teacher's decision to use one of the programs was associated with subjective norms and perceived instrumentality (refers to whether the curriculum meets the teachers' primary planning concerns such as time, instructions and anticipated student reactions). A teacher's decision to use a particular curriculum was most strongly related to curriculum-specific beliefs about instrumentality, social norms, and financial costs. The finding of limited impact of teachers' perceptions of the feasibility and importance of student learning outcomes fits with other research on teacher planning behavior, which shows that teacher planning is guided by program content and activities rather than by program objectives. Teacher planning appears to be directed by the teacher's estimated ability to maximize students' participation and enjoyment (C. M. Clark & Peterson, 1986; Shavelson & Stern, 1981).

Based on our review of teachers' intentions to provide HIV education, we hypothesized that targeting the following determinants would be important to facilitate adoption and implementation of our program:

- Knowledge of the program characteristics including a strong perception of the innovative program's advantages
- A perception that the program is easy to implement
- A perception that the youth would like it
- Knowledge of how to acquire the program

- Skills to easily implement the program
- Confidence in their ability to implement the program

Implementation Support

The adoption and implementation plan for postevaluation diffusion included written materials to make teachers aware of the program and its characteristics. The reach of written materials was enhanced by addressing information to individual teachers and to their subject departments as Stokking and Leenders (1992) suggested and by stimulating teacher collaboration. We used brochures with role models who demonstrated short-term benefits, effective use, and positive student participation and learning. In order to facilitate program implementation, we linked our program to a national teacher-training program that was specific to the performance objectives and to a large degree based on social learning techniques. Readers should note that we did not make these efforts for the research evaluation implementation but only for the program's national postevaluation diffusion, which this chapter does not discuss.

Step 6: Generating an Evaluation Plan

Examples from the evaluation of this program are included in Chapter Ten.

Evaluation Model and Questions

We were able to evaluate program outcomes in a quasi-experimental field experiment that included fifty-one secondary schools (H. P. Schaalma et al., 1996). Because our program was intended to reduce sexual risk behavior among young adolescents and because prevalence of sexual risk behavior among these young people is quite low, the emphasis of the program evaluation was on the changes in cognitions and skills. Therefore, evaluation questions related to program effects on behavior, health, and quality-of-life indicators were beyond the scope of our demonstration project.

In addition to expected program effects, we were interested in students' and teachers' evaluation of the program. Does the program match students' reality? Do students like working with the program? Do they perceive it as personally valuable? Does it match teaching practice? Do teachers like working with it? Do they perceive the program as an improvement on their classes on sexuality and AIDS and HIV prevention? Furthermore, we were interested in the way that teachers implemented the various strategies.

Outcome Evaluation Design and Results

We evaluated the potential program outcomes using a pretest and posttest comparison group design (H. P. Schaalma et al., 1996). Participating schools were matched in pairs on the basis of school type, participating grade levels (nine and ten), religious affiliation, degree of urbanization, number of participating students, boy-girl ratio, proportion of ethnic minorities, and qualifications of participating teachers. Within these pairs, schools were randomly assigned to the experimental or the comparison condition. Experimental schools provided education about HIV, STIs, and prevention by using the program; comparison schools provided education about HIV, STIs, and prevention as they had in the past.

Fifty-four schools from a stratified random sample of 415 schools for lower secondary education agreed to participate in the study (13 percent). Nineteen were Catholic schools; twelve were Protestant schools; twenty-one were nonreligious schools; and two schools had a mixed religious affiliation. Three schools were excluded from the analyses because they failed to provide either baseline or follow-up data. In total, seventy-seven teachers participated in the study; thirty-nine were male, thirty-eight female. Most were teachers of health education (38 percent), biology (23 percent), or social studies (19 percent). Students were requested to complete a questionnaire in their classroom about one month before the education on HIV, STIs, and prevention was provided (baseline assessment). They had to complete a comparable second questionnaire four to eight weeks after the education had been given (follow-up assessment). The teachers supervised completion of the questionnaires. The questionnaire was to a large extent based on a model of behavioral determinants distinguishing attitude, social influence, and self-efficacy beliefs (H. Schaalma et al., 1993).

The baseline questionnaire was completed by 3,142 students; the follow-up questionnaire by 2,786 students. The final participating study sample consisted of fifty-one schools and all students whose baseline and follow-up questionnaires the schools could correctly match by school, class, date of birth, mother's initials, and father's occupation (N = 2,430; 77 percent of baseline sample). Unavailability for follow-up was primarily due to absenteeism, transfer to other schools, or missing data on matching variables.

Multilevel regression analyses of students' baseline and follow-up questionnaires revealed that our program had a significant favorable impact on students' HIV and STI knowledge, on their beliefs and intentions regarding consistent use of condoms, and on their sexual risk-taking behavior. The program produced its most pronounced effects within the area of knowledge and attitudes. The changes in perceived social influences, self-efficacy beliefs, intentions, and sexual risk-taking were smaller but still significant. Figure 11.3 presents the effect sizes from the evaluation study.

FIGURE 11.3. EFFECT SIZES.

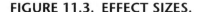

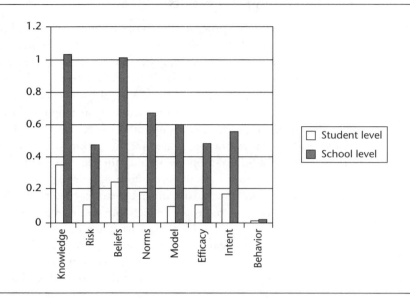

Process Evaluation

In addition to the effect evaluation, the program was subject to a process evaluation. A survey among 1,481 students showed that we managed quite well to match the program to students' perception of their environment. About 75 percent of the students evaluated the program as informative, good, and clear. Only 10 percent of them evaluated the program as difficult and unpleasant, and about 25 percent judged it boring. The student magazine, especially, was positively evaluated: 69 percent of the students evaluated the magazine as attractive, 43 percent as beautiful, 82 percent as informative, 76 percent as good, 83 percent as clear-cut, 8 percent as difficult, and 21 percent as boring. The video was also positively evaluated, although to a lesser degree: 58 percent evaluated the video as attractive, 59 percent as informative, 58 percent as good, 63 percent as clear, 19 percent as lifelike, and 30 percent as boring.

A survey among thirty-eight teachers revealed that we also managed quite well to match the program to teachers' wishes, needs, and opportunities. Most teachers liked the suggested program lessons (82 percent); most of them had the impression that their students had liked the lessons (84 percent); and most of them perceived the program as an improvement on their classes on the prevention of HIV and AIDS and STIs (76 percent). Most teachers evaluated the program as well organized (92 percent), realistic (90 percent), comprehensive (84 percent), applicable in heterogeneous groups of students (68 percent), and superior to other programs (61 percent). However, most teachers also evaluated the length of the program as too long (74 percent). Opinions about the time required for class organization and preparation were mixed. Despite this positive evaluation of the program, teachers' perceptions of the program's impact on their students' sexual behavior were only moderately positive.

In addition to this survey, three other methods were used for process evaluation: classroom observations were conducted using a matrix-sampling procedure; twenty-three teachers who completed the program were individually interviewed; and implementation of the program was monitored by means of structured teacher self-reports. Teachers recorded the number of lessons, the activities they had executed, teaching time per lesson and per activity, and the pace of the lessons and activities. These self-reports revealed that 97 percent of the teachers had implemented the lesson on HIV and STI knowledge and risk perception (average instruction time, AIT, was seventy-six minutes); 96 percent implemented the lesson on attitudes toward safe sex and condom use (AIT, sixty-five minutes); 96 percent implemented the lesson on values, social influences, and communication skills (AIT, sixty-five minutes); and 90 percent implemented the lesson on assertiveness and refusal skills (AIT, sixty minutes). These self-reports also revealed positive reactions to the pace of the lessons and most of the basic program activities. Notably, only a few teachers implemented the homework assignments that addressed buying condoms (25 percent) and interviewing shopkeepers who sell condoms (13 percent).

On the basis of the results of these evaluation activities, we further matched the program to classroom practice. We excluded some of the exercises that none of the teachers had used and adjusted other exercises in accordance with teachers' comments and suggestions. Because the video turned out to be too long, it was reedited. In addition, we somewhat simplified video-viewing exercises.

Summary

The results of the program evaluation showed that a well-planned development process may improve the quality of HIV- and STI-prevention practice. In comparison with previous programs, our program produced a significantly larger increase in students' knowledge about HIV and STIs; greater changes in their attitudes, perceived social influences, self-efficacy, and intentions regarding consistent condom use; and a more favorable behavioral change regarding the prevention of HIV and STIs.

But program development is just a start. To contribute to the prevention of a further spread of HIV and other STIs, the program has to be implemented on a large scale. Research has revealed that a widespread diffusion of innovative school-based HIV- and STI-prevention programs requires strategies that go beyond current mass media promotion activities (Paulussen et al., 1994, 1995). Funding agencies, however, are slow to recognize the importance of widespread diffusion. Despite little financial support, we were able to develop a brochure based on persuasive communication and social modeling, and Dutch secondary schools finally adopted our program.

This chapter may inadvertently suggest that Intervention Mapping goes through the protocol in only one direction. However, this chapter's more or less straight-line presentation is only for the sake of clarity. In practice, Intervention Mapping goes back and forth again and again, and sometimes it even goes two steps forward and three steps back. The protocol leads the planning team to reconsider decisions it has made time and again, and one strength of Intervention Mapping is that it keeps the development process well organized despite its iterative nature.

CHAPTER TWELVE

ASTHMA MANAGEMENT FOR INNER-CITY CHILDREN

The Partners in School Asthma Management Program

Christine Markham, Shellie Tyrrell, Ross Shegog, María Fernández, and L. Kay Bartholomew

Reader Objectives

- Specify behavioral factors and environmental conditions related to chronic disease
- Develop matrices for environmental conditions
- Use theory to specify behavioral performance objectives
- Consider computer technology as a program vehicle

Asthma is a common chronic disease in childhood and a priority for efforts to improve care and control because of its high rates of morbidity, mortality, and health care expenditures (Mannino et al., 1998). While the prevalence of asthma is reported to be 6 percent to 8 percent among children under eighteen years of age, it may be much higher among children living in urban areas, particularly among minority children and those with low socioeconomic status (N. M. Clark et al., 2002; Joseph, Foxman, Leickly, Peterson, & Ownby, 1996).

Asthma has a negative impact on the quality of life and functioning of many children (Centers for Disease Control and Prevention [CDC], 2001a). It can affect school performance and is a leading cause of school absence (Diette et al., 2000;

This work was supported by the National Heart, Lung, and Blood Institute, National Institutes of Health, Contract No. NOI-HR-56079.

Newacheck & Halfon, 2000). Authors have found a relation between asthma and school attendance and academic performance (Fowler, Davenport, & Garg, 1992; Lieu et al., 2002). The school setting is a target for asthma intervention because it may offer unique opportunities to reach children with asthma who have not been diagnosed or who have poor control of their symptoms and limited access to medical care. However, the school setting can also be a cause of asthma problems related to exposure to environmental allergens and irritants or inadequate nursing or medical services for proper medication administration and management of acute symptoms (National Heart, Lung, and Blood Institute [NHLBI], 1997). Although national guidelines emphasize the need for collaboration between the family, school, and health care team, the school has sometimes been left out (NHLBI, 1997). For example, families may not report the child's condition to the school, provide a copy of a written action plan, or assure that medication is available. Schools may not have knowledge or resources to limit exposure to irritants such as outdoor air pollution, create adequate indoor air exchange, and eliminate common indoor asthma triggers.

In this chapter we describe how we used the Intervention Mapping process to develop and implement the Partners in School Asthma Management program, a school-based, multicomponent program for inner-city children with asthma. The program was a demonstration project to develop and test a feasible model for elementary schools nationwide. The project goals were to identify children with asthma and to develop partnerships with families and physicians to provide appropriate asthma care.

Perspectives

The Partners in School Asthma Management program is unique in that it emphasizes the management of asthma-related environmental factors in addition to the behaviors of children, parents, and physicians involved in managing asthma. This program addresses change at the individual level (child), interpersonal level (family, physician, school nurse, and other school personnel), and organizational level (school environment, school district policies and practices). The resulting program has four components: case finding, asthma self-management education for the child and family, a linkage system for physician care, and school environmental intervention.

The program represents innovations in asthma management because it uses interactive computer technology to individualize self-management education. This computer program (CD-ROM) allowed us to teach children using their unique asthma symptoms, triggers, and treatment characteristics. Further, this program uses self-regulatory theory to specify performance objectives and to enable the explicit teaching of self-regulatory processes.

Intervention Mapping Step 1: Needs Assessment

The asthma needs assessment was done according to the PRECEDE model and began with documentation of the scope and seriousness of the rising number of asthma cases and the impact on health and quality of life of certain populations (L. W. Green & Kreuter, 1999, 2005). From the perspectives of self-management or secondary prevention, we also asked: What behaviors and environmental factors are related to better management of asthma and better health and quality-of-life outcomes? The needs-assessment model for asthma was presented in Chapter Two.

Asthma-Related Health and Quality-of-Life Issues

At the time of our program development, asthma morbidity and mortality rates had been rising. The NHLBI expert panel's report (1991) noted an increase in the prevalence of asthma among people less than twenty years of age. The rate rose from approximately thirty-five cases per one thousand persons in 1980 to a rate of approximately fifty cases per one thousand in 1987. A report from the Centers for Disease Control and Prevention (CDC) (1996) established that the asthma death rate among children five to fourteen years of age almost doubled between 1980 and 1993, from 1.7 deaths per million to 3.2.

A study by Crain and colleagues (1994) reported an asthma prevalence (8.6 percent) among inner-city children in the Bronx, New York, twice the typical estimated rate for all U.S. children. Many studies have implicated urban residency, minority status, and lower socioeconomic status as risk factors for increased prevalence of asthma (Crain, et al.; Wood, Hidalgo, Prihoda, & Kromer, 1993). Poor and minority populations, particularly African Americans, living in urban areas have experienced a disproportionately high prevalence of asthma and an increase in morbidity and mortality compared to whites (CDC, 1996; Crain et al., 1994; Cunningham, Dockery, & Speizer, 1996; Gergen & Weiss, 1990; Weitzman, Gortmaker, & Sobol, 1990). Depending on age, African Americans are three to five times more likely than Caucasians to die from asthma (NHLBI, 1991). In a study conducted by Cunningham and colleagues (1996) among 1,416 Caucasian and African American children, race was found to be a significant predictor of the diagnosis of asthma. After adjustment for the demographic and environmental factors, being African American was a significant predictor of active, diagnosed asthma. The study by Crain and colleagues (1994) also showed that the cumulative prevalence of asthma was significantly higher among Hispanics and children from the lowest-income families from the Bronx, New York. The study by Wood and colleagues (1993) found that children with lower socioeconomic status exhibited an excess of severe asthma as well as a greater amount of functional morbidity, such as school absenteeism.

Of chronic childhood diseases, asthma is the leading cause of school absenteeism and poor academic performance (Pope, Patterson, & Burge, 1993; W. R. Taylor & Newacheck, 1992). It has been estimated that children with asthma average 7.6 school days absent, compared with 2.5 days for children without asthma (Fowler, Davenport, & Garg, 1992). Asthma is also responsible for more than five hundred thousand emergency room visits each year (K. B. Weiss, Gergen, & Hodgson, 1992). Asthma hospitalization rates for 1979 were 1.73 per one thousand among infants to seventeen-year-olds, and by 1987 that rate had increased to 2.57 per one thousand (Gergen & Weiss, 1990). Data from the 1988 National Health Interview Survey on Child Health also showed that poor children have diminished accessibility to appropriate health services and higher rates of asthma morbidity, as measured by hospitalization and bed days (Halfon & Newacheck, 1993).

Environment

The risk factors for asthma are multifactorial, comprising genetic susceptibility, early history of pulmonary problems, poor medical management, and environmental factors such as indoor and outdoor aeroallergen and irritant exposure (NHLBI, 1991; C. B. Sherman, Tosteson, Tager, Speizer, & Weiss, 1990; Weitzman et al., 1990). Sensitivity to specific allergens is quite common among persons with asthma, and estimates are that as many as 80 percent of children with asthma have some allergic hypersensitivity to aeroallergens (Burrows, Martinez, Halonen, Barbec, & Cline, 1989; Gergen & Turkeltaub, 1992; Platts-Mills, 1994; Pollart, Chapman, Fiocoo, Rose, & Platts-Mills, 1989). Because children spend most of their time indoors, the home and school environments are important sources of allergen exposure for children with asthma. Asthma has been significantly associated with reactivity to house dust mites, mold, cockroaches, cat dander, and pollens (Gergen & Turkeltaub, 1992; Ingram et al., 1995; Kang, Johnson, & Veres-Thorner, 1993; Platts-Mills, 1994; Platts-Mills, Pollart, & Squillace, 1997; Rosenstreich et al., 1997). For example, in inner-city residents of Chicago, both indoor and outdoor aeroallergen sensitivity was observed in 75 percent of children less than fifteen years of age with asthma, and sensitivity to cockroach allergens was observed in 59 percent of children less than fifteen years (Kang et al., 1993). A study of inner-city houses in Atlanta found significant levels of either mite or cockroach allergens in 86 percent of homes (Call, Smith, Morris, Chapman, & Platts-Mills, 1992). These types of studies are only now being conducted in schools, but the same conditions are thought to exist (Tortolero et al., 2002).

Environmental tobacco smoke has been consistently reported to cause increased lower respiratory infections and increased risk for asthma and asthma exacerbations in children (Emerson et al., 1994; A. B. Murray & Morrison, 1989; Overpeck & Moss, 1991; Samet, Cain, & Leaderer, 1991). A study by Cuijpers, Swaen, Wesseling, Stumans, and Wouters (1995) found passive smoking (during a child's entire life) to be significantly correlated with impairments to all spirometry parameters tested. Smoking in the child's environment should be eliminated, as it has been shown to be an irritant to airways (Hovell et al., 1994). The National Cooperative Inner-City Asthma Study showed that exposure to environmental tobacco smoke is common among inner-city children with asthma: 59 percent reported at least one smoker in the home. Additionally, at the study's baseline testing, 48 percent of children had a cotinine/creatine ratio above 30 ng/mg, a level of significant exposure to tobacco smoke in the last twenty-four hours (Kattan et al., 1997).

Irritants include strong odors such as outside air pollution, paint fumes, chalk, perfume, scented talcum powder, hair sprays, and pesticides (Pope et al., 1993; Swanson & Thompson, 1994). Pesticides must be used with caution in the indoor environment because unsuspected surface contamination of pesticides may occur through air transport through venting ducts, which can become repeated point sources of contamination (U.S. Environmental Protection Agency [EPA], 1995). A steady supply of uncontaminated outside air is recommended by many indoor air studies to keep allergens and irritants to a minimum and carbon dioxide levels to less than one thousand parts per million (Ruhl, Chang, Halpern, & Gershwin, 1993; U.S. Environmental Protection Agency (EPA), Indoor Air Division, 1991). The air ventilation recommendations from the 1989 American Society of Heating, Refrigerating, and Air-Conditioning Engineers Standard 62 for classrooms is fifteen cubic feet per minute.

To confirm suspected asthma-related environmental conditions in local schools, we conducted environmental surveys in sixty elementary schools and dust sampling and allergen assays in a subsample of twenty schools in a Southeast Texas city. Especially high levels of dust-mite allergens and mold were found in many schools, and moderate levels of cockroach allergens were found in some schools. The presence of environmental irritants was also a problem in many schools. Factors that seemed to underlie these conditions included high humidity, poor ventilation, dirty heating, ventilation, and air conditioning systems, and water and carpet damage (Tortolero et al., 2002; Tyrrell, 2000; Abramson et al., 2000).

Eliminating exposure to allergens and irritants has been identified as an important factor in managing asthma in children. Recommendations for control of indoor allergens such as dust mites, cockroaches, and mold include regular vacuum cleaning, washing bedding and stuffed animals weekly and at a high temperature, removing carpet, and reducing humidity. Extensive cleaning and dust-proofing have been shown to reduce asthma symptoms and medication requirements (Bahir et al., 1997; A. B. Murray, 1988; Peroni, Boner, Vallone, Antolini, & Warner, 1994; Sarsfield, Gowland, Toy, & Normal, 1974). Although it has been shown that rigorous measures can reduce allergen levels and symptoms, most of these measures are difficult for families and schools to accomplish. There has been little research on allergens and irritants in inner-city elementary schools or on recommendations for the reduction of these contaminants in the school environment (Dungy, Kozak, Gallup, & Galant, 1986; Neuberger et al., 1991; Norback, Torgen, & Edling, 1990). No studies were available at the time of this program development on school environmental intervention to reduce asthma morbidity. Investigations and recommendations for one elementary school in Kansas City were reported in 1991; however, this investigation focused on sick-building syndrome and did not look at allergens in the school environment, nor were all the irritants investigated specific to asthma (Neuberger, et al., 1991).

Asthma Management

The cornerstone of good medical management of asthma is appropriate pharmacological therapy to control the airway inflammation that underlies asthma episodes (Global Initiative for Asthma, 1995; NHLBI, 1991, 1997). For acute exacerbation, bronchodilators act quickly to relieve constriction and the accompanying cough, chest tightness, and wheezing. However, bronchodilators are not recommended as the only treatment for persistent moderate to severe asthma (NHLBI, 1991). Recent studies strongly suggest that anti-inflammatory agents, particularly inhaled corticosteroids, are the most effective medications in controlling persistent asthma (Britton, Earnshaw, & Palmer, 1992; Djukanovic et al., 1992; Global Initiative for Asthma, 1995; Juniper et al., 1990; Salmeron et al., 1989). In spite of the fact that asthma treatment guidelines from the National Institutes of Health were publicized and widely disseminated to primary care physicians and specialists in 1991 and 1997, there are still misconceptions among physicians about optimal pharmacological therapy; and as a result, anti-inflammatory agents may be underused (Finkelstein et al., 1995; NHLBI, 1991, 1997). In particular, Latino and African American children aged one to six years are less likely than non-Hispanic whites to have used either beta agonists or steroids prior to hospitalization for asthma or to be prescribed a nebulizer on discharge (Finkelstein et al., 1995). Inner-city minority children are not very likely to be treated with anti-inflammatory medications; the reported rates vary from 11 percent to 17 percent of children with moderate to severe asthma (Homer et al., 1996; Huss et al., 1994; Lieu et al., 1997). Furthermore, even though written action plans with medication schedules and criteria have been shown to be associated with lower hospitalizations and emergency department visits, they are seldom provided to patients and families (Dawson, Van Asperen, Higgins, Sharpe, & Davis, 1995; Wasilewski et al., 1996).

Many urban minority children with asthma may be unable to obtain appropriate diagnosis or treatment for asthma (Crain et al., 1994). For example, in a survey of Baltimore public school children, 32 percent of first graders and 43 percent of sixth graders with asthma had received care in emergency rooms rather than from a consistent primary health care provider (Mak, Johnston, Abbey, & Talamo, 1982). Among African Americans, 44 percent used the emergency room as the primary source of care compared with 24 percent of whites, and those using emergency rooms also reported a greater number of school days missed (Mak, Johnston, Abbey, & Talamo, 1982). Wood and colleagues (1993) indicated that Mexican American parents were more likely to use emergency department services as the primary source of care than were non-Hispanics.

Even though school nurses are in a position to assist the child and family with adherence to asthma medications and to serve as a liaison with primary health care personnel to obtain appropriate care for asthma, their role is largely overlooked by families and physicians. Case-finding data from the Partners in School Asthma Management program showed that 62 percent of students identified as having asthma or having symptoms of asthma were unknown to the school nurse (Bartholomew et al., 1999). This finding means that a large number of students who develop asthma symptoms during the school day are unable to receive timely treatment to reduce or prevent more serious exacerbations.

Child and family behavior should play a crucial role in asthma management. However, the foregoing discussion should make it clear that, without environmental support, families cannot do their part to manage asthma. In general, families need support to recognize asthma symptoms and to take steps to prevent symptoms' onset or escalation. These steps include following prescription guidelines for use of routine control (preventive) medications and relief medications for symptoms or episodes; avoiding and controlling indoor and outdoor irritants and allergens; and maintaining a medical care relationship for the primary care of asthma. These behaviors require time and commitment from the child and family. For example, to manage indoor irritants, parents must protect their children from environmental tobacco smoke, and older children must do their part to avoid it. Because children at different ages have different capacities to manage their own daily treatment regimens, another important asthma-management behavior is the transfer of specific responsibilities from parent to child as the child matures.

Needs Assessment Summary

Based on the increasing prevalence of asthma in inner-city children of color and on the burden of the disease in this group, we focused our intervention on these children. We targeted from the health and quality-of-life factors the following program objectives: reduced hospitalizations, emergency room visits, daytime and nighttime symptoms, and increased school attendance and performance. The needs assessment made it clear that the greatest impact on health and quality of life would occur from a combination of enhancing self-management skills and changes in the child's environment, including the medical care environment. These environmental changes are necessary in order for the parent and child to be able to do their parts to manage asthma. Therefore, in this project we focused on children and their immediate context—parents, physicians, and schools—to bring about behavioral and environmental change.

Step 2: Matrices of Change Objectives

In the needs assessment we identified environmental conditions that needed changing, such as inadequate medical care and the presence of asthma triggers in the child's physical surroundings at home and school. We also identified the role of parents and children in asthma self-management. For comprehensive program development, we had two sets of planning matrices: the at-risk group (that is, the child and the parents) and the child's interpersonal and organizational environment (that is, medical care and school). Because elementary school children depend to some extent on their parents to manage asthma, parents were considered together with the children in the at-risk group; and because of their role in medical care, parents were considered to be part of the interpersonal environment as well. To accommodate this complexity, we first discuss the behavior, performance objectives, determinants, and matrices for the child; then we discuss the environmental change, performance objectives, and matrices at the interpersonal levels (medical care change) and organizational levels (school environment change).

Matrices for the At-Risk Group

The first task in developing matrices of change objectives for the at-risk group is to specify the exact behaviors that are to be influenced by an intervention.

Behavior and Performance Objectives. In the needs assessment, we identified such asthma-specific behaviors as identifying triggers and taking medication; but, as we began to develop the intervention, we elaborated our conceptualization of behaviors using theories of self-regulation. We developed two categories of behaviors: asthma-specific behaviors such as taking preventive medication, removing environmental triggers, and taking medication to deal with an episode or exacerbation; and the broader self-regulatory processes of monitoring behavior and symptoms, comparing with a standard, identifying a problem, and trying and evaluating a solution (Clark & Starr-Schneidkraut, 1994; Creer, 1990; Kotses, Stout, McConnaughy, Winder, & Creer, 1996; Thoresen & Kirmil-Gray, 1983; Creer, 2000a, 2000b). When we combined these asthma-specific and self-regulatory behaviors, we had a more comprehensive picture of what was required for effective asthma self-management as well as a self-regulatory framework to guide the children's application of asthma-specific behaviors.

We then designed a conceptual framework that would integrate both types of processes, reduce redundancy, and expose any gaps in the delineation of behaviors. Figure 12.1 is an asthma decision tree that combines both types of asthma self-management behaviors. The self-regulatory behaviors of goal setting, monitoring, problem identification, solution identification, action, and evaluation are represented to the left of the framework. These behaviors are the processes by which asthma-specific behaviors such as taking medicine, monitoring peak flow, or avoiding triggers take place. For example, monitoring asthma involves the child watching his or her overall condition. The asthma decision tree in Figure 12.1 shows that the child uses asthma-specific skills, such as peak-flow measurement, to monitor for symptoms. The child also monitors the environment for triggers and monitors his or her behavior with respect to taking medications as prescribed and keeping medical appointments.

Using this comprehensive picture of what is involved in asthma management, we combined asthma-specific behaviors with self-regulatory processes in order to create performance objectives. In order to narrow the scope of the target behaviors, we collapsed self-regulation to three steps (monitoring and problem identification, solution development, and action) and prioritized the categories of behavior as symptom resolution, asthma control, and trigger avoidance. Table 12.1 presents the first level of performance objectives for the child and family, and the following example shows the level of detail in the performance objectives:

1.a. Monitor objectively using a peak-flow meter
    1.a.1. Set a schedule for peak-flow monitoring
    1.a.2. Obtain a peak-flow meter
    1.a.3. Put the mouthpiece between the lips and blow hard until all the air possible is released
    1.a.4. Repeat three times
    1.a.5. Record the highest number

FIGURE 12.1. ASTHMA SELF-MANAGEMENT BEHAVIORAL FRAMEWORK.

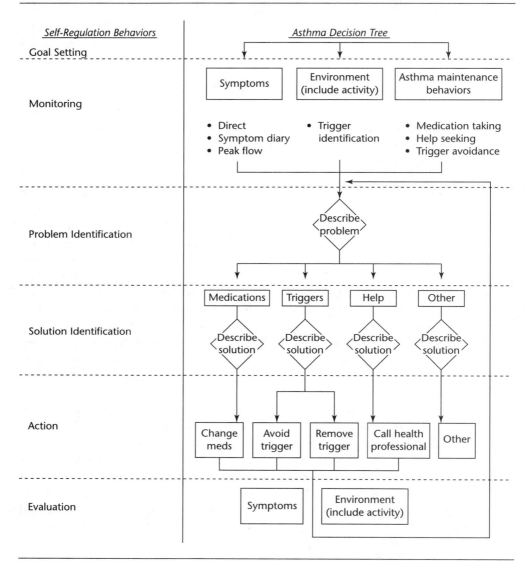

Source: Bartholomew, Shegog, and others, 2000. Reprinted from *Patient Education and Counseling, 39*(2–3), "Watch, Discover, Think, and Act: A model for patient education program development," copyright 2000, with permission of Elsevier.

TABLE 12.1. PERFORMANCE OBJECTIVES CHILD AND PARENT.

PO.1. Monitor symptoms of asthma and compare to personal standard

PO.2. Monitor symptoms and compare to personal standard symptoms using objective measures (such as a peak-flow meter)

PO.3. Monitor for personal environmental triggers

PO.4. Monitor self-management efforts and compare to personal standard

PO.5. Identify when a problem exists (with any of the above)

PO.6. Implement solutions:

    PO.6.1. Keep regular appointments with health care providers

    PO.6.2. Refer to asthma action plan

    PO.6.3. Maintain chronic medication as prescribed

    PO.6.4. Maintain normal exercise level

    PO.6.5. Make medication adjustments, including administration of rescue medication (based on symptoms, environment, or both) as prescribed

    PO.6.6. Avoid or remove asthma triggers

    PO.6.7. Call health care professional in acute situation

    PO.6.8. Communicate with family members and with health care providers

PO.7. Evaluate actions and return to monitoring

Determinants of Child and Parent Asthma Management. Our next step was to discover important and changeable factors associated with asthma management. Using primarily Social Cognitive Theory (SCT) as our conceptual framework, and using the literature regarding other self-management interventions, we specified such internal determinants as behavioral capability, skills, self-efficacy, and outcome expectations (Bandura, 1986). *Behavioral capability* is the procedural knowledge for the various performance objectives. *Self-efficacy* is the confidence that the children and parents have for each task, and *outcome expectations* are what they expect to occur as a result of their performance. Self-efficacy is expected to be related to the initiation of the performance objectives and persistence in making the changes (Bandura, 1986). Other factors chosen were knowledge, attributions, and perceptions of seriousness and chronicity. An *external determinant* is something outside the individual, such as reinforcement (Bandura, 1986). These included patient-provider interaction such as teaching and reinforcement of self-management skills, cultural orientation to illness and health care, and income and socioeconomic status (N. M. Clark, 1989; N. M. Clark, Rosenstock, et al., 1988; D. Evans et al., 1987; Kotses, Lewis, & Creer, 1990; Manson, 1988; McNabb, Wilson-Pessano, & Jacobs, 1986; Wissow, Gittelsohn,

Szklo, Starfield, & Mussman, 1988). We added attributions to our list of determinants from the needs assessment because of their demonstrated interaction with self-management for other chronic illnesses and health problems (Hospers, Kok, & Strecher, 1990; Kuttner, Delamater, & Santiago, 1990; Weiner, 1985). We wanted the child's attributions of success to be internal and attributable to effort: "Working with my parents, doctor, and school nurse, I can control my own asthma. I don't need grown-ups to do it for me."

At this step we also had to decide whether to differentiate the population on one or more descriptive variables. The decision was based on whether performance objectives or their determinants would vary for subgroups of the at-risk population. Based on the needs assessment, we wanted the program to reach both African American and Hispanic American inner-city youth, and therefore we needed to decide whether there was evidence that the determinants or desired behaviors were different in these two ethnic groups. Must we influence different sets of determinants? Or do we simply need to vary the strategies to be culturally acceptable? In other words, at this point in the planning process, do we have an ethnocentric intervention or a multiethnic one? Based on our needs assessment, we had no evidence that behaviors or determinants were different for the two groups of children; therefore, we did not differentiate. We did need to address ethnic differences in program design, including graphics and messages, to ensure that the program would be acceptable and appealing.

Another consideration in determining how to differentiate the population was the age range of six to eleven years of children who were potential program participants. This age group includes significant variation in cognitive, social, and emotional development. However, because all these children manage asthma as a team with parents, we decided that the performance objectives were not so different that they could not be handled with different versions of the same program rather than with different matrices and potentially different programs. See Step 4 for a description of the two versions (one for grades one through three and another for grades four and five).

Change Objectives. The next task was to create the matrix of change objectives for the behavioral conditions. Conceptually, the matrix represents the change necessary to influence the child's asthma self-management behavior. To form the matrix, we entered the performance objectives on the left side of the table and the determinants across the top. Table 12.2 shows both personal determinants (those within the child) and external determinants (those in the child's environment that are related to the specific performance objectives). We assessed each cell of the matrix to judge whether the determinant was likely to influence the performance objective and wrote change objectives in the appropriate cells. For example, in the cell in Table

12.2 where the performance objective "monitor for symptoms of asthma" is paired with the personal determinant "self-efficacy," we asked the question, What needs to change regarding self-efficacy for the child to be able to use a peak-flow meter? Answers to this question include the learner's experience of enhanced self-efficacy that he or she can do the actions necessary to observe symptoms.

Matrices at the Interpersonal and Organizational Levels

The first task for creating matrices at the environmental level involves specifying exactly what needs to change and who in the environment is responsible for that change.

Agents and Performance Objectives. The goals for environmental change were identified from the needs assessment and included changes in medical care (interpersonal level) and in the school environment (organizational level). We worked with a school district advisory committee to understand what environmental changes were feasible for the schools.

Needed changes in medical care focused on appropriate diagnosis of asthma and asthma severity using the National Asthma Education and Prevention Program guidelines; prescription of both rescue and control medications when necessary; use of an asthma action plan; and increased communication between the patient, family, school nurse, and physician based on the plan (NHLBI, 1991). Three agents were needed to perform these changes: the school nurse, the parent, and the physician. Performance objectives related to medical care changes are presented in Table 12.3.

Based on the needs assessment, the planning team determined that the following changes were needed in the school's physical environment: eliminating the allergens of mold, dust mites, cockroaches, and rodents; eliminating pollutants such as strong odors and their sources; eliminating contaminants that enter the building through the air-handling systems or originate in the systems; and increasing the circulation of fresh air in the building. Organizational-level environmental change agents or decision makers (school personnel) were then differentiated to include principals, plant operators, and teachers. The environmental conditions of concern in the schools are the same for all school personnel identified at the organizational level; however, performance objectives differ because of the aspects each is able to control. Table 12.4 takes one environmental change and compares performance objectives for plant operators, principals, and teachers.

Determinants and Matrices. Just as we did in developing the matrices for the child's change objectives, we used SCT to specify both internal and external

TABLE 12.2. MATRIX FOR CHILDREN WITH ASTHMA (SAMPLE CELLS).

Performance Objectives (Children)	Personal Determinants					External Determinants	
	Perceived Susceptibility and Seriousness	Behavioral Capability	Skills and Self-Efficacy	Outcome Expectations	Attributions	Physician and Parent Behavior	Reinforcement
PO.1. Monitor for symptoms of asthma	PSS.1.a. Describe asthma as a serious disease that does not go away PSS.1.b. Describe own asthma as involving inflammation in the lungs—can't be seen but is always there	BC.1.a. Identify possible personal symptoms of asthma BC.1.b. Identify early symptoms and late symptoms	SSE.1.a. Demonstrate comparing current respiratory status to baseline SSE.1.b. Express confidence in recognizing symptoms	OE.1.a. Expect that by monitoring symptoms asthma control can be better OE.1.b. Expect that action can be taken to prevent asthma episodes if symptoms are monitored	A.1.a. Attribute ability to monitor for asthma symptoms to self ("Children can tell when they have symptoms.") A.1.b. Attribute failure to monitor symptoms to temporary state or unstable causes ("I can get back to monitoring.")	PPB.1.a. Parents remind child to use peak-flow meter. PPB.1.b. Parents assist younger children with direct observation and peak flow.	R.1.a. Parents, physicians, and intervention reinforce for monitoring for asthma symptoms.
PO1.1. Monitor objectively using a peak-flow meter	PSS.1.1.a. State that asthma episodes can be serious	BC.1.1.a. List personal peak-flow numbers that are congruent with asthma	SSE.1.1.a. Demonstrate using a peak-flow meter	OE.1.1.a. Expect that peak-flow meter will allow early detection of decline and episode prevention	A.1.1.a. Attribute ability to use peak-flow meter to self	PPB.1.1.a. Parents and physicians look at and discuss peak-flow numbers.	R.1.1.a. Parents and physicians look at and discuss peak-flow numbers.
PO.1.2. Set a schedule for peak-flow monitoring	PSS.1.2.a. State that asthma is serious enough to monitor regularly and to catch decline in lung function early	BC.1.2.a. Describe schedule for peak-flow monitoring BC.1.2.b. Plan when to measure peak-flow in daily schedule	SSE.1.2.a. Express confidence that can fit peak-flow monitoring into current schedule	OE.1.1.a. Expect that monitoring peak flow on a certain schedule will result in the ability to predict and prevent asthma episodes	A.1.2.a. Attribute ability to use peak-flow on a schedule to self A.1.2.b. Attribute difficulties in keeping to a schedule to unstable causes		R.1.2.a. Parents congratulate child for keeping to schedule.

	PSS	BC	SSE	OE	A	PPB	R
PO1.3. Obtain a peak-flow meter	PSS.1.3.a. Think asthma is serious enough to monitor and to catch decline in function early	BC.1.3.a. Describe the uses of a peak-flow meter	SSE.1.3.a. Express confidence to negotiate with physician for a peak-flow meter				
PO1.4. Perform correct peak-flow technique		BC.1.4.a. Describe the steps of using a peak-flow meter	SSE.1.4.a. Demonstrate correct technique SSE.1.4.b. Express confidence in ability to obtain and use a correct number			PPB.1.4.a. Physicians teach peak-flow technique. PPB.1.4.b. Parents teach use of peak-flow meter.	R.1.4.a. Parents, school nurses, and physicians reinforce correct technique.
PO2. Take control (anti-inflammatory) medication	PSS.2.a. See the inflammatory process as serious, as needing to be controlled	BC.2.a. Describe purpose of control medications (meds) BC.2.b. Identify types of asthma meds BC.2.c. State when to use each asthma med	SSE.2.a. Demonstrate correct procedure for use of inhaler SSE.2.b. Express confidence that can use inhaler correctly	OE.2.a. Expect control meds to reduce episodes OE.2.b. Expect few side effects OE.2.c. Expect to be able to decrease control meds with doctor	A.2.a. See asthma as something that can be controlled by own efforts A.2.b. See lack of asthma control as due to inadequate meds	PPB.2.a. Physicians prescribe control (anti-inflammatory) meds. PPB.2.b. Parents give child control meds.	
PO2.1. Take control medication according to asthma action plan	PSS.2.1.a. Recognize that control meds should be taken according to plan, not symptoms		SSE.2.1.a. Demonstrate how to take meds according to action plan SSE.2.1.b. Express confidence in ability to take meds according to action plan	OE.2.1.a. Expect meds to work better if taken as prescribed	A.2.1.a. Expect to be able to follow action plan A.2.1.b. Attribute failure to temporary state	PPB.2.1.a. Physicians give action plan with section prescribing control meds.	
PO2.2. Continue control medications when symptoms are not present	PSS.2.2.a. Recognize that control meds should be taken according to plan, not symptoms	BC.2.2.a. Recognize that control meds are to manage inflammation that cannot be seen or felt	SSE.2.2.a. Express confidence in ability to take meds even when not having symptoms	OE.2.2.a. Expect meds to work better if taken as prescribed		PPB.2.2.a. Physicians write clear instructions about when to take meds on action plan.	R.2.2.a. Physicians, parents, school nurses, and intervention reinforce taking meds.

TABLE 12.3. PERFORMANCE OBJECTIVES FOR MEDICAL CARE CHANGE.

Parents	Physicians	School Nurses
Obtain asthma action plan and have completed by physician	Use National Asthma Education and Prevention Program (NAEPP) assessment and severity guidelines to diagnose identified students	Ensure that children have functional asthma action plans and proper medications at school
Get prescriptions filled		Review action plans with children and parents
Take completed action plan, inhaler, spacer, and peak-flow meter (if needed) to school nurse	Prescribe long-term control medicines and quick relief medicines according to severity	Assist children to use inhaler and spacer or nebulizer correctly
Work with child, physician, school nurse, teachers, and other school personnel to identify, avoid, and remove child's triggers	Identify concerns patients and families might have about being diagnosed with asthma and educate them regarding this diagnosis	Assist children to use peak-flow meter correctly
Give all medications as ordered	Agree on treatment goals with patients and families	Administer routine medications
Help child use peak-flow meter and to determine child's personal best	Explain how to discover triggers and how to avoid them	Respond to asthma episodes and administer relief medications as needed
Clean inhalers, spacers, and nebulizers properly	Explain to patients how to watch for early warning signs and asthma symptoms	Manage school environment to remove triggers and help children avoid triggers
Record details of asthma episodes to share with physician	Follow up with patients on performance of asthma action plan	Review performance of action plans with children, parents, and physicians
Keep all follow-up physician appointments	Ensure that children complete physician visits	
Talk with school nurse and physician about asthma problems as they arise		

determinants for the performance of the environmental agents (Bandura, 1986). For example, behavioral capability would be related to the physician setting a goal or to the plant operator identifying and removing sources of allergens and irritants. Self-efficacy is the confidence that the agents experience for each task, and outcome expectations are what the agents expect to occur as a result of their performance. An external determinant is something outside the individual, such as reinforcement (Bandura, 1986). The actions in environmental cleanup should be a source of negative reinforcement (that is, if removing an aversive stimulus, in this case, sources of respiratory irritants and illness results in increased health or

TABLE 12.4. PLANT OPERATOR, PRINCIPAL, AND TEACHER ENVIRONMENTAL CHANGE PERFORMANCE OBJECTIVES (PARTIAL).

Plant Operators	Principals	Teachers
Plant operators prevent air contaminants from entering the school building.	*Principals ensure that air contaminants are prevented from entering the building.*	*Teachers monitor building for signs that air contaminants are entering building or causing children to have asthma symptoms.*
Appraise air-handling units for nearby contaminants	Relocate holding area for buses, loading dock, and so on, if near outdoor air intake or windows	Report children with asthma symptoms to school nurse and note time of day and potential exposures
Clear outdoor air intakes of nearby pollutant sources and debris	Ensure that plant operators and other personnel are keeping air intakes clear of nearby pollutant sources (such as mold) and debris	Report odors to principal
Check filter for clogs or gaps		Routinely check air handling system in classroom
Replace filters every three months (including hard-to-reach units)	Work with district to schedule and change filters in all air handling units every three months	Notice and report outside sources of contaminants to the principal
Install local exhausts and seal off returns in area of activities that emit odors	Work with district and contractors during activities that emit odors to ensure that local exhausts are temporarily installed, returns are sealed off in areas, and work is done during unoccupied times	
Schedule activities that emit odors during unoccupied times		
Relocate dumpsters or incinerators fifty feet from any air intake		
Secure openings on exterior of building for rodent or bird entry (especially along roofline and crawl space)	Work with plant operators to relocate dumpsters or incinerators that are near air supplies or windows (should be fifty feet from any air intake)	
Schedule painting, roofing, and pest control to unoccupied times	Ensure that openings on exterior of building are secured to prevent rodent or bird entry (especially along roofline and crawl space)	
Close outdoor air damper for reroofing		
Maintain drain traps to prevent odorous dry traps by pouring water down floor drains once per week; run water in sinks and flush unused toilets once per week	Schedule painting, roofing, maintenance and pest control to unoccupied times	
	Ensure that outdoor air dampers are closed during reroofing	
Evaluate if above action items are completed consistently	Ensure drain trap maintenance	
	Evaluate if above action items are completed consistently and compliment plant operator for completed items	
	Add items to plant operators' job descriptions and evaluations	

in feelings of doing the right thing). For example, a teacher removes potted plants with mold in them from underneath the classroom air-intake, thereby decreasing the spread of mold spore and, consequently, her allergy symptoms and those of the children. Sometimes there is a significant time lag between the removal of the contaminant and improvement in health. Therefore, to be reinforcing, the contingencies may need to be pointed out to the environmental agents. Other reinforcements include those from the social environment, such as approval expressed by the principal for the plant operator's efforts. Other external determinants at the organizational level include the availability of unscented products, such as cleaners, and equipment that helps eliminate contaminants, such as vacuum cleaners with HEPA filters. The school district advisory committee meetings, along with other interviews, were crucial in identifying availability of appropriate products. For example, we found that a plant operator must have unscented germicides available for order through the school district warehouse if he or she is to be able to discontinue using bleach (a strong-scented cleaner) inside the school building. External determinants for physician practice included office policy and barriers, particularly length of visits for asthma.

At the interpersonal level, these determinants were crossed with performance objectives in matrices for physicians, school nurses, and parents. Table 12.5 shows an example from a physician's matrix. At the organizational level, determinants were crossed with performance objectives for plant operators, school principals, and teachers. Table 12.6 shows an example from a plant-operator matrix.

Step 3: Theory-Informed Methods and Practical Strategies

The third step in Intervention Mapping is to delineate theoretical methods and match them with practical strategies, making sure to specify methods to affect each change objective. Tables 12.7, 12.8, and 12.9 present selected methods and strategies that were identified for the program objectives at the individual, interpersonal, and organizational levels.

Step 4: Program Design

The actual development of the program components and materials requires incorporating all of the chosen methods and strategies in ways that fit with the context of the intervention and the preferences of the intended participants.

TABLE 12.5. MATRIX AT THE INTERPERSONAL LEVEL: PHYSICIANS (PARTIAL).

Performance Objectives (Physicians)	Personal Determinants			External Determinants	
	Behavioral Capability	Skills and Self-Efficacy	Outcome Expectations	Barriers	Office Policy
PO.1. Agree on treatment goals with patients and families PO.1.1. Determine families' goals for asthma management (ask what patients would like to do but can't because of asthma)	BC.1.1.a. Describe how including children's input in goal setting leads to greater compliance	SSE.1. Express confidence and demonstrate ability to determine appropriate treatment goals from patient information	OE.1. Believe that creating patient treatment goals leads to better control of asthma	B.1.a. Allow enough time per scheduled exam to educate patients about optimal expectations and to set treatment goals with them B.1.b. Have interpreter readily available	OP.1. Have printed materials available that explain general treatment goals that patients and families should strive for and expect to achieve
PO.1.2. Explain physician's goals for managing asthma to families (such as children should sleep through the night, have no or minimal emergency department (ED) visits or days absent from school, feel well, and have near-normal lung function)	BC.1.2. List reasons to treat persistent asthma as a chronic illness	SSE.1.2. Express confidence in being able to persuade parents and children that good function is possible when asthma is well treated	OE.1.2. Expect that good treatment will produce the outcomes described		
PO.1.3. Note the family's goals in each child's action plan	BC.1.3.a. Show familiarity with action plan BC.1.3.b. Describe characteristics of an effective goal	SSE.1.3. Express confidence in being able to use plan at each visit	OE.1.3. Believe that using plan will enable child and parents to better manage asthma	B.1.3.a. Allow time to complete action plan B.1.3.b. Allow time in schedule to review goals at each visit	OP.1.3.a. Have action plans in each child's chart ahead of asthma visit OP.1.3.b. Have action plans accessible in every exam room

TABLE 12.6. MATRIX AT THE ORGANIZATIONAL LEVEL: PLANT OPERATOR (PARTIAL).

Performance Objectives (Plant Operators)	Personal Determinants				External Determinants	
	Behavioral Capability	Self-Efficacy and Skills	Outcome Expectations	Reinforcement	Policy and Availability of Resources	
PO.1. Prevent air contaminants from entering school building	BC.1.a. Describe how to appraise air-handling rooms and exhaust fans BC.1.b. Describe ten procedures to prevent air contaminants from entering the school building BC.1.c. Describe type of filters to use BC.1.d. Describe how to change filters	SSE.1.a. Express confidence in ability to investigate air-handling systems SSE.1.b. Demonstrate filter change	OE.1.a. Believe that protecting children and staff from airborne contaminants will improve their health OE.1.b. Expect that the principal will appreciate efforts to improve air quality	R.1.a. Principals praise plant operator for efforts to improve air quality. R.1.b. District officials respond positively to efforts to improve air quality.	P.1.a. Custodial crew policy reflects the need for compliance with proper air ventilation standards. P.1.b. All heating, ventilation, and air conditioning system parts are available for immediate replacement when necessary.	
PO.2. Remove existing air contaminants from building	BC.2.a. Describe how to appraise air-handling units and rooms BC.2.b. Describe ten items to check for contaminants BC.2.c. Describe how to remove mold and other contaminants from the building	SSE.2.a. Express confidence in and demonstrate ability to investigate air-handling systems and rooms for air contaminants	OE.2.a. Believe the importance of having clean, well-running ventilation systems for clean air and therefore good health	R.2.a. Principals check systems and praise plant operators for good conditions.	P.2.a. District officials respond rapidly with requests for parts and help with cleaning.	

TABLE 12.7. BRAINSTORMING METHODS AND STRATEGIES FOR CHILD AND PARENT MATRIX.

Methods from Theory	Examples of Practical Strategies
Goal setting	Asthma action plan
Modeling	Character in computer game is learning to manage asthma.
	Coach in computer game has managed asthma.
Skill training	Computer game simulation teaches self-regulatory skills and asthma-specific skills.
	Video clips in game teach psychomotor skills.
Self-monitoring	Game includes asthma action plan.
	Character in the game monitors asthma status.
Persuasive communication	Coach in computer game encourages player.
Cues to action	Asthma action plan serves as cue to action.
Reinforcement	Computer game provides symptom feedback, score, and certificates of congratulation.
	Computer game provides feedback on each child's game progress so that physicians can socially reinforce children.
Attribution training	Coach is an older child who successfully manages asthma.
	Child is encouraged throughout game to manage asthma.
	Characters in game model managing their own asthma and are reinforced with symptom reduction.

Review of Asthma-Management Programs

Before beginning to work on this new program, we reviewed the literature on health education and promotion interventions for asthma. Educational programs to enhance self-management of childhood asthma have had some impact on the following variables: anxiety about asthma, children's responsibility for asthma management, school attendance, school performance, acute episodes of reactive airways, and medical costs (N. M. Clark, Feldman, Evans, Duzey, et al., 1986; N. M. Clark, Feldman, Evans, Levison, et al., 1986; N. M. Clark, Feldman, Evans, Wasilewski, & Levison, 1984; Creer et al., 1988; Fireman, Friday, Gira, Viethaler, & Michaels, 1981; Hindi-Alexander, 1984; C. E. Lewis, Rachelefsky, Lewis, de la Seta, & Kaplan, 1984; McNabb et al., 1986; Parcel & Nader, 1977; Parcel, Nader, & Tiernan, 1980; Wilson-Pessano et al., 1987). The development process for these

TABLE 12.8. BRAINSTORMING METHODS AND STRATEGIES FOR THE INTERPERSONAL LEVEL MATRICES.

Methods from Theory	Examples of Practical Strategies		
	Parents	Physicians	School Nurses
Goal setting	Asthma action plan	Asthma action plan	Asthma action plan
Persuasive communication	Narrator in video encourages parent to take child to physician. Project staff and school nurses encourage parents to take children to physicians.	Narrator in video encourages physicians to use asthma action plans to increase patients' adherence with self-management.	Project staff members encourage nurses to implement program to decrease students' symptoms and absenteeism.
Modeling	Role models in video show parent and child discussing asthma action plan with physician. Role models in video show parent and child reviewing action plan at home and placing it in a prominent position.	Role model in video shows physician examining child for asthma and using National Asthma Education and Prevention Program (NAEPP) guidelines to diagnose severity. Role model in video shows physician discussing asthma action plan with families.	At in-service training, respiratory therapists model correct techniques for using inhalers, spacers, and peak-flow meters. At in-service training, project staff members model school nurse interaction with child on computer game.
Cues to action	Children bring home action plans and videos from school. Project staff members or school nurses call parents about action plans.	Project staff members mail action plans and videos to physicians. Physicians are directed to place action plans in children's medical charts.	Project staff members deliver log sheets to record interactions with students.
Self-monitoring	Asthma action plan		Nurses record interaction with students on log sheets.
Skill training	Videotape models step-by-step use of the action plan.	Video provides detailed information on how to use NAEPP guidelines to diagnose asthma and asthma severity. Video provides detailed instructions on how to complete asthma action plan.	At in-service training, school nurses practice correct techniques for using inhalers, spacers, and peak-flow meters. At in-service training, school nurses role-play discussing action plan with parents and physician.
Reinforcement	Project staff and school nurses provide feedback on children's asthma management at school.	Parents and school nurses provide feedback to physicians on children's asthma management.	Project staff members and school district personnel recognize nurses' efforts.

TABLE 12.9. BRAINSTORMING METHODS AND STRATEGIES FOR THE ORGANIZATIONAL LEVEL.

Methods from Theory	Examples of Practical Strategies			
	Principals	Plant Operators	Teachers
Goal setting	Environmental action committee agreement	Environmental action committee agreement	Environmental action committee agreement
Skill training	At environmental action committee meetings, project staff members teach ways to identify and remove irritants and allergens from the school building and grounds. Project staff members provide feedback on actions taken.	At training, speakers and project staff demonstrate proper cleaning and prevention techniques. Project staff members provide feedback on actions taken.	At teacher in-service, project staff members present steps to identify and remove irritants and allergens in the classroom. Project staff members provide feedback on actions taken.
Consciousness raising	At meetings of principals and superintendents, data are presented concerning levels of irritants and allergens found in schools. Individualized environmental "school report cards" give information on irritants and allergens in general and on specific problems identified in school buildings and grounds. At environmental action committee meetings, members (including principals) brainstorm solutions to identified problems and identify additional problematic conditions.	At training, project staff members provide educational materials on irritants and allergens. Plant operators participate in brainstorming sessions to identify problems and solutions under the control of custodial staff. Individualized environmental "school report cards" give information on irritants and allergens in general and inform of specific problems identified in school building and grounds. At environmental action committee meetings, members (including the plant operators) brainstorm solutions to identified problems and identify additional problematic conditions.	At teacher in-services, project staff members provide educational materials and information on irritants and allergens in the classroom. Teachers participate in brainstorming sessions to generate solutions. Individualized environmental "school report cards" give information on irritants and allergens in general and inform of specific problems identified in school building and grounds. At environmental action committee meetings, members (including teachers) brainstorm solutions to identified problems and identify additional problematic conditions.

TABLE 12.9. BRAINSTORMING METHODS AND STRATEGIES FOR THE ORGANIZATIONAL LEVEL, Cont'd.

Methods from Theory	*Examples of Practical Strategies*		
	Principals	Plant Operators	Teachers
Modeling	At environmental action committee meetings, project staff members presented testimonials of other elementary schools encountering problematic conditions and trying solutions.	At plant operator trainings, plant operators give testimonials of problems encountered in the schools and solutions used to reduce irritants and allergens.	Teacher in-services include testimonials of teachers who have encountered and remedied problematic conditions.
		Pest control worker for district gives testimonials on pest control strategies.	
		Project staff members provide demonstrations of proper cleaning techniques.	
Facilitation	Project staff members work with district on policy change.	Project staff members facilitate purchase orders and maintenance requests at the district level.	
Persuasive communication	Project staff members encourage principals to ensure follow-through on items from environmental action committee agreements.	Project staff members encourage plant operators to follow-through on needed purchase orders identified from environmental action committee agreements.	Project staff members encourage teachers to remove irritants and allergens from classrooms.
			Teachers are reminded of the risks to staff and student health if removal not done consistently.

and other programs has contributed greatly to the understanding of asthma management. However, the volume of program objectives and related lessons may deter health care providers or school personnel from using them to teach children and parents. Also, at the time we developed our program, the programs did not deal directly with change in the child's school environment. Furthermore, most approaches to asthma self-management were not easily individualized; they required that all children learn the same skills, regardless of individual characteristics or asthma-management needs. Little was known about which intervention components contribute to behavior change and thereby to the noted outcomes (Creer, Kotses, & Wigal, 1992). Some programs are group oriented; others make little or no use of information about the child's asthma precipitants, prescribed treatment, or orientation to self-management of asthma. Furthermore, there has been minimal success in implementing these programs within schools or medical care practices. Based on this review, we knew that we wanted a program with the following characteristics:

- Can be individualized and tailored to use the child's own data and meet the specific needs of a child and family
- Is designed to help a child progress to more advanced asthma management
- Is able to be implemented in a variety of settings
- Includes a tie to the child's medical care
- Includes a direct environmental change component

Program Components and Support Materials

After reviewing the strategies and change objectives, we determined that there should be three primary program components: child self-management, a linkage system with physician care, and a school environment intervention. Because we knew that the program was to be implemented in an inner-city school setting, we also had to consider the constraints and limitations that this setting placed on program design. Inner-city schools usually lack resources of space, personnel, and discretionary funds; therefore, the program had to fit into the school setting with minimum interruption to regular school activities, minimum burden for school personnel, and minimum cost to the school administration.

Child Self-Management Training Component. The principal delivery mechanism for the child self-management component was a computer program that was tailored to the individual children's characteristics. The computer program was a game that stimulated children's interest and allowed them to identify with role models from their own ethnic group, African American or Hispanic. We expected reading skills of some of the children to be below grade level. Furthermore, some of the children spoke only Spanish, according to estimated enrollment in English as a second language classes in the school district. In order to accommodate ethnic differences, children could choose attractive Hispanic or African American, male or female, character role models who were about twelve years of age and coach role models who were about sixteen years of age. School nurses could help the child choose whether to play the game in English or Spanish.

The theme and title of the program, Watch, Discover, Think, and Act, is based on the self-regulatory sequence and is depicted as icons in the program. The icons guide the children to watch (monitor), discover (identify problems and causes), think (decide on solutions), and act (act to solve the problem). A screen from the computer game was presented in Figure 8.1. These themes are repeated in feedback to the child and in the asthma action plan. The scope and sequence of the computer program is four computer-simulated venues in which children must manipulate their characters to manage asthma: home, community, school, and the fantasy castle (Shegog et al., 2001; Bartholomew, Gold, et al., 2000; Bartholomew, Shegog, et al., 2000). The school nurse enters information about the child's own triggers, symptoms, and medications. As the game progresses through the scenes and venues, the learner manages asthma by avoiding or eliminating triggers, taking control and relief medications, visiting the doctor, and making doctors appointments for checkups.

The major contextual theme in the computer program is the mission to the castle of Dr. Foulair. In addition to managing their asthma, children collect items required on their mission to liberate an air-cleaning machine from the menacing castle of the inventor-turned-bad guy. Once in the castle, the learner must continue to manage asthma in the face of very unusual obstacles and asthma triggers. Fantasy and adventure-game playing in education have been reported to motivate learners (L. E. Parker & Lepper, 1992).

We were interested in using computer-assisted instruction for this health intervention program in order to tailor the intervention to each child's asthma symptoms and triggers. Even with this delivery method in mind, however, we had to determine theoretical methods that could produce change in the determinants we had specified in the matrix. Methods used in the computer self-management program were modeling, skill training, goal setting, self-monitoring, persuasive communication, reinforcement, cues to action, and attribution training (see Table 12.7).

Symbolic modeling was chosen as a principal method to elicit change in the child's knowledge and skills, self-efficacy, outcome expectations, and attributions (Bandura, 1986). The models—the child's chosen character and coach in the computer program—were used to teach skills and to reinforce the child's asthma management, thereby enhancing self-efficacy and outcome expectations. The models also illustrated that asthma-management behavior is internal, controllable, and unstable in terms of attribution for failure (Weiner, 1985). The role models remind the children that personal effort plays the major role in the management of asthma, that self-management begins with them, and that asthma is something they can control. Further, when self-management failure occurs, it is controllable and unstable; it can be avoided in the future.

Reinforcement occurs throughout the computer program by vicarious reinforcement of the program role models, by simulated symptom reduction for the character in the game, and by accumulated points. The program also generates a report of the child's progress to stimulate reinforcement by parents and health care providers. The asthma action plan is also designed to elicit social reinforcement for the child's self-management behavior until the desired behavior becomes an internally reinforced part of the daily routine. Goal setting as a part of the asthma action plan is a means to improve the behavioral change effort, persistence, and concentration (E. A. Locke & Latham, 1990; V. J. Strecher et al., 1995).

Physician Linkage Component. The principal delivery mechanism for the physician linkage component is the asthma action plan, which we developed at a low reading level in English and Spanish. Once completed by the child's physician, the action plan provides written, individualized guidelines for the child's asthma care. Action plans were sent home to the parent with an accompanying video, which modeled taking the plan to the physician and reviewing it with the school nurse. A short video was mailed to children's homes to persuade parents of the importance of having the child's physician complete an action plan. The video included modeling of parents making a physician appointment, discussing the action plan with the physician, and reviewing the plan at home with the child. The video also provided modeling for interaction between the parent and school nurse discussing the action plan and medication use at school. The project staff and school nurses used persuasive communication and reinforcement strategies to encourage parents to work with the physician on the action plan.

If the child was under a physician's care, an action plan and physician-training video were also mailed to the physician's office. The physician was instructed to place the action plan in the child's medical records chart for completion at the next office visit. The school nurse was also able to fax an action plan to the child's physician and request that the information be completed.

Video was also used as a vehicle for delivering program components that were designed to change physician behavior. The video modeled physicians using National Asthma Education and Prevention Program guidelines to judge asthma severity and to monitor asthma symptoms objectively. The video also emphasized the use of a written asthma action plan to increase adherence for self-management.

School nurses play a central role in the intervention to link children to medical care; therefore, project staff provided nurses with modeling and guided practice related to use of medication and peak-flow meters, communication with parents and physicians to evaluate the effectiveness of action plans, and effective communication with students to increase self-management skills. Cues to action, such as medication logs and computer player logs, were provided to prompt the school nurse to implement program activities.

Because many families participating in the study lacked a primary care provider or medical health insurance, the school nurse and project staff also assisted families in identifying free or low-cost medical services and to apply for Medicaid or other assistance. Project staff contacted families by telephone and by meetings at school to encourage participation. Once completed action plans were obtained from the physician, the school nurse retained a copy of each plan at the school and periodically reviewed it with the child, family, and physician to determine its effectiveness in reducing asthma exacerbations.

School Environmental Change. Included in the environmental change intervention were the following:

- School-level environmental action committees
- Feedback of environmental survey data on a school report card
- Trainings for plant operators and teachers
- District-level policy change
- Facilitation of purchasing and maintenance at the district level

Raising the awareness of school personnel toward the potential harm of allergens and irritants to asthmatics was paramount. To accomplish this awareness, school committees were established and comprised the principal, plant operator, school nurse, and a teacher. Individualized school conditions were reported to the committees on environmental report cards that summarized the findings of allergens, irritants, and carbon dioxide levels found during the environmental survey. The cards had four columns: three columns contained general information on irritants and allergens, school findings, and low-cost action recommendations; and one column was for documenting item completion. This report card was laminated in banner size, and action committees were encouraged to display it in the school as a document to monitor improvement and show commitment (Figure 12.2).

The committees set goals and established an environmental action committee agreement. To enable school personnel to obtain the skills and self-efficacy to implement the agreement, we trained plant operators in the steps for identification of allergens and irritants and removal techniques. At training sessions for

FIGURE 12.2. ENVIRONMENTAL REPORT CARD.

Should You Improve Moisture and Mold Conditions?

Air Facts	School Findings	Action Recommendations	Identify and Complete Action Tasks — Needs to Be Completed?
• Many people have allergic reactions to mold. • Mold can hide from sight but not usually from smell, since mold spores give off a strong moldy, musty smell. • Where there is moisture there is usually mold. Mold and mildew can grow almost anywhere that offers a food source and a small amount of moisture, whether from leaks, spills, or condensation.	Percent of classrooms surveyed with: • Mold smell . . . . 83.3 • Visible mold . . . . 0 (usually on ceiling or floor tiles, around HVAC systems, or in/around cabinets) • Mold in the HVAC . . . . . . 50 • Visible water damage . . . . . 20 Other areas in your school where mold is detected: Standing water next to the school building? ☐ yes ☐ no Evidence of moisture found in the exterior walls of the building? ☐ yes ☐ no Mold or mildew on the exterior of the building? ☐ yes ☐ no	• Use the enclosed *Checklist to Detect Mold and Signs of Moisture, Leaks, or Spills* to identify problems • Use proper cleaning practices on floors—using standard of no mold is acceptable. • Fix leaks immediately (call district contact person: _____ Phone number: _____ if needed for extra fast service.) • Remediate wet materials or dry rapidly • Wash outside or inside mold from buildings with a bleach-borax solution—including T-buildings • Fill in drainage ditches with dirt or landscaping—do not allow standing water around buildings—including T-buildings • Use anti-mold paints—do not paint over mold	 ☐ yes ☐ no By _____ Done ☐ ☐ yes ☐ no By _____ Done ☐ ☐ yes ☐ no By _____ Done ☐ ☐ yes ☐ no By _____ Done ☐ ☐ yes ☐ no By _____ Done ☐ ☐ yes ☐ no By _____ Done ☐

plant operators and teachers, role models from each group provided testimonials about their problems and solutions. project staff provided checklists for inspecting air-handling systems; checklists for identifying and removing mold, moisture, leaks, and spills; clipboards; and face masks. At action committee meetings, project staff encouraged school policy to be changed when needed to reflect action recommendations, such as enforcing a no-food rule in classrooms to reduce cockroaches and other pests.

The project staff helped schools overcome barriers by working on policy at the district level (such as developing suppliers of environmentally friendly items) and helped speed purchase orders and requests for maintenance through the district procedures.

Teachers at each school were provided an in-service workshop in which they were updated on environmental conditions, informed of children enrolled in the study in their classes, and trained to identify and remove triggers of asthmatic children. Materials provided to teachers included asthma trigger information, checklists to inspect air-handling systems, checklists to identify and remove allergens and irritants from the classrooms, and a list of recommended products for the classroom.

Program Scope and Sequence

Each of the program components had a scope and sequence, but they also were coordinated into an overall program scope and sequence. The intervention was implemented at thirty elementary schools over twenty-four months. The sequence of program activities is depicted in Table 12.10.

Pretesting

The computer game *Watch, Discover, Think, and Act* (Bartholomew, Gold, et al., 2000; Bartholomew, Shegog, et al., 2000) was tested by children with asthma six to twelve years of age prior to final production and implementation. Determination was made as to whether children could understand the program directions and information and whether they could follow the watch, discover, think, and act self-regulatory process. Estimates were made as to how well the child made decisions and how engaged the child was in the process.

Materials such as the asthma action plan were reviewed by members of the school district advisory committee, participating school nurses, and physicians on the research team. Spanish-language focus groups were held before translation to explore commonly used words to describe asthma, and back translation (see Chapter Eight) of Spanish language materials was conducted.

TABLE 12.10. PROGRAM SCOPE AND SEQUENCE.

	Quarter 1	Quarter 2	Quarter 3	Quarter 4	Quarters 5–8
School environmental change	Survey of schools Meeting between superintendent and principals	District advisory committee	Environmental report card School environmental committee District advisory committee	Training of plant operators, teachers, and principals Repeat meetings of school environmental committees	Continuation of school environmental committees and district advisory committee meetings Facilitation of purchasing and facilities' services at the district level
Self-management training		Survey of asthma symptoms School nurse training on computer	Computer game playing Action plan sent home with video Phone calls to parents	Computer game playing Phone calls to parents of symptomatic children	Continuation of computer game playing and phone calls to parents of symptomatic children
Physician linkage		Action plan and video to physicians Action plan to home Nurse training on action plans	Letter to physicians	Letter and repeat action plan mailing	

Step 5: Adoption and Implementation

Even though plans for assuring the adoption of the program are begun very early in a project, they are more easily discussed in detail at this stage when the program components have been fully described.

Linkage System

The fifth step in Intervention Mapping involves developing a plan to ensure program adoption and implementation by identifying adopters and implementers, defining potential barriers, developing a linkage system, and preparing an implementation plan. Because Partners in School Asthma Management was to be implemented in an elementary school setting, the first part of creating a linkage system was to include school district personnel on the program development team to represent their perspectives of asthma management and the realities of working in schools. The school district advisory committee played an important role in conceptualizing program development and implementation and assisted in identifying additional school district personnel who would be instrumental for program adoption. The school district advisory committee consisted of directors and personnel from the departments of health and medical services, risk management, environmental affairs, construction management, and health education and curriculum development, as well as a school nurse, elementary school principal, and parent advocate. The advisory committee provided insight into the culture and practice of the school district community.

Program Adopters and Implementers

To identify program adopters and implementers, we conducted a series of meetings, first with the school district area superintendents and then with elementary school principals in each of the school district areas. Often principals expressed interest in the program but indicated that they would leave the decision to their school nurses. From these meetings and later meetings with nurses, we hypothesized that adoption and implementation would be influenced by the following factors:

- Ease and low cost of implementation
- Outcome expectations such as perceived student benefits and better health for staff
- Lack of increased burden for school personnel
- No fear of negative publicity from the environmental intervention
- The feeling of doing something good for children with asthma

The school nurse was the key adopter as well as implementer of the program, and we addressed our recruitment efforts to the nurses with the messages that the program would be easy to implement, they would get help with the computer, the environment could benefit, and children and staff would possibly be healthier. In addition, in order to reduce the burden placed on the school nurse to implement the computerized self-management component, project staff trained school parent volunteers to assist children in playing the game. Each participating school was provided with a computer with CD-ROM capability, specifically for program implementation, to reduce administrative costs and to alleviate competition for limited computer resources. To minimize disruption of the child's academic activities, it was recommended that students play the game during ancillary periods or during their regular computer class period.

Step 6: Monitoring and Evaluation

The sixth step in Intervention Mapping involves developing a plan for monitoring and evaluation that makes use of the previously executed planning. The Partners in School Asthma Management program described in this chapter was evaluated in a randomized controlled trial conducted in sixty elementary schools in a large urban school district in southeast Texas. We evaluated the program in terms of its effect on cognitive and behavioral impact variables and health and quality-of-life outcome variables. The evaluation model is included in Figure 12.3.

Eight hundred thirty-five children with diagnosed asthma or probable asthma as identified by a case-finding process were enrolled in the study. The students were predominantly Hispanic and African American, and most lived in households with income of less than $20,000 per year. Students were followed for three years. Results showed that children in the intervention group had higher self-efficacy and knowledge scores related to asthma management at posttest compared to children in the comparison group. They also reported higher levels of self-management for avoiding triggers, exercise pretreatment, and home episode self-management. Although asthma symptoms did decline significantly over time, health outcomes related to hospitalizations, emergency room visits, and school outcomes were not significantly different between children in the intervention and control groups.

Process evaluation data can help to explain these outcomes. Process data indicate that two components of the multicomponent program were very well implemented; however, one was more difficult to execute. We were able to deliver the computerized self-management training to all children enrolled in the intervention. School nurses' offices were appropriate sites for this intervention, but our hope of enhancing the role of the nurse in students' asthma management was not realized. The school environmental survey was also conducted in all schools and

FIGURE 12.3. EVALUATION MODEL.

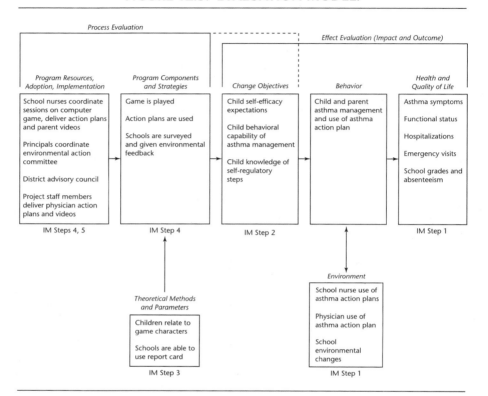

served to increase the asthma awareness of teachers and administrators. To some extent we were able to implement environmental changes by working at the school level and at the district level for policy change.

However, we were not able to change the behavior of health care providers; nor were we able to enhance partnerships between families, school nurses, and health care providers. One problem was the inconsistent nature of the care that these inner-city children received. Although we identified their health care providers, we could not be sure that a child had the same provider from one month to the next. We had very little response from our communications with physicians and suspect that we did not influence the parents' care-seeking behavior or the physicians' management strategies.

These findings underscore the need for future school-based asthma-management programs to be linked to appropriate medical care. One area in need of continued research is the patient-physician linkage in promotion of guideline-congruent behavior on the part of physicians, patients, and families.

CHAPTER THIRTEEN

THEORY AND CONTEXT IN PROJECT PANDA: A PROGRAM TO HELP POSTPARTUM WOMEN STAY OFF CIGARETTES

Patricia Dolan Mullen, Carlo C. DiClemente, and L. Kay Bartholomew

Reader Objectives

- Apply theory and evidence to define the intervention focus
- Develop and use design documents to communicate message intent
- Use context of participant group to improve intervention salience

Just as a life-threatening disease often sparks an individual to modify health-related behaviors, pregnancy also motivates women and their partners to make lifestyle changes (Johnson, McCarter, & Ferencz, 1987; Kruse, LeFevre, & Zweig, 1986). Although most changes are appropriate only for the duration of the pregnancy, some, such as smoking cessation, would confer health benefits to the woman and her child if the woman maintained them. Further, although the media often portrays pregnancy through idealized images of happiness and family harmony, it is a highly tumultuous experience for most women and has predictable stages and concerns. Fathers who are in a relationship with the woman are typically engaged a little later, but they also undergo an intense and broadly recognizable experience during the pregnancy and period immediately after the birth.

Project PANDA was funded by the National Cancer Institute (CA-27821 and 2R25CA57712-06).

An estimated one-third of smokers quit sometime during pregnancy, usually in the first trimester (Floyd, Rimer, Giovino, Mullen, & Sullivan, 1993; Mullen, 1999; Quinn, Mullen, & Ershoff, 1991), and there have been numerous evaluations of programs to promote smoking cessation during this time (Dolan-Mullen, Ramirez, & Groff, 1994; Mullen & Ramirez, 2001). Interventions with parents who smoked had not been very effective. One study conducted in pediatrics offices about the same time as Project Parents and Newborns Developing and Adjusting (PANDA) found a small increase in self-reported cessation by mothers who smoked and a larger increase when the intervention was with a woman who had stopped smoking during pregnancy and whose intervention message was not to resume smoking (Wall, Severson, Andrews, Lichtenstein, & Zoref, 1995). However, at the time we developed the PANDA intervention, there had been no reports of programs to improve the rate of maintenance of cessation postpartum.

This chapter is a case study of using Intervention Mapping to create Project PANDA, a program to decrease rates of return to smoking among pregnant women who had stopped smoking (Mullen, DiClemente, Carbonari, Nicol, Sockrider, & Richardson et al., 1997; Mullen, 2004). The project is a good example of an explicit, rational approach to intervention design and is a particularly good model of the use of both theory and evidence very early in the design process to define the problem. The case also highlights the importance of understanding the context of the target groups and of designing messages to increase the intervention's salience by addressing the context in addition to the health risk. Finally, Project PANDA illustrates the successful use of detailed design documents to communicate message intent to the producers of program materials.

Perspectives

This case study is a good example of using theory to define the behavior of interest and of embedding the behavior in its context.

Using Theory to Define the Problem

The case provides an example of the role of reasoning with theory and evidence in the delineation of the actual problem to be solved. We discuss in detail the analysis by Mullen and colleagues (Mullen, Quinn, & Ershoff, 1990), which the team later elaborated (Stotts, DiClemente, Carbonari, & Mullen, 1996; Stotts, DiClemente, Carbonari, & Mullen, 2000; Mullen, 2004), that went beyond the interpretation that the problem of women who returned to smoking after having quit during pregnancy was a problem of relapse (Marlatt & Gordon, 1985). Had these women really relapsed? Thinking of them as relapsers implies that they had intended to quit for good. But Mullen had worked with Ershoff and Quinn on a pregnancy smoking-cessation trial in a health maintenance organization (HMO) in Los Angeles, and when they followed up six months postpartum with women who had successfully quit smoking, they heard statements from the women indicating no such resolve (Ershoff, Mullen, & Quinn, 1989; Mullen, Quinn, & Ershoff, 1990). Many of the women who returned to smoking right after the birth said they had not planned to quit for good. Virtually every woman who reported having returned to smoking added "but I never smoke around the baby (Mullen, Richardson, Quinn, & Ershoff, 1997, p. 328). Thus, Mullen initiated the collaboration with DiClemente, co-developer of the Transtheoretical Model (TTM), reasoning that the model could accommodate women who might be in various stages with respect to postpartum smoking even though they had abstained from smoking for several months at least. The TTM encompassed relapse prevention, but its broader view of the change process allowed us to gain some evidence about that process for these women.

Understanding the Importance of the Context

A second issue that this case study explicates well is the importance of the context of the pregnant women who are at risk for returning to smoking postpartum. What are the women's interests? Are they interested in changes in their bodies, in their relationships, in babies? Are they interested in future changes in daily schedules, jobs, and careers? Are they interested in creating an environment for a new baby? Is the possibility of return to cigarette smoking in this list of women's concerns? If it is, it may be only a vague concern. The PANDA development team reviewed lay and scientific literature to distill a list of the issues that may be of concern to women and their partners during the phases of pregnancy (Tables 13.1 and 13.2 give examples of these concerns). For example, at twenty-eight weeks the couple may be participating together in prepared childbirth-classes, and they may begin to communicate more about the baby. Women report an upsurge in conflict with their partners (Saunders & Robins, 1987). Nesting, the feeling of wanting to provide a special place for the baby and family, also begins about this time (Joffe, 1989). Later, both the mother and father develop anxiety about the birth, with the man more focused on threats to the woman's well-being and the mother more focused on the baby (Arizmendi & Affonso, 1987).

Mullen and DiClemente then based the intervention on the mothers' concerns as a framework for including messages designed to promote continued abstinence from smoking. This case study is an excellent example of consideration of context, because the planning team was concerned from the project's very

TABLE 13.1. CONCERNS OF WOMEN AND THEIR PARTNERS DURING PREGNANCY.

Before the Birth		
28 Weeks	**34 Weeks**	**36 Weeks**
Prepared childbirth classes: messages on labor and delivery, little on emotional or relationship transition (Imle, 1990).	Woman focuses on labor and delivery.	Anxiety increases (Drake, Verhuist, & Fawcett, 1988).
"Nesting" begins for both parents (Joffe, 1989).	Beginning of worry about well-being of baby at birth; partner worries about woman's health and safety.	Physical discomfort might lessen when baby engages.
Beginning focus on woman's "bigness" (Arizmendi & Affonso, 1987)	Increase in communication between partners; increased conflict (Saunders & Robins, 1987)	Focus may narrow to delivery (Joffe, 1989).
Woman feels better but anticipates having "old" body back.	Poignancy about loss of couplehood	Focus intensifies on time until delivery. ("Haven't you had the baby yet?")
Baby becomes more of a reality for partner.	Partner participates in plans for birth of the baby; not anticipating decrease in opportunities for participation.	Planning for and fantasizing about going to hospital
	Motivated to learn infant caretaking skills (Bliss-Holtz, 1988)	Arranging for help with the newborn
	Physical discomforts heighten.	Little information about recovery from delivery

beginning about how difficult it might be to get the women to attend to messages about the problem of return to smoking. However, the issue of context should be an important focus in all intervention development.

Intervention Mapping Step 1: Needs Assessment

In the needs assessment, the team reviewed the epidemiologic evidence for this problem and also conceptualized the problem using theory.

Epidemiologic Analysis

Approximately 20 percent of pregnant women smoke during pregnancy (U.S. Department of Health and Human Services, Office on Smoking and Health, 1980). In 1994 more than fourteen million U.S. women ages fifteen to forty-five were

TABLE 13.2. CONCERNS OF WOMEN AND THEIR PARTNERS AFTER THE BIRTH.

	After the Birth	
Immediately Postpartum	**Two Weeks Postartum**	**Six Weeks Postpartum**
Woman focused on physical recovery.	Mother home alone with baby; mother thinking about whether to return to work.	Feeling more competent as a mother
Sleep deprivation and possible depression	Baby is separate entity; mother and baby's health now separate.	New schedule challenges from returning to work
Demand to learn many new skills		Negotiating child care
Overwhelmed and out of control	Partner might feel loss of woman.	Six-week checkup for mother
Lack of instrumental role for partner	Focus of healthcare on baby; mother has lost supportive relationship with obstetrician.	May resume sexual intercourse
Extended family at home to "help"		Breastfeeding often discontinued at this point
Attention on baby, not mother	First well-baby checkup	Trauma of returning to work; emotional separation, longing, and guilt (Lewis & Cooper, 1987)
Learning who infant is	Baby begins to have a schedule.	
Some movement back to old self	Still sleep-deprived but venturing out of the house	Return to old environment and smoking cues
Surprised at how far from old self		Second well-baby checkup
Partner might feel left out		Peak of baby's crying

smokers; eight hundred thousand to one million of these women become pregnant each year. As with smoking generally, smoking during pregnancy is much more prevalent in women who are unmarried and have low income and education (Stockbauer & Land, 1991; U.S. Department of Health and Human Services, Office on Smoking and Health).

In the industrialized world, cigarette smoking is the most powerful known determinant of fetal growth retardation, affecting 22 percent to 36 percent of all cases (Wen, Goldenberg, Cutter, Hoffman, & Cliver, 1989). The relationship between smoking and low birth weight is one of the most consistent findings in the epidemiology literature. Maternal smoking also is recognized as a significant risk factor for preterm birth (Wen et al., 1989), sudden infant death syndrome (Malloy, Hoffman, & Peterson, 1992; Malloy, Kleinman, Land, & Schramm, 1988), spontaneous abortion (Windham, Swan, & Fenter, 1992), cleft palate or cleft lip, and mental retardation and impaired school performance (Cook, Peterson, & Moore, 1990; Lieberman, Gremy, Lang, & Cohen, 1994; U.S. Department of Health and Human Services, Office on Smoking and Health, 1980).

It is well established that smoking increases risk for lung and heart disease, cancer, and stroke as the most serious and prevalent problems (U.S. Department of Health and Human Services, Office on Smoking and Health, 1980, 1984a, 1984b, 1985). The prospect of hastening quitting in such a relatively young group is particularly important in light of these effects on the health of the woman herself.

Environmental tobacco smoke (ETS) has been consistently reported to cause increased respiratory infections and risk for asthma and asthma exacerbation in children (Emerson et al., 1994; A. B. Murray & Morrison, 1989; Overpeck & Moss, 1991; Samet, Cain, & Leaderer, 1991). A study by Cuijpers, Swaen, Wesseling, Stumans, and Wouters (1995) found ETS during a child's entire life to be significantly correlated with impairments to all spirometry parameters tested, and others have argued that smoking in the child's environment is an irritant to airways and should be eliminated (Hovell et al., 1994). A study of urban children with asthma showed that exposure to ETS is common; 59 percent of subjects' parents reported at least one smoker in the home. Additionally, at the study's baseline testing, 48 percent of children had a cotinine/creatinine ratio above 30 ng/mg, a level indicating significant exposure to ETS in the last twenty-four hours (Huss et al., 1994).

The Behavior: Quitting During Pregnancy and the Problem of Return to Smoking

Many female smokers stop smoking early in pregnancy, either on their own or with assistance. As many as 40 percent of women who smoked prior to the pregnancy stop spontaneously by the time of their first visit for prenatal care (Quinn et al., 1991; Secker-Walker et al., 1995; Woodby, Windsor, Snyder, Kohler, & DiClemente, 1999). Brief counseling of five to fifteen minutes along with pregnancy-oriented self-help materials almost doubles validated cessation over the 5 percent to 15 percent cessation rate that would have occurred with regular visits to a physician after the first visit (Dolan-Mullen et al., 1994; Mullen & Ramirez, 2001). Smoking cessation for pregnancy is important because it benefits the baby. However, it is disappointing to know that 63 percent to 73 percent of mothers return to smoking within six months after the birth, putting the infant at risk for the effects of ETS and themselves back on the track to severe health consequences (Fingerhut, Kleinman, & Kendrick, 1990; Mullen et al., 1990; Pirie et al., 1992; Mullen, Richardson, et al., 1997). Viewed as relapse, these rates are very similar to those measured for other addictive behaviors—including heroin—after the end of a treatment program (Hunt, Barnett, & Branch, 1971) (see Figure 13.1).

FIGURE 13.1. RELAPSE CURVES.

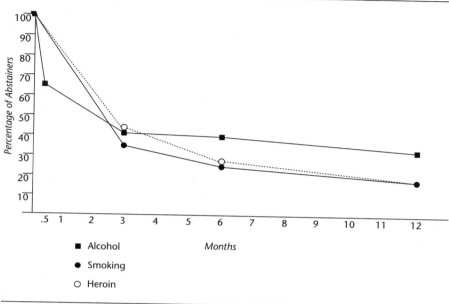

Source: Hunt, Barnett, and Branch, 1971.

Factors Related to the Return to Smoking

At the time we were planning this intervention, findings from cross sectional, prospective, and qualitative studies suggested several predictors of postpartum smoking, including not completely abstaining from it ("taking puffs") during pregnancy; having a partner, friends, and family who smoke; having been more addicted before pregnancy; having lower self-efficacy in midpregnancy about maintaining cessation postpartum; and quitting but neglecting to use coping strategies to resist the temptation to smoke. Study findings have been mixed with respect to level of smoking before the pregnancy as a predictor of postpartum smoking. Another issue, dissatisfaction with weight loss after the birth, has been shown to have a relationship to postpartum smoking, and postpartum exercise may be a protective factor (Mullen, Richardson, et al., 1997; Pirie et al., 1992; Severson, Andrews, Lichtenstein, Wall, & Zoref, 1995).

In addition to reviewing the literature, we used quantitative and qualitative data from interviews with women who had achieved biochemically validated cessation six months after the birth (Ershoff et al., 1989; Mullen et al., 1990;

Mullen, Richardson, et al., 1997). We also conducted focus groups with women and men in childbirth preparation classes and with pregnant women who had smoked prior to pregnancy and with their partners. Women and men were in separate groups with leaders of the same gender. We administered mail surveys once in mid- to late pregnancy and again about six weeks after delivery to women who had been smokers before their pregnancy and to their partners. The surveys addressed perceptions of pregnancy, perceived social support, sources of stress, concerns, and behavior change stimulated by the pregnancy (Pollak & Mullen, 1997; Richardson, Mullen, & DiClemente, 1993; Stotts, et al., 1996; Taylor, Richardson, & Mullen, 1993). In the course of data collection, we learned that women were not sure about the seriousness of ETS or at what distance or under what conditions the baby is actually exposed.

The women noted the benefits of smoking: it helps them control stress, concentrate, and take off the weight they still had by six weeks postpartum. Interestingly, although others have investigated concern about gestational weight gain and postpartum weight loss as predictors of smoking cessation and postpartum return to smoking (McBride, Pirie, & Curry, 1992), smoking intervention trials with pregnant women had not measured cessation's effect on weight gain. Data collected during the PANDA trial established that white, non-Hispanic women with singleton pregnancies (that is only one fetus) who stop smoking gain more weight (36.6 pounds; SD = 14.5) than do continuing smokers (28.9 pounds; SD = 11.7). Smoking cessation was associated with a lower risk of gaining too little (relative risk = 0.47; 95 percent confidence interval 0.27–0.81) using authoritative standards (Institute of Medicine, 1990) but also with gaining too much weight by those same standards (relative risk = 1.74; 95 percent confidence interval 0.1.21–2.51) (Mongoven, Dolan-Mullen, Groff, Nicol, & Burau, 1996). And the excessive gainers were 3.1 times as likely to give birth to babies weighing more than four thousand grams. The latter group may also be more likely to retain excess weight after the pregnancy and to have a higher lifetime risk of obesity. More thought should thus be given to the role that a smoking-cessation intervention can play in limiting excessive pregnancy weight gain and supporting return to normal weight through a nutritious diet and physical activity.

Significantly, most women did not view quitting during pregnancy as a success. When we framed their stopping as a success, their attributions were to external, temporary causes (that is, the baby, nausea). Further, new mothers expressed increased stress from such factors as sleep deprivation, dissatisfaction with slow postpartum weight loss, return to cues for smoking such as caffeine and alcohol consumption, and the perception that important others no longer disapproved of their smoking once the pregnancy was over.

Both from the literature and from our conversations with women who quit during pregnancy, we found that the role of the partner was important to returning to smoking postpartum. A partner who smoked created not only social pressure but also a presence of stimuli for smoking and a ready access to cigarettes. Lastly, it was apparent that intervention should start in late pregnancy. Half of those women who would return to smoking by six months had already returned by the sixth postpartum week. The six-week postpartum checkup by the obstetrician-gynecologist was too late, and for many mothers, so was the first pediatric visit.

How to Define the Problem: A Problem of Relapse or a Problem of Change?

We have recounted how Mullen came to understand the problem as more complex than relapse alone. This shift was an important one in describing desired behavior change and performance objectives; it would have profound effects on hypothetical determinants of performance. The relapse prevention model (Figure 13.2) seems to show that common reasons for relapse would relate to the presence of temptation or stimuli to smoke and the presence or absence of a coping

FIGURE 13.2. RELAPSE PREVENTION MODEL: A COGNITIVE-BEHAVIORAL MODEL OF THE RELAPSE PROCESS.

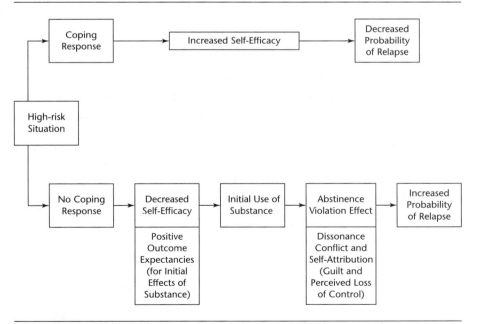

Source: Marlatt and Gordon, 1985.

response for dealing with the temptation (Marlatt & Gordon, 1985). It was clear that the women had reasons for return to smoking that spanned a much broader conceptual range than just temptation and coping.

Thus we found that some women reported not intending to quit for good, believing that smoking is safe after birth if they keep smoke away from the baby. Others said that they "hoped" they wouldn't go back to smoking, although they had no specific plan to enable abstinence. Another group expressed resolve to make this quit "for good," although it was clear that even though they may have spent six months "in action," they had not been tested in the same way that smokers in the general population would have been.

Using stages of change from the TTM, we explored in more depth whether the women were conceptually in the action stage (having quit smoking) or were distributed over the earlier stages of precontemplation and contemplation with respect to abstaining from postpregnancy smoking. We based this analysis on what the women said about quitting during pregnancy and the processes they had used to quit, as well as on an emerging staging algorithm tailored for pregnancy. For example, women who had "really quit" probably would no longer be grappling with beliefs about the harm that cigarettes could cause themselves and their children, but some of these women were unconvinced about these issues. Real quitters would have high self-efficacy, determined at least partially by attributing successful quitting more to internal, stable causes: "I am the type of person who can give up cigarettes" (Marlatt & Gordon, 1985; Prochaska, Velicer, DiClemente, & Fava, 1988,) and not to unstable, external causes.

In other words, women who had really quit smoking would have used many of the change processes that Prochaska, DiClemente, and colleagues (C. C. DiClemente et al., 1991; Prochaska, Velicer, DiClemente, & Fava, 1988; Prochaska, Velicer, Guadagnoli, Rossi, & DiClemente, 1991) described. Processes of change in the TTM are described in the following way: experiential processes peak in the contemplation stage, and behavioral processes peak in the preparation, or early action, stage (Prochaska et al., 1988, 1991). In the contemplation stage, higher levels of experiential processing cause the pros of smoking to become less important than the cons of smoking. Yet in an analysis of the survey data from this project compared with similar data for women who were not pregnant, pregnant women who quit smoking were seen as having lower use of experiential and behavioral processes than the comparison group in the action stage (Stotts et al., 1996).Thus, based on process use and self-efficacy, those women seemed to be in contemplation for abstaining from smoking postpartum.

These considerations led us to conclude that the TTM was an appropriate conceptual framework and that relapse prevention could be subsumed within it. Further, we were intrigued with the successful coping path of the relapse prevention model and saw that it had received less attention than unsuccessful coping had (Mullen, Pollak, & Kok, 1999). We also recognized the ambiguity of the role of attributions on the success path and of the general lack of salience of success, particularly among women (Deaux & Farris, 1977; Reno, 1981) (see Figure 13.3). In discussing with pregnant women the reason for quitting, we were reminded that individual women may perceive the same reason for success quite differently. For example, one woman may view quitting for the baby's sake as temporary and another as permanent. Researchers who study attributions have adopted the convention of asking respondents for their perceptions (for example, Russell's Causal Dimension Scale) (Russell, 1982). Intervention planners considering a reattribution component also need to clarify the meaning of frequently mentioned reasons. They might try, as we did, to define nonsmoking during pregnancy as a success, by giving relevant information, for example: "Only one in five women in this clinic has been able to stop smoking." Because most pregnant women who stop smoking find it easy, a persuasive statement we used was: "It will never be easier." Another example of attribution retraining (Fosterling, 1985) would be promoting an ambiguous reason, the baby as a permanent rather than temporary reason, for example: "You are giving your baby a good start. Continuing to be a nonsmoker can help avoid unnecessary illness for your baby and inconvenient doctoral visits and worry for you." We also learned that stable success attritions

FIGURE 13.3. STAGES, PROCESSES OF CHANGE, AND EVIDENCE THAT WOMEN MIGHT NOT BE QUITTERS.

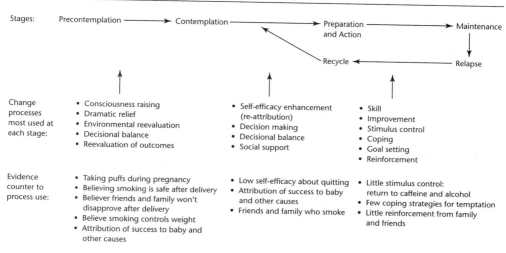

seem to affect smoking through self-efficacy. In other words, attribution of success to more stable causes increases confidence in one's ability to maintain a behavior change. Other interventionists might consider including success attributions when designing programs that contribute to maintenance after initial behavior change.

Under the conceptual framework of the TTM, the purpose of the program was to help women who had merely stopped smoking temporarily to stop smoking permanently. We hypothesized that among women not smoking at twenty-eight weeks of pregnancy, there would be precontemplators, contemplators, and women in action. (Preparation was included in action.) And even those women with six or more months of continuous abstaining from smoking were not classified as being in the maintenance stage, because of lower process use and less exposure to usual temptations.

Because the standard algorithm for staging smoking cessation was not applicable, a stepped approach to staging postpartum smoking was used in which women were first differentiated by assessing their personal goal for postpartum smoking. We expected the majority of women to report their goal to be continued abstinence, the socially acceptable response but unlikely, according to previous studies described above. Thus, to separate them further, womens' perceived likelihood of smoking postpartum was evaluated. This item is conceptualized as a type of efficacy expectation—a combination of both their confidence to abstain from smoking (self-efficacy) and the barriers or temptations that might interfere with abstinence. Figure 13.4 depicts the algorithm used to stage the women for staying off cigarettes postpartum.

Conclusions and Program Objectives

The focal factors from the needs assessment were the following:

- Moving women across the stages of change instead of assuming they were in the action phase
- Viewing men as important environmental influences who would need their own program
- Turning stopping for pregnancy into permanent cessation, focusing on the woman rather than ETS

Based on the needs assessment, program objectives for the women's program were as follows:

- Decrease return to smoking at twelve months postpartum by 10 percentage points

FIGURE 13.4. STAGE OF CHANGE FOR POSTPARTUM SMOKING.

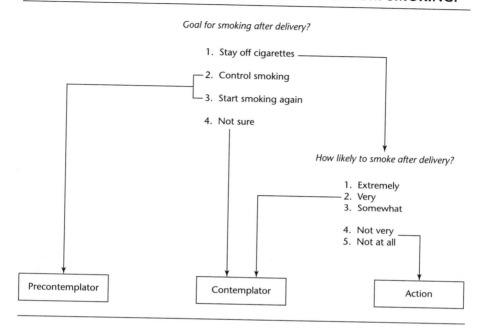

• Decrease infant ETS exposure by increasing nonsmoking by parents and other household members and by decreasing smoking in the home by parents who continued to smoke

Because of the important association of the prevalence of smoking in women's social networks (particularly their partners) with the likelihood of their return to smoking and with infant ETS exposure, we focused the program on men as well as women. The association of quitting and smoking by friends and family is ubiquitous in the smoking literature; yet interventions to increase social support through buddy contracts, tip sheets for quitters to give to significant others, and other such interventions had not produced the hoped-for results (Cohen et al., 1988). Thus, because the pregnancy presumably would be a time when some smoking fathers might be motivated to stop, Mullen and DiClemente decided that the intervention for fathers should be focused on quitting if the father was a smoker. This focus would have another benefit, because mothers are the number-one source of ETS if they are smokers, but fathers who smoke are a significant source as well. Thus, one program objective for the men was to decrease the percentage of partners who smoke.

Step 2: Matrices of Change Objectives

We had two major behavior-change objectives for both women and their partners. The women were to abstain from smoking and protect the infant from ETS. The men who smoked were to quit smoking; all the men were to protect the infant from ETS. Women and men were staged with respect to these objectives; they were in precontemplation, contemplation, or action. They were also differentiated by time-point in the transition from pregnancy to parenthood. Table 13.3 shows the groups after the population was differentiated.

Because of their primary role in the environment for the women's smoking and because of their efforts at ETS control, we considered men a primary group for ETS and a secondary group for quitting. Further, we wanted men to provide instrumental, appraisal, and emotional social support to help the women cope with postpartum stress and temptations to smoke (see Table 13.3).

Based on the TTM, there is one performance objective for each stage for the two behaviors (refraining from smoking and controlling ETS). For example, the performance objective for women in the contemplation stage for smoking is: move to the action stage for remaining abstinent from cigarettes after the birth. For women in the action stage, the performance objective is: continue to remain abstinent from cigarettes after the birth. Table 13.3 illustrates that, technically, every person × each pregnancy stage × behavior × stage of change is a separate matrix because the behaviors and determinants are different. This breakdown results in twenty-seven matrices. However, each matrix has only one performance objective, and few determinants or factors were hypothesized to influence the performance objective. Tables 13.4, 13.5, and 13.6 are sample matrices. We chose determinants with guidance from theory (from the change processes of the TTM in Figure 13.3 and from evidence). For example, Table 13.4 includes the decisional balance as an important determinant for moving from precontemplation to contemplation; whereas Table 13.5 includes attribution, decisional balance, skills, and social support as hypothesized determinants for moving from contemplation to action. Each matrix also includes notations about the salient pregnancy issues that will interact with the determinants.

Step 3: Methods and Strategies

Processes of change have been proposed as mechanisms that people use to get themselves from one stage of change to another (see Table 3.3). For example, for people to move from precontemplation to contemplation, they need to become

TABLE 13.3. TARGET POPULATION DIFFERENTIATION.

Pregnancy Transition

	29–30 Weeks	32–34 Weeks	34–36 Weeks	Immediate Postpartum	Two Weeks Postpartum	Six Weeks Postpartum
Women	Smoking: Precontemplator Contemplator	Smoking: Contemplator	Smoking: Contemplator	Smoking: Action	Smoking: Action	Smoking: Action
		Environmental Tobacco Smoke (ETS) Control: Contemplator	ETS Control: Action	ETS Control: Action	ETS Control: Action	ETS Control: Action
Men	Smoking: Precontemplator Contemplator	Smoking: Contemplator	Smoking: Contemplator	Smoking: Contemplator	Smoking: Contemplator	Smoking: Contemplator
	ETS Control: Precontemplator Contemplator	ETS Control and Social Support: Contemplator Action	ETS Control and Social Support: Action	ETS Control and Social Support: Action	ETS Control and Social Support: Action	ETS Control and Social Support: Action

TABLE 13.4. SAMPLE MATRIX FOR SMOKING AND ETS, WOMEN PRECONTEMPLATORS, 29 TO 30 WEEKS.

Performance Objectives (Women)	Determinants	
	Attribution	**Awareness and Decisional Balance**
PO.1. Smoking: Women move to the contemplation stage of remaining abstinent from cigarettes after the birth.	A.1.a. View stopping smoking as a success A.1.b. View self as the kind of person who can successfully give up cigarettes	ADB.1.a. Believe that smoking is bad for self and baby ABD.1.b. Notices negative responses to smoking ABD.1.c. Develop ideas about long-term benefits of not smoking for self ABD.1.d. Describe how smoking is bad for the baby after birth ABD.1.e. Describe possible improvements in health and self-image
PO.2. Environmental tobacco smoke (ETS) Control: Women move to the contemplation stage of protecting the infant from environmental tobacco smoke.	A.2. See self as the kind of person who would (and can) protect her child from environmental tobacco smoke	ABD.2. Increase awareness of effects of ETS on infants and children

Pregnancy issues: Beginning childbirth classes, many messages on labor and delivery, beginning to think about having old body back, baby becomes more of a reality for the partner, nesting begins for both parents

more aware through consciousness raising, dramatic relief, environmental reevaluation, and increased perception of risks and benefits. They need to begin to tip the scales toward the pro side of making a change. To enable movement from contemplation to action, the experiential processes continue to tip the decisional balance with reevaluation of self that focuses on important benefits and positive outcomes. Promoting movement between these stages must also include processes to enhance self-efficacy, such as building skills and trying out the new behavior. Social support becomes important at this point. As a person moves firmly into action, he or she continues to build skills, enhance self-efficacy, and exert control over the environment.

Table 13.7 presents some of the theoretical methods and practical strategies used to correspond with the stage-of-change segments of the target groups for Project PANDA. For example, to raise their awareness of the benefits of not smoking and of protecting their baby from ETS, fathers first had to see themselves as important to

TABLE 13.5. SAMPLE MATRIX FOR SMOKING AND ETS, WOMEN CONTEMPLATORS, 32 TO 34 WEEKS.

	Determinants					External
	Personal					
Performance Objectives (Women)	Attribution	Self-Efficacy	Decisional Balance	Skills	Social Support	
PO.1. Smoking: Women move to the action stage of remaining abstinent from cigarettes after the birth.	A.1.a. View stopping smoking as a success based on stable characteristics of self A.1.b. View self as the kind of person who can successfully give up cigarettes	SE.1.a. Express confidence for remaining off cigarettes postpartum SE.1.b. Express confidence in maintaining relations where smoking has been a shared activity SE.1.c. Express confidence in returning to normal postpartum without smoking	DB.1.a. Notice negative responses to smoking DB.1.b. Develop long-term benefits of not smoking for self		SS.1. Partners do not smoke around woman pre- or postpartum.	
PO.2. Environmental tobacco smoke (ETS) Control: Women move to the action stage of protecting the infant from environmental tobacco smoke. PO.2.1. Deal with visitors and relatives who smoke PO.2.2. Make house smoke free PO.2.3. Choose smoke-free environments outside of the home	A.2. See self as the kind of person who would (and can) protect her child from ETS	SE.2.1.a. Express confidence in asking family members not to smoke SE.2.1.b. Express confidence in asking partners not to smoke in the house SE.2.1.c. Express confidence in asking friends not to smoke around baby SE.2.1.d. Express confidence in making house smoke free SE.2.1.e. Express confidence in negotiating non-smoking seats in venues outside the house	DB.2.a. Increase awareness of effects of ETS on infants and children DB.2.b. See stress of negotiating smoke-free environments as less negative than infant exposure	S.2. Demonstrate negotiating with partner, friends, and family members for not smoking around baby	SS.2.a. Partners negotiate about a smoke-free environment. SS.2.b. Partners begin to help develop smoke-free house rules.	

Pregnancy issues: Focusing more on labor and delivery, beginning to worry about the birth and the health of the baby, increased communication between couple, poignancy about loss of couplehood

TABLE 13.6. SAMPLE MATRIX FOR MEN CONTEMPLATORS FOR QUITTING SMOKING AND ACTION FOR ETS AND SOCIAL SUPPORT, 32 TO 34 WEEKS.

Performance Objectives	Determinants	Change Objectives
Quitting Smoking Contemplation PO.1. Partners move to the action stage for quitting smoking.	Attribution Self-Efficacy Decisional Balance	A.1. View self as the kind of person who can successfully give up cigarettes SE.1. Express confidence in giving up smoking DB.1. Notice negative response to smoking DB.2. Increase awareness of effects of environmental tobacco smoke (ETS) on infants and children DB.3. Increase awareness of self as smoking role model for children and of self as an instrumental parent
ETS and Social Support Action PO.2. Partners protect child from ETS. PO.2.1. Work with partners to make house smoke free PO.2.2. Deal with friends and relatives regarding smoke-free house PO.2.3. Refrain from smoking around the woman or child PO.2.4. Choose smoke-free environments outside of the house	Skills Self-Efficacy Stimulus Control Coping	S.2.1. Discuss how to make home smoke free S.2.2. Practice routine for dealing with friends and relatives S.2.3. Practice leaving the home environment to smoke S.2.4. List places outside of home that will be avoided with family SE.2.2.a. Express confidence in asking family not to smoke SE.2.2.b. Express confidence in asking friends not to smoke around baby SE.2.3. Express confidence in not smoking in the house SC.2. Display cues for smoke-free house C.2. Have plans for how to cope with friends and family for not smoking around the baby or in the house

Pregnancy issues: Beginning to worry about the birth and the woman's health and safety, participation in plans for the birth, not anticipating postpartum changes in participation, motivated to learn infant caretaking

TABLE 13.7. METHODS AND STRATEGIES FOR PROJECT PANDA.

Theoretical Methods	Practical Strategies: Women	Practical Strategies: Men
To Move from Precontemplation to Contemplation		
Persuasion of the benefits of not smoking Persuasion of risks of smoking Persuasion of the costs of smoking and the costs of a new baby Persuasion of the risks of environmental tobacco smoke (ETS) to baby Modeling reattribution training	Newsletter article on risks and benefits Newsletter messages about attribution for quitting	Articles pairing general parenting competence and expectation of being a participatory father with protecting baby from ETS Videotape modeling of moving to the role of fatherhood as one that gets healthier and protects the infant Article stressing the benefits of taking care of health—consider quitting
To Move from Contemplation to Action		
Modeling for reattribution training Promoting decisional balance shift Skill building Encouraging social support from partner and others Providing cues for environmental control	Attribution article on becoming a good parent—including ETS protection Article on skill-building for dealing with stress without cigarettes Persuasive articles about environmental control Signs for environmental control Letter from the baby to reinforce environmental control	Newsletter articles teaching social support strategies and how to cope well enough to give support Articles with attribution messages—the type of fathers who will protect baby Skill building for environmental control Article and videotape models stressing fathers as role models for their children
To Support Action and Move Toward Maintenance		
Skill building for coping with relapse temptations Skill building for environmental control and social support Modeling coping Social comparison Skill training for coping with negative feelings Modeling problem solving	Videotape with role model of coping with temptation, recycling from relapse Newsletter role-model story—preventing relapse Newsletter skill-training—coping with stress Newsletter articles to model a coping mom versus a mastery mom—enhance self-efficacy and lower stress Newsletter skill training article for coping with negative feeling Video modeling for enhancing social support Newsletter article encouraging building social support	Newsletter article with skill building for problem solving Articles with skill building for stress management Skill building for infant protection

the baby. Articles in the first newsletter for fathers delivered these messages about the importance of fathers to their children. Figure 13.5 shows one of these articles.

We designed this program for delivery in managed care settings, which now provide a large part of the prenatal care in the United States. In the health maintenance organization (HMO) setting in which the program would initially be implemented and evaluated, the average prenatal visit with a health care provider

FIGURE 13.5 EXAMPLE OF METHOD DELIVERY—NEWSLETTER.

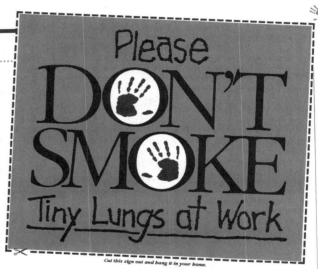

THE SMOKE-FREE ZONE

Creating your own zone

You know the effects of passive smoke aren't good for you or your baby, but how about friends and family? Smoking is a habit people do without thinking. Often they will light up whenever they feel like it, whether or not you and your baby are present. To keep you and your baby smoke-free, you will need to take action.

First decide what "smoke-free" means. How big of a smoke-free zone do you need? Certainly, babies shouldn't be in a closed car or in the same room with someone smoking. But what about the next room? Or a house where someone has been smoking? Scientific studies tell us that the byproducts of cigarette smoke don't leave an area as quickly as we might think. Practical experience tells us the same thing. Airlines switched from no-smoking sections to a ban on smoking because cigarette smoke affected passengers throughout the plane.

Protecting your zone

Often a "no smoking" sign is enough to communicate the message that you don't want smoking in your house or car. Some smokers, however, may have to be told what your rules are. Say, for example, "I'd like you to smoke outside," or "I really feel tempted to smoke right now, and I want to remain a nonsmoker, so please don't smoke around me."

Friends and relatives

To her neighbor who was about to take a pack of cigarettes out of her purse, Amelia said: "If you want to smoke, please smoke on the balcony. There's a chair and an ashtray, and when you're finished, we'll have the iced tea I'm making."

Some situations are more complicated. Mothers we have talked to say that discouraging smoking by members of their husband's family, and in someone else's house, is especially touchy. They

suggest a private talk before the visit or strategies like keeping the baby in another room. If the smokers are your partner's friends or family, maybe you can suggest that he talk to them.

Partner

We all know perfectly well that the most difficult situation in the no-smoke battle is having a husband or partner who smokes. His smoking may make it hard for you not to smoke. And, of course, smoking fathers are a big source of smoke exposure for their babies. Although to quit smoking entirely is best for him, he has to make that decision. While he is still smoking, you will need to be assertive, factual, and firm. Let him know how much you value his company. Don't be judgmental about his smoking habit or get into arguments. Focus on finding a solution together. Ask him how he would keep some part of the house smoke-free. Perhaps the

establishment of a smoking area is one solution. The best place is outside. The garage or a room with the door closed is next-best.

After the birth of their twins, Amelia's husband decided he could not quit smoking. But, agreeing that protecting the babies was the priority, he smoked on the patio when he needed a cigarette. He worked on old cars in the garage, which they agreed to designate as a second smoking area.

Working together on solutions seems to be best for both partners. After establishing a smoke-free routine with family and friends, you will find that visits will be more enjoyable because both you and your visitors will be more relaxed.

Keeping you and your baby smoke-free takes effort. You will need to be assertive. Most mothers find they have hidden stores of strength when it comes to protecting their children.

Cut this sign out and hang it in your home.

was scheduled for seven minutes. Early in the project, developers recognized that counseling for maintaining abstinence from smoking probably could not fit within these time constraints. Therefore, we decided to use the mediated delivery mechanisms of newsletters and videotapes mailed to program participants at home. In checking with various types of videotape rental businesses, we estimated that more than 90 percent of U.S. households have access to VCRs and that this rate could be expected to hold in this employed population. Further, the men who participated in focus groups expressed a preference to have their own materials (versus sharing materials with the woman) mailed directly to them (versus having the women deliver these to them).

Step 4: Program Design

The challenge of this step of program development is to translate the planning up to this point into a creative, deliverable program with a defined scope and sequence. Chapter Eight explains that program design documents are needed to communicate product characteristics within a design team and especially to production people or vendors who may not have participated in the planning process. One of the defining characteristics of Project PANDA development was our careful use of design documents. Figure 13.6 shows a flow diagram for the preparation of the newsletters (the design document for which is shown in Figure 8.4), and Figure 13.5 shows part of an article from a final newsletter.

The video writer–producer, in addition to creating the design documents for the two videotapes that were part of the intervention, participated with the development team in conducting focus groups. In this way she heard the concerns of women and their partners firsthand. We recommend involving outside vendors in as much of the planning and target group communication process as is possible and practical. Seeing and hearing the potential program participants convey much more than reading through design documents alone. Even so, being in the entire process and communicating with the priority group often does not take the place of working from a design document.

In pretesting the Project PANDA materials, we wanted to verify how much of our intent to respond to the women's pregnancy context we had been able to operationalize. We wanted to confirm, for example, how much of the "airtime" in the videotapes and how much of the copy in the newsletters had been devoted to smoking and how much had been devoted to supportive topics for the new mothers and fathers. Figures 13.7 and 13.8 are graphs that show the percentage of time per minute devoted to smoking in the men's and women's videotape. The men's tape, which came to the men early in the program sequence, when we expected them to be in the early stages of change for smoking cessation and for protecting

FIGURE 13.6. FLOW DIAGRAM FOR NEWSLETTER PREPARATION.

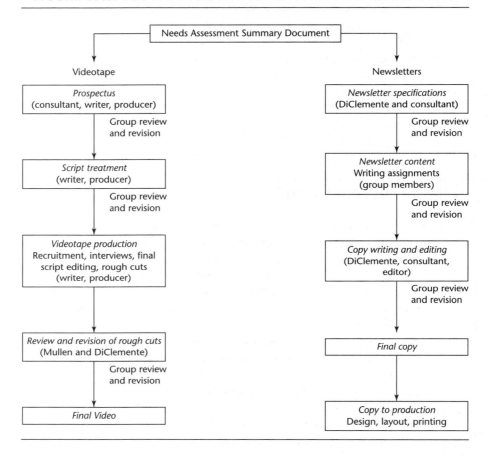

the baby from ETS, did not mention smoking until the tenth minute and focused on smoking in only six of eighteen minutes of tape. The women's tape was delivered when most of the women were hypothesized to be in the action stage of continued abstinence and when the temptations to return to smoking immediately postpartum were particularly high. The women's tape focused almost entirely on smoking (twelve of nineteen minutes had a smoking focus), whereas the newsletters that preceded the tape were heavily devoted to pregnancy issues.

FIGURE 13.7. PERCENTAGE OF SMOKING FOCUS IN MEN'S VIDEO.

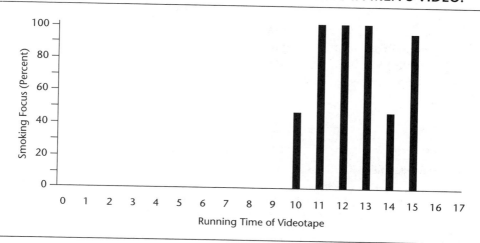

FIGURE 13.8. PERCENTAGE OF SMOKING FOCUS IN WOMEN'S VIDEO.

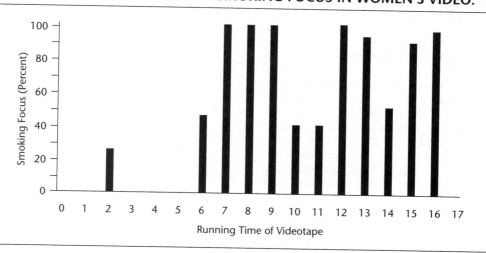

To pretest the Project PANDA materials, we engaged a panel of men and another of women from the target groups to review and respond to materials. The newsletters were presented in an almost-finished format with response boxes at the end of each article (Figure 13.9). Because each article, rather than each newsletter, was intended to have a specific impact, we wanted the panel members' responses to specific newsletter segments.

FIGURE 13.9. PRETESTING NEWSLETTER.

Familiar Faces, Familiar Routines

About this time, most new mothers feel more like their old selves and are going back to their usual activities. They are no longer getting the special treatment of pregnancy and the first few weeks after giving birth they are feeling the demands of job and family.

Reentering life as it was before brings special challenges. You changed because you gave birth and are now responsible for another, very needy human being. In pregnancy, you were more conscious of your body and how you treated it; you ate more healthful foods; and you stopped smoking.

Although most women would like to stick to these healthy patterns, it's easy to drift back into the old ones. Now is the time to make a conscious decision about what you want for yourself. Don't expect this to be easy, because old habits arise with old routines. For example, your partner and co-workers probably didn't expect you to smoke along with them while you were pregnant. But now they may think there's no reason for you not to.

Women who went through this process tell us that drinking juice or water during coffee breaks with co-workers reduces the temptation to smoke. Another technique is keeping both hands busy with handwork such as needlepoint, which interferes with smoking but promotes conversation.

Tell people what you've decided to do, but don't judge them. One mother who returned to work told us, "It's easy to act self-righteous about changing my habits and get down on others for continuing to smoke or eat unhealthy foods. But I remember how hard and slow the change was for me. It doesn't give me the license to judge someone else for the choices they make. Reminding myself of this helps me think twice before I reach for a cigarette or for another doughnut at the office."

Circle the appropriate number.

This article:

A. Was not interesting	Was moderately interesting	Was very interesting
1	2	3
B. Was not easy to understand	Was moderately easy to understand	Was very easy to understand
1	2	3
C. Did not apply to my life	Moderately applied to my life	Very much applied to my life
1	2	3
D. Included information that was not helpful	Included information that was moderately helpful	Included information that was very helpful
1	2	3

We reviewed videotapes at the rough-cut stage. As we discussed in Chapter Eight, the women's tape required significant changes because the role-model material that the video producer abstracted from interviews was overly focused on mastery rather than coping. We needed to reedit to find material that was closer to the psychological and physical state of a newly delivered woman who was trying to stay off cigarettes.

Step 5: Implementation

Project PANDA entailed entirely mediated intervention components—newsletters and videotapes. However, the women's managed care plan mailed components to the homes of the women and their partners. Therefore, an advisory committee from the care plans worked with the project to review intervention development and facilitate implementation.

Step 6: Evaluation

The evaluation model is presented in Figure 13.10. For this project the evaluation of the validity of the hypothetical determinants was explored in a pilot project rather than in the randomized trial of smoking abstinence. Therefore, in the model, process extends to the determinants box and includes consideration of self-efficacy, the influence of attributions on self-efficacy, stress, social support, and use of the change processes.

In the process evaluation, we looked at the implementation of the project through telephone interviews with the women. We asked whether they and their partners received the videos and newsletters (women, 96 percent; partners, 90 percent) and whether they read all the newsletters (women, 78 percent; partners, 59 percent) and watched the videos (women, 66 percent; men, 59 percent). We also explored aspects of the intervention components in terms of how well they met our assumptions about methods and strategies. During the evaluation of the PANDA intervention, Stotts, Carbonari, and Mullen (2000) asked women in late pregnancy their stage of change for continued abstinence from smoking after the birth. This survey confirmed our idea of the women's perspective. For this analysis women were classified into one of three stages of change for postpartum smoking cessation described in Figure 13.4. After examining predictors, it was evident that a behavioral challenge might usefully separate women classified as being in action (the general smoking algorithm uses a "quit attempt in the past year" criterion). Thus, reporting a puff of a cigarette since intake, was included to further separate women in preparation from those truly in the action stage of change. The

FIGURE 13.10. PROJECT PANDA EVALUATION LOGIC MODEL.

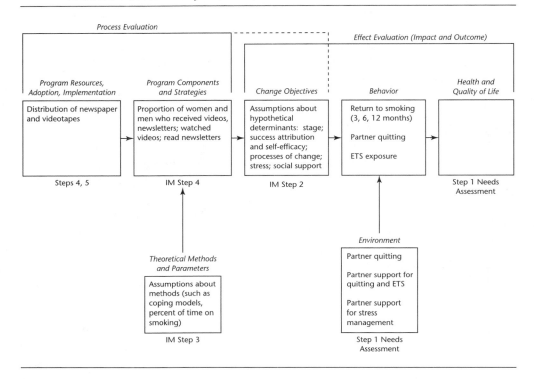

algorithm is mutually exclusive so that all pregnant quitters were classified in only one stage as follows: 24 precontemplators (9.4 percent), 58 contemplators (22.7 percent), 94 preparation stage (36.7 percent), and 80 action stage (31.3 percent). Stage differences were found on exposure to other smokers in the environment, with precontemplators reporting more smoke exposure than the other three groups. The percentage of women who returned to smoking after the delivery was highest in the precontemplation stage and decreased with each subsequent stage. Results lend support for the stages of change for postpartum smoking (Stotts et al., 2000).

As the evaluation model (Figure 13.10) indicates, the main outcome variable being measured is whether the woman is smoking at six weeks and at three, six, and twelve months. The measure in the woman is self-report with urine cotinine validation in a subsample; and at twelve months postpartum, there was a 10 percentage-point difference in point prevalence abstinence favoring the intervention group (Mullen, DiClemente, et al., 1997; Mullen, 2004). Women were also asked to report on their partners' smoking without the validation measure, and there appears to be an impact on partner smoking (DiClemente et al., 1998; Mullen, 2004). The other outcome measure is ETS protection, which is being measured by the placement of nicotine monitors in the room where the family reports spending the most time, and this variable did not show a difference.

Summary

Project PANDA is a good example of using theory to define the behavior of interest for a health education and promotion program and to tailor interventions to create change in the behavior. Had program developers Mullen and DiClemente adopted the most obvious approach to addressing return to smoking among women who had quit postpartum (that is, relapse prevention), they would have had a very different program. And in these differences, the program would have lacked messages for a majority of the women (that is, the precontemplators and contemplators for staying off cigarettes).

In addition, Project PANDA is a model for getting to know the priority group for a program and using members' input throughout program development. From the very beginning of thinking about the program, when the development team heard clues to an early stage of change and the lack of use of the change processes, through the target group pretesting of the intervention materials, this project was guided by the women and men it sought to help.

CHAPTER FOURTEEN

CULTIVANDO LA SALUD

María Fernández, Alicia Gonzales, Guillermo Tortolero-Luna, Sylvia Partida, and L. Kay Bartholomew

Reader Objectives

- Describe the use of community-based planning methods
- Develop performance objectives for lay health workers
- Develop performance objectives, training, and materials for program adoption and implementation

Hispanics represent 13.3 percent of U.S. residents and are the nation's fastest growing minority group, increasing from 22.4 million in 1990 to 39.9 million in 2003. This increase represents a growth almost four times that of the total U.S. population (R. R. Ramirez & Cruz, 2003; United States Census Bureau & Bernstein, 2004). Within the United States, Hispanics who reside in the West and South are mainly of Mexican origin, and counties with the highest proportions of Hispanics (about 80 percent) are found along the Texas-Mexico border (Texas Department of State Health Services, 2003a, 2003b). When compared with non-Hispanics, Texas Hispanics (particularly those living along the Texas-Mexico border) are younger, have lower educational levels, experience higher poverty and unemployment rates, and have insufficient access to primary health care services (Larson, 2002).

Approximately 4.2 million migrant and seasonal farm workers live in the United States, and many reside along the U.S.-Mexico border (National Center for Farmworker Health, 2002). Along the border, farmworkers often live in *colonias*. *Colonias* are unincorporated, unzoned, and rural or semirural communities characterized by substandard housing; and they lack such basic infrastructure as access to public drinking water or wastewater systems (U.S. Department of Health and Human Services, Health Resources and Services Administration [HRSA], 2005). Approximately 432,000 people (many of them farmworkers) live in twelve hundred *colonias* on the Texas and New Mexico borders. Many *colonia* residents, particularly farmworkers, experience both cultural and logistic barriers to health care service, including poverty, mobility, low literacy, English-language deficiency, and lack of access to health care providers (Coughlin, Uhler, Richards, & Wilson, 2003; National Center for Farmworker Health, 2002). Because of these many barriers, farmworkers often do not obtain health care services, particularly for prevention or early detection such as cancer screening.

Cancer is the second leading cause of death among Hispanic adults in the United States; and the most commonly diagnosed cancers among Hispanics are prostate, colon and rectum, lung, and breast (among women) (American Cancer Society, 2003). Hispanic women are the least likely of all racial and ethnic groups to have Pap tests, mammography, and clinical breast exams (CBE) (American Cancer Society; Gotay & Wilson, 1998; Hubbell, Mishra, Chavez, & Valdez, 1997). Underuse of screening among Hispanic women may contribute to lower survival rates for breast and cervical cancers. Mortality from breast cancer increased twice that of non-Hispanic whites (approximately an 82 percent increase in Hispanics between the periods from 1958 to 1962 and 1983 to 1987) (Ries et al., 2002). Hispanic women have twice the incidence rate of cervical cancer compared with non-Hispanic white women, and some of the highest mortality rates in the United States are observed along the Texas-Mexico border area (American Cancer Society, 2003; Devessa et al., 1999; Ries et al., 2002). Screening for breast and cervical cancer among Hispanics is lower than among non-Hispanic whites, and the disparity is even greater among low-income and border residents (Coughlin et al., 2003).

Despite the burden of cancer and disparities in screening practices among Hispanics, few screening interventions have been developed for these populations. In their literature review of 245 intervention studies of cervical cancer screening, Marcus and Crane (1998) identified only a few developed for Hispanic women. Similarly, information about effective interventions for breast cancer screening among diverse populations is limited (Bonfill, Marzo, Pladevall, Marti, & Emparanza, 2001; Legler et al., 2002). This paucity of relevant interventions suggests a need for carefully planned programs that identify specific determinants of screening and use the most appropriate change strategies in order to increase screening behaviors among Hispanics.

In this chapter we describe how the Intervention Mapping process was used to develop and implement Cultivando la Salud (CLS) (Cultivating Health), an intervention to increase breast and cervical cancer screening for U.S. Hispanic farmworker women. The program was developed by the National Center for Farmworker Health, Inc. (NCFH), an organization dedicated to addressing farmworkers' health care needs, in collaboration with the Center for Health Promotion and Prevention Research, University of Texas Health Science Center at Houston, School of Public Health.

Perspectives

Cultivando la Salud provides an excellent example of the use of participatory community-based planning, lay health workers as an intervention strategy and delivery channel, and early planning for adoption and implementation.

Community-Based Planning

This case provides an example of a community-based participatory process. The CLS planning team established a coalition to advise program planners and participate in planning decisions. These community members participated in development by providing suggestions concerning performance objectives, determinants of screening, intervention methods and strategies, and program messages and materials. This chapter illustrates how this frequent and continued community participation assisted planners in identifying important and changeable determinants of the screening behaviors and helped them select messages and strategies that would be most acceptable, appealing, and appropriate for farmworker women.

Lay Health Workers: Intervention Strategy and Delivery Channel

This case illustrates the use of the lay health worker model as a delivery channel for the intervention. (In Spanish the lay health worker is referred to as a *promotora de salud* or simply *promotora*. In this chapter, we will use the Spanish term.) The *promotora* is, however, more than just a channel. The model represents a strategy for operationalizing theoretical methods such as those described in the Social Cognitive Theory (SCT) (Bandura, 1986). These include interpersonal communication, verbal persuasion, facilitation, and modeling. Through her interaction with the priority population, the *promotora* serves as a model of a person who has successfully completed screening. She also uses the program material as she discusses the importance of screening with participants and helps women access low-cost screening services and make appointments with providers. The impact of the health promotion program then depends on both the strategies and materials that the *promotora* helps deliver (for example, video messages, pamphlets, role-playing activities) and her ability to motivate and facilitate screening behavior through her interaction with the farmworker woman.

Program Adoption and Implementation

CLS provides an example of the consideration, early in the planning process, of program adopters and implementers and the development of program components specifically designed to enable adoption and implementation. Planners considered specific performance objectives and determinants that would enable reliable and efficient adoption and delivery of the program; they then developed strategies to address these objectives. Intervention Mapping Step 5 describes the adopters and implementers, provides example matrices, and describes program components directed at adoption and implementation behaviors.

Intervention Mapping Step 1: Needs Assessment

In this section, we describe the process for the needs assessment and the findings for each element of the PRECEDE planning model.

Planning Group

Through the innovative application of human, technical, and information resources, NCFH is dedicated to addressing the health care needs and health status of farmworkers and their families as they follow the harvest. NCFH convened a planning group that included university faculty and members of a coalition known as the National Cancer Coalition. Key members of the coalition were *promotoras* who were current or former farmworkers and individuals from migrant health centers, national cancer organizations, and farmworker communities. Representatives from the following organizations participated in the coalition: American Cancer Society; U.S. National Cancer Institute; La Clinica de Cariño–Hood River, Oregon; Texas Department of Health; the Cancer and Chronic Disease Consortium, El Paso, Texas; Brownsville Community Health Center, Brownsville, Texas; and Hudson River Health Care, Peekskill, New York. The National Cancer Coalition worked with NCFH to provide input during the planning process and to assist in the development and testing of program materials. The members reviewed performance objectives, determinants of screening, and ideas for proposed methods and strategies and provided feedback about the appeal, acceptability, and cultural appropriateness of specific messages and materials.

Needs-Assessment Methods

This case study exemplifies a program planning effort in which there are few data about the health and quality-of-life problems, behaviors and environmental conditions, and determinants of breast and cervical cancer screening in Hispanic farmworker women. Therefore, we reviewed the literature on screening in Hispanic women in general and collected new data to provide information about the health problem, risk behaviors and environmental conditions, and determinants influencing breast and cervical cancer screening among Hispanic farmworker women.

The U.S. federal definition of *farmworker* is an individual whose principal employment at least 51 percent of the time is in agriculture and who has been so employed within the last twenty-four months (Larson, 2002). We defined our priority population more broadly to include all Hispanic women who had personally or whose immediate family members had done farm work for at least five years at any time during their lives. We assumed that the issues related to cancer screening were similar for all women living in farmworker communities whether or not they met the federal definition. However, because there may be special concerns among women who work in the fields, we also considered the specific behaviors, environmental conditions, and determinants that may be unique to women who traveled to perform farm work each year. The needs-assessment methods included an extensive review of the literature, focus groups, in-depth interviews, and a face-to-face survey.

Focus Groups. We conducted five focus group sessions in January 1999 with farmworker women aged fifty years and older. Two groups were conducted with farmworker women who had not had a mammogram or a Pap test in the previous two years (nonadherent to screening guidelines), two with women who had received a mammogram and a Pap test in the previous two years (adherent to screening guidelines), and a fifth group with both adherent and nonadherent women. Women were recruited to the focus groups by posting flyers in *colonias* that included a telephone number that those who were interested in participating could call. Program planners conducted the focus groups using an interview guide that covered the health topics, health care services, prevention, cancer, and cancer screening. The focus groups were audiotaped, professionally transcribed, and analyzed in Spanish to identify themes.

Survey. Based on findings from the literature review and focus groups, we developed and administered a survey instrument to a sample of two hundred women aged fifty years and older (mean age 60.7, SD 9.7) living in several *colonias* in the Texas Lower Rio Grande Valley (LRGV). *Promotoras* affiliated with community and migrant health centers in the LRGV recruited women door-to-door. They assessed eligibility, obtained informed consent, and conducted the interview. See Table 14.1 for the demographic characteristics of the survey participants.

TABLE 14.1. DEMOGRAPHIC CHARACTERISTICS OF SURVEY PARTICIPANTS.

	N	Percent
Sociodemographic Variables		
Age		
50—59 years	115	57.5
60—69 years	47	23.5
70 years—over	38	19.0
Income		
< $10,000	147	74.5
≥ $10,000	48	25.5
Marital Status		
Married	129	64.5
Not married	71	35.5
Education		
≤ 6 years	161	81.5
≥ 7 years	36	18.5
Place of Birth		
United States	44	22.0
Mexico	156	78.0
Length in United States		
< 20 years	52	27.3
≥ 20 years	120	62.8
Entire life	19	9.9

The survey addressed the following constructs: self-efficacy, perceived susceptibility, subjective norms, decisional balance, cancer knowledge, and attitudes about cancer. The independent effects of these constructs on mammography and Pap test screening behaviors were assessed while controlling for sociodemographic and access-to-care variables (Palmer, Fernandez, Tortolero-Luna, Mullen, & Gonzales, 2005).

Health and Quality of Life

The literature review revealed cancer-related health disparities among Hispanic women, particularly those who were poor and living in border counties. Breast cancer incidence and mortality among Hispanics remains lower than among non-Hispanics; however, breast cancer is the most common cancer among Hispanic women, and they have experienced an almost twofold increase in mortality over the last decades (Devessa et al., 1999). Hispanic women have considerably higher incidence and mortality rates of cervical cancer than do non-Hispanic White women (incidence: 16.2 vs. 7.3 per one hundred thousand; mortality 3.6 vs. 2.5 per one hundred thousand) (Ries et al., 2002). Rates were even higher among Hispanic women living in the LRGV counties: incidence 18.7 per one hundred thousand vs. 8.2 and mortality 6.2 per one hundred thousand vs. 3.4 per one hundred thousand, respectively (Texas Department of State Health Services, 2005b).

The focus group findings helped identify quality-of-life concerns related to cancer. The program planners had initially thought that cancer screening might not be an important health interest for these women given their many needs and responsibilities, such as taking care of their families and ensuring that they have the basic needs of food, water, and shelter. However, we found that the women were very concerned about cancer, feared receiving a cancer diagnosis and recounted numerous stories of friends and family members who had died from the disease. Primary concerns were that cancer would mean that they would be unable to work or take care of their families. The prospect of being a burden to their families and social isolation were also concerns. Many people, particularly older women, living in *colonias* can become socially isolated if they are confronted with chronic illness. Furthermore, women expressed concern that a diagnosis of cancer might require travel to the referral hospital for indigent patients in Texas (several hundred miles from the LRGV) and would result in separation from family members and friends. Travel between the LRGV and the hospital also represents a real deportation danger for those women who are undocumented, because the U.S. Border Patrol often sets up checkpoints on the route.

Behavior and Environment

The primary behaviors identified in the needs-assessment model were low utilization of breast and cervical cancer screening. Although between 1995 and 2002, an overall high percentage of all women aged eighteen or older with an intact uterine cervix reported ever having a Pap test (94.1 percent to 95.2 percent) (Centers for Disease Control and Prevention, 2003), these trends were not seen among women with less than a high school education, women in the lowest income groups, women without health insurance, and Hispanics. About 85 percent of Hispanic women forty years of age and older living in border counties and 71 percent of Hispanic women fifty years and older living in the LRGV reported ever having had a Pap test (Coughlin et al., 2003; Gonzales, Saavedra-Embesi, Fernandez, & Tortolero-Luna, 2001). Weighted estimates from Behavioral Risk Factor Surveillance Surveys (BRFSS) (1999–2000) in border counties indicated that 26.4 percent of Hispanic women reported not having a Pap test in the previous three years versus 11.7 percent of non-Hispanic women in the same counties (Coughlin et al., 2003). In two recent studies that the authors conducted as part of this project, 34.6 percent and 40 percent of low-income Hispanic women fifty years and older reported no Pap test in the previous three years and 54 percent and 66 percent reported no mammogram within the previous year (Gonzales et al., 2001; Gonzales, Fernandez, & Saavedra-Embesi, 2003).

Findings from the survey indicated much lower levels of breast and cervical cancer screening among women in our sample than among other Hispanics elsewhere in Texas and nationally. For example, only about half (51.5 percent) of women from the LRGV sample reported mammography screening within the previous two years as compared with 69.4 percent of non-Hispanic whites in Texas and 59.7 percent of Hispanics in Texas, based on 1997 and 1998 BRFSS data (Bolen et al., 2000).

Important environmental conditions that are negatively associated with breast and cervical cancer screening include lack of physician referral, lack of health insurance, cost, lack of access to health care, no regular place of care, restrictive work policies, rigid clinic payment policies, and poor transportation (Chavez, Cornelius, & Jones, 1986; Chavez, Hubbell, Mishra, & Valdez, 1997; Fernandez, Tortolero-Luna, & Gold, 1998; Harlan, Bernstein, & Kessler, 1991; Harmon, Castro, & Coe, 1996; Hayward, Shapiro, Freeman, & Corey, 1988; Hubbell, Waitzkin, Mishra, Dombrink, & Chavez, 1991; Otero-Sabogal, Stewart, Sabogal, Brown, & Perez-Stable, 2003; Perez-Stable, Sabogal, & Otero-Sabogal, 1995; Rimer et al., 1996; Wilcher, Gilbert, Siano, & Arredondo, 1999).

Results from our focus groups revealed that even women who did use health care services did not typically receive recommendations or referrals from their health care providers to obtain screening. Women also mentioned difficulty accessing screening because of cost and inability to visit the clinics or screening facilities during regular hours of operation. These findings provided evidence of environmental conditions that may be negatively affecting cancer screening at both the interpersonal (providers) and the organizational (clinic) levels. Additionally, we found that the women had low access to a regular source of care and lack of insurance (Palmer et al., 2005).

Determinants of the Risk Behavior

The planning team used empirical data, theoretical literature, and the collection of new data to develop a refined list of determinants (Table 14.2).

Both internal and external factors negatively influence breast and cervical cancer screening among Hispanic women. Psychosocial factors negatively influencing Pap test screening include embarrassment, discomfort during examinations, a low level of acculturation, fatalism, language barriers, distrust of physicians, lack of child care, fear of the procedure and the results, concern about confidentiality, lack of knowledge, and perceived discrimination (Coronado, Thompson, Koepsell, Schwartz, & McLerran, 2004; Fernandez et al., 1998; Fernandez-Esquer, Espinoza, Ramirez, & McAlister, 2003; Otero-Sabogal et al., 2003; Suarez et al., 1997). Low self-efficacy, low acculturation, lack of knowledge, perceived norms regarding screening, fear of finding cancer, and embarrassment were related to decreased mammography screening (C. Morgan, Park, & Cortes, 1995; A. S. O'Malley, Kerner, Johnson, & Mandelblatt, 1999).

We found few studies on the factors influencing screening behaviors among farmworker women. Two studies of migrant farmworkers in Wisconsin found low levels of knowledge about screening and fatalistic attitudes toward cancer (Lantz, Dupuis, Reding, Krauska, & Lappe, 1994; Lantz & Reding, 1994). Another study reported that cervical cancer knowledge and Pap test screening behavior were low among farmworker women; 44 percent had never heard of a Pap test (Hooks et al., 1996). Fear of the disease and pain associated with cancer, fear of the medical system, and the belief that only God can determine whether someone gets cancer were cited as additional barriers to cancer-screening services reported among a farmworker population (Goldsmith and Sisneros, 1996).

Several external factors such as lack of social support, lack of physician referral, inadequate health insurance coverage, low access to health care services and regular care, cost, restrictive and inflexible workplace policies, strict clinic payment policies, lack of transportation, lack of partner approval, and few social ties have also been shown to influence breast and cervical cancer screening (Bazargan, Bazargan, Farooq, & Baker, 2004; Coronado et al., 2004; Fox & Stein, 1991; NCFH, 2002; M. S. O'Malley, Earp, & Harris, 1997; V. M. Taylor, Taplin,

TABLE 14.2. IDENTIFYING DETERMINANTS OF UNDERUTILIZATION OF BREAST AND CERVICAL CANCER SCREENING.

Original Provisional List	Additions From Empirical Literature	Additions From Theory	Additions From New Data
Personal Determinants			
Embarrassment	Low perceived risk of breast and cervical cancer	Intention to obtain screening (Theory of Planned Behavior)	Perception of time constraints
Lack of knowledge about screening guidelines	Fear of radiation	Subjective norms (Theory of Planned Behavior)	Competing priorities
Fear of cancer	Fatalism		Partner objection to screening
Misconceptions about cancer	Perceived group norms	Perceived barriers to screening (Health Belief Model)	Cancer misconceptions
Low perceived benefits	Uncomfortable examinations	Perceived susceptibility (Health Belief Model)	Use of folk healing practices common
High perceived barriers	Low acculturation		Low self-efficacy
Low perceived risk	Language barriers	Self-efficacy (Social Cognitive Theory)	Belief that cancer leads to death
	Distrust of physicians		
	Fear of the procedure	Decisional balance (Transtheoretical Model)	
	Fear of the results/finding cancer		
	Concerns about confidentiality		
	Lack of knowledge		
	Perceived discrimination		
	Low self-efficacy for screening		
	Perceived social norms		
External Determinants			
Lack of services	Acculturation		Cultural norms
High cost of services	Lack of knowledge		Social support
Lack of health insurance	Low perceived norms		
No provider referral	Fear of finding cancer		
Transportation problems			
Lack of child care			
Language barriers			

Urban, White, & Peacock, 1995; Otero-Sabogal et al., 2003; Urban, Anderson, & Peacock, 1994). We have mentioned some of these factors in the description of environmental conditions that are negatively associated with screening. Later in the process, we determined which of these factors remained as environmental conditions and thus required their own matrices and which were external determinants.

The theoretical literature provided some additional evidence, particularly regarding the strength of the association between identified constructs and risk behaviors. Some studies, although not exclusively of Hispanic women, measured constructs that were more specifically theory-based. Perceived susceptibility from the Health Belief Model (HBM) has been found to be associated with mammography (J. D. Allen, Sorensen, Stoddard, Colditz, & Peterson, 1998; Bastani et al., 1994; Janz & Becker, 1984); self-efficacy from SCT has been found to be associated with both mammography and Pap testing (J. D. Allen et al., 1998; Kurtz, Given, Given, & Kurtz, 1993), and subjective norms from the Theory of Planned Behavior (TPB) were found to be associated with the intention to complete mammography screening (J. D. Allen et al., 1998; Fishbein & Ajzen, 1975; Montaño, Thompson, Taylor, & Mahloch, 1997).

To better understand mammography and Pap test screening in this population we used the Transtheoretical Model (TTM). The TTM, developed by DiClemente, Prochaska, and colleagues, involves a number of dimensions, including stages of change, processes of change, decisional balance (pros and cons), and self-efficacy (C. C. DiClemente & Prochaska, 1985; Prochaska, Velicer, DiClemente, & Fava, 1988). The pros (perceived positives or benefits) and cons (perceived negatives or barriers) are much like the HBM constructs of benefits and barriers of a target behavior are associated with adoption of the behavior (M. H. Becker, 1974a, 1974b; Janz & Becker, 1988). Decisional balance is a summary index of the pros and cons (Velicer, DiClemente, Prochaska, & Brandenburg, 1985). Precontemplators have a negative decisional balance, reflecting the weight of reasons not to change while persons in action and maintenance have a positive decisional balance. Contemplators are somewhere in between with approximately the same number of pros and cons (Rakowski et al., 1992; Rakowski, Fulton, & Feldman, 1993). Two studies using the TTM to study mammography screening found that as stage of adoption proceeds from not being screened to being screened on a regular schedule, decisional balance becomes more favorable (Rakowski et al., 1992; Rakowski et al., 1993). In a study examining multiple cancer-screening behaviors in a low-income minority community, decisional balance had a strong positive relationship with cancer-screening practices, including Pap test screening (Rakowski et al., 1993; Rimer et al., 1996).

Community Capacity

The communities identified for implementation of the CLS program had several strengths that made such a program's success more likely. Among these were familiarity with and acceptance of the *promotora* model, community clinics with existing *promotora* programs, and the availability of low-cost screening through clinics that had National Breast and Cervical Cancer Early Detection Program funding administered through the state health department. Additionally, the existence of well-defined neighborhoods (*colonias*) was also considered a strength. Although these *colonias* often had little infrastructure and often lacked even basic services, the community itself was typically united. In fact, some *colonias* had a history of community organizing to lobby for basic services. Residents clearly identify with their *colonia*, partly because they often have strong family ties within *colonias*. This can occur because families frequently pool resources to buy property and then build homes. It was common, therefore, to find individuals who lived next door or very close to other family members. During the implementation of the CLS project, the cohesiveness and personal relationships between women within *colonias* accelerated the dissemination of the program. Women spread the word about the program and would often organize intervention groups at informal community leaders' homes. This made better use of the *promotora's* time because she could reach several women during one educational session.

Step 2: Matrices of Change Objectives

The tasks involved with the development of matrices include stating the health promoting behaviors and environmental conditions, adding specificity to the behaviors by creating performance objectives, choosing evidence-informed determinants of the performance, and combining these elements.

Health-Promoting Behavior and Environmental Conditions

The health-promoting behaviors were obtaining a mammogram, a CBE, and a Pap test to decreases morbidity and mortality attributable to breast and cervical cancer.

The environmental conditions that influence the participant's ability to obtain the screening behaviors of interest included making mammography and Pap test clinic services more available to women (organizational level).

Performance Objectives

The next task in Step 2 was to develop performance objectives that specified what the participants needed to do in order to obtain a mammogram and a Pap test and what the agents in the environment (for example, clinic director, receptionist, outreach coordinator) needed to do to bring about the desired change in services. The performance objectives for each of these behaviors included making an appointment for the screening, going to the clinic or screening facility to have the screening, and obtaining the results and any necessary follow-up care. The performance objectives for the environmental conditions included clinic directors seeking funds for screening programs, physicians and other providers referring patient for mammograms, and clinic directors facilitating transportation to screening.

Determinants

The identification in the needs assessment of factors negatively influencing mammography, CBE, and Pap test screening also often revealed the determinants of the health-related behaviors. For example, we found that compared with women who were adherent to recommended screening guidelines, nonadherent women had lower levels of self-efficacy; influencing self-efficacy might be important to promote screening.

Focus groups information came not only from the nonadherent women, who provided information about barriers to screening, but also from the groups of adherent women who gave us insight into why some women did complete screening. Adherent women mentioned such factors as the outcome expectation of having peace of mind after completing screening, wanting to comply with doctor recommendations (subjective norms), and knowledge about screening guidelines.

Matrices

To develop the matrices, we listed proposed determinants of the health-related behaviors across the top of a matrix and the performance objectives in the left column. Within the matrix cells, we wrote change objectives based on the question, What do participants need to change related to the determinant in order to accomplish the performance objective? The matrices for mammography and Pap test screening are shown in Tables 14.3 and 14.4.

The planning team's approach to environmental matrix development was twofold:

1. Identify the environmental agents, such as clinic directors, outreach coordinators, receptionists, and providers, responsible for proposed changes

2. Develop specific performance objectives essential to bringing about the desired environmental condition

In-depth interviews with clinic staff (including outreach coordinators and providers) helped the planning team identify the determinants that influenced these performance objectives, which are designed to bring about organizational change. See Table 14.5 for the matrix of environmental change objectives.

Community input was important during this stage. Program planners invited review of the matrices by members of the National Cancer Coalition and by individuals in the priority populations, including a clinic outreach worker, *promotoras*, and others. We asked reviewers to recommend changes in performance objectives, determinants, and change objectives, and we used their comments to refine the matrices. For Step 3 we also enlisted the assistance of women from the priority community to provide advice about which types of intervention methods and strategies would be most appropriate and appealing to women in the community.

Step 3: Methods and Strategies

Working with the Farmworker Women

During the needs-assessment phase, the farmworker women also identified methods and strategies that would be well received by the priority community. For example, women mentioned that they received most of their health information from family and friends, from *promotoras*, and from their providers. They also talked about how others had convinced them to get screened and how they had convinced others to do the same. Based on this information, we identified several potential methods such as verbal persuasion, modeling, and mobilization of social support. These findings complemented information available from the theoretical literature.

Identifying and Choosing Theoretical Methods

In this step we organized all of the change objectives by the relevant determinants so that we could begin brainstorming methods and matching them with sets of change objectives (Table 14.6). We included a column in the table where we could note ideas about program components and materials that would deliver the methods strategies.

We then examined the theoretical and empirical literature for evidence of methods and strategies that might be appropriate for us to use according to the type of determinant they influence. For example, modeling is an example of a

TABLE 14.3. MAMMOGRAPHY MATRICES FOR FARMWORKER WOMEN.

Performance Objectives	Personal Determinants						External Determinants	
	Knowledge	Outcome Expectations	Perceived Barriers and Benefits	Attitude[1]	Self-Efficacy	Perceived Social Norms	Social Support	Availability and Accessibility

Behavior: Women Will Obtain a Mammogram

Performance Objectives	Knowledge	Outcome Expectations	Perceived Barriers and Benefits	Attitude[1]	Self-Efficacy	Perceived Social Norms	Social Support	Availability and Accessibility
PO.1. Call to schedule an appointment	K.1. Describe where to call and where to go	OE.1. Expect to obtain an appointment when they call for one	PBB.1. List a greater number of benefits than barriers to scheduling appointment for a mammogram.	A.1. Believe their role is to request mammography if their doctors have not recommended it	SE.1.a. Express confidence in calling and scheduling appointments SE.1.b. Express confidence in setting aside time to obtain a mammogram	PSN.1. Believe that other women like themselves schedule mammograms or ask doctors for referrals	SS.1 Friends and family members encourage them to schedule appointments.	AA.1.a. Clinics arrange convenient appointment times. AA.1.b. Providers make referrals for mammograms.
PO.2. Obtain a mammogram	K.2.a. Discuss what cancer is and why it is a health threat K.2.b. Describe mammography screening recommendations K.2.c. Describe the important reasons to detect cancer early	OE.2. Expect that obtaining a regular mammogram will result in better chances of surviving cancer if they develop it	PBB.2.a. List a greater number of benefits than barriers to mammography screening PBB.2.b. Describe mammography procedure and express lack of fear and low expectation of pain	A.2.a. Believe that treatment can be effective in curing breast cancer A.2.b. Discuss being optimistic about prognosis of cancer detected early A.2.c. Describe the pain of the test as minimal or bearable	SE.2. Express confidence in obtaining mammograms	PSN.2. Believe that other women like themselves obtain mammograms	SS.2. Friends or family members accompany them to appointments.	AA.2. Clinics facilitate appointment times.

PO.3. Obtain results of the mammogram and get follow-up care as necessary	K.2.d. Recognize the importance of obtaining previous films if next mammogram will be by a different provider K.2.e. Explain that treatment is available K.2.f. Describe how to get to a screening facility K.2.g. Describe mammography procedure K.3.a. Describe where to call for mammography results K.3.b. Describe what a mammogram can show	OE.3.a. Expect to be given the results when they ask for them OE.3.b. Expect that they can obtain follow-up for questionable results OE.3.c. Expect that they can obtain effective treatment for results that show cancer	PBB.3. Express benefits of knowing results of a mammogram	A.2.d. Express low or manageable levels of embarrassment A.2.e. Express low levels of fear and expectation of pain A.3. Describe the relief of knowing that nothing is wrong or being able to get treatment for something that is wrong	SE.3.a. Express confidence in being able to obtain results SE.3.b. Express confidence in being able to understand the results	PSN.3. Believe that other women like themselves can get mammography results	SS.3.a. Friends and family members remind them to get results. SS.3.b. Friends and family members ask them about the results. SS.3.c. Friends and family members accompany them to needed follow-up.	AA.3. Clinics clarify how and when to obtain results.

[1] Fear of detection, fear of procedure, and belief that cancer is incurable are strong attitudinal factors found in the assessment.

TABLE 14.4. PAP TEST MATRICES FOR FARMWORKER WOMEN.

		Personal Determinants					External Determinants	
Performance Objectives	Perceived Barriers and Benefits	Knowledge	Attitude[1]	Outcome Expectations	Perceived Social Norms[2]	Self-Efficacy	Social Support	Access and Availability
Behavior: Women Will Obtain a Pap Test								
PO.1. Schedule a Pap test appointment	PBB.1. Express more benefits than barriers to setting a time for an appointment for Pap test	K.1.a. Recognize their own need for a Pap test (that it is past due) K.1.b. Identify locations where Pap test screening is offered	A.1.a. Believe it is important to schedule a Pap test A.1.b. Believe it is their responsibility to schedule a Pap test	OE.1. Expect to obtain an appointment by calling a clinic	PSN.1. Believe that other women like themselves call to schedule appointments for Pap tests	SE.1. Feel confident to schedule a Pap test appointment	SS.1. Friends and family members encourage them to schedule an appointment.	AA.1.a. Pap test appointments are easily available from clinic. AA.1.b. Providers recommend Pap test screening.
PO.2. Obtain a Pap Test	PBB.2.a. Express greater benefits than barriers to Pap test screening PBB.2.b. Report low levels of embarrassment about Pap test screening PBB.2.c. Recognize that female providers are available PBB.2.d. Recognize the right to ask for a female nurse or companion to be present during the procedure	K.2.a. Describe what cervical cancer is and why it is a health threat K.2.b. Describe Pap test recommendations K.2.c. Discuss the probability of preventing cervical cancer through detection and treatment of precancerous lesions K.2.d. Discuss the fact that treatment is available	A.2.a. Believe that getting a Pap test regularly is important A.2.b. Believe that Pap tests can help prevent cervical cancer by detecting changes before they become cancerous A.2.c. Believe that a yearly Pap test can find cancer early so that treatment can be effective in curing cancer	OE.2. Expect that obtaining regular Pap tests will increase their chances in curing cervical cancer if they develop it	PSN.2. Believe that other women like themselves obtain Pap tests	SE.2.a. Express confidence in obtaining a Pap test SE.2.b. Feel confident that they will understand what the doctor is doing and why	SS.2. Ask partners, friends, or family members to remind them to get a Pap test	AA.2. Clinics provide assistance with transportation.

		K.2.e. Describe the Pap test procedure	A.2.d. Express optimism about prognosis of early detected cancer A.2.e. Believe that protecting themselves against cervical cancer through Pap test screening is important for them and for their families A.2.f. View Pap test as a routine medical procedure					AA.3.a. Clinic providers explain abnormal results in a way women can understand. AA.3.b. Clinics provide rapid appropriate follow-up.
PO.3. Follow-up on a Pap test with abnormal results	PBB.3. Express greater benefit than barriers to follow-up	K.3.a. Discuss the types of results that are possible and what kinds of treatment can be necessary K.3 b. Recognize that they will be notified if a test is abnormal	A.3. Believe that following up on an abnormal result is important to themselves and their families	OE.3. Expect that by following up they can obtain a good treatment outcome	PSN.3. Believe that other women like them would follow up an abnormal result	SE.3.a. Feel confident in understanding the results of a Pap test SE.3.b. Express confidence in obtaining follow-up care	SS.3. Partners, friends, or family members accompany women to follow-up.	

[1]Fear of detection of cancer and belief that cancer is incurable are strong attitudinal factors found in the assessment.

[2]A strong cultural factor from the needs assessment was embarrassment.

TABLE 14.5. MATRICES FOR CLINICS FOR PAP TESTS AND MAMMOGRAPHY.

Performance Objectives	Knowledge	Outcome Expectations	Perceived Barriers and Benefits	Attitude[1]	Perceived Practice Norms and Standards of Care
Environmental Change: Mammograms and Pap Tests Will Be Easily Accessible to Farmworker Women					
PO.1.1. Clinic directors seek funds for screening programs. PO.1.2. Explore becoming a screening site by contacting department of health PO.1.3. Negotiate low-cost screening with providers PO.1.4. Establish policy of providing Pap test for women unable to pay	K.(1.1–1.4.).a. Describe excess morbidity and mortality for farmworker women from breast and cervical cancer K.(1.1–1.4).b. Describe inadequate screening rates K.1.1. Describe process for acquiring funding	OE.1.1.a. Expect that acquiring funding for screening will prevent cervical cancer and save treatment costs OE.1.1.b. Expect that acquiring funding will increase early detection of breast cancer	PBB.(1.1–1.4).a. Describe funding and service as worth the hassles of reporting and paperwork PBB.(1.2–1.4).b. Plan how to cope with demand when monies run out	A.(1.1–1.4). Describe cancer screening as a very important part of taking care of their population	PPN.1.1. Recognize that other clinics that serve this population access funds for screening
PO.2.1. Receptionists ascertain farmworker status. PO.2.2. *Promotoras* provide farmworker women with eligibility assessment.	K.2.1.a. Describe how ascertaining farmworker status can benefit the clinic K.2.1.b.Describe the definition of farmworker and the pointers for scheduling appointments for patients who are farmworkers K.2.2.a. Describe how providing eligibility assessment can benefit the clinic K.2.2.b. List the criteria for eligibility for various programs	OE.2.1. Expect that clinics will value ascertaining framworker status OE.2.2. Expect that clinics will value eligibility assessment	PBB.2.1. List benefits of making time to ask the patients questions to ascertain farmworker status PBB.2.2. Believe they can make the time to perform eligibility assessment	A.2.1. Believe that it is important and it is their role to assess farmworker status among clients A.2.2. Argue that their role includes eligibility assessment	PPN.2.1. Discuss with other clinics how they ascertain farmworker status among their clients PPN.2.2. Believe that other clinics provide eligibility assessment among their farmworker clients

PO.3.1. Physicians and other providers make referrals for mammograms. PO.3.2. Clinic directors establish referral and tracking systems in clinics. PO.3.3. Outreach coordinators identify screening programs for farmworker women.	K.(3.1–3.3).a. Describe excess morbidity and mortality from breast cancer in this population; K.(3.1–3.3).b. Describe referral sources and funding mechanisms; K.3.1.c. Discuss how to make a motivational referral	OE.(3.1–3.2).a. Expect that making a referral will result in completed mammography; OE.(3.1–3.2).b. Expect that access to screening programs will increase rates; OE.3.3. Expect that help with insurance will increase coverage and increase rates	PBB.3.1.a. Believe that they can overcome barriers (time, language) to provide a recommendation; PBB.3.1.b. Believe that the benefits of recommending screening now outweigh the barriers; PBB.3.3. Believe that identifying low- or no-cost programs is important to facilitate screening	A.3.1. Physicians believe that providing recommendations are an important part of the care they provide.	PPN.3.1. Recognize that other providers meet guidelines for mammography referral
PO.4.1. Clinic directors facilitate transportation to screening. PO.4.2. Establish contract with mobile screening to serve women in *colonias*	K.4.1.a. Recognize transportation as a barrier to screening for some women	OE.4.1. Expect that women will use transportation services to get screened; OE.4.2. Believe that collaboration with a mobile van will result in a higher rate of screening	PBB.(4.1–4.2). Believe that providing these services is worth the trouble because women need them	A.(4.1–4.2). Believe that providing access is an important part of the clinic's role in serving the community	PPN.4.1. Recognize that other clinics and screening programs provide support to address transportation barriers; PPN.4.2. Recognize that other clinics collaborate with mobile screening programs
PO.5.1. Clinic directors ensure that appointments are readily accessible and hours are convenient. PO.5.2. Clinic directors coordinate provider schedules so that a bilingual provider is available convenient hours or provide for a professional interpreter.	K.5.1. Recognize that appointment availability and times are barriers for some women; K.5.2. Describe the need for bilingual staff given the high percentage of Spanish-only speakers in catchment area	OE.5.1. Expect that women will use the service when it is accessible; OE.5.2. Expect that providing bilingual providers and interpreters will enhance care	PBB.5.1. Believe that providing accessible appointments and convenient hours is worth the trouble; PBB.5.2. Believe that the benefits of providing bilingual staff and interpreter's services outweigh the potential barriers	A.5.1. Believe that it is the clinic's responsibility to accommodate community accessibility needs; A.5.2. Believe that good communication with patients is essential to provide good care	PPN.5.1. Recognize that other clinics and service organizations provide flexible plans to enhance access

[1]Fear of detection, fear of procedure, and belief that cancer is incurable are strong attitudinal factors found in the assessment.

TABLE 14.6. METHODS, STRATEGY, AND PROGRAM.

Change Objectives	Method	Strategy	Program Component
OE.1, OE.2, OE.3.a, OE.3.b, OE.3.c, SE.1.a, SE.1.b, SE.2, SE.3.a, SE.3.b, PSN.1, PSN.2, PSN.3	Modeling	Modeling of woman scheduling an appointment, obtaining mammogram, and receiving results	Breast cancer screening video (mammography segment)
A.1, A.2.a, A.3.b, A.3.c, OE.2, PBB.1, PBB.2.a, PBB.2.b, PBB.3	Verbal persuasion	*Promotora* to use convincing language and encouraging remarks	Flip chart
K.1, K.2.f, K.3.a, SE.2, SE.3.a	Individual education and counseling	*Promotora* to provide list of screening sites with directions	Printed materials Call for Health number
		Promotora to explain key information using flip chart	Flip chart
PSN.1, PSN.2, PSN.3, SE.1.a, SE.1.b, SE.2, SE.3.a, SE.3.b	Modeling	Testimonials	Breast cancer screening video

theoretical method that influences self-efficacy and outcome expectations (Bandura, 1986). We proposed using *promotoras* as role models and as a way to deliver program strategies including role-model stories of women who had detected cancer early and survived (influencing perceived social norms and outcome expectations). Additionally, program materials were designed to deliver strategies and messages based on such methods as information transmission, persuasion, and facilitation (Bandura, 1986).

Selecting Practical Strategies

The planning team generated ideas about strategies in two ways: (1) by brainstorming and documenting ideas about strategies, materials, and delivery channels throughout the planning process; (2) and by thinking about each method that was selected and deciding on specific strategies that could operationalize that method. For example, one strategy was to use a role model who would overcome the women's barriers to ultimately carrying out the target behaviors. We noted the popularity of *telenovelas* or soap opera–type stories among women in the priority community, particularly among women the priority population (fifty years and older).

In Latin America *telenovelas* are extremely popular, and Miguel Sabido has been a pioneer of entertainment educational *telenovelas* in Mexico. Between 1975 and 1997 Sabido produced at least seven educational *telenovelas* based on social cognitive and other theories that addressed issues such as family planning, adult education and literacy, and street children (E. M. Rogers & Antola, 1985; Sabido, 1989; Singhal & Rogers, 1999). The planning group decided to develop short *telenovela*-type scenarios that would be delivered on videotapes and flip charts. The team also considered several important methods such as using role models in the development of video segments. The story lines for the *telenovelas* included women addressing barriers, talking to health care providers, engaging in screening behaviors, and getting support from family members and friends.

The development of a video that included role-model stories; illustrations and descriptions of female anatomy, cancer, and the screening tests; discussion about the barriers to and benefits of screening; testimonials from cancer survivors; and other strategies and messages was a major focus during this phase of the project. We also developed other small media materials including a flip chart and informational brochures and flyers that contained information about screening facilities. The flip chart had many of the same elements (role-model stories, descriptions and images about the screening tests, a discussion about barriers and benefits, and so on) as the video. The video, however, focused on addressing objectives that were better met with moving visual media (such as demonstration of breast self-exam and modeling of good communication with the provider).

From a programmatic perspective, the central strategy was the use of *promotoras*. The *promotora* model is a peer health education model first developed in Latin America. *Promotoras* typically promote healthy living by educating community members in a culturally appropriate manner and by facilitating the connection between community members and health and human services. Although the effectiveness of *promotora* programs have typically been measured in terms of their ability to affect short-term outcomes, such as changing health knowledge, attitudes, and beliefs, some long-term outcomes have also been reported (for example reduction of infant mortality) (Meister, Warrick, de Zapien, & Wood, 1992). *Promotora* programs have been effectively used to educate Hispanics about prenatal care, cardiovascular health, and cancer screening. Morris, Felkner, and McLean (1994) found that it is possible to motivate Hispanic women to obtain Pap screening by using community health workers and informal, active encouragement as tools for motivation. According to Navarro and colleagues (1995), the identification of natural helpers (see Chapter Four) in the Hispanic community and their subsequent training in interventions using culturally appropriate educational materials provides a viable approach for increasing the use of cancer-screening tests in Hispanic women of low socioeconomic and acculturation levels.

Although the use of *promotoras* to deliver educational materials and messages to the community may be seen as a channel for the intervention, we describe the *promotora* model also as a strategy because it is the *promotoras* who operationalize selected methods. For example, using modeling and verbal persuasion to influence change objectives related to self-efficacy and outcome expectations, *promotoras* themselves modeled appropriate screening behaviors and discussed their experiences with other women. They also provided encouraging messages and reinforcement for women who were taking initial steps toward completing screening. *Promotoras* also offered facilitation services such as helping women enroll in special screening programs, apply for health insurance, identify low- or no-cost screening services, and schedule appointments. *Promotoras* could also be considered a health promotion channel because they were able to deliver other educational materials, such as the video and flip chart, pamphlets, and informational materials about screening resources in the community.

Step 4: Program

In Step 4, guided by the matrices and ideas about methods and strategies, the planning team developed specific messages and overall content for each program component (Table 14.7). This table facilitated our producing design documents for each of the program elements.

Working with the Farmworker Women

The planning team worked closely with community members to develop culturally appropriate program components and messages. We first looked closely at the data to understand the words farmworker women used to describe cancer, screening, lumps in the breast, and other important concepts. We then conducted additional interviews with farmworker women and *promotoras* to gather preferences for pictures, graphics, and wording for messages. Community members participating in these interviews noted that they preferred photographs to drawings. They also preferred images of people similar to themselves rather than images of models or movie stars.

As development of video scripts and messages proceeded, the National Cancer Coalition reviewed materials to assure that members of the priority community could easily understand them. All of the materials, which included audio and

TABLE 14.7. DEVELOPING
PROGRAM COMPONENTS AND MESSAGES.

Change Objectives	Program Components	Content and Messages
P.O.2. Obtain a mammogram Determinant: Knowledge, Attitude K.2.g. Describe mammography procedures A.2.d. Express low or manageable levels of embarrassment	Video Flip chart Discussion	Feel free to ask for a female nurse or assistant to be present during the exam Demonstrate the procedures and place an emphasis on the respect for modesty Role-model stories: women who obtained a mammogram discuss their initial embarrassment and their decision to get the screenings anyway because of the importance of early detection. Role-model story: another woman says she thought that she would feel very embarrassed, but the actual exam was not as embarrassing as she thought it would be. The woman says that while she was having the mammogram the doctor explained everything she was doing, and it went by very quickly. Now the woman goes every year.
P.O.1. Call to schedule an appointment Determinant: Self-Efficacy SE.1.a. Express confidence in calling and scheduling appointments SE.1.b. Express confidence in setting aside time to obtain a mammogram	Discussion Video	*Promotora* role-plays with participants calling and scheduling appointments. *Promotora* sends many "you can do it" messages throughout presentation. Shows a woman like herself scheduling a mammogram with her doctor and shows the doctor's positive response
P.O.2. Obtain a mammogram Determinant: Self-Efficacy SE.2. Express confidence in obtaining mammograms	Discussion Video Flip chart	*Promotora* sends many "you can do it" messages throughout presentation. The video and flip chart show a farmworker obtaining a mammogram.
P.O.3. Obtain results of the mammogram and get follow-up care as necessary	Discussion Video Flip chart	*Promotora* role-plays with participant(s) calling and obtaining results of a mammogram. *Promotora* sends many "you can do it" messages throughout presentation.

TABLE 14.7. DEVELOPING
PROGRAM COMPONENTS AND MESSAGES, Cont'd.

Change Objectives	Program Components	Content and Messages
Determinant: Self-Efficacy SE.3.a. Express confidence in being able to obtain results SE.3.b. Express confidence in being able to understand what will happen and the results	Pamphlet	The video and flip chart will show the actual mammogram. During the exam, the technician or doctor will explain everything that is going on. The farmworker (actor) will obtain the results of her mammogram and ask questions about them, and the health care provider will respond. The pamphlet will show possible results of these tests.
P.O.1. Call to schedule and appointment Determinant: Social Support SS.1. Friends and family members encourage them to schedule an appointment for a mammogram.	Video	Video of a woman's daughter encouraging her mother to get a mammogram
P.O.2. Obtain a mammogram Determinant: Social Support SS.2. Friends or family members accompany them to appointments.	Discussion	*Promotora* talks to woman about including her family in her commitment to call and schedule a mammogram.
P.O.3. Obtain the results of the mammogram and get follow-up care as necessary Determinant: Social Support SS.3.a. Friends and family members remind them to check on their results.	Discussion	*Promotora* will tell the woman to let a friend or family member know when she has her appointment scheduled and when she should expect the results. She should ask that person to remind her to get the results.
P.O.1. Call to schedule an appointment Determinant: Barriers and Benefits	Video Discussion Pamphlet	The video shows a woman getting a mammogram with no apparent discomfort. Later, the video will show the woman talking to her friend describing how she felt during the procedure.

TABLE 14.7. DEVELOPING
PROGRAM COMPONENTS AND MESSAGES, Cont'd.

Change Objectives	Program Components	Content and Messages
BB.1.a. Describe procedure and express lack of fear and low expectation of pain BB.1.b. List a greater number of benefits than barriers to scheduling appointment for a mammogram		She will say that she felt some pressure, but the mammogram did not really hurt. The video will include statements from women describing how easy it was to call and make the appointment. She shows that she had the list the promotora gave her of everything she would need for the appointment and what to ask for.
P.O.2. Obtain a mammogram Determinant: Barriers and Benefits BB.2.a. List a greater number of benefits than barriers to obtaining mammography screening	Video Flip chart	The video will include statements from women describing some of the common barriers to screening, such as lack of time, fear of finding cancer, fear of the test itself, and embarrassment. Then the women will talk about how they overcame those problems. The *promotora* asks the woman to make a list of all of the reasons she should have a mammogram and another list about the reasons she does not want to go or feels that it would be difficult to get one (barriers). According to the list the woman has made, the *promotora* will offer suggestions about overcoming these barriers. The *promotora* will have a script (on the flip chart) to help her know what to say in response to the barriers mentioned.

visual messages, were designed to be appropriate for individuals with low or no literacy skills. Additionally, because *promotoras* delivered the information directly or through small media materials (such as videotape), exposure to the program materials did not require reading skills. However, the terminology and messages had to be ones that the participants could easily understand. Hence, the planning team paid close attention to the literacy level of the materials and confirmed the understanding of these materials by means of pilot testing.

Some members of the National Cancer Coalition who had experience developing materials for low-literacy audiences provided detailed feedback to ensure that members of the priority community would easily understand the messages. To ensure the cultural appropriateness of materials, the team read parts of the script to women to verify that scenarios and language included in the script were appropriate and reflected the way women in the community communicated with each other. Their feedback allowed us to make changes before production of the video and to avoid costly postproduction changes.

Wherever possible, we used actual farmworker women in the video. When we needed to use actors (for example, in *telenovela* scenes with specific scripting), we solicited feedback about the women about their preferences and who they felt was most like them. A documentary-style video, however, requires featuring people from the community in order to appeal to the priority population. In the CLS video, farmworker women with no training as actors were seen giving a testimonial and making a decision about screening. Whether or not community members participate as actors in a video, however, is not as important as ensuring that they can identify with the characters in the video. We used techniques of behavioral journalism to ensure that this was the case (A. McAlister & Fernandez, 2001). This technique allowed us to use the exact words of farmworker women in the testimonials and in role-model stories included in the flip chart and the video.

All materials were developed and produced in both English and Spanish. They also incorporated graphics and step-by-step guidance; and they addressed farmworker-specific topics such as arranging travel, facing language barriers, and taking time off work. Our materials were the first to be designed for audiences of very low literacy, and they filled a gap in farmworker and migrant health education.

Scope and Sequence

The scope of this program included the delivery of the health education messages and materials during two one-on-one *promotora* visits with women in the priority communities. During the first session, the *promotora* would determine whether the woman was due for mammography, CBE, Pap test screening, or any combination of these. If she was due, the *promotora's* primary concern was to motivate the woman to obtain screening and help facilitate access. If the woman had obtained screening as recommended, the *promotora* would still offer the educational session to encourage continued regular screening. During the first visit, the *promotora* would show the woman the flip chart and the video and talk with her about any specific barriers she encounters as she considers screening. The *promotora* would then set up another appointment to visit the woman. During the second visit, the *promotora* would show the woman any materials she had not seen during the first visit and help the woman make an appointment for screening.

Consistent with traditional lay health worker services, the CLS *promotoras* often provided information and facilitation services such as identifying modes of transportation to the clinics and low- and no-cost services and helping women apply for insurance coverage, if they were eligible.

Design Documents

Table 14.6 illustrates one of the early design documents that guided our development of program materials. From each component of this document, we compiled content and draft messages to be included in the program's video, flip chart, pamphlet, and information handouts. We then elaborated the content and refined the messages for each, continually checking that the materials clearly addressed each component's change objectives. Tables 14.8 and 14.9 illustrate portions of design documents at two stages of video development: the draft of ideas about video scenes and relevant content to be covered and a section of the video treatment.

TABLE 14.8. VIDEO SCENES.

Videos: two (one English, one Spanish)

Cast: Five to six Latina women, various bit parts, extras

Opening Scene: The video begins at the fields at the end of a long day's work. As many of the workers leave for the day, four or five female farmworkers are talking by their cars. One of the women (Woman Number One) has just come back to work after a long absence. The other women ask her how she is. Woman Number One explains that she was being treated for breast cancer, but she is fine now. The group begins to talk about cancer. Some of them have questions, some bring up various fears and myths (that cancer is contagious, it is caused by bumps or bruises, and so on). They realize they should know more about cancer and their health. Woman Number Two promises to call and speak to a local *promotora* about cancer detection and treatment. Several of the women know the *promotora* and want to meet with her as well. They all agree to set up a meeting.

Promotora *Scene:* A women in the group tells story about her mother dying. Other women listen.

Content:

- Testimonial of a woman saying she never thought breast cancer would happen to her, but now she knows anyone can get it

- Understanding what cancer and breast cancer are, what are the risks, and why they are health threats

- Understanding that any woman can develop breast cancer

Call for Health Number Scene: Woman using the Call for Health number

Content:

- The woman uses the call for health number and asks about a nearby clinic. She calls the clinic and speaks to the *promotora.*

- *Promotora* explains how to use the number.

- Where to call for health flyer and key chain

TABLE 14.8. VIDEO SCENES, Cont'd.

Continuation Scene: Several days later, it's lunch time. The women gather at the edge of the field for lunch. The *promotora* arrives, and they begin to talk. The *promotora* leads the meeting, but all of the women participate. Some of the women are more knowledgeable than others and help answer questions or introduce information. Some women bring up barriers, and other women talk about overcoming them. The discussion is very positive and upbeat. Woman Number One shares her experience and gives the message that women can survive breast cancer.

Lunch with Promotora *Scene:* Women in the group have lunch with the *promotora.*

Content:

- Testimonial of woman who was diagnosed with breast cancer and has been treated and cured. The woman gives messages such as, "I thought that cancer could not be cured, but I am proof that it can. I had never had a mammogram before, but my friend encouraged me to get one. I'm so glad I did because they found the cancer when it was small and easier to treat. They removed the lump, and now I am fine."

- Express confidence in ability to obtain the CBE and the mammogram. *Promotora* sends many "you can do it" messages throughout the presentation.

- Mammography screening recommendations: have your breasts examined by a doctor or nurse practitioner every year.

- If someone in your family has had breast cancer, or you have had breast cancer before, you might need to have breast exams and mammograms more often. Ask your doctor how often you need these exams.

- Understanding CBE screening recommendations: all women should have their breasts examined by a doctor or nurse every year.

- CBE, or a breast exam by a doctor, and mammography are two ways to find breast cancer when it is early stage and easy to cure. Doctors can find lumps that are very small when they examine breasts. Mammograms can find lumps as small as a grain of rice. These exams work better when done regularly and correctly. The smaller the cancer is when it is found, the easier it is to treat and cure.

- Importance of early detection: treatment for breast cancer is more successful if the cancer is found when it is small and has not spread. Also, if the cancer is found when it is small, it is more likely that the doctor can treat it by removing just the breast lump. If the cancer has spread further, more of the breast must be removed. Finding cancer early can help save your breast and your life.

- Effectiveness of treatment: breast cancer can be cured. Out of every ten women, nine survive breast cancer when it is found early.

TABLE 14.9. VIDEO TREATMENT.

Preliminary Video Scenes

Cast: Four women

Scene 1: Lunch in the field

The video begins at the fields as the women are headed for their lunch break. A woman named Teresa joins them. The women ask Teresa where she was this morning. Teresa explains that she was at the clinic getting her annual exam and check for cancer. The group has a lot of questions about the exams for Teresa, and Teresa explains to them briefly about them until it flashes back to Scene 2: The annual exam.

Ana, Linda, and Margarita are sitting around opening their lunch bags having a conversation about getting ready for lunch.

Ana: I'm tired. I was ready for lunch.

Linda: Me too, I was hungry! So where's Teresa, she always eats with us, and I haven't seen her today.

(Teresa enters.)

Ana: Hello Teresa! We were just talking about you. Where have you been?

Teresa: I went to the health center for my Pap test this morning. You know, the test for cancer. And while I was there the doctor examined my breasts and explained to me the importance of the Pap test and the clinical breast exam.

Linda: A test for cancer. What's that?

Teresa: It's an exam that all women over the age of eighteen should get every year. It is a simple test to see if you have cancer in the cervix or neck of the uterus. The Pap test can even find changes before they become cancer.

Ana: How do you know all this?

Teresa: The doctor talked to me about the importance of the exams.

Ana: Why are they so important?

Teresa: Because they can help you find cancer early.

Ana: But I thought if you had cancer, you'd die.

Teresa: Not if it's found early. It can be treated, and you can survive it.

Linda: And how do you get breast cancer? I heard that you can get breast cancer from bumps and bruises to the breasts.

Teresa: No, you can't get breast cancer from bumps and bruises.

Margarita: I heard that breast cancer is contagious. You can catch it from someone who has it.

Teresa: It's not like a cold; you can't catch breast cancer from anyone.

Ana: So, what about the breast exam you mentioned? What is that?

Program Materials

The program's theme was *Cultivando la salud* (cultivating health), and it expressed a culturally significant message to farmworker women. During the formative phase, we received many positive comments about both the theme and the logo (see Figure 14.1). We referred to the final program materials, which aimed to influence screening behaviors among women in the priority population, as the breast and cervical cancer toolbox because these materials represented tools that the *promotora* would have at her disposal when conducting educational sessions. The toolbox included a teaching guide, flip chart, video, brochures, and other resource information.

FIGURE 14.1. PROGRAM LOGO.

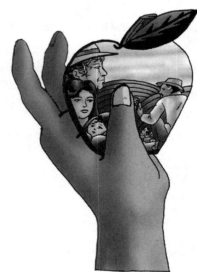

Source: Cultivando la Salud is a program of the National Center for Farmworker Health, Inc.

The Flip Chart and Video. The flip chart and video provided basic information about breast and cervical cancer and about screening recommendations and messages to increase knowledge, influence attitudes, provide cues, and facilitate access to screening services. The flip chart (a large spiral-bound book that could be held or set up on a table) contained photographs and illustrations on one side and information and messages for the *promotora* on the other side. The *promotora* referred to this written information (in English and Spanish) as she described each section.

Pamphlets. The toolbox included Spanish-language educational pamphlets from the American Cancer Society and the National Cancer Institute. The pamphlets are free of charge and were made available for *promotoras* to distribute.

Resource Information. The outreach coordinator at the health centers compiled lists of resources that gave locations of breast and cervical cancer screening facilities, phone numbers, contact individuals, hours of operation, and cost. Other material such as referral information, maps, and bus schedules were also included in the toolbox.

Pilot Testing

We solicited feedback from the priority population and from the National Cancer Coalition during the development of these materials. We also conducted a formal pilot test to obtain in-depth information concerning the relevance, acceptability, appropriateness, understandability, and potential impact of the program materials.

We selected pilot-test sites—health centers or clinics—based on the following:

- Experience in developing and implementing a lay health worker program
- Existence of a lay health worker program in the health center
- Knowledge of breast and cervical cancer
- Availability of a high proportion of farmworker women aged fifty years and older living in the clinic catchment area
- Existence of the National Breast and Cervical Cancer Early Detection Program-funded mammography and Pap test services within twenty miles of the clinic

We developed the following research questions to guide the pilot-test design:

- Do the methods and materials address the specific change objectives outlined during the intervention development process?

- Are the methods and materials theoretically based?
- Are the methods and materials appropriate for farmworker women (that is, culturally sensitive, appropriate for low-literacy skills)?
- Do the materials address barriers specific to Hispanic farmworker women that influence breast and cervical cancer screening behavior (for example, fear of detection, embarrassment, lack of time, fear of procedure)?
- Do farmworker women find the materials appropriate and appealing?

During the pilot phase, *promotoras* visited women and conducted educational sessions using the draft materials. Upon completion of the sessions, the planning team conducted six focus groups: two with *promotoras* who had participated in the pilot test and four with farmworker women who had received the education. Based on feedback from the groups, planning team members refined the messages, altered specific language, improved production quality of the flip chart, and edited the video.

We compared content of the materials to the matrices from Step 2 to ensure that they were consistent with determinants of breast and cervical cancer screening for this population and addressed the specific change objectives.

Step 5: Adoption and Implementation

Identifying Potential Program Users

Early in the development effort, we enlisted the participation of the members of various program user groups to serve on the National Cancer Coalition, described earlier. These members included intended program users such as clinic directors, outreach coordinators, lay health workers, and community members. Essentially, this group, in addition to its advisory function throughout program development, formed our linkage system (E. M. Rogers, 1995).

Although different clinics may have varying titles for these positions, program adopters were generally individuals who made decisions about new programs and resources to use for activities. Program implementers included individuals responsible for community outreach, education, coordination of lay health programs, and similar activities. Implementers also included individuals who would deliver the educational sessions to women in the priority population (the CLS lay health workers).

Performance Objectives for Adoption, Implementation, and Sustainability

To specify performance objectives for program adoption, implementation, and sustainability, we relied on information gathered during our formative work, input from the linkage system (that is, the National Cancer Coalition), and additional information obtained through new interviews with potential program adopters (clinic directors, clinical coordinators) and implementers (outreach coordinators, *promotoras*). Through these structured interviews, we were able to identify specific performance objectives that would lead to the successful adoption and implementation of the program.

These data helped answer the following questions:

- What does the individual (adopter) need to do in order to successfully adopt the program?
- What does the implementer (that is, the outreach coordinator or lay health worker) need to do to successfully implement the program?

These answers led to development of performance objectives. To adopt the CLS program, clinic directors had to become familiar with its goals and parameters of implementation, obtain clinic and community buy-in, and make a commitment to support a lay health worker program. The clinic outreach coordinators needed to identify, recruit, and train *promotoras;* supervise their educational activities; and develop locally relevant referral information. Performance objectives for lay health workers detailed the activities they needed to perform, including participant recruitment, home visitation, program materials use, visit documentation, and assistance to women in obtaining screening appointments. All of the performance objectives are included in the matrix (Tables 14.10 and 14.11).

Determinants and Matrices

In order to develop appropriate methods and strategies to increase adoption and implementation behaviors, we identified, as in Steps 2 and 3, relevant determinants and subsequently developed change objective matrices to guide the development of materials. To do this we began with existing data from *promotoras* and outreach coordinators, and we conducted two additional focus groups with clinic staff. We asked participants about likely barriers and facilitators of adoption and implementation and then asked them to suggest strategies to overcoming the barriers. Tables 14.7 and 14.8 provide portions of the adoption and implementation matrices for program users.

Because the *promotoras* were from the priority communities and often had similar levels of knowledge and barriers regarding screening, their matrices included many of the same performance objectives, determinants, and change objectives as the matrices for the intended program recipients. The *promotora* matrices also included objectives related to implementation activities.

TABLE 14.10. SAMPLE CHANGE OBJECTIVES FOR ADOPTION AND IMPLEMENTATION CLINICS.

Performance Objectives (Clinic directors)	and Awareness	Knowledge Social Norms	Perceived Expectations	Outcome Attitudes
		Personal Determinants		
PO.1. Adopts Cultivando La Salud Program	K.1.a. Recognize this program as available K.1.b. Recognize that the program will provide resources to the clinic K.1.c. Describe the program as promoting breast and Pap screening for farmworker women over fifty K.1.d. Describe the program as developed from extensive work with the community	PSN.1. Describe other clinics as using this program	OE.1. Expect that, if they use this program, rates of screening will rise	A.1.a. Describe breast and cervical cancer morbidity and mortality as a real problem for farmworker women A.1.b. Argue for increasing screening for farmworker women A.1.c. Describe the program as being better than what they have now, fitting with current services, able to be tried without much risk, not too complex
PO.2. Establish and support *promotora* program PO.2.1. Obtain staff buy-in PO.2.2. Obtain community buy-in		PSN.2. Describe other clinics in the area as using *promotora* programs successfully	OE.2. Reflect that *promotoras* can effectively engage women to participate in clinic services OE.2.1. Reflect that staff members will accept the program if given the opportunity to talk about *promotoras*, needs and resources, program goals, and agency support OE.2.2. Reflect that involving community leaders in planning will help develop a program that communities will accept	A.2.a. Describe *promotora* programs as building ties to the community A.2.b. Describe *promotoras* as a credible source of health information

TABLE 14.11. IMPLEMENTATION MATRIX FOR *PROMOTORAS*.

| | Personal Determinants | | | | | External Determinants |
Performance Objectives (*Promotoras*)	Knowledge	Skills and Self-efficacy	Attitudes	Perceived Social Norms	Outcome Expectations	Social Support
P.O.1. Adopt the role of lay health worker	K.1.a. Describe the role of the lay health worker K.1.b. Describe the challenges involved with being a lay health worker	SSE.1. Express confidence in adopting and fulfilling the role of *promotora*	A.1. Believe that becoming a *promotora* is an important contribution to the community	PSN.1. Recognize that other community women have become *promotoras*	OE.1. Expect that if they adopt the *promotora* role they will be successful at providing education to the community	SS.1. Existing *promotoras* encourage new *promotoras* and express their availability to help them.
P.O.2. Locate farmworker women ages fifty and over P.O.2.1. Post flyers P.O.2.2. Identify community leaders to help with recruitment P.O.2.3. Go door to door in health center neighborhood P.O.2.4. Contact and work with community centers, churches, schools, migrant Head Start program, and local migrant councils	K.2.a. Describe the neighborhoods in which farmworker women reside K.2.b. Compare the needs of farmworker women to other women K.2.4. Identify community centers, churches, and other locations to conduct community education	SSE.2. Express confidence in locating farmworker women SSE.2.4. Express confidence in making contact with community centers, churches, Head Start programs, and migrant councils	A.2. Explain that locating farmworker women is an important part of the *promotora* role	PSN.2. Recognize that successful *promotoras* target at-risk groups such as farmworker women	OE.2. Explain that locating and educating farmworker women will result in improvements in the health of the community OE.2.4. State that collaborating with churches, community centers, and other organizations will help them locate farmworker women	SS.2. Outreach coordinators provide encouragement and logistic support to *promotoras* in their effort to locate farmworkers. SS.2.4. Other *promotoras* will provide contacts and assistance in locating farmworker women.
P.O.3. Conduct home and community group visits P.O.3.1. Develop a safety plan for home visits P.O.3.2. Plan community sessions with manager of community site	K.3. Describe the proper protocol for conducting home visits K.3.1. Describe safe ways to conduct home visits K.3.2. Describe points to discuss with manager of community site	SSE.3.a. Demonstrate how to approach women during home visits SSE.3.b. Express confidence in conducting a home visit SSE.3.1. Express confidence in conducting a safe home visit	A.3. Explain that home visits are an effective way of reaching farmworker women	PSN.3. Recognize that other respected *promotoras* conduct home visits and community educational sessions	OE.3.a. State that if they follow the protocol they will be welcomed into the homes of farmworker women OE.3.2. State that if they follow a good safety plan they will be safe during home visits	SS.3.a. Other *promotoras* accompany new *promotoras* on home site visits. SS.3.b. Family members express support and help at home so that *promotora* can conduct home and community group visits.

Methods and Strategies

Methods selected to influence adoption and implementation objectives included modeling, guided practice, social support, and reinforcement. The activities in Step 5 led to the development of a program manual for potential program adopters and a program curriculum for training lay health workers. The manual included program goals and objectives, evidence of effectiveness, and an overview of program materials. It also included support materials for managing a lay health worker program, such as

- A job description for a *promotora*
- Guidelines for *promotora* recruitment
- Training tips for management about maintenance of lay health worker programs
- Encounter forms to collect program participation data
- A sample staffing plan and budget
- Program evaluation tools

The planning team used the matrices to develop a curriculum for clinic staff to use as they trained *promotoras* and to make decisions about methods and strategies for the training. Clinic staff trained *promotoras* over three days using the curriculum. The curriculum included twelve lessons each with an outline and notes for the trainer, suggested activities, handouts, and resource materials.

The breast and cervical cancer teaching guide was another component that we developed to facilitate program implementation. The teaching guide provided *promotoras* with the necessary information to carry out an educational session and with options for structuring the sessions depending on time and location. The guide outlined specific messages for the *promotora* to communicate, for example, one teaching guide included points to cover in a discussion of the video. The *promotora* was encouraged to play the video and then to talk with the women about how relevant the topics were to their lives, potential barriers to screening, and questions that the video may have provoked.

Program Implementation

We initially implemented the program over three months in two cities, Eagle Pass, Texas, and Merced, California. We first trained two staff members from each participating health center on the management and content of the CLS program. Following the train-the-trainer workshop, the planning team attended and observed the *promotora* training. Eagle Pass, Texas, recruited five *promotoras;* and Merced, California, recruited two *promotoras*. For three months following the training, *promotoras* were responsible for conducting education sessions with farmworker women, fifty years of age and older. Each *promotora* was employed for fifteen hours per week. The intervention consisted of a minimum of two individual contacts with each woman. If a third session was conducted, it was done in a small group setting.

Step 6: Evaluation Planning

Our program evaluation built directly on the preceding steps of Intervention Mapping, because we had specified intended program outcomes, intermediate or mediator variables, change objectives, and methods and strategies. We had developed evaluation questions at each step in the process.

Program Outcome Evaluation Questions

Because it would be impossible within the time frame of our study to assess long-term health and quality-of-life outcomes, such as decreased incidence and mortality due to cervical cancer and breast cancer, we developed questions that addressed the behaviors and environmental conditions. The primary objective of the evaluation was to assess the effectiveness of the CLS program in increasing breast and cervical cancer screening behavior among farmworker women fifty years and older. The primary outcome evaluation questions addressed the effectiveness of the program in:

- Increasing mammography completion rates among a cohort of farmworker women fifty years and older who were previously nonadherent to mammography screening guidelines?
- Increasing CBE completion among a cohort of farmworker women fifty years and older who were previously nonadherent to CBE screening guidelines?
- Increasing Pap test completion rates among a cohort of farmworker women aged fifty years and older who were previously nonadherent to Pap test screening guidelines?

Evaluation Questions Based on the Matrix: Mediator Variables

Secondary aims were related to the intermediate impact (or mediator) variables derived from the matrices. These aims were to increase knowledge, attitudes, self-efficacy, intention, and other factors related to breast and cervical cancer screening. We expected that the program would have an impact on these determinants and that these changes would in turn influence the adoption of the screening behaviors. For example, some of the evaluation questions that we based on the matrix asked how effectively the intervention did the following:

- Increase knowledge about breast and cervical cancer and screening procedures
- Increase favorable attitudes and beliefs (pros) and decrease negative attitudes and beliefs (cons) about breast and cervical cancer screening
- Increase perceived susceptibility to breast and cervical cancer
- Reduce the perception of barriers to breast and cervical cancer screening
- Increase self-efficacy to obtain mammography, CBE, and Pap test screening
- Increase outcome expectations about obtaining screening (CBE, mammography, Pap)
- Increase intentions to obtain regular mammography, CBE, and Pap test screening

Although some existing measures of salient determinants (for example, perceived risk) had already been developed, program planners used Intervention Mapping matrices to develop measurement instruments to assess these determinants.

Process Evaluation

The process evaluation design included an assessment at each intervention level to ensure that the program was implemented as planned. The assessment also allowed us to acquire sufficient information so that program outcomes could be linked with program implementation activities and levels of exposure.

We used the results in Steps 3 and 4 to formulate program process indicators. Questions asked during the formative phases of the project included those designed to gauge the appropriateness and relevance of methods and strategies selected and satisfaction, understanding of messages, and positive emotional reactions of the farmworker women to the program components. We also collected additional information using focus groups and in-depth interviews after the program had been delivered as part of the overall evaluation design.

We developed additional process indicators to assess fidelity and reach of the program using Step 5. These measures assessed all intervention levels and acquired sufficient information so that program outcomes could be linked with program implementation activities. Process measures included the following:

- An observation checklist completed by program staff to determine the completeness and fidelity of *promotora* training conducted by health centers
- A log in which site coordinators could record women enrolled in the program and visits made by the *promotora* to each woman

- An encounter form on which the *promotora* could record information about each visit, for example, length, topics covered, and referrals to screening sites
- An observation checklist for the supervisor to use when accompanying the *promotora* on home visits

Finally, we conducted weekly phone calls with site supervisors to assess program implementation.

Evaluation Design and Findings

We conducted an intervention trial to test the program's effectiveness on increasing screening and influencing intermediate impact variables (for example, knowledge, attitudes). Two community intervention sites (Eagle Pass, Texas, and Merced, California) and two comparison sites (Anthony, New Mexico, and Watsonville, California) participated in the study. Consistent with principles of community participatory research, we hired community members to gather the data. They participated in a two-day training session and then began data collection activities in the *colonias* in their areas. The program effectively increased both mammography and Pap test screening among farmworker women. Among women who were previously nonadherent to mammography screening guidelines, 40.8 percent of the intervention group and 29.9 percent of the comparison group completed screening. Among women with no recent history (in the previous three years) of a Pap test, 39.5 percent of intervention group and 23.6 percent of the comparison group completed screening. Results provide important information about the effectiveness of a community-based intervention for increasing breast and cervical cancer screening among low-income Hispanic women, specifically farmworkers, along with evidence of the effectiveness of an intervention based on the lay health worker model.

Program Status

The planning team is now in the dissemination phase of the CLS program. The NCFH received additional funding from the U.S. Centers for Disease Control and Prevention and the Susan G. Komen Foundation to provide training to migrant health clinics interested in adopting the training. There has been an overwhelmingly positive response about the program, and many clinics and lay health worker groups have requested the CLS program. We continue to refine and adapt the materials according to additional feedback and in response to changes in screening recommendations. At the same time, we are exploring ways to accelerate the program's adoption across the many migrant and community health centers nationwide.

REFERENCES

Abbema, E. A., Van Assema, P., Kok, G. J., De Leeuw, E., & De Vries, N. K. (2004). Effect evaluation of a comprehensive community intervention aimed at reducing socioeconomic health inequalities in The Netherlands. *Health Promotion International, 19,* 141–156.

Abel, E., Darby, A. L., & Ramachandran, R. (1994). Managing hypertension among veterans in an outpatient screening program. Journal of the American Academy of Nurse Practitioners, 6(9), 413–419.

Abraham, C., Sheeran, P., & Johnston, M. (1998). From health beliefs to self-regulation: theoretical advances in the psychology of action control. *Psychology and Health, 13,* 569–591.

Abrams, D., Abraham, C., Spears, R., & Marks, D. (1990). AIDS invulnerability: Relationships, sexual behavior, and attitudes among 16- to 19-year-olds. In P. Aggleton, P. Davies, & G. Hart (Eds.), *AIDS: Individual, cultural, and policy dimensions* (pp. 35–51). London: Falmer Pres.

Abramson, S. L., Shegog, R., Bartholomew, L. K., Sockrider, M. M., Czyzewski, D. I., & Mullen, P. D. (2000). Conceptual basis of an expert system to promote asthma self-management support behavior of asthma health care providers. Unpublished manuscript.

ActKnowledge & the Aspen Institute Roundtable. (2003). Making sense: Reviewing program design with theory of change. Retrieved November 23, 2004, from http://www.theoryof change.org

Adams, H. P., Jr., Brott, T. G., Furlan, A. J., Gomez, C. R., Grotta, J., Helgason, C. M., et al. (1996). Guidelines for thrombolytic therapy for acute stroke: a supplement to the guidelines for the management of patients with acute ischemic stroke. A statement for healthcare professionals from a Special Writing Group of the Stroke Council, American Heart Association. *Circulation, 94,* 1167–1174.

Adams, J., & White, M. (2004). Why don't stage-based activity promotion interventions work? *Health Education Research, 20,* 237–243.

Adams, R. J., Fuhlbrigge, A., Finkelstein, J. A., Lozano, P., Livingston, J. M., Weiss, K. B., et al. (2001). Use of inhaled anti-inflammatory medication in children with asthma in managed care settings. *Archives of Pediatrics and Adolescent Medicine, 155,* 501–507.

Aday, L. A. (1996). *Designing and conducting health surveys* (2nd ed.). San Francisco: Jossey-Bass.

Agars, J., & McMurray, A. (1993). An evaluation of comparative strategies for teaching breast self-examination. *Journal of Advanced Nursing, 18*(10), 1595–1603.

Airhihenbuwa, C. O. (1994). Health promotion and the discourse on culture: Implications for empowerment. *Health Education Quarterly, 21,* 345–353.

Airhihenbuwa, C. O., Kumanyika, S. K., TenHave, T. R., & Morssink, C. B. (2000). Cultural identity and health lifestyles among African Americans: a new direction for health intervention research? *Ethnicity and Disease, 10,* 148–164.

Ajzen, I. (1988). *Attitudes, personality and behavior.* Chicago: Dorsey Press.

Ajzen, I. (1991). The theory of planned behavior. *Organizational Behavior and Human Decision Processes, 50,* 179–211.

Ajzen, I. & Madden, T. J. (1986). Prediction of goal-directed behavior: Attitudes, intentions, and perceived behavioral control. *Journal of Experimental Social Psychology, 22,* 453–474.

Alan Guttmacher Institute (2004). *U.S. teenage pregnancy statistics: Overall trends, trends by race and ethnicity and state-by-state information.* New York & Washington: Alan Guttmacher Institute.

Albers, G. W., Amarenco, P., Easton, J. D., Sacco, R. L., & Teal, P. (2004). Antithrombotic and thrombolytic therapy for ischemic stroke: the Seventh ACCP Conference on Antithrombotic and Thrombolytic Therapy. *Chest, 126,* 483S-512S.

Albers, G. W., Bates, V. E., Clark, W. M., Bell, R., Verro, P., & Hamilton, S. A. (2000). Intravenous tissue-type plasminogen activator for treatment of acute stroke: The Standard Treatment with Alteplase to Reverse Stroke (STARS) study. *JAMA: Journal of the American Medical Association, 283,* 1145–1150.

Albers, G. W., Easton, J. D., Sacco, R. L., & Teal, P. (1998). Antithrombotic and thrombolytic therapy for ischemic stroke. *Chest, 114,* 683s–698s.

Alberts, M. J., Bertels, C., & Dawson, D. V. (1990). An analysis of time of presentation after stroke. *JAMA: Journal of the American Medical Association, 263,* 65–68.

Alcoe, S. Y., Wallace, D. G., & Beck, B. M. (1990). Ten years later: An update of the case for teaching breast self-examination. *Canadian Journal of Public Health, 81*(6), 447–449.

Alderson, P., Green, S., & Higgins, J.P.T. (2004). Cochrane reviewers' handbook 4.2.2. The Cochrane Library. Retrieved July 5, 2005, from http://www.cochrane.dk/cochrane/handbook/hbook.htm

Alewijnse, D., Mesters, I. E., Metsemakers, J. F., & van den Borne, B. (2002). Program development for promoting adherence during and after exercise therapy for urinary incontinence. *Patient Education and Counseling, 48,* 147–160.

Alinsky, S. D. (1969). *Reveille for radicals.* Chicago: University of Chicago Press.

Alinsky, S. D. (1972). *Rules for radicals.* New York: Random House.

Allegrante, J. P., & Roizen, M. F. (1998). Can net-present-value economic theory be used to explain and change health-related behaviors? *Health Education Research, 13,* i–iv.

Allegrante, J. P., & Sleet, D. A. (2004). *Derryberry's educating for health: A foundation for contemporary health education practice.* San Francisco: Jossey-Bass.

Allen, D. B., & Bergman, A. B. (1976). Social learning approaches to health education: Utilization of infant auto restraint devices. *Pediatrics, 58,* 323–328.

Allen, J., & Bellingham, R. (1994). Building supportive cultural environments. In M. P. O'Donnell & J. S. Harris (Eds.), *Health promotion in the workplace* (2nd ed., pp. 204–216). Albany, NY: Delmar Thomson Learning Publishers.

Allen, J. D., Sorensen, G., Stoddard, A. M., Colditz, G., & Peterson, K. (1998). Intention to have a mammogram in the future among women who have underused mammography in the past. *Health Education Behavior, 25,* 474–488.

Allen, R., & Kraft, C. (1984). The importance of cultural variables in program design. In M. P. O'Donnell & T. H. Ainsworth (Eds.), *Health promotion in the workplace* (1st ed., pp. 69–95). New York: Wiley.

Allensworth, D., Lawson, E., Nicholson, L., & Wyche, J. (Eds.) and Committee on Comprehensive School Health Programs in Grades K-12. (1997). *Schools and health: Our nation's investment.* Washington, DC: National Academy of Science.

Altman, D. G. (1995a). Strategies for community health intervention: Promises, paradoxes, pitfalls. *Psychosomatic Medicine, 57,* 226–233.

Altman, D. G. (1995b). Sustaining interventions in community systems: On the relationship between researchers and communities. *Health Psychology, 14,* 526–536.

Altman, D. G., Balcazar, F. E., Fawcett, S. B., Seekins, T. M., & Young, J. Q. (1994). *Public health advocacy: Creating community change to improve health.* Palo Alto, CA: Stanford Center for Research in Disease Prevention.

Altschuler, A., Somkin, C. P., & Adler, N. E. (2004). Local services and amenities, neighborhood social capital, and health. *Social Science and Medicine, 59,* 1219–1229.

American Academy of Neurology, Quality Standards Subcommittee (1996). Practice advisory: Thrombolytic therapy for acute ischemic stroke—summary statement. *Neurology, 47,* 835–839.

American Cancer Society (2003). *Cancer facts and figures for Hispanics/Latinos 2003–2005.* Retrieved February 21, 2005, from http://www.cancer.org/downloads/STT/CAFF2003 HispPWSecured.pdf

American Psychological Association. (2001). *Publication manual of the American Psychological Association* (5th ed.). Washington, DC: Author.

American Psychological Association, Commission on Youth and Violence (1993). *Violence and youth: Psychology's response. Vol. 1: Summary report of the American Psychological Association commission on violence and youth.* Washington D.C.: Author.

American Society of Heating, Refrigerating, and Air-Conditioning Engineers. (1989). *Standard 62–1989. Ventilation for acceptable indoor air quality.* Atlanta, GA: Author.

American Urological Association (2000). Prostate-specific antigen (PSA) best practice policy. *Oncology, 14,* 267–268, 280.

Ammerman, A., Washington, C., Jackson, B., Weathers, B., Campbell, M., Davis, G., et al. (2002). A church-based nutrition intervention designed for cultural appropriateness, sustainability, and diffusion. *Health Promotion Practice, 3,* 286–301.

Anderson, E. (1990). Neighborhood effects on teenage pregnancy. In C. Jencks & P. E. Peterson (Eds.), *The urban underclass* (pp. 375–390). Washington, DC: Brookings Institution.

Anderson, J. R. (1983). A spreading activation theory of memory. *Journal of Verbal Learning and Verbal Behavior, 22,* 261–295.

Andreasen, A. R. (1995). *Marketing social change: Changing behavior to promote health, social development, and the environment.* San Francisco: Jossey-Bass.

Arizmendi, T. G., & Affonso, D. D. (1987). Stressful events related to preganancy and postpartum. *Journal of Psychosomatic Research, 31,* 743–756.

Armitage, C. J. (2004). Evidence that implementation intentions reduce dietary fat intake: a randomized trial. *Health Psychology, 23,* 319–323.

Atkin, C. K., & Freimuth, C. (1989). Formative evaluation research in campaign design. In R. E. Rice & C. K. Atkin (Eds.), *Public communication campaigns* (pp. 131–150). Thousand Oaks, CA: Sage.

Averch, H. A. (1994). The systematic use of expert judgment. In J. S. Wholey, H. P. Hatry, & K. E. Newcomer (Eds.), *Handbook of practical program evaluation* (1st ed., pp. 293–309). San Francisco: Jossey-Bass.

Averett, S. L., Rees, D. I., & Argys, L. M. (2002). The impact of government policies and neighborhood characteristics on teenage sexual activity and contraceptive use. *American Journal of Public Health, 92,* 1773–1778.

Awofeso, N. (2003). The healthy cities approach—reflections on a framework for improving global health. *Bulletin of the World Health Organization, 81,* 222–223.

Azzimondi, G., Bassein, L., Fiorani, L., Nonino, F., Montaguti, U., Celin, D., et al. (1997). Variables associated with hospital arrival time after stroke: Effect of delay on the clinical efficiency of early treatment. *Stroke, 28,* 537–542.

Backer, T. E. (2000). The failure of success: Challenges of disseminating effective substance abuse prevention programs. *Journal of Community Psychology, 28,* 363–373.

Bahir, A., Goldberg, A., Mekori, Y. A., Confino-Cohen, R., Morag, H., Rosen, Y., et al. (1997). Continuous avoidance measures with or without acaricide in dust mite–allergic asthmatic children. *Annals of Allergy, Asthma, and Immunology, 78,* 506–512.

Bakeman, R., McCray, E., Lumb, J. R., Jackson, R. E., & Whitley, P. N. (1987). The incidence of AIDS among blacks and Hispanics. *Journal of the National Medical Association, 79,* 921–928.

Baker, D. W., Gazmararian, J. A., Williams, M. V., Scott, T., Parker, R. M., Green, D., et al. (2002). Functional health literacy and the risk of hospital admission among Medicare managed care enrollees. *American Journal of Public Health, 92,* 1278–1283.

Baker, D. W., Parker, R. M., Williams, M. V., & Clark, W. S. (1998). Health literacy and the risk of hospital admission. *Journal of General Internal Medicine, 13,* 791–798.

Baker, D. W., Parker, R. M., Williams, M. V., Clark, W. S., & Nurss, J. (1997). The relationship of patient reading ability to self-reported health and use of health services. *American Journal of Public Health, 87,* 1027–1030.

Baker, D. W., Williams, M. V., Parker, R. M., Gazmararian, J. A., & Nurss, J. (1999). Development of a brief test to measure functional health literacy. *Patient Education and Counseling, 38,* 33–42.

Baker, S. P., O'Neill, M., Ginsburg, M. J., & Li, G. (1992). *The injury fact book.* New York: Oxford University Press.

Balderman, B. (1995). *Buying creative services.* Lincolnwood, IL: NTC Publishing Group.

Bandura, A. (1986). *Social foundations of thought and action: A social cognitive theory.* Englewood Cliffs, NJ: Prentice Hall.

Bandura, A. (1990). Perceived self-efficacy in the exercise of control over AIDS infection. *Evaluation and Program Planning, 13,* 9–17.

Bandura, A. (1997). *Self-efficacy: The exercise of control.* New York: W. H. Freeman & Co.

Baranowski, T., Anderson, C., & Carmack, C. (1998). Mediating variable framework in physical activity interventions. How are we doing? How might we do better? *American Journal of Preventive Medicine, 15,* 266–297.

Baranowski, T., Klesges, L. M., Cullen, K. W., & Himes, J. H. (2004). Measurement of outcomes, mediators, and moderators in behavioral obesity prevention research. *Preventive Medicine, 38*(Suppl), S1–13.

Baranowski, T., Lin, L. S., Wetter, D. W., Resnicow, K., & Hearn, M. D. (1997). Theory as mediating variables: Why aren't community interventions working as desired? *Annals of Epidemiology, 7,* s89–s95.

Baranowski, T., Perry, C. L., & Parcel, G. S. (2002). How individuals, environments, and health behavior interact: Social cognitive theory. In K. Glanz, F. M. Lewis, & B. K. Rimer (Eds.), *Health behavior and health education: Theory, research, and practice* (3rd ed., pp. 165–184). San Francisco, CA: Jossey-Bass.

Baranowski, T., & Stables, G. (2000). Process evaluation of the 5-a-day projects. *Health Education and Behavior, 27,* 157–166.

Bargh, J. A., & Chartrand, T. L. (1999). The unbearable automaticity of being. *American Psychologist, 54,* 462–479.

Barlow, J., Wright, C., Sheasby, J., Turner, A., & Hainsworth, J. (2002). Self-management approaches for people with chronic conditions: A review. *Patient Education and Counseling, 48,* 177–187.

Baron, R. M., & Kenny, D. A. (1986). The moderator-mediator variable distinction in social psychological research: An overview. *Journal of Personality and Social Psychology, 51,* 1073–1182.

Barsan, W. G., Brott, T. G., Broderick, J. P., Haley, E. C., Levy, D. E., & Marler, J. R. (1993). Time of hospital presentation in patients with acute stroke. *Archives of Internal Medicine, 153,* 2558–2561.

Bartholomew, L. K. (2004). Development and evaluation of messages to address safety and adverse event concerns about influenza vaccination among adults. (Special Interest Project [SIP] 11). University of Texas Health Science Center at Houston (SIP Grant U 48 DP 000057-01). Centers for Disease Control and Prevention.

Bartholomew, L. K., Bettencourt, J., McQueen, A., Perez, C., Greisinger, T., & Vernon, S. (2005). Development of a multi-media Transtheoretical Model-based program to promote colon cancer screenings. Unpublished manuscript.

Bartholomew, L. K., Czyzewski, D. I., Parcel, G. S., Swank, P. R., Sockrider, M. M., Mariotto, M. J., et al. (1997). Self-management of cystic fibrosis: Short-term outcomes of the Cystic Fibrosis Family Education Program. *Health Education and Behavior, 24,* 652–666.

Bartholomew, L. K., Czyzewski, D. I., Swank, P. R., McCormick, L., & Parcel, G. S. (2000). Maximizing the impact of the Cystic Fibrosis Family Education Program: Factors related to program diffusion. *Family and Community Health, 22,* 27–47.

Bartholomew, L. K., Gold, R. S., Parcel, G. S., Czyzewski, D. I., Sockrider, M. M., Fernandez, M., et al. (2000). Watch, Discover, Think, and Act: Evaluation of computer-assisted instruction to improve asthma self-management in inner-city children. *Patient Education and Counseling, 39,* 269–280.

Bartholomew, L. K., Koenning, G., Dahlquist, L., & Barron, K. (1994). An educational needs assessment of children with juvenile rheumatoid arthritis. *Arthritis Care and Research, 7,* 136–143.

Bartholomew, L. K., Parcel, G. S., Seilheimer, D. K., Czyzewski, D., Spinelli, S. H., & Congdon, B. (1991). Development of a health education program to promote the self-management of cystic fibrosis. *Health Education Quarterly, 18,* 429–443.

Bartholomew, L. K., Parcel, G. S., Swank, P. R., & Czyzewski, D. I. (1993). Measuring self-efficacy expectations for the self-management of cystic fibrosis. *Chest, 103,* 1524–1530.

Bartholomew, L. K., Seilheimer, D. K., Parcel, G. S., Spinelli, S. H., & Pumariega, A. J. (1989). Planning patient education for cystic fibrosis: Application of a diagnostic framework. *Patient Education and Counseling, 13,* 57–68.

Bartholomew, L. K., Selwyn, B. J., Livoti-Debellis, M. A., Chronister, K., Sablotne, E., Abrams, C., & Hodgson, H. (2005). Using qualitative and quantitative methods to develop persuasive messages for influenza vaccination. Unpublished manuscript.

Bartholomew, L. K., Shegog, R., Parcel, G. S., Gold, R. S., Fernandez, M., Czyzewski, D. I., et al. (2000). Watch, Discover, Think, and Act: A model for patient education program development. *Patient Education and Counseling, 39,* 253–268.

Bartholomew, L. K., Sockrider, M. M., Seilheimer, D. K., Czyzewski, D. I., Parcel, G. S., & Spinelli, S. H. (1993). Performance objectives for the self-management of cystic fibrosis. *Patient Education and Counseling, 22,* 15–25.

Bartholomew, L. K., Tortolero, S., Sockrider, M. M., Markham, C., Abramson, S., Fernandez, M., et al. (1999, April). *Screening children for asthma: Results from 60 elementary schools.* Paper presented at the meeting of the American Thoracic Society, San Diego, CA.

Basara, L. R., & Juergens, J. P. (1994). Patient package insert readability and design 2. *American Pharmacy, 34,* 48–53.

Basch, C. E. (1987). Focus group interview: An underutilized research technique for improving theory and practice in health education. *Health Education Quarterly, 14,* 411–448.

Basch, C. E. (1989). Preventing AIDS through education: Concepts, strategies, and research priorities. *Journal of School Health, 59,* 296–300.

Basen-Engquist, K., Coyle, K. K., Parcel, G. S., Kirby, D., Banspach, S. W., Carvajal, S. C., et al. (2001). Schoolwide effects of a multicomponent HIV, STD, and pregnancy prevention program for high school students. *Health Education and Behavior, 28,* 166–185.

Basen-Engquist, K., Masse, L. C., Coyle, K., Kirby, D., Parcel, G. S., Banspach, S. et al. (1999). Validity of scales measuring the psychosocial determinants of HIV/STD-related risk behavior in adolescents. *Health Education Research, 14,* 25–38.

Basen-Engquist, K., O'Hara-Tompkins, N. M., Lovato, C. Y., Lewis, M. J., Parcel, G. S., & Gingiss, P. L. (1994). The effect of two types of teacher training on implementation of Smart Choices: A tobacco prevention curriculum. *Journal of School Health, 64,* 334–339.

Basen-Engquist, K. & Parcel, G. S. (1992). Attitudes, norms, and self-efficacy: A model of adolescents' HIV-related sexual risk behavior. *Health Education Quarterly, 19,* 263–277.

Bass, P. F., III, Wilson, J. F., & Griffith, C. H. (2003). A shortened instrument for literacy screening. *Journal of General Internal Medicine, 18,* 1036–1038.

Bastani, R., Maxwell, A. E., Carbonari, J., Rozelle, R., Baxter, J., & Vernon, S. (1994). Breast cancer knowledge, attitudes, and behaviors: A comparison of rural health and non-health workers. *Cancer Epidemiology, Biomarkers and Prevention, 3,* 77–84.

Batson, C. D. (1991). *The altruism question: Toward a social-psychological answer.* Mahwah, NJ: Erlbaum.

Batson, C. D., Polycarpou, M. P., Harmon-Jones, E., Imhoff, H. J., Mitchener, E. C., Bednar, L. L., et al. (1997). Empathy and attitudes: Can feeling for a member of a stigmatized group improve feelings toward the group? *Journal of Personality and Social Psychology, 72,* 105–118.

Bauer, K. W., Yang, Y. W., & Austin, S. B. (2004). "How can we stay healthy when you're throwing all of this in front of us?" Findings from focus groups and interviews in middle schools on environmental influences on nutrition and physical activity. *Health Education and Behavior, 31,* 34–46.

Baum, F. E., & Ziersch, A. M. (2003). Social capital. *Journal of Epidemiology and Community Health, 57,* 320–323.

Bauman, K. E., Foshee, V. A., Ennett, S. T., Hicks, K., & Pemberton, M. (2001). Family matters: A family-directed program designed to prevent adolescent tobacco and alcohol use. *Health Promotion Practice, 2,* 81–96.

Bauman, L. J., & Adair, E. G. (1992). The use of ethnographic interviewing to inform questionnaire construction. *Health Education Quarterly, 19,* 9–23.

Bauman, L. J., Wright, E., Leickly, F. E., Carin, E., Kurszon-Moran, D., Wade, S. L., et al. (2002). Relationship of adherence to pediatric asthma morbidity among inner-city children. *Pediatrics, 110,* p. e6.

Baumeister, R. F., & Vohs, K. D. (2004). *Handbook of self-regulation; research, theory, and applications.* New York: The Guilford Press.

Bayne-Smith, M., Fardy, P. S., Azzollini, A., Magel, J., Schmitz, K. H., & Agin, D. (2004). Improvements in heart health behaviors and reduction in coronary artery disease risk factors in urban teenaged girls through a school-based intervention: The PATH program. *American Journal of Public Health, 94,* 1538–1543.

Bazargan, M., Bazargan, S. H., Farooq, M., & Baker, R. S. (2004). Correlates of cervical cancer screening among underserved Hispanic and African-American women. *Preventive Medicine, 39,* 465–473.

Beaulieu, L. J. (2002). Mapping the assets of your community: A key component for building local capacity (Civic Engagement: Southern Rural Development Center Series No. 227). Retrieved April 6, 2005, from http://srdc.msstate.edu/publications/227/227_asset_mapping.pdf

Beaver, K., & Luker, K. (1997). Readability of patient information booklets for women with breast cancer. *Patient Education and Counseling, 31,* 95–102.

Becker, A. B. (2002). Challenges to treatment goals and outcomes in pediatric asthma. *Journal of Allergy and Clinical Immunology, 109,* S533-S538.

Becker, M. H. (1974a). The Health Belief Model and personal health behavior. *Health Education Monographs, 2,* 324–508.

Becker, M. H. (1974b). The Health Belief Model and sick role behavior. *Health Education Monographs, 2,* 409–419.

Beeker, C., Kraft, J., & Goldman, R. (2001). Strategies for increasing colorectal cancer screening among African Americans. *Journal of Psychosocial Oncology, 19,* 113–132.

Beeker, C., Kraft, J. M., Southwell, B. G., & Jorgensen, C. M. (2000). Colorectal cancer screening in older men and women: Qualitative research findings and implications for intervention. *Journal of Community Health, 25,* 263–278.

Begley, C. E., Fourney, A., Elreda, D., & Teleki, A. (2002). Evaluating outcomes of HIV prevention programs: Lessons learned from Houston, Texas. *AIDS Education and Prevention, 14,* 432–443.

Bell, D. E. (1982). Regret in decision making under uncertainty. *Operations Research, 21,* 961–981.

Bender, B. G. (2002). Overcoming barriers to nonadherence in asthma treatment. *The Journal of Allergy Clinical Immunology, 109,* S554–S559.

Bennis, W. G., Benne, K. D., & Chin, R. (Eds.). (1969). *The planning of change* (2nd ed.). New York: Holt, Rinehart, and Winston.

Bental, D. S., Cawsey, A., & Jones, R. (1999). Patient information systems that tailor to the individual. *Patient Education and Counseling, 36,* 171–180.

Berg, B. L. (1989). *Qualitative research methods for the social sciences.* Boston: Allyn and Bacon.

Berg, B. L. (2003). *Qualitative research methods for the social sciences* (5th ed.). Boston: Allyn & Bacon.

Berkman, L. S., & Glass, T. G. (2000). Social integration, social networks, social support and health. In L. S. Berkman & I. Kawachi (Eds.), *Social epidemiology* (pp. 137–173). New York: Oxford University Press.

Berkman, L. S., & Kawachi, I. (2000). *Social epidemiology.* New York: Oxford University Press.

Berwick, D. M. (2003). Disseminating innovations in health care. *JAMA: Journal of the American Medical Association, 289,* 1969–1975.

Best, A., Moor, G., Holmes, B., Clark, P. I., Bruce, T., Leischow, S., et al. (2003). Health promotion dissemination and systems thinking: Towards an integrative model. *American Journal of Health Behavior, 27*(Suppl 3), S206–S216.

Beyer, J. M., & Trice, H. M. (1978). *Implementing change: Alcoholism policies in work organizations.* New York: Free Press.

Biener, L., & Siegel, M. (2000). Tobacco marketing and adolescent smoking: More support for a causal inference. *American Journal of Public Health, 90,* 407–411.

Bird, J., Otero-Sabogal, R. A., Ha, N.-T., & McPhee, S. (1996). Tailoring lay health worker interventions for diverse cultures: Lessons learned from Vietnamese and Latina communities. *Health Education Quarterly, 23,* S105–S122.

Bishop-Townsend, V. (1996). STDs: Screening, therapy and long-term implications for the adolescent patient. *International Journal of Fertility and Menopausal Studies, 41,* 109–114.

Bloom, S. S. (1956). *Taxonomy of education objectives. Handbook I: Cognitive domain.* New York: McKay.

Boekaerts, M., Pintrich, P. R., & Zeidner, M. (2001). *Handbook of self-regulation.* New York: Academic Press.

Boer, H., & Seydel, E. R. (1996). Protection motivation theory. In M. Conner & P. Norman (Eds.), *Predicting health behaviour: Research and practice with social cognition models* (pp. 95–120). Buckingham, England, and Philadelphia: Open University Press.

Bolen, J. C., Rhodes, L., Powell-Griner, E. E., Bland, S. D., Holtzman, D., Division of Adult and Community Health, et al. (2000). State-specific prevalence of selected health behaviors, race and ethnicity: Behavioral risk factor surveillance system, 1997. *MMWR Surveillance Summaries, 49,* 1–60.

Bonfill, X., Marzo, M., Pladevall, M., Marti, J., & Emparanza, J. I. (2001). Strategies for increasing women participation in community breast cancer screening. *Cochrane Database of Systematic Reviews, 1,* CD002943.

Bordieu, P. (1986). The forms of capital. In *The handbook of theory and research for the sociology of education* (pp. 241–258). New York: Greenwood Press.

Borkan, J. M., & Neher, J. O. (1991). A developmental model of ethnosensitivity in family practice training. *Family Medicine, 23,* 212–217.

Borkan, J. M., Quirk, M., & Sullivan, M. (1991). Finding meaning after the fall: Injury narratives from elderly hip fracture patients. *Social Science and Medicine, 33,* 947–957.

Bornstein, R. (1989). Exposure and affect: Overview and meta-analysis of research. *Psychological Bulletin, 106,* 265–289.

Bouman, M., Maas, L., & Kok, G. (1998). Health education in television entertainment—Medisch Centrum West: a Dutch drama serial. *Health Education Research, 13,* 503–518.

Bowditch, J. L., & Buono, A. F. (1994). *A primer on organizational behavior* (3rd ed.). New York: Wiley.

Boyer, C. B., Shafer, M. A., & Tschann, J. M. (1997). Evaluation of a knowledge- and cognitive-behavioral skills—building intervention to prevent STDs and HIV infection in high school students. *Adolescence, 32,* 25–42.

Bracht, N., Finnegan, J. R., Rissel, C., Weisbrod, R., Gleason, J., Corbett, J., & Veblen-Mortenson, S. (1994). Community ownership and program continuation following a health demonstration project. *Health Education Research: Theory and Practice, 9*(2), 243–255.

Bracht, N., & Kingsbury, L. (1990). Community organization principles in health promotion: A five-stage model. In N. Bracht (Ed.), *Health promotion at the community level* (1st ed., pp. 66–88). Thousand Oaks, CA: Sage.

Bradford, L. P. (1976). *Making meetings work: A guide for leaders and group members.* San Diego, CA: University Associates.

Brager, G. A., & Holloway, S. (1978). *Changing human service organizations: Politics and practice.* New York: Free Press.

Braithwaite, R. L., Bianchi, C., & Taylor, S. E. (1994). Ethnographic approach to community organization and health empowerment. *Health Education Quarterly, 21,* 407–416.

Brandon, P. R. (1992). State-level evaluations of school programs funded under the Drug-Free Schools and Communities. *Journal of Drug Education, 22*(1), 25–36.

Bratina, P., Greenberg, L., Pasteur, W., & Grotta, J. C. (1995). Current emergency department management of stroke in Houston, Texas. *Stroke, 26,* 409–414.

Brawley, L. R., & Culos-Reed, S. N. (2000). Studying adherence to therapeutic regimens: overview, theories, recommendations. *Controlled Clinical Trials, 21,* 156S–163S.

Brennan, F. A., & Fink, S. V. (1997). Health promotion, social support, and computer networks. In R. L. Street, W. R. Gold, T. Manning, & R. L. Street, Jr. (Eds.), *Health promotion and interactive technology: Theoretical applications and future directions* (pp. 157–169). Mahwah, NJ: Erlbaum.

Brennan, P., Ripich, S., & Moore, S. (1991). The use of home-based computers to support persons living with AIDS/ARC. *Journal of Community Health Nursing, 8,* 3–14.

Brink, S. G., Basen-Engquist, K. M., O'Hara-Tompkins, N. M., Parcel, G. S., Gottlieb, N. H., & Lovato, C. Y. (1995). Diffusion of an effective tobacco prevention program. Part 1: Evaluation of the dissemination phase. *Health Education Research, 10,* 283–295.

Briss, P. A., Mullen, P. D., & Hopkins, D. P. (2005). Methods used for reviewing evidence and linking evidence to recommendations in the Community Guide. In S. Zaza, P. A. Briss, & K. W. Harris (Eds.), *The guide to community preventive services: What works to promote health?* New York: Oxford University Press.

Briss, P., Rimer, B., Reilley, B., Coates, R. C., Lee, N. C., Mullen, P. D., et al. (2004). Promoting informed decisions about cancer screening in communities and healthcare systems. *American Journal of Preventive Medicine, 26,* 67–80.

Briss, P. A., Rodewald, L. E., Hinman, A. R., Shefer, A. M., Strikas, R. A., Bernier, R. R., et al. (2000). Reviews of evidence regarding interventions to improve vaccination coverage in children, adolescents, and adults: The task force on community preventive services. *American Journal of Preventive Medicine, 18,* 97–140.

Briss, P. A., Zaza, S., Pappaioanou, M., Fielding, J., Wright-De Aguero, L., Truman, B. I., et al. (2000). Developing an evidence-based guide to community preventive services—methods: The task force on community preventive services. *American Journal of Preventive Medicine, 18,* 35–43.

Britton, M. G., Earnshaw, J. S., & Palmer, J. B. (1992). A 12-month comparison of salmeterol with salbutamol in asthmatic patients. *European Respiratory Journal, 5,* 1062–1067.

Brock, D. J. (1996). Population screening for cystic fibrosis. *Current Opinion in Pediatrics, 8*(6), 635–638.

Brown, R., & Ogden, J. (2004). Children's eating attitudes and behavior: A study of the modeling and control theories of parental influence. *Health Education Research, 19,* 261–271.

Brown, S. J., Lieberman, D. A., Germeny, B. A., Fan, Y. C., Wilson, D. M., & Pasta, D. J. (1997). Education video game for juvenile diabetes self-care: Results of a controlled trial. *Medical Informatics, 22,* 77–89.

Brownson, R. C., Baker, E. A., Housemann, R. A., Breannan, L. K., & Bacak, S. J. (2001). Environmental and policy determinants of physical activity in the United States. *American Journal of Public Health, 91,* 1995–2003.

Brownson, R. C., Chang, J. J., Eyler, A. A., Ainsworth, B. E., Kirtland, K. A., Saelens, B. E., et al. (2004). Measuring the environment for friendliness toward physical activity: A comparison of the reliability of 3 questionnaires. *American Journal of Public Health, 94,* 473–483.

Brownson, R. C., Eriksen, M. P., Davis, R. M., & Warner, K. E. (1997). Environmental tobacco smoke: Health effects and policies to reduce exposure. *Annual Reviews of Public Health, 18,* 163–185.

Brug, J., Campbell, M., & Van Assema, P. (1999). The application and impact of computer-generated personalized nutrition education: A review of the literature. *Patient Education and Counseling, 36,* 145–156.

Brug, J., Glanz, K., Van Assema, P., Kok, G., & van Breukelen, G. J. (1998). The impact of computer-tailored feedback and iterative feedback on fat, fruit, and vegetable intake. *Health Education and Behavior, 25,* 517–531.

Brug, J., Hospers, H. J., & Kok, G. (1997). Differences in psychosocial factors and fat consumption between stages of change for fat reduction. *Psychology and Health, 12,* 719–727.

Brug, J., Oenema, A., & Campbell, M. (2003). Past, present, and future of computer-tailored nutrition education. *American Journal of Clinical Nutrition, 77,* 1028S–1034S.

Brug, J., Oenema, A., & Ferreira, I. (in press). Theory, evidence, and intervention mapping to improve behavioral nutrition and physical activity interventions. *International Journal of Behavioral Nutrition and Physical Activity.*

Brug, J., Schols, A., & Mesters, I. (2004). Dietary change, nutrition education and chronic obstructive pulmonary disease. *Patient Education and Counseling, 52,* 249–257.

Brug, J., Steenhuis, I., Van Assema, P., & De Vries, H. (1996). The impact of a computer-tailored nutrition intervention. *Preventive Medicine, 25,* 236–242.

Brug, J., Van Assema, P., Kok, G., Lenderink, T., & Glanz, K. (1994). Self-rated dietary fat intake: Association with objective assessment of fat, psychosocial factors and intention to change. *Journal of Nutrition Education, 26,* 218–223.

Brugman, E., Goedhart, H., Vogels, T., & Van Zessen, G. (1995). *Jeugd en sex* [Youth and sex]. Utrecht, The Netherlands: SWP.

Bryant, F. B., & Wortman, P. M. (1984). Methodological issues in the meta-analysis of quasi-experiments. In W. H. Yeaton & P. M. Wortman (Eds.), *New directions for program evaluation: No. 24. Issues in data synthesis.* San Francisco: Jossey-Bass.

Buchner, D. A., Carlson, A. M., & Stempel, D. A. (1997). Patterns of anti-inflammatory therapy in the post-guidelines era: A retrospective claims analysis of managed care members. *American Journal of Managed Care, 3,* 87–93.

Bull, F. C., Kreuter, M. W., & Scharff, D. P. (1999). Effects of tailored, personalized and general health messages on physical activity. *Patient Education and Counseling, 36,* 181–192.

Bull, S. S., Gillette, C., Glasgow, R. E., & Estabrooks, P. (2003). Work site health promotion research: To what extent can we generalize the results and what is needed to translate research to practice? *Health Education and Behavior, 30,* 537–549.

Bunton, R., Murphy, S., & Bennett, P. (1991). Theories of behavioral change and their use in health promotion: Some neglected areas. *Health Education Research, 6,* 153–162.

Burdine, J. N., & McLeroy, K. R. (1992). Practitioners' use of theory: Examples from a workgroup. *Health Education Quarterly, 19,* 331–340.

Burgher, M. S., Rasmussen, V. B., & Rivett, D. (1999). *The European Network of Health Promoting Schools: The alliance of education and health.* Copenhagen, Denmark: World Health Organization.

Burgoon, M. (1989). Messages and persuasive effects: Review of issues in message-effects research in the social influence literature. In J. J. Bradac (Ed.), *Message effects in communication science* (pp. 129–164). Thousand Oaks, CA: Sage.

Burkhart, P. V., Dunbar-Jacob, J. M., Fireman, P., & Rohay, J. (2002). Children's adherence to recommended asthma self-management. *Pediatric Nursing, 28,* 409–414.

Burrows, B., Martinez, F. D., Halonen, M., Barbec, R. A., & Cline, M. G. (1989). Association of asthma and serum IgE levels and skin test reactivity to allergens. *New England Journal of Medicine, 320,* 271–277.

Butterfoss, F. D., & Kegler, M. C. (2002). Toward a comprehensive understanding of community coalitions: Moving from practice to theory. In R. J. DiClemente, R. A. Crosby, & M. C. Kegler (Eds.), *Emerging theories in health promotion practice and research: Strategies for improving public health* (1st ed., pp. 157–193). San Francisco: Jossey-Bass.

Butz, A. M., Eggleston, P., Huss, K., Kolodner, K., & Rand, C. (2000). Nebulizer use in inner-city children with asthma: Morbidity, medication use, and asthma management practices. *Archives of Pediatrics and Adolescent Medicine, 154,* 984–990.

Cabana, M. D., Ebel, B. E., Cooper-Patrick, L., Powe, N. R., Rubin, H. R., & Rand, C. S. (2000). Barriers pediatricians face when using asthma practice guidelines. *Archives of Pediatrics and Adolescent Medicine, 154,* 685–693.

Cabana, M. D., Slish, K. K., Lewis, T. C., Brown, R. W., Nan, B., Lin, X., et al. (2004). Parental management of asthma triggers within a child's environment. *Journal of Allergy and Clinical Immunology, 114,* 352–357.

Caburnay, C. A., Kreuter, M. W., & Donlin, M. J. (2001). Disseminating effective health promotion programs from prevention research to community organizations. *Journal of Public Health Management and Practice, 7,* 81–89.

Caffarella, R. (1985). *Planning programs for adult learners: A practical guide for educators, trainees, and staff developers.* San Francisco: Jossey-Bass.

Caldwell, C. H., Wright, J. C., Zimmerman, M. A., Walsemann, K. M., Williams, D., & Isichei, P. A. (2004). Enhancing adolescent health behaviors through strengthening nonresident father-son relationships: A model for intervention with African-American families. *Health Education Research, 19,* 644–656.

Call, R. S., Smith, T. F., Morris, E., Chapman, M. D., & Platts-Mills, T. A. (1992). Risk factors for asthma in inner-city children. *Journal of Pediatrics, 121,* 862–866.

Cameron, L. D., & Leventhal, H. (2003). *The self-regulation of health and illness behavior.* New York: Routledge.

Cameron, R., Jolin, M. A., Walker, R., McDermott, N., & Cough, M. (2001). Linking science and practice: Toward a system for enabling communities to adopt best practices for chronic disease prevention. *Health Promotion Practice, 2,* 35–42.

Campbell, M., Fitzpatrick, R., Haines, A., Kinmonth, A. L., Sandercock, P., Spiegelhalter, D., et al. (2000). Framework for design and evaluation of complex interventions to improve health. *British Medical Journal, 321,* 694–696.

Campbell, M. K., DeVellis, B. M., Strecher, V. J., Ammerman, A. S., DeVellis, R. F., & Sandler, R. S. (1994). Improving dietary behavior: The effectiveness of tailored messages in primary care settings. *American Journal of Public Health, 84*(5), 783–787.

Campbell, M. K., Tessaro, I., DeVellis, B., Benedict, S., Kelsey, K., Belton, L., et al. (2000). Tailoring and targeting a worksite health promotion program to address multiple health behaviors among blue-collar women. *American Journal of Health Promotion, 14,* 306–313.

Campbell, M. K., Tessaro, I., DeVellis, B., Benedict, S., Kelsey, K., Belton, L., et al. (2002). Effects of a tailored health promotion program for female blue-collar workers: Health works for women. *Preventive Medicine, 34,* 313–323.

Canadian Public Health Association. (1998). *Plain-language forms for seniors: A guide for the public, private and not-for-profit sectors.* Ottawa: National Literacy and Health Program and Canadian Public Health Association.

Cancer Research Center and Centers for Disease Control (1994). *Beyond the brochure: Alternative approaches to effective health communication.* Denver: AMC Cancer Research Center.

Caplan, L. R., Mohr, J. P., Kistler, J. P., & Koroshetz, W. (1997). Should thrombolytic therapy be the first-line treatment for acute ischemic stroke? Thrombolysis—not a panacea for ischemic stroke. *New England Journal of Medicine, 337,* 1309–1310.

Capraro, R. M., & Caparro, M. M. (2002). Treatments of effect sizes and statistical significance tests in textbooks. *Educational and Psychological Measurement, 62,* 771–782.

Carney, O., McIntosh, J., & Worth, A. (1996). The use of the Nominal Group Technique in research with community nurses. *Journal of Advanced Nursing, 23,* 1024–1029.

Carroll, J. S. (1978). The effects of imagining an event on expectations for the event: An interpretation in terms of the availability heuristic. *Journal of Experimental Social Psychology, 14,* 88–96.

Castro, F. G., Elder, J., Coe, K., Tafoya-Barraza, H. M., Moratto, S., Campbell, N., et al. (1995). Mobilizing churches for health promotion in Latino communities: Compañeros en la Salud. *Journal of National Cancer Institute Monographs, 18,* 127–135.

Catania, J. A., Kegeles, S. M., & Coates, T. J. (1990). Towards an understanding of risk behavior: An AIDS risk reduction model (ARRM). *Health Education Quarterly, 17,* 53–72.

Cavanaugh, N., & Cheney, K. S. (2002). Community collaboration: A weaving. *Journal of Public Health Management and Practices, 8,* 13–20.

Centers for Disease Control and Prevention. (1994a). *Preventing tobacco use among young people: A report of the Surgeon General* (Report No. 017–001–00491–0). Atlanta: Centers for Disease Control and Prevention, National Center for Chronic Disease Prevention and Health Promotion, Office on Smoking and Health.

Centers for Disease Control and Prevention. (1994b). *HIV/AIDS Surveillance Report, 43,* 659.

Centers for Disease Control and Prevention. (1996). Asthma mortality and hospitalization among children and young adults-United States, 1980–1993. *Morbidity and Mortality Weekly Report, 45,* 350–353.

Centers for Disease Control and Prevention. (1999). U.S. HIV and AIDS cases reported through December 1999. *HIV/AIDS Surveillance Report, 11,* 1–44.

Centers for Disease Control and Prevention. (1999). *Best Practices for Comprehensive Tobacco Control Programs—August 1999.* Atlanta GA: U.S. Department of Health and Human Services,

Centers for Disease Control and Prevention, National Center for Chronic Disease Prevention and Health Promotion, Office on Smoking and Health.

Centers for Disease Control and Prevention. (1999). *Tobacco advertising and promotion fact sheet.* Retrieved July 7, 2005, from http://www.cdc.gov/tobacco/sgr/sgr_2000/factsheets/factsheet_advertising.htm

Centers for Disease Control and Prevention. (2001a). Asthma: 10 million school days lost each year. *Chronic Disease Notes and Reports, 14,* 18.

Centers for Disease Control and Prevention (2001b). BRFSS trends data: Nationwide vs. Texas. No pap smear within 3 years. *Behavioral Risk Factor Surveillance System.* Retrieved March 21, 2005, from http://apps.nccd.cdc.gov/brfss/Trends/trendchart_c.asp?state_c=TX&state=US&qkey=10070&SUBMIT1=Go

Centers for Disease Control and Prevention (2001c). Tracking the hidden epidemics: Trends in STDs in the United States 2000. Retrieved March 25, 2005, from http://www.cdc.gov/nchstp/dstd/Stats_Trends/Trends2000.pdf

Centers for Disease Control and Prevention (2003). BRFSS trends data: Nationwide vs. Texas. No Pap smear within 3 years. Retrieved February 22, 2005 from http://apps.nccd.cdc.gov/brfss/Trends/trend chart_c.asp?state_TX&state=US&qkey=10070&SUBMIT1=Go

Centers for Disease Control and Prevention (2004). Cases of HIV infection and AIDS in the United States, 2003. *HIV/AIDS Surveillance Report.* Retrieved February 23, 2005,from http://www.cdc.gov/hiv/stats/2003SurveillanceReport.pdf

Centers for Disease Control and Prevention (2004). Quality of life as a new public health measure: Behavioral risk factor surveillance system, 1993. *Morbidity and Mortality Weekly Report, 43,* 375–380.

Centers for Disease Control and Prevention (2005). CDC recommends [Searchable storehouse of on-line documents]. Retrieved February 9, 2005, from http://www.phppo.cdc.gov/CDCREcommends/AdvSearchV.asp

Centers for Disease Control and Prevention (2005). School health index: A self-assessment and planning guide. Centers for Disease Control. Retrieved January 25, 2005, from http://apps.nccd.cdc.gov/SHI/pdf/Elementary.pdf

Centers for Disease Control and Prevention, Agency for Toxic Substances, & Disease Registry Committee on Community Engagement (1997). Principles of community engagement: CDC/ATSDR Committee on Community Engagement. Retrieved from http://www.cdc.gov/phppo/pce/

Centers for Disease Control and Prevention, AIDS Community Demonstration Projects Research Group (1999). Community-level HIV intervention in 5 cities: Final outcome data from the CDC AIDS community demonstration projects. *American Journal of Public Health, 89,* 336–345.

Centers for Disease Control and Prevention & Oak Ridge Institute for Science and Education. (2003). Cdcynergy: Your guide to effective health communication (Version 3.0) [Computer software]. Atlanta, GA: Author.

Center for Pediatric Research (1997). *Materials for Coalition Training Institute.* Norfolk, VA: Eastern Virginia Medical School.

Centerwall, B. S. (1993). Television and violent crime. *Public Interest, 111,* 56–71.

Chaffe, S. H., & Roser, C. (1986). Involvement and the consistency of knowledge, attitudes, and behavior. *Communication Research, 13,* 373–399.

Chaiken, S. (1987). The heuristic model of persuasion. In M. P. Zanna, J. M. Olsen, & C. P. Herman (Eds.), *Social influence* (pp. 3–39). Mahwah, NJ: Erlbaum.

Chambers, K. B., & Rew, L. (2003). Safer sexual decision making in adolescent women: perspectives from the conflict theory of decision-making. *Issues in Comprehensive Pediatric Nursing, 26,* 129–143.

Champion, V. L., Ray, D. W., Heilman, D. K., & Springston, J. K. (2000). A tailored intervention for mammography among low-income African-American women. *Journal of Psychosocial Oncology, 18,* 1–13.

Chartrand, T. L., & Bargh, J. A. (1999). The chameleon effect: The perception-behavior link and social interaction. *Journal of Personality & Social Psychology, 76,* 893–910.

Chaskin, R. J., Brown, P., Venkatesh, S., & Vidal, A. (2001). *Building community capacity.* New York: Aldine de Gruter.

Chavez, L. R., Cornelius, W. A., & Jones, O. W. (1986). Utilization of health services by Mexican immigrant women in San Diego. *Women and Health, 11,* 3–20.

Chavez, L. R., Hubbell, F. A., Mishra, S. I., & Valdez, R. B. (1997). The influence of fatalism on self-reported use of Papanicolaou smears. *American Journal of Preventive Medicine, 13,* 418–424.

Chavis, D. M., & Wandersman, A. (1990). Sense of community in the urban environment: A catalyst for participation in community development. *American Journal of Community Psychology, 18,* 55–81.

Cheatham, A., & Shen, F. (2003). Community-based participatory research with Cambodian girls in Long Beach, CA. In M. Minkler & N. Wallerstein (Eds.), *Community-based participatory research for health* (pp. 316–331). San Francisco: Jossey-Bass.

Chen, H. T. (1990). Evaluating with sense: The theory-driven approach. *Evaluation Review, 3,* 283–302.

Chew, L. D., Bradley, K. A., Flum, D. R., Cornia, P. B., & Koepsell, T. D. (2004). The impact of low health literacy on surgical practice. *American Journal of Surgery, 188,* 250–253.

Chiang, L. C., Huang, J. L., & Lu, C. M. (2003). Educational diagnosis of self-management behaviors of parents with asthmatic children by triangulation based on PRECEDE-PROCEED model in Taiwan. *Patient Education and Counseling, 49,* 19–25.

Choi, W. S., Ahluwalia, J. S., Harris, K. J., & Okuyemi, K. (2002). Progression to established smoking: The influence of tobacco marketing. *American Journal of Preventive Medicine, 22,* 228–233.

Chu, C., Breucker, G., Harris, N., Stitzel, A., Gan, X., Gu, X., et al. (2000). Health-promoting workplaces: International settings development. *Health Promotion International, 15,* 155–167.

Clark, C. M., & Peterson, P. L. (1986). Teachers' thought processes. In M. C. Wittrock (Ed.), *Third handbook of research on teaching.* (pp. 255–296). New York: Macmillan.

Clark, N. M. (1989). Asthma self-management education: Research and implications for clinical practice. *Chest, 95,* 1110–1113.

Clark, N. M. (2003). Management of chronic disease by patients. *Annual Review of Public Health, 24,* 289–313.

Clark, N. M., Brown, R., Joseph, C. L., Anderson, E. W., Liu, M., Valerio, M., et al. (2002). Issues in identifying asthma and estimating prevalence in an urban school population. *Journal of Clinical Epidemiology, 55,* 870–881.

Clark, N. M., Feldman, C. H., Evans, D., Duzey, O., Levison, M. J., Wasilewski, Y., et al. (1986). Managing better: Children, parents, and asthma. *Patient Education and Counseling, 8,* 27–38.

Clark, N. M., Feldman, C. H., Evans, D., Levison, M. J., Wasilewski, Y., & Mellins, R. B. (1986). The impact of health education on frequency and cost of health care use by low-income children with asthma. *Journal of Allergy and Clinical Immunology, 78,* 108–115.

Clark, N. M., Feldman, C. H., Evans, D., Wasilewski, Y., & Levison, M. J. (1984). Changes in children's school performance as a result of education for family management of asthma. *Journal of School Health, 54,* 143–145.

Clark, N. M., Gong, M., Schork, M. A., Evans, D., Roloff, D., Hurwitz, M., et al. (1998). Impact of education for physicians on patient outcomes. *Pediatrics, 101,* 831–836.

Clark, N. M., Gong, M., Schork, M. A., Kaciroti, N., Evans, D., Roloff, D., et al. (2000). Long-term effects of asthma education for physicians on patient satisfaction and use of health services. *European Respiratory Journal, 16,* 15–21.

Clark, N. M., Janz, N. K., Dodge, J. A., Schork, M. A., Wheeler, J.R.C., Liang, J., et al. (1997). Self-management of heart disease by older adults. *Research on Aging, 19,* 362–382.

Clark, N. M., Janz, N. K., Dodge, J. A., & Sharpe, P. A. (1992). Self-regulation of health behavior: The "Take PRIDE" program. *Health Education Quarterly, 19*(3), 341–354.

Clark, N. M., & Nothwehr, F. (1997). Self-management of asthma by adult patients. *Patient Education and Counseling, 32,* S5–20.

Clark, N. M., Rakowski, W., Ostrander, L., Wheeler, J. R., Oden, S., & Keteyian, S. (1988). Development of self-management education for elderly heart patients. *Gerontologist, 28,* 491–494.

Clark, N. M., Rosenstock, I. M., Hassan, H., Evans, D., Wasilewski, Y., Feldman, C., & Mellins, R. B. (1988). The effect of health beliefs and feelings of self-efficacy on self-management behavior of children with chronic disease. *Patient Education and Counseling, 11,* 131–139.

Clark, N. M., & Starr-Schneidkraut, N. J. (1994). Management of asthma by patients and families. *American Journal of Respiratory and Critical Care Medicine, 194,* S54–S66.

Clark, N. M., & Zimmerman, B. J. (1990). A social cognitive view of self-regulated learning about health. *Health Education Research, 5,* 371–379.

Cleary, T. J., & Zimmerman, B. (2000). Self-regulation empowerment program: A school-based program to enhance self-motivated cycles of student learning. *Psychology in the Schools, 41,* 537–550.

Cobb, R. W., & Elder, C. D. (1983). *Participation in American politics: The dynamics of agenda-building* (2nd ed.). Baltimore: Johns Hopkins University Press.

Cochrane, A. L. (1971). *Effectiveness and and efficiency.* London: The Nuffield Provincial Hospitals Trust. Cited in Aday, L. A., Begley, C. E., Lairson, D. R., and Slater, C. H. (1998). *Evaluating the healthcare system: Effectiveness, efficiency, and equity.* (p. 51). Chicago: Health Administration Press.

Cohen, J. (1988). *Statistical power analysis for the behavioral sciences.* Mahwah, NJ: Erlbaum.

Cohen, J. (1992). A proper primer. *Psychological Bulletin, 112,* 155–159.

Cohen, J. E., Milio, N., Rozier, R. G., Ferrence, R., Ashley, M. J., & Goldstein, A. O. (2000). Political ideology and tobacco control. *Tobacco Control, 9,* 263–267.

Cohen, S., & Lichtenstein, E. (1990). Partner behaviors that support quitting smoking. *Journal of Consulting and Clinical Psychology, 58,* 304–309.

Cohen, S., Lichtenstein, E., Kingsolver, K., Mermelstein, R., Baer, J. S., & Kamarck, T. W. (1988). Social support interventions for smoking cessation. In B. H. Gottlieb (Ed.), *Marshaling social support: Formats, processes, and effects* (pp. 211–240). Newbury Park, CA: Sage.

Coleman, J. S. (1990). *Foundations of social theory.* Cambridge, MA: Harvard University Press.

Commendador, K. A. (2003). Concept analysis of adolescent decision making and contraception. *Nursing Forum, 38,* 27–35.

Commers, M., Gottlieb, N. H., Kok, G. (2005). How to change environments for health. Unpublished manuscript.

Connell, J., & Kubisch, A. (1996). *Applying A Theories of Change approach to the evaluation of comprehensive community initiatives: Progress, prospects, and problems. Roundtable on comprehensive community initiatives for children and families.* Retrieved March 23, 2005, from http://www. aspeninstitute.org/site/c.huLWJeMRK.pH/b.612045/k.4BA8Roundtable_on_ Community_Change.htm

Connelly, J. (2001). Critical realism and health promotion: effective practice needs an effective theory. *Health Education Research, 16,* 115–119.

Conner, M., & Norman, P. (1996). *Predicting health behaviour: Research and practice with social cognition models.* Buckingham, England: Open University Press.

Conner, M., & Sparks, P. (1996). The theory of planned behaviour and health behaviours. In M. Conner & P. Norman (Eds.), *Predicting health behaviour: Research and practice with social cognition models* (pp. 121–162). Buckingham, England: Open University Press.

Cook, T. D., & Campbell, D. T. (1979). *Quasi-experimentation: Design and analysis issues for field settings.* Boston: Houghton Mifflin.

Cook, P. S., Peterson, R. C., & Moore, D. T. (1990). *Alcohol, tobacco, and other drugs may harm the unborn.* (Report No. DHHS (ADM) 90-1711). Rockville, MD: U.S. Department of Health and Human Services.

Cooley, M. E., Moriarty, H., Berger, M. S., Selm-Orr, D., Coyle, B., & Short, T. (1995). Patient literacy and the readability of written cancer educational materials 10. *Oncology Nursing Forum, 22,* 1345–1351.

Cooper, H., & Hedges, L. V. (1994). *The handbook of research synthesis.* New York: Russell Sage Foundation.

Corby, N. H., Enguidanos, S. M., & Kay, L. S. (1996). Development and use of role model stories in a community-level HIV risk reduction intervention. *Public Health Reports, 111,* 54–58.

Coronado, G. D., Thompson, B., Koepsell, T. D., Schwartz, S. M., & McLerran, D. (2004). Use of pap test among Hispanics and non-Hispanic whites in a rural setting. *Preventive Medicine, 38,* 713–722.

Cortina, J. M., & Nouri, H. (2000). *Effect sizes for ANOVA designs.* New York: Russell Sage Foundation.

Costa, F. M., Jessor, R., Fortenberry, J. D., & Donovan, J. E. (1996). Psychosocial conventionality, health orientation, and contraceptive use in adolescence. *Journal of Adolescent Health, 18,* 404–416.

Costa, M. (1995). Needs assessment and community development. In J. Rothman, J. L. Erlich, J. E. Tropman, & U. Cox (Eds.), *Strategies of community intervention* (pp. 257–266). Itasca, IL: F. E. Peacock.

Costa, M. (2001). Needs assessment and community development. In J. Rothman, J. L. Erlich, & J. E. Tropman (Eds.), *Strategies of community intervention: Macro practice* (6th ed.). Belmont, CA: Wadsworth.

Cottrell, L. (1977). The competent community. In R. L. Warren (Ed.), *New perspectives on the American community: A book of readings.* (3rd ed.). Chicago: Rand McNally College Publishing Company.

Coughlin, S. S., Uhler, R. J., Richards, T., & Wilson, K. M. (2003). Breast and cervical cancer screening practices among Hispanic and non-Hispanic women residing near the United States–Mexico border, 1999–2000. *Family and Community Health, 26,* 130–139.

Coulton, C. (1995). Using community-level indicators of children's well-being in comprehensive community initiatives. In J. Connell, A. Kubisch, L. Schorr, & C. Weiss (Eds.), *New approaches to evaluating community initiatives* (pp. 173–200). Washington, DC: The Aspen Institute.

Counsell, C. (1997). Formulating questions and locating primary studies for inclusion in systematic reviews. *Annals of Internal Medicine, 127,* 380–387.

Cox, D. J., Gonder-Frederick, L., Julian, D. M., & Clarke, W. (1994). Long-term follow-up evaluation of blood glucose awareness training. *Diabetes Care, 17,* 1–5.

Coyle, K., Basen-Engquist, K., Kirby, D., Parcel, G., Banspach, S., Collins, J., et al. (2001). Safer choices: reducing teen pregnancy, HIV, and STDs. *Public Health Reports, 116*(Suppl. 1), 82–93.

Coyle, K., Basen-Engquist, K., Kirby, D., Parcel, G., Banspach, S., Harrist, R., et al. (1999). Short-term impact of safer choices: a multicomponent, school-based HIV, other STD, and pregnancy prevention program. *Journal of School Health, 69,* 181–188.

Coyle, K., Kirby, D., Parcel, G., Basen-Engquist, K., Banspach, S., Rugg, D., et al. (1996). Safer Choices: a multicomponent school-based HIV/STD and pregnancy prevention program for adolescents. *Journal of School Health, 66,* 89–94.

Coyle, S. L. (1998). Women's drug use and HIV risk: findings from NIDA's Cooperative Agreement for Community-Based Outreach/Intervention Research Program. *Women and Health, 27,* 1–18.

Crain, E. F., Weiss, K. B., Bijur, P. E., Hersh, M., Westbrook, L., & Stein, R. E. (1994). An estimate of the prevalence of asthma and wheezing among inner-city children. *Pediatrics, 94,* 356–362.

Cramer, M. E., Mueller, K. J., Harrop, D. (2003). Comprehensive evaluation of a community coalition: A case study of environmental tobacco smoke reduction. *Public Health Nursing. 20,* 464–477.

Craun, A. M., & Deffenbacher, J. L. (1987). The effects of information, behavioral rehearsal, and prompting on breast self-exams. *Journal of Behavioral Medicine, 10*(4), 351–365.

Creer, T. L. (1990). Strategies for judgment and decision making in the management of childhood asthma. *Pediatric Allergy and Immunology, 4,* 253–264.

Creer, T. L. (1991). The application of behavioral procedures to childhood asthma: Current and future perspectives. *Patient Education and Counseling, 17,* 9–22.

Creer, T. L. (2000a). Self-management and the control of chronic pediatric illness. In D. Drotar (Ed.), *Promoting adherence to medical treatment in chronic childhood illness* (pp. 95–128). Mahwah, NJ: Erlbaum.

Creer, T. L. (2000b). Self-management of chronic illness. In M. Boekaerts, P. R. Pintrich, & M. Zeidner (Eds.), *Handbook of self-regulation* (pp. 601–629). New York: Academic Press.

Creer, T. L., Backial, M., Burns, K. L., Leung, P., Marion, R. J., Miklich, D. R., et al. (1988). Living with asthma: I. Genesis and development of a self-management program for childhood asthma. *Journal of Asthma, 25,* 335–362.

Creer, T. L., Kotses, H., & Wigal, J. K. (1992). A second-generation model of asthma self-management. *Pediatric Allergy and Immunology, 6,* 143–165.

Cuijpers, C., Swaen, G., Wesseling, G., Stumans, F., & Wouters, E. E. (1995). Adverse effects of the indoor environment on respiratory health in primary school children. *Environmental Research, 68,* 11–23.

Cullen, K. W., Bartholomew, L. K., & Parcel, G. S. (1997). Girl Scouting: An effective channel for nutrition education. *Journal of Nutrition Education, 29,* 86–91.

Cullen, K. W., Bartholomew, L. K., Parcel, G. S., & Kok, G. (1998). Intervention Mapping: Use of theory and data in the development of a fruit and vegetable nutrition program for Girl Scouts. *Journal of Nutrition Education, 30,* 188–195.

Cullinane, P. M., Hyppolite, K., Zastawney, A. L., & Friedman, R. H. (1994). Telephone-linked communication: Activity counseling and tracking for older patients. *Journal of General Internal Medicine, 9,* 86.

Cummings, T. G., & Worley, C. G. (1993). *Organization development and change* (5th ed.). Eagan, MN: West Publishing.

Cunningham, J., Dockery, D., & Speizer, F. (1996). Race, asthma, and persistent wheeze in Philadelphia schoolchildren. *American Journal of Public Health, 86,* 1406–1409.

Curry, S. J., McBride, C., Grothaus, L. C., Louie, D., & Wagner, E. H. (1995). A randomized trial of self-help materials, personalized feedback, and telephone counseling with non-volunteer smokers. *Journal of Consulting and Clinical Psychology, 63,* 1005–1014.

Curry, S. J., Wagner, E. H., & Grothaus, L. C. (1991). Evaluation of intrinsic and extrinsic motivation interventions with a self-help smoking cessation program. *Journal of Consulting and Clinical Psychology, 59,* 318–324.

Curtis, S., & Jones, J. R. (1999). Is there a place for geography in the analysis of health inequality? In M. Bartley, D. Blane, & G. D. Smith (Eds.), *The sociology of health inequalities* (pp. 85–112). Cambridge, MA: Blackwell.

Cystic Fibrosis Foundation (1995). *Cystic Fibrosis Foundation Patient Registry: 1995 data report.* Bethesda, MD: Cystic Fibrosis Foundation.

D'Angelo, S. L. (2001). Approaches to problems of adherence. In M. Bluebond-Langner, B. Lask, & D. B. Angst (Eds.), *Psychosocial aspects of cystic fibrosis* (pp. 361–379). New York: Oxford University Press.

Daniels, W. R. (1986). *Group power I: A manager's guide to using task-force meetings.* Erlanger, KY: Pfeiffer.

Davis, T. C., Crouch, M. A., Long, S. W., Jackson, R. H., Bates, P., George, R. B., et al. (1991). Rapid assessment of literacy levels of adult primary care patients 2. *Family Medicine, 23,* 433–435.

Davis, T. C., Crouch, M. A., Wills, G., Miller, S., & Abdehou, D. M. (1990). The gap between patient reading comprehension and the readability of patient education materials. *Journal of Family Practice, 31,* 533–538.

Dawson, K. P., Van Asperen, P., Higgins, C., Sharpe, C., & Davis, A. (1995). An evaluation of the action plans of children with asthma. *Journal of Pediatrics and Child Health, 31,* 21–23.

Day, R. S., Nakamori, M., & Yamamoto, S. (2004). Recommendations to develop an intervention for Japanese youth on weight management. *The Journal of Medical Investigation, 51,* 154–162.

Deaux, K., & Farris, E. (1977). Attributing causes for one's own performance: The effects of sex, norms, and outcome. *Journal of Research in Personality, 11*(1), 59–72.

de Haes, W. F. (1987). Looking for effective drug education programs: Fifteen years' exploration of the effects of different drug education programs. *Health Education Research, 2,* 433–438.

de Leeuw, E. (2000). Beyond community action: Communication arrangements and policy networks. In B. D. Poland, L. W. Green, & I. Rootman (Eds.), *Settings for health promotion: Linking theory and practice* (pp. 287–300). Thousand Oaks, CA: Sage.

De Moor, C., Baranowski, T., Cullen, K. W., & Nicklas, T. (2003). Misclassification associated with measurement error in the assessment of dietary intake. *Public Health Nutrition, 6,* 393–399.

De Vries, H., & Backbier, E. (1994). Self-efficacy as an important determinant of quitting among pregnant women who smoke: The phi-pattern. *Preventive Medicine, 23,* 167–174.

De Vries, H., Backbier, E., Dijkstra, M., van Breukelen, G., Parcel, G., & Kok, G. (1994). A Dutch social influence smoking prevention approach for vocational school students. *Health Education Research, 9,* 365–374.

De Vries, H., Backbier, E., Kok, G., & Dijkstra, M. (1995). The impact of social influences in the context of attitude, self-efficacy, intention and previous behavior as predictors of smoking onset. *Journal of Applied Social Psychology, 25,* 237–257.

De Vries, H., & Dijkstra, M. (1989). Non-smoking, your choice, a Dutch smoking prevention programme. In C. James, I. Balding, & D. Harris (Eds.), *World yearbook of education* (pp. 20–31). London: Kogan Page.

De Vries, H., Weijts, W., Dijkstra, M., & Kok, G. (1992). The utilization of qualitative and quantitative data for health education program planning, implementation, and evaluation: A spiral approach. *Health Education Quarterly, 19,* 101–115.

Dede, C., & Fontana, L. (1995). Transforming health education via new media. In L. M. Harris (Ed.), *Health and the new media: Technologies transforming personal and public health* (pp. 163–183). Mahwah, NJ: Erlbaum.

Delbecq, A. L. (1983). The Nominal Group as a technique for understanding the qualitative dimensions of client needs. In R. A. Bell (Ed.), *Assessing health and human service needs* (pp. 191–209). New York: Human Sciences Press.

Delbecq, A., Van de Ven, A. H., & Gustafson, D. H. (1975). *Group techniques for program planning: A guide to nominal and delphi processes.* Glenview, IL: Scott, Foresman.

Delichatsios, H. K., Friedman, R. H., Glanz, K., Tennstedt, S., Smigelski, C., Pinto, B. M., et al. (2001). Randomized trial of a "talking computer" to improve adults' eating habits. *American Journal of Health Promotion, 15,* 215–224.

Denzin, N., & Lincoln, Y. (1998). *Collecting and interpreting qualitative data* (2nd ed.). Thousand Oaks, CA: Sage.

Derry, S. J. (1984). Effects of an organizer on memory for prose. *Journal of Educational Psychology, 76,* 98–107.

Desvousges, W. H. & Frey, J. H. (1989). Integrating focus groups and surveys: Examples from environmental risk studies. *Journal of Official Statistics, 5,* 349–363.

Deutsches Cochrane Zentrum [*The German Cochrane Center*]. (1999). *Verfassen, Aktualisieren und Verbreiten systematischer Übersichtsarbeiten in der Medizin* [Preparing, maintaining and promoting the accessibility of systematic reviews of the effects of health care interventions]. Retrieved January 4, 1999, from http://www.update-software.com/ccweb/default.html

DeVellis, R. F. (1991). *Scale development: Theory and applications.* Thousand Oaks, CA: Sage.

Devers, K. J. (1999). How will we know "good" qualitative research when we see it? Beginning the dialogue in health services research. *Health Services Research, 34,* 1153–1188.

Devessa, S. S., Grauman, D. G., Blot, W. J., Pennello, G., Hoover, R. N., & Fraumeni, J. F. (1999). *Atlas of cancer mortality in the United States, 1950–1994 (NIH 99–4564).* Washington, D.C.: United States Printing Office.

Dewar, A., White, M., Posade, S. T., & Dillon, W. (2003). Using nominal group technique to assess chronic pain, patients' perceived challenges and needs in a community health region. *Health Expectations, 6,* 44–52.

Dey, J. (1999). *Grounding grounded theory: Guidelines for qualitative inquiry.* San Diego, CA: Academic Press.

Dickersin, K. (1997). How important is publication bias? A synthesis of available data. *AIDS Education and Prevention, 9,* 15–21.

DiClemente, C. C., Marinilli, A. S., Singh, M., & Bellino, L. E. (2001). The role of feedback in the process of health behavior change. *American Journal of Health Behavior, 25,* 217–227.

DiClemente, C. C., Mullen, P. D., Pollak, K. I., Sockrider, M. M., & Stotts, A. L. (March 1998). *Intervention effects on pregnant quitters' partners' smoking.* Paper presented at the Society of Behavioral Medicine Annual Meeting, New Orleans, LA.

DiClemente, C. C., & Prochaska, J. O. (1985). Process and stages of self-change: Coping and competence in smoking behavioral change. In S. Shiffman & T. A. Wells (Eds.), *Coping and substance abuse* (pp. 319–343). New York: Academic Press.

DiClemente, C. C., & Prochaska, J. O. (1998). Toward a comprehensive Transtheoretical Model of change. In W. Miller & N. Heather (Eds.), *Treating addictive behaviors* (pp. 3–24). New York: Plenum Press.

DiClemente, C. C., Prochaska, J. O., Fairhurst, S. K., Velicer, W. F., Velasquez, M. M., & Rossi, J. S. (1991). The process of smoking cessation: an analysis of precontemplation, contemplation, and preparation stages of change. *Journal of Consulting and Clinical Psychology, 59,* 295–304.

DiClemente, R. J., Crosby, R. A., & Kegler, M. C. (2002). *Emerging theories in health promotion practice and research: Strategies for improving public health* (1st ed.). San Francisco: Jossey-Bass.

Diette, G. B., Markson, L., Skinner, E. A., Nguyen, T. T., Algatt-Bergstrom, P., & Wu, A. W. (2000). Nocturnal asthma in children affects school attendance, school performance, and parents' work attendance. *Archives of Pediatrics and Adolescent Medicine, 154,* 923–928.

Diette, G. B., Skinner, E. A., Markson, L. E., Algatt-Bergstrom, P., Nguyen, T. T., Clark, R. D., et al. (2001). Consistency of care with national guidelines for children with asthma in managed care. *The Journal of Pediatrics, 138,* 59–64.

Dijker, A. J., Kok, G., & Koomen, W. (1996). Emotional reactions to people with AIDS. *Journal of Applied Social Psychology, 26,* 731–748.

Dijkstra, A., & De Vries, H. (1999). The development of computer-generated tailored interventions. *Patient Education and Counseling, 36,* 193–203.

Dijkstra, A., De Vries, H., & Roijackers, J. (1998). Long-term effectiveness of computer-generated tailored feedback in smoking cessation. *Health Education Research, 13,* 207–214.

Dijkstra, A., De Vries, H., Roijackers, J., & van Breukelen, G. (1998a). Tailoring information to enhance quitting in smokers with low motivation to quit: Three basic efficacy questions. *Health Psychology, 17,* 513–519.

Dijkstra, A., De Vries, H., Roijackers, J., & van Breukelen, G. (1998b). Tailored interventions to communicate stage-matched information to smokers in different motivational stages. *Journal of Consulting and Clinical Psychology, 66,* 549–557.

Dillman, D. (2000). *Mail and internet surveys: The tailored design method* (2nd ed.). New York: Wiley.

DiMatteo, M. R., & DiNicola, D. D. (1985). *Achieving patient compliance: The psychology of the medical practitioner's role.* New York: Pergamon Press.

Dimeff, L. A., & Marlatt, G. A. (1998). Preventing relapse and maintaining change in addictive behaviors. *Clinical Psychology-Science and Practice, 5,* 513–525.

Djukanovic, R., Wilson, J. W., Britten, K. M., Wilson, S. J., Walls, A. F., Roche, W. R., et al. (1992). Effect of an inhaled corticosteroid on airway inflammation and symptoms in asthma. *American Review of Respiratory Disease, 145,* 669–674.

Doak, C. C., Doak, L. G., & Root, J. H. (1996). *Teaching patients with low literacy skills* (2nd ed.). Philadelphia: Lippincott.

Dodge, J. K., Janz, N. K., & Clark, N. M. (2002). The evolution of an innovative heart disease management program for older women: Integrating quantitative and qualitative methods in practice. *Health Promotion Practice, 3,* 30–42.

Dodge, K., & Cole, J. (1987). Social information processing factors in reactive and proactive aggression in children's peer groups. *Journal of Personality and Social Psychology, 53,* 1146–1158.

Dolan-Mullen, P., Ramirez, G., & Groff, J. Y. (1994). A meta-analysis of randomized trials of prenatal smoking cessation interventions. *American Journal of Obstetrics and Gynecology, 171*(5), 1328–1334.

Dollahite, J., Thompson, C., & McNew, R. (1996). Readability of printed sources of diet and health information. *Patient Education and Counseling, 27,* 123–134.

Donahue, J. G., Fuhlbrigge, A. L., Finkelstein, J. A., Fagan, J., Livingston, J. M., Lozano, P., et al. (2000). Asthma pharmacotherapy and utilization by children in three managed care organizations. *Journal of Allergy Clinical Immunology, 106,* 1108–1114.

D'Onofrio, C. N., Moskowitz, J. M., & Braverman, M. T. (2002). Curtailing tobacco use among youth: evaluation of project 4-health. *Health Education and Behavior, 29,* 656–682.

Donovan, J. E., Jessor, R., & Costra, F. M. (1991). Adolescent health behavior and conventionality-unconventionality: An extension of problem-behavior theory. *Health Psychology, 10,* 52–61.

Drummond, M. F., O'Brien, B., Stoddart, G. L., & Torrance, G. W. (1997). *Methods for the economic evaluation of health care programmes* (2nd ed.). Oxford, England: Oxford University Press.

Drummond, N., Abdalla, M., Beattie, J.A.G., Buckingham, J. K., Lindsay, T., Osman, L. M., et al. (1994). Effectiveness of routine self-monitoring of peak flow in patients with asthma. *British Medical Journal, 308,* 564–567.

Drury, J., & Reicher, S. (2005). Explaining enduring empowerment: A comparative study of collective action and psychological outcomes. *European Journal of Social Psychology, 35,* 35–58.

Duhl, L. (1990). *The social entrepreneurship of change.* New York: Pace University Press.

Duhl, L. (2004). Transitions and paradigms. *Journal of Epidemiological Community Health, 58,* 806–807.

Dungy, C. I., Kozak, P. P., Gallup, J., & Galant, S. P. (1986). Aeroallergen exposure in the elementary school setting. *Annals of Allergy, 56,* 218–221.

Dutton, J. P., Posner, B. A., Smigelski, C., & Friedman, R. H. (1995). Lowering of total serum cholesterol through the use of DietAid? A telecommunications system for dietary counseling. *Annals of Behavioral Medicine, 17,* S088.

Eagly, A. H., & Chaiken, S. (1993). *The psychology of attitudes.* Ft. Worth, TX: Harcourt, Brace, Jovanovich.

Earp, J. A., & Ennett, S. T. (1991). Conceptual models for health education research and practice. *Health Education Research, 6,* 163–171.

Earp, J. A., & Ory, M. G. (1979). The effects of social support and health professionals' home visits on patient adherence to hypertension regimens. *Preventive Medicine, 8,* 155–165.

Edwards, B., & McCarthy, J. D. (2004). Resources and social movement mobilization. In D. A. Snow, S. A. Soule, & H. Kriesi (Eds.), *The Blackwell companion to social movements* (pp. 116–152). Oxford, England: Blackwell.

Eertmans, A., Baeyens, F., & Van den Bergh, O. (2001). Food likes and their relative importance in human eating behavior: Review and preliminary suggestions for health promotion. *Health Education Research, 16,* 443–456.

Eggleston, P. A., Malveaux, F. J., Butz, A. M., Huss, K., Thompson, L., Kolodner, K., et al. (1998). Medications used by children with asthma living in the inner city. *Pediatrics, 101,* 349–354.

Eiser, C., Patterson, D., & Tripp, J. H. (1984). Illness experience and children's concepts of health and illness. *Child: Care, Health & Development, 10*(3), 157–162.

el-Askari, G., Freestone, J., Irizarry, C., Kraut, K. L., Mashiyama, S. T., Morgan, M. A., et al. (1998). The Healthy Neighborhoods Project: A local health department's role in catalyzing community development. *Health Education and Behavior, 25,* 146–159.

El-Bassel, N., Ivanoff, A., Schilling, R. F., Borne, D., & Gilbert, L. (1997). Skills building and social support enhancement to reduce HIV risk among women in jail. *Criminal Justice and Behavior, 24,* 205–223.

Elder, J. P., Geller, E. S., Hovell, M. F., & Mayer, J. A. (1994). *Motivating health behavior.* Albany, NY: Delmar.

Elliott, S. J., O'Loughlin, J., Robinson, K., Eyles, J., Cameron, R., Harvey, D., et al. (2004). Conceptualizing dissemination research and activity: The case of the Canadian Heart Health Initiative. *Health Education and Behavior, 30,* 267–282.

Emerson, J. A., Wahlgren, D., Hovell, M. R, Meltzer, S. B., Zakarian, J. M., & Hofstetter, C. R (1994). Parent smoking and asthmatic children's exposure patterns: A behavioral epidemiology study. *Addictive Behaviors, 19,* 677–689.

Eng, E., & Hatch, J. W. (1991). Networking between agencies and black churches: The lay health education model. *Prevention in Human Services, 10,* 123–146.

Eng, E., & Parker, E. (1994). Measuring community competence in the Mississippi Delta: The interface between program evaluation and empowerment. *Health Education Quarterly, 21,* 199–220.

Eng, E., & Parker, E. (2002). Natural helper models to enhance a community's health and competence. In R. J. DiClemente, R. A. Crosby, & M. C. Kegler (Eds.), *Emerging theories in health promotion practice and research: Strategies for improving public health* (1st ed.). San Francisco: Jossey-Bass.

Eng, E., & Smith, J. (1995). Natural helping functions of lay health advisors in breast cancer education. *Breast Cancer Research and Treatment, 35,* 23–29.

Eng, E., & Young, R. (1992). Lay health advisors as community change agents. *Family and Community Health, 15,* 24–40.

Engels, R. C., & Willemsen, M. (2004). Communication about smoking in Dutch families: Associations between anti-smoking socialization and adolescent smoking-related cognitions. *Health Education Research, 19,* 227–238.

Epstein, L. H., & Wing, R. R. (1987). Behavioral treatment of childhood obesity. *Psychological Bulletin, 101,* 331–342.

Eriksen, M. P., & Gottlieb, N. H. (1998). A review of the health impact of smoking control at the workplace. *American Journal of Health Promotion, 13,* 83–104.

Eron, L. D., Huesmann, L. R., Lefkowitz, M. M., & Walder, L. O. (1996). Does television violence cause aggression? In *Criminal careers: Vol. 2. The international library of criminology, criminal justice, and penology* (pp. 311–321). Aldershot, England: Dartmouth Publishing Company Limited.

Ershoff, D. H., Mullen, P. D., & Quinn, V. P. (1989). A randomized trial of a serialized self-help smoking cessation program for pregnant women in an HMO. *American Journal of Public Health, 79*, 182–187.

Escobedo, L. G., Chorba, T. L., Remington, P. L., Anda, R. F., Sanderson, L., & Saidi, A. A. (1991). State laws and the use of car seat belts [Letter]. *New England Journal of Medicine, 325*, 1586–1587.

Estrada, C. A., Hryniewicz, M. M., Higgs, V. B., Collins, C., & Byrd, J. C. (2000). Anticoagulant patient information material is written at high readability levels. *Stroke, 31*, 2966–2970.

Estrada, C. A., Martin-Hryniewicz, M., Peek, B. T., Collins, C., & Byrd, J. C. (2004). Literacy and numeracy skills and anticoagulation control. *American Journal of the Medical Sciences, 328*, 88–93.

Evans, D., Clark, N. M., Feldman, C. H., Rips, J., Kaplan, D., Levison, M. J., et al. (1987). A school health education program for children with asthma aged 8–11 years. *Health Education Quarterly, 14*, 267–279.

Evans, R. I., Getz, J. G., & Raines, B. S. (1991, August). *Theory-guided models on prevention of AIDS in adolescents.* Paper presented at the meeting of the Science Weekend at the American Psychological Association, San Francisco, CA.

Evans, R. I., Getz, J. G., & Raines, B. S. (1992, April). *Applying social inoculation concepts to prevention of HIV/AIDS in adolescents: Just say no is obviously not enough.* Paper presented at the Society of Behavioral Medicine, New York.

Evans, R. I., Rozelle, R. M., Mittelmark, M. B., Hansen, W. B., Bane, A. L., & Havis, J. (1978). Deterring the onset of smoking in children: Knowledge of immediate physiological effects and coping with peer pressure, media pressure, and parent modeling. *Journal of Applied Social Psychology, 8*, 126–135.

Evans, R. I., Smith, C. K., & Raines, B. S. (1984). Deterring cigarette smoking in adolescents: A psychosocial-behavioral analysis of an intervention strategy. In A. Baum, J. Singer, & S. Taylor (Eds.), *Social psychological aspects of health* (pp. 301–318). Mahwah, NJ: Erlbaum.

Farley, C., Otis, J., & Benoit, M. (1997). Evaluation of a four-year bicycle helmet promotion campaign in Quebec aimed at children ages 8 to 12: Impact on attitudes, norms and behaviours. *Canadian Journal of Public Health, 88*, 62–66.

Farrington, D. P. (1995). The development of offending and antisocial behavior from childhood: Key findings from the Cambridge study in delinquent development. *Journal of Child Psychology and Psychiatry, 36*, 929–964.

Fawcett, S. B. (1991). Some values guiding community research and action. *Journal of Applied Behavior Analysis, 24*, 621–636.

Fawcett, S. B., Francisco, V. T., Schultz, J. A., Berkowitz, B., Wolff, T. J., & Nagy, G. (2000). The Community Tool Box: a Web-based resource for building healthier communities. *Public Health Reports, 115*, 274–278.

Fawcett, S. B., Paine-Andrews, A., Francisco, V. T., Schultz, J. A., Richter, K. P., Lewis, R. K., et al. (1995). Using empowerment theory in collaborative partnerships for community health and development. *American Journal of Community Psychology, 23*, 677–697.

Fazio, R. H. (2001). On the automatic activation of associated evaluations: An overview. *Cognition and Emotions, 15*, 115–141.

Feighery, E., & Rogers, T. (1989). *Building and maintaining effective coalitions.* Palo Alto, CA: Health Promotion Resource Center, Stanford Center for Research in Disease Prevention.

Feldmann, E., Gordon, N., Brooks, J. M., Brass, L. M., Fayad, P. B., Sawaya, K., et al. (1993). Factors associated with early presentation of acute stroke. *Stroke, 24*, 1805–1810.

Fellin, P. (1995). Understanding American communities. In E. J. Rothman, I. Erlich, & J. Tropman (Eds.), *Strategies of community intervention* (5th ed., pp. 114-129)). Itasca, IL: Peacock.

Fenner, F., Henderson, D. A., Arita, I., Jezek, Z., & Ladnyi, I. D. (1988). Lessons and benefits. In *Smallpox and its eradication* (pp. 10–14). Geneva, Switzerland: World Health Organization.

Fernandez, M. E., Bartholomew, L. K., Lopez, A., Tyrrell, S., Czyzewski, D., & Sockrider, M. M. (2000, Nov.). *Using intervention mapping in the development of a school-based asthma management intervention for Latino children and families: The FAMILIAS Project.* Boston: American Public Health Association.

Fernandez, M. E., Bartholomew, L. K., Sockrider, M. M., Czyzewski, D. I., Abramson, S., Linares, A., et al. (2000, May). *Development of an asthma management program for Latino children in Houston using Intervention Mapping.* Washington, DC: 15th National Conference on Chronic Disease Prevention and Control.

Fernandez, M. E., Gonzales, A., Tortolero-Luna, G., Partida, S., Bartholomew, L. K. (2005). Using intervention mapping to develop a breast and cervical cancer screening program for Hispanic farmworkers: Cultivanda la salud. *Health Promotion Practice, 6*, 394–404.

Fernandez, M. E., Tortolero-Luna, G., & Gold, R. S. (1998). Mammography and pap test screening among low-income foreign-born Hispanic women in the USA. *Cadernos de Saúde Pública, 14*, 133–147.

Fernandez-Esquer, M. E., Espinoza, P., Ramirez, A. G., & McAlister, A. L. (2003). Repeated Pap smear screening among Mexican-American women. *Health Education Research, 18*, 477–487.

Fetterman, D. M., Kaftariau, S. J., & Wandersman, A. (1996). *Empowerment evaluation: Knowledge and tools for self-assessment and accountability.* Thousand Oaks, CA: Sage.

Fingerhut, L. A., Kleinman, J. C., & Kendrick, J. S. (1990). Smoking before, during, and after pregnancy. *American Journal of Public Health, 80*(5), 541–544.

Finkelstein, J. A., Brown, R. W., Schneider, L. C., Weiss, S. T., Quintana, J. M., Goldmann, D. A., et al. (1995). Quality of care for preschool children with asthma: The role of social factors and practice setting. *Pediatrics, 95*, 389–394.

Fireman, P., Friday, G. A., Gira, C., Vierthaler, W. A., & Michaels, L. (1981). Teaching self-management skills to asthmatic children and their parents in an ambulatory care setting. *Pediatrics, 68*, 341–348.

Fiscella, K., Franks, P., Gold, M. R., & Clancy, C. M. (2000). Inequality in quality: addressing socioeconomic, racial, and ethnic disparities in health care. *JAMA: Journal of the American Medical Association, 283*, 2579–2584.

Fishbein, M. (1995). Developing effective behavior change interventions: Some lessons learned from behavioral research. In T. E. Backer, S. L. David, & G. Soucey (Eds.), *Reviewing the behavioral science knowledge base on technology transfer* (pp. 246–261). National Institute on Drug Abuse (NIDA) Monograph 155. Washington, DC: U.S. Department of Health and Human Services.

Fishbein, M. (1996). Great expectations, or do we ask too much from community-level interventions? [Editorial]. *American Journal of Public Health, 86*, 1075–1076.

Fishbein, M., & Ajzen, I. (1975). *Belief, attitude, intention and behavior: An introduction to theory and research.* Reading, MA: Addison-Wesley.

Fishbein, M., Triandis, H. C., Kanfer, F. H., Becker, M., Middlestadt, S. E., & Eichler, A. (2001). Factors influencing behavior and behavior change. In A. Baum, T. A. Revenson, & J. E. Singer (Eds.), *Handbook of health psychology* (pp. 3–17). Mahwah, NJ: Erlbaum.

Fisher, E. B., Jr., Auslander, W., Sussman, L., Owens, N., & Jackson-Thompson, J. (1992). Community organization and health promotion in minority neighborhoods. *Ethnicity and Disease, 2*, 252–272.

Fisher, E. B., Strunk, R. C., Sussman, L. K., Arfken, C., Sykes, R., Munro, J., et al. (1995). Acceptability and feasibility of a community approach to asthma management: The Neighborhood Asthma Coalition. *Journal of Asthma, 33*, 367–383.

Fisher, E. B., Jr., Sussman, L. K., Arfken, C., Harrison, D., Munro, J., Sykes, R. K., et al. (1994). Targeting high-risk groups: Neighborhood organization for pediatric asthma management in the Neighborhood Asthma Coalition. *Chest, 106*, 248S–259S.

Fisher, J. D., Fisher, W. A., Bryan, A.D., & Misovich, S. (1998). *School-based interventions change HIV risk behavior in inner-city minority youth.* Storrs, CT: University of Connecticut, Department of Psychology, Center for HIV Intervention and Prevention.

Fisher, R. (1997). Social action community organization: Proliferation, persistence, roots and prospects. In M. Minkler (Ed.), *Community organizing and community building for health.* New Brunswick, NJ: Rutgers University Press.

Fisher, R., & Kling, J. (1991). Popular mobilization in the 1990s: Prospects for the new social movements. *New Politics, 3*, 71–84.

Fisher, R., & Ury, W. (1991). *Getting to yes: Negotiating agreement without giving in* (2nd ed.). New York: Penguin Books.

Fishman, S. (1997). *The copyright handbook: How to protect and use written works* (4th ed.). Berkeley, CA: Nolo Press.

Flay, B. R. (1985). Psychosocial approaches to smoking prevention: A review of findings. *Health Psychology, 4*, 449–488.

Flay, B. R. (1986). Efficacy and effectiveness trials and other phases of research in the development of health promotion programs. *Preventive Medicine, 15*, 451–474.

Flay, B. R., Brannon, B. R., Johnson, C. A., Hansen, W. B., Ulene, A. L., Whitney-Saltiel, D. A., et al. (1988). The television, school, and family smoking prevention and cessation project. I: Theoretical basis and program development. *Preventive Medicine, 17*, 585–607.

Flesch, R. F. (1974). *The art of readable writing (25th anniversary ed.).* New York: Harper & Row.

Floyd, D. L., Prentice-Dunn, S., & Rogers, R. W. (2000). A meta-analysis of research on protection motivation theory. *Journal of Applied Social Psychology, 30*, 407–429.

Floyd, R. L., Rimer, B. K., Giovino, G. A., Mullen, P. D., & Sullivan, S. E. (1993). A review of smoking in pregnancy: Effects on pregnancy outcomes and cessation efforts. *Annual Review of Public Health, 14*, 379–411.

Flynn, B. S., Goldstein, A. O., Solomon, L. J., Bauman, K. E., Gottlieb, N. H., Cohen, J. E., et al. (1998). Predictors of state legislators' intentions to vote for cigarette tax increases. *Preventive Medicine, 27*, 157–165.

Fogelholm, R., Murros, K., Rissanen, A., & Ilmavirta, M. (1996). Factors delaying hospital admission after acute stroke. *Stroke, 27*, 398–400.

Foltz, A., & Sullivan, J. (1996). Reading level, learning presentation preference, and desire for information among cancer patients 1. *Journal of Cancer Education, 11*, 32–38.

Forrest, R., & Kearns, A. (2001). Social cohesion, social capital and the neighborhood. *Urban Studies, 38*, 2125–2143.

Forsyth, A. D., & Carey, M. P. (1998). Measuring self-efficacy in the context of HIV risk reduction: Research challenges and recommendations. *Health Psychology, 17,* 559–568.

Forsyth, D. R. (1998). *Group dynamics* (3rd ed.). Belmont, CA: Wadsworth.

Fortenberry, J. D., Costa, F. M., Jessor, R., & Donovan, J. E. (1997). Contraceptive behavior and adolescent lifestyles: A structural modeling approach. *Journal of Research on Adolescence, 7,* 307–329.

Foster, D. R., & Rhoney, D. H. (2002). Readability of printed patient information for epileptic patients. *Annals of Pharmacotherapy, 36,* 1856–1861.

Fosterling, F. (1985). Attributional training; A review. *Psychological Bulletin, 98,* 495–512.

Fowler, M. G., Davenport, M. G., & Garg, R. (1992). School functioning of U.S. children with asthma. *Pediatrics, 90,* 939–944.

Fox, C. L., Forbing, S. E., & Anderson, P. S. (1988). A comprehensive approach to drug-free schools and communities. *Journal of School Health, 58*(9), 365–369.

Fox, S. A., & Stein, J. A. (1991). The effect of physician-patient communication on mammography utilization by different ethnic groups. *Medical Care, 29,* 1065–1082.

Frank, G. C., Vaden, A., & Martin, J. (1987). School health programs: Child nutrition programs. *Journal of School Health, 57*(10), 451–460.

Freimuth, V. S. (1985). Developing the public service advertisement for nonprofit marketing. In R. Belk (Ed.), *Advances in nonprofit marketing* (pp. 55–95). Greenwich, CT: JAI Press.

Freire, P. (1973a). *Education for critical consciousness.* New York: Seabury Press.

Freire, P. (1973b). *Pedagogy of the oppressed.* New York: Seabury Press.

Freudenberg, N., Eng, E., Flay, B., Parcel, G., Rogers, T., & Wallerstein, N. (1995). Strengthening individual and community capacity to prevent disease and promote health: In search of relevant theories and principles. *Health Education Quarterly, 22,* 290–306.

Friedman, R. H. (2000). Automated telecounseling for screening mammography. Grant Number: 5R01CA084447–04. National Institutes of Health. Retrieved February 2, 2004, from http://crisp.cit.nih.gov/crisp/CRISP_LIB.

Friedman, R. H., Kazis, L. E., Jette, A., Smith, M. B., Stollerman, J. E., & Torgerson, J., et al. (1996). A telecommunications system for monitoring and counseling patients with hypertension: Impact on medication adherence and blood pressure control. *American Journal of Hypertension, 9,* 285–292.

Friedman, R. H., Stollerman, J. E., Mahoney, D. M., & Rozenblyum, L. (1997). The virtual visit: Using telecommunications technology to take care of patients. *JAMA: Journal of the American Medical Informatics Association, 4,* 413–425.

Friis, R. H., & Sellers, T. A. (2004). *Epidemiology for public health practice* (3rd ed.). Boston: Jones and Bartlett.

Fry, E. (1977). Fry's readability graph: Clarification, validity, and extension to level 17. *Journal of Reading, 21,* 242–252.

Fulk, J., & Boyd, B. (1991). Emerging theories of communication in organizations. *Journal of Management, 17,* 407–446.

Funk, J. B., & Buchman, D. D. (1995). Video game controversies. *Pediatric Annals, 24,* 91–94.

Gadotti, M. (1994). *Reading Paulo Freire: His life and work.* Albany, NY: State University of New York Press.

Gage, A. J. (1998). Sexual activity and contraceptive use: the components of the decision making process. *Studies in Family Planning, 29,* 154–166.

Gagne, R. M., Briggs, L. J., & Wagner, W. W. (1992). *Principles of instructional design.* Orlando, FL: Harcourt Brace Jovanovich.

Gamson, W. A. (2004). Bystanders, public opinion, and the media. In D. A. Snow, S. A. Soule, & H. Kriesi (Eds.), *The Blackwell companion to social movements* (pp. 242–261). Oxford, England: Blackwell.

Ganster, D. C., & Victor, B. (1988). The impact of social support on mental and physical health. *British Journal of Medical Psychology, 61*(Pt 1), 17–36.

Gebhardt, W. A., Kuyper, L., & Greunsven, G. (2003). Need for intimacy in relationships and motives for sex as determinants of adolescent condom use. *Journal of Adolescent Health, 33,* 154–164.

Gedney, K., & Fultz, P. (1988). *The complete guide to creating successful brochures.* Brentwood, NY: Asher-Gallant Press.

Gentry, E. M., & Jorgensen, C. M. (1991). Monitoring the exposure of "America Responds to AIDS" PSA campaign. *Public Health Reports, 106,* 651–655.

Gerald, L. B., Redden, D., Turner-Henson, A., Feinstein, R., Hemstreet, M. P., Hains, C., et al. (2002). A multi-stage asthma screening procedure for elementary school children. *Journal of Asthma, 39,* 29–36.

Gergen, P. J., & Turkeltaub, E. C. (1992). The association of individual allergen reactivity with respiratory disease in a national sample: Data from the second National Health and Nutrition Examination Survey (NHANES II), 1976 to 1980. *Journal of Allergy and Clinical Immunology, 90,* 579–588.

Gergen, P. J., & Weiss, K. B. (1990). Changing patterns in hospitalizations among children: 1979–1987. *JAMA: Journal of the American Medical Association, 264,* 1688–1692.

Gibson, P. G., Powell, H., Coughlan, J., Wilson, A. J., Abramson, M., Haywood, P., et al. (2003). Self-management education and regular practitioner review for adults with asthma. *Cochrane Database of Systematic Reviews, 2,* CD001117.

Gielen, A. C., McDonald, E. M., Wilson, M.E.H., Hwang, W. T., Serwint, J. R., Andrews, J. S., et al. (2002). Effects of improved access to safety counseling, products, and home visits on parents' safety practices: Results of a randomized trial. *Archives of Pediatrics and Adolescent Medicine, 156,* 33–40.

Gielen, A. C., & Sleet, D. (2003). Application of behavior-change theories and methods to injury prevention. *Epidemiologic Reviews, 25,* 65–76.

Gilbert, D. T., Fiske, S. T., & Lindzey, G. (1998). *The handbook of social psychology* (4th ed., Vol. 2). Boston: McGraw-Hill.

Gilmore, G. D., & Campbell, M. D. (1996). *Needs assessment strategies for health education and health promotion* (2nd ed.). Madison, WI: Brown & Benchmark.

Gilmore, G. D., Campbell, M. D., & Becker, B. L. (1989). *Needs assessment strategies for health education and health promotion.* Madison, WI: Brown and Benchmark.

Gilpin, E. A., Distefan, J. M., & Pierce, J. P. (2004). Population receptivity to tobacco advertising/promotions and exposure to anti-tobacco media: Effect of Master Settlement Agreement in California: 1992–2002. *Health Promotion Practice, 5,* 91S–98S.

Gingiss, P. L., Gottlieb, N. H., & Brink, S. G. (1994). Increasing teacher receptivity toward use of tobacco prevention education programs. *Journal of Drug Education, 24,* 163–176.

Ginsburg, K. R., Menapace, A. S., & Slap, G. B. (1997). Factors affecting the decision to seek health care: The voice of adolescents. *Pediatrics, 100,* 922–930.

Glanz, K., Lewis, F. M., & Rimer, B. K. (1990). Theory, research, and practice in health education: Building bridges and forging links. In K. Glanz, F. M. Lewis, & B. K. Rimer (Eds.), *Health Behavior and Health Education: Theory, Research, and Practice.* (1st ed.). San Francisco: Jossey-Bass.

Glanz, K., Lewis, F. M., & Rimer, B. K. (1997). *Health behavior and health education: Theory, research, and practice* (2nd ed.). San Francisco: Jossey-Bass.

Glanz, K., Lewis, F. M., & Rimer, B. K. (2002). *Health behavior and health education: Theory, research and practice* (3rd ed.). San Francisco: Jossey-Bass.

Glasgow, R., Marcus, A. C., Bull, S. S., & Wilson, K. M. (2004). Disseminating effective cancer screening interventions. *Cancer, 101,* 1239–1250.

Glasgow, R. E., Klesges, L. M., Dzewaltowski, D. A., Bull, S. S., & Estabrooks, P. (2004). The future of health behavior change research: What is needed to improve translation of research into health promotion practice? *Annals of Behavioral Medicine, 27,* 3–12.

Glasgow, R. E., Lando, H., Hollis, J., McRae, S. G., & La Chance, P. A. (1993). A stop-smoking telephone help line that nobody called. *American Journal of Public Health, 83,* 252–253.

Glasgow, R. E., Lichtenstein, E., & Marcus, A. C. (2003). Why don't we see more translation of health promotion research to practice? Rethinking the efficacy-to-effectiveness transition. *American Journal of Public Health, 93,* 1261–1267.

Glasgow, R. E., Toobert, D. J., Hampson, S. E., Brown, J. E., Lewinson, P. M., & Donnelly, J. (1992). Improving self-care among older patients with type II diabetes: The "Sixty Something . . ." study. *Patient Education and Counseling, 19*(1), 61–74.

Glasgow, R. E., Vogt, T. M., & Boles, S. M. (1999). Evaluating the public health impact of health promotion interventions: The RE-AIM framework. *American Journal of Public Health, 89,* 1322–1327.

Glazer, H. R., Kirk, L. M., & Bosler, F. E. (1996). Patient education pamphlets about prevention, detection, and treatment of breast cancer for low-literacy women. *Patient Education and Counseling, 27,* 185–189.

Global Initiative for Asthma. (1995). Workshop report: *Global strategy for asthma management and prevention.* Available from http://www.ginasthma.com//GuidelineItem.asp?intId=819

Glover, J. A., Ronning, R. R., & Bruning, R. H. (1990). *Cognitive psychology for teachers.* New York: MacMillian.

Glynn, S. M., & Britton, B. (1984). Supporting readers' comprehension through effective text design. *Educational Technology, 24,* 40–43.

Godden, D. R., & Baddeley, A. D. (1975). Context-dependent memory in two natural environments: In land and underwater. *British Journal of Psychology, 66,* 325–331.

Godin, G., Fortin, C., Michaud, F., Bradet, R., & Kok, G. (1997). Use of condoms: Intention and behavior of adolescents living in juvenile rehabilitation centers. *Health Education Research, 12,* 289–300.

Godin, G., & Kok, G. (1996). The theory of planned behavior: A review of its applications to health-related behaviors. *American Journal of Health Promotion, 11,* 87–98.

Godin, G., Savard, J., Kok, G., Fortin, C., & Boyer, R. (1996). HIV seropositive gay men: Understanding adoption of safe sexual practices. *AIDS Education and Prevention, 8,* 529–545.

Goebel, J. B., Copps, T. J., & Sulayman, R. F. (1984). Infant car seat usage. Effectiveness of a postpartum educational program. *Journal of Obstetrical, Gynecologic, and Neonatal Nursing, 13,* 33–36.

Goeppinger, J., & Baglioni, A. J., Jr. (1985). Community competence: A positive approach to needs assessment. *American Journal of Community Psychology, 13,* 507–523.

Gold, M. R., Siegel, J. E., Russell, L. B., & Weinstein, M. C. (1996). *Cost-effectiveness in health and medicine.* New York: Oxford University Press.

Goldberg, J., Rudd, R. E., & Dietz, W. (1999). Using three data sources and methods to shape a nutrition campaign. *Journal of the American Dietetic Association, 99,* 717–722.

Goldman, R., Hunt, M. K., Allen, J. D., Hauser, S., Emmons, K., Maeda, M., et al. (2003). The life history interview method: Applications to intervention development. *Health Education and Behavior, 30,* 564–581.

Goldsmith, D. F., & Sisneros, G. C. (1996). Cancer prevention strategies among California farmworkers: Preliminary findings. *Journal of Rural Health, 12,* 343–348.

Gollwitzer, P. M. (1999). Implementation intentions: Strong effects of simple plans. *American Psychologist, 54,* 493–503.

Gonzales, A., Fernandez, M., & Saavedra-Embesi, M. (2003). *Cultivando la salud: Breast and cervical cancer replication and dissemination program, final report.* Buda, TX: National Center for Farmworker Health.

Gonzales, A., Saavedra-Embesi, M., Fernandez, M., & Tortolero-Luna, G. (2001). *Cultivando la salud: Breast and cervical cancer replication and dissemination program, pilot report.* Buda, TX: National Center for Farmworker Health.

Goodman, D. C., Lozano, P., Stukel, T. A., Chang, C., & Hecht, J. (1999). Has asthma medication use in children become more frequent, more appropriate, or both? *Pediatrics, 104,* 187–194.

Goodman, D. T. (1998). Using the empowerment model to develop sex education for Native Americans. *Journal of Sex Education and Therapy, 23,* 135–144.

Goodman, R. M. (2000). Bridging the gap in effective program implementation: From concept to application. *Journal of Community Psychology, 28,* 309–321.

Goodman, R. M., McLeroy, K. R., Steckler, A. B., & Hoyle, R. H. (1993). Development of level of insitutionalization scales for health promotion programs. *Health Education Quarterly, 20,* 161–178.

Goodman, R. M., Smith, D. W., Dawson, L., & Steckler, A. (1991). Recruiting school districts into a dissemination study. *Health Education Research, 6,* 373–385.

Goodman, R. M., Speers, M. A., McLeroy, K., Fawcett, S., Kegler, M., Parker, E., et al. (1998). Identifying and defining the dimensions of community capacity to provide a basis for measurement. *Health Education and Behavior, 25,* 258–278.

Goodman, R. M., & Steckler, A. (1989). A model for the institutionalization of health programs. *Family and Community Health, 11,* 63–78.

Goodman, R. M., Steckler, A., Hoover, S., & Schwartz, R. (1993). A critique of contemporary community health promotion approaches: Based on a qualitative review of six programs in Maine. *American Journal of Health Promotion, 7,* 208–220.

Goodman, R. M., Steckler, A., & Kegler, M. C. (1997). Mobilizing organizations for health enhancement: Theories of organizational change. In K. Glanz, F. M. Lewis, & B. K. Rimer (Eds.), *Health behavior and health education: Theory, research, and practice* (2nd ed., pp. 287–312). San Francisco: Jossey-Bass.

Goodson, P., Gottlieb, N. H., & Smith, M. M. (1999). Put prevention into practice. Evaluation of program initiation in nine Texas clinical sites. *American Journal of Preventive Medicine, 17,* 73–78.

Gotay, C. C., & Wilson, M. E. (1998). Social support and cancer screening in African American, Hispanic, and Native American women. *Cancer Practice, 6,* 31–37.

Gottlieb, B. H. (1985). Social networks and social support: An overview of research, practice, and policy implications. *Health Education Quarterly, 12,* 5–22.

Gottlieb, N. H., Goldstein, A. O., Flynn, B. S., Cohen, E. J., Bauman, K. E., Solomon, L. J., et al. (2003). State legislators' beliefs about legislation that restricts youth access to tobacco products. *Health Education and Behavior, 30,* 209–224.

Gottlieb, N. H., Huang, P. P., Blozis, S. A., Guo, J. L., & Murphy, S. M. (2001). The impact of Put Prevention into Practice on selected clinical preventive services in five Texas sites. *American Journal of Preventive Medicine, 21,* 35–40.

Gottlieb, N. H., Lovato, C. Y., Weinstein, R., Green, L. W., & Eriksen, M. P. (1992). The implementation of a restrictive worksite smoking policy in a large decentralized organization. *Health Education Quarterly, 19,* 77–100.

Goumans, M., & Springett J. (1997). From projects to policy: "Healthy Cities" as a mechanism for policy change for health? *Health Promotion International,12*(24), 311–322.

Graeff, J. A., Elder, J. P., Booth, E. M. (1993). *Communication for health and behavior change: A developing country perspective.* San Francisco: Jossey-Bass.

Greathouse, L. W., Hahn, E. J., Okoli, C.T.C., Warnick, T. A., & Riker, C. A. (2005). Passing a smoke-free law in a pro-tobacco culture: A multiple streams approach. *Policy, Politics, & Nursing Practice, 5,* 211–220.

Green, J. (2000). The role of theory in evidence-based health promotion practice. *Health Education Research, 15,* 125–129.

Green, J., & Tones, K. (1999). For debate. Towards a secure evidence base for health promotion. *Journal of Public Health, 21,* 133–139.

Green, L. W. (1986). Theory of participation: A qualitative analysis of its expression in national and international health policies. In W. B. Ward (Ed.), *Advances in health education and health promotion* (pp. 211–236). Greenwich, CT: JAI Press.

Green, L. W. (2001). From research to best practices in other settings and populations. *American Journal of Health Behavior, 25,* 165–178.

Green, L. W., & Frankish, C. J. (1994). Theories and principles of health education applied to asthma. *Chest, 106,* 219S–230S.

Green, L. W., Glanz, K., Hochbaum, G. M., Kok, G., Kreuter, M. W., Lewis, F. M., et al. (1994). Can we build on, or must we replace, the theories and models in health education? *Health Education Research, 9,* 397–404.

Green, L. W., Gottlieb, N., & Parcel, G. (1991). Diffusion theory extended and applied. In W. B. Ward and F. M. Lewis (Eds.), *Advances in health education and promotion, Vol. 3.* (pp. 91–117). Philadelphia: Kingsley.

Green, L. W., & Kreuter, M. W. (1991). *Health promotion planning: An educational and environmental approach.* (2nd ed.) Mountain View, CA: Mayfield.

Green, L. W., & Kreuter, M. W. (1999). *Health promotion planning: An educational and ecological approach* (3rd ed.). Mountain View, CA: Mayfield.

Green, L. W., & Kreuter, M. W. (2002). Fighting back or fighting themselves? Community coalitions against substance abuse and their use of best practices. *American Journal of Preventive Medicine, 23,* 303–306.

Green, L. W., & Kreuter, M. W. (2005). *Health program planning: An educational and ecological approach* (4 ed.). New York: McGraw-Hill.

Green, L. W., Kreuter, M. W., Deeds, S. G., & Partridge, K. B. (1980). *Health education planning: A diagnostic approach.* Mountain View, CA: Mayfield.

Green, L. W., & Lewis, F. M. (1986). *Measurement and evaluation in health education and health promotion.* Mountain View, CA: Mayfield.

Green, L. W., Richard, L., & Potvin, L. (1996). Ecological foundations of health promotion. *American Journal of Health Promotion, 10,* 270–281.

Greenbaum, T. L. (1988). *The practical handbook and guide to focus group research.* Lexington, MA: Lexington Books.

Greene, J. C. (1988). Stakeholder participation and utilization in program evaluation. *Evaluation Review, 15,* 471–481.

Greiner, K. A., Li, C., Kawachi, I., Hunt, D. C., & Ahluwalia, J. S. (2004). The relationships of social participation and community ratings to health and health behaviors in areas with high and low population density. *Social Science and Medicine, 59,* 2303–2312.

Grissom, R. J., & Kim, J. J. (2005). *Effect size for research: A broad practical approach.* Mahwah, NJ: Erlbaum.

Gronlund, E. E. (1978). *Stating objectives for classroom instruction* (2nd ed.). New York: Macmillan.

Grootaert, C., & van Bastelaer, T. (2002). *Understanding and measuring social capital* (1st ed.). Washington, DC: The World Bank.

Guide to Community Preventive Services: Systematic reviews and evidence based recommendations (2004). Retrieved March 3, 2005, from http://www.thecommunity guide.org

Guidry, J. J., Fagan, P., & Walker, V. (1998). Cultural sensitivity and readability of breast and prostate printed cancer education materials targeting African Americans. *Journal of the National Medical Association, 90,* 165–169.

Gustafson, D. H., Bosworth, K., Chewning, B., & Hawkins, R. P. (1987). Computer-based health promotion: Combining technological advances with problem-solving techniques to effect successful health behavior changes. *Annual Review of Public Health, 8,* 387–415.

Gustafson, D. H., Wise, M., McTavish, F., Taylor, I., Wolberg, W., Stewart, I., et al. (1993). Development and pilot evaluation of a computer-based support system for women with breast cancer. *Journal of Psychosocial Oncology, 11,* 69–93.

Haglund, B.J.A., Finer, D., Tillgren, P., & Pettersson, B. (1996). *Creating supportive environments for health.* Geneva, Switzerland: World Health Organization.

Hale, J. L., & Dillard, J. P. (1995). Fear appeals in health promotion campaigns: Too much, too little, just right? In E. Maibach & R. L. Parrott (Eds.), *Designing health messages: Approaches from communication theory and public health practice.* Thousand Oaks, CA: Sage.

Halfon, N., & Newacheck, P. (1993). Childhood asthma and poverty: Differential impacts and utilization of health services. *Pediatrics, 91,* 56–61.

Hall, A., & Wellman, B. (1985). Social networks and social support. In S. Cohen & L. Syme (Eds.), *Social support and health.* New York: Academic Press.

Hall, G. E., & Loucks, S. F. (1978). *Innovation configurations: Analyzing the adaptations of innovations.* Austin, TX: University of Texas, Research and Development Center for Teacher Education.

Hamilton, M. A., & Hunter, J. E. (1998). A framework for understanding meta-analyses of the persuasion literature. In M. Allen & R. W. Preiss (Eds.), *Persuasion: Advances through meta-analysis* (pp. 1–28). Cresskill, NJ: Hampton Press.

Hamilton, R. J., & Ghatala, E. (1994). *Learning and instruction.* New York: McGraw-Hill.

Hammond, D., Fong, G. T., McDonald, P. W., Brown, K. S., & Cameron, R. (2004). Graphic Canadian cigarette warning labels and adverse outcomes: Evidence from Canadian smokers. *American Journal of Public Health, 94,* 1442–1445.

Hancock, T., & Duhl, L. (1986). *Healthy Cities: Promoting health in the urban context.* Copenhagen, Denmark: World Health Organization Europe.

Hancock, T., & Minkler, M. (1997). Community health assessment or healthy community assessment: Whose community? Whose health? Whose assessment? In M. Minkler (Ed.), *Community organizing and community building* (pp. 139–156). New Brunswick, NJ: Rutgers University Press.

Handy, S. L., Boarnet, M. G., Ewing, R., & Killingsworth, R. E. (2002). How the built environment affects physical activity: Views from urban planning. *American Journal of Preventive Medicine, 23,* 64–73.

Harachi, T. W., Abbott, R. D., Catalano, R. F., Haggerty, K. P., & Fleming, C. B. (1999). Opening the black box: Using process evaluation measures to assess implementation and theory building. *American Journal of Community Psychology, 27,* 711–731.

Hardeman, W., Johnston, M., Johnston, D. W., Bonetti, D., Wareham, N. J., & Kinmonth, A. L. (2002). Application of the theory of planned behavior in behavior change interventions: A systematic review. *Psychology & Health, 17,* 123–158.

Harlan, L. C., Bernstein, A. B., & Kessler, L. G. (1991). Cervical cancer screening: Who is not screened and why? *American Journal of Public Health, 81,* 885–890.

Harmon, M. P., Castro, F. G., & Coe, K. (1996). Acculturation and cervical cancer: knowledge, beliefs, and behaviors of Hispanic women. *Women and Health, 24,* 37–57.

Harrison, J. A., Mullen, P. D., & Green, L. W. (1992). A meta-analysis of studies of the Health Belief Model with adults. *Health Education Research, 7,* 107–116.

Havelock, R. G. (1971). *Planning for innovation through dissemination and utilization of knowledge.* Ann Arbor, MI: University of Michigan, Institute for Social Reseach, Center for Research on Utilization of Scientific Knowledge.

Hawe, P., & Shiell, A. (2000). Social capital and health promotion: a review. *Social Science and Medicine, 51,* 871–885.

Hawkins, R. P., Pingree, S., Gustafson, D. H., Boberg, E. W., Bricker, E., McTavish, F., et al. (1997). Aiding those facing health crises: The experience of the CHESS Project. In *Health promotion and interactive technology: Theoretical applications and future directions* (pp. 79–102). Mahwah, NJ: Erlbaum.

Hayward, R. A., Shapiro, M. F., Freeman, H. E., & Corey, C. R. (1988). Who gets screened for cervical and breast cancer? Results from a new national survey. *Archives of Internal Medicine, 148,* 1177–1181.

Hearth-Holmes, M., Murphy, P. W., Davis, T. C., Nandy, I., Elder, C. G., Broadwell, L. H., et al. (1997). Literacy in patients with a chronic disease: Systemic lupus erythematosus and the reading level of patient education materials 1. *Journal of Rheumatology, 24,* 2335–2339.

Heath, E. M., & Coleman, K. J. (2003). Adoption and institutionalization of the Child and Adolescent Trial for Cardiovascular Health (CATCH) in El Paso, Texas. *Health Promotion Practice, 4,* 157–164.

Heaney, C. A., & Israel, B. A. (2002). Social networks and social support. In K. Glanz, F. M. Lewis, & B. K. Rimer (Eds.), *Health behavior and health education: Theory, research and practice* (3rd ed., pp. 185–209). San Francisco: Jossey-Bass.

Heinen, M. M., Bartholomew, L. K., Wensing, L. K., van de Kerkhof, P., & van Achterberg, T. (2005). Supporting compliance and healthy lifestyles in leg ulcer patients: Systematic development of the Lively Legs program for dermatology outpatient clinics. *Patient Education and Counseling.*

Heitzmann, C. A., & Kaplan, R. M. (1988). Assessment of methods for measuring social support. *Health Psychology, 7,* 75–109.

Helman, C. G. (1990). *Culture, health and illness* (2nd ed.). London: Butterworth Heinemann.

Henderson, K. A., & Ainsworth, B. E. (2000). Sociocultural perspectives on physical activity in the lives of older African American and American Indian women: A cross-cultural activity participation study. *Women and Health, 31,* 1–20.

Hendrickx, L. (1991). *How versus how often.* Groningen, The Netherlands: Van Denderen.

Hendrickx, L., Vlek, C., & Oppewal, H. (1989). Relative importance of scenario information and frequency information in the judgment of risk. *Acta Psychologica, 72,* 463.

Hennessy, C. H., Moriarty, D. G., Zack, M. M., Scherr, P. A., & Brackbill, R. (1994). Measuring health-related quality of life for public health surveillance. *Public Health Reports, 109,* 665–672.

Herek, G. M., & Capitanio, J. P. (1998). Symbolic prejudice or fear of infection? A functional analysis of AIDS-related stigma among heterosexual adults. *Basic and Applied Social Psychology, 20,* 230–241.

Hersey, J. C., Klibanoff, L. S., Lam, D. J., & Taylor, R. L. (1984). Promoting social support: The impact of California's "Friends Can Be Good Medicine" campaign. *Health Education Quarterly, 11,* 293–311.

Hill, J. (1997). A practical guide to patient education and information giving. *Bailliere's Clinical Rheumatology, 11,* 109–127.

Hindi-Alexander, M. C. (1984). Evaluation of a family asthma program. *Allergy and Clinical Immunology, 74,* 505–510.

Hirsch, B. J., & DuBois, D. L. (1992). The relation of peer social support and psychological symptomatology during the transition to junior high school: A two-year longitudinal analysis. *American Journal of Community Psychology, 20*(3), 333–347.

Hochbaum, G. M., Sorenson, J. R., & Lorig, K. (1992). Theory in health education practice. *Health Education Quarterly, 19,* 295–313.

Hoefnagels, C., & Mudde, A. (2000). Mass media and disclosures of child abuse in the perspective of secondary prevention: Putting ideas into practice. *Child Abuse and Neglect, 24,* 1091–1101.

Hoelscher, D. M., Evans, A., Parcel, G. S., & Kelder, S. H. (2002). Designing effective nutrition interventions for adolescents. *Journal of the American Dietetic Association, 102,* S52–S63.

Hoelscher, D. M., Feldman, H. A., Johnson, C. C., Lytle, L. A., Osganian, S. K., Parcel, G. S., et al. (2004). School-based health education programs can be maintained over time: Results from the CATCH Institutionalization study. *Preventive Medicine, 38,* 594–606.

Hogan, B. E., Linden, W., & Najarian, B. (2002). Social support interventions: Do they work? *Clinical Psychology Review, 22,* 381–440.

Hogan, J. A., Baca, I., Daley, C., Garcia, T., Jaker, J., Lowther, M., et al. (2003). Disseminating science-based prevention: Lessons learned from CSAP's CAPTs. *Journal of Drug Education, 33,* 233–243.

Holcomb, C., & Ellis, J. (1978). Measuring the readability of selected patient education materials: The CLOSE procedure. *Health Education, 9,* 8.

Holmbeck, G. N. (1997). Toward terminological, conceptual, and statistical clarity in the study of mediators and moderators: Examples from the child-clinical and pediatric psychology literatures. *Journal of Consulting and Clinical Psychology, 65,* 599–610.

Holmes, P., Neville, D., Donovan, C., & MacDonald, C. A. (2001). The Newfoundland and Labrador Heart Health Program dissemination story: The formation and functioning of effective coalitions. *Promotion and Education*(Suppl. 1), 8–12.

Holtgrave, D. R., Tinsley, B. J., & Kay, L. S. (1995). Encouraging risk reduction: A decision-making approach to message design. In E. Maibach & R. L. Parrott (Eds.), *Designing health messages: Approaches from communication theory and public health practice* (pp. 24–40). Thousand Oaks, CA: Sage.

Homer, C. J., Szilagyi, P., Rodewald, L., Bloom, S. R., Greenspan, P., Yazdgerdi, S., et al. (1996). Does quality of care affect rates of hospitalization for childhood asthma? *Pediatrics, 98,* 18–23.

Hooks, C., Ugarte, C., Silsby, J., Brown, R., Weinman, J., Fernandez, G., et al. (1996). Obstacles and opportunities in designing cancer control communication research for farmworkers on the Delmarva Peninsula. *Journal of Rural Health, 12,* 332–342.

Hosey, G. M., Freeman, W. L., Stracqualursi, F., & Gohdes, D. (1990). Designing and evaluating diabetes education material for American Indians. *Diabetes Educator, 16,* 407–414.

Hospers, H. J., Harterink, P., van den Hoek, K., & Veenstra, J. (2002). Chatters on the Internet: A special target group for HIV prevention. *AIDS Care, 14,* 539–544.

Hospers, H. J., Kok, G., Harterink, P., & de Zwart, O. (2005). A new meeting place: Chatting on the Internet, e-dating, and sexual risk behavior among Dutch men who have sex with men. *AIDS, 19,* 1097–1101.

Hospers, H. J., Kok, G., & Strecher, V. J. (1990). Attributions for previous failures and subsequent outcomes in a weight reduction program. *Health Education Quarterly, 17,* 409–415.

Hou, S. I., Fernandez, M. E., Baumler, E., & Parcel, G. S. (2002). Effectiveness of an intervention to increase pap test screening among Chinese women in Taiwan. *Journal of Community Health, 27,* 277–290.

Hou, S. I., Fernandez, M. E., & Parcel, G. S. (2004). Development of a cervical cancer educational program for Chinese women using Intervention Mapping. *Health Promotion Practice, 5,* 80–87.

Hough, J. F. (1999, March). *"Healthy Days" measures and data: New tools for population surveillance and research. Disability surveillance using the BRFSS disability module.* Paper presented at the Ninth Prevention Research Centers Conference, Atlanta, GA.

House, J. S., Umberson, D., & Landis, K. R. (1988). Structures and processes of social support. *Annual Review of Sociology, 14,* 293–318.

Hovell, M. P., Meltzer, S. B., Zakarian, J. M., Wahlgren, D. R., Emerson, J. A., Hofstetter, C. R., et al. (1994). Reduction of environmental tobacco smoke exposure among asthmatic children: A controlled trial. *Chest, 106,* 440–446. (Published erratum in *Chest, 107,* 1480.)

Howell, J. M., & Higgins, C. A. (1990). Champions of technological innovations. *Administrative Science Quarterly, 35,* 317–341.

Hubbell, F. A., Mishra, S. I., Chavez, L. R., & Valdez, R. B. (1997). The influence of knowledge and attitudes about breast cancer on mammography use among Latinas and Anglo women. *Journal of General Internal Medicine, 12,* 505–508.

Hubbell, F. A., Waitzkin, H., Mishra, S. I., Dombrink, J., & Chavez, L. R. (1991). Access to medical care for documented and undocumented Latinos in a southern California county. *The Western Journal of Medicine, 154,* 414–417.

Huberman, A. M., & Miles, M. B. (1984). *Innovation up close: How schools improvement works.* New York: Plenum Press.

Huberman, A. M., & Miles, M. B. (1994). Data management and analysis methods. In N. K. Denzin & Y. S. Lincoln (Eds.), *Handbook of qualitative research* (pp. 428–444). Thousand Oaks, CA: Sage.

Hugentobler, M. K., Israel, B. A., & Schurman, S. J. (1992). An action research approach to workplace health: Integrating methods. *Health Education Quarterly, 19,* 55–76.

Hunt, M. K., Lederman, R., Potter, S., Stoddard, A., & Sorensen, G. (2000). Results of employee involvement in planning and implementing the Treatwell 5-a-Day work-site study. *Health Education and Behavior, 27,* 223–231.

Hunt, W. A., & Barnett, & Branch, L. G. (1971). Relapse rates in addiction programs. *Journal of Clinical Psychology, 27*(4), 455–456.

Hunter, J. E., & Schmidt, F. L. (1996). Cumulative research knowledge and social policy formulation: The critical role of meta-analysis. *Psychology, Public Policy, and Law, 2,* 324–347.

Hunter, J. E., & Schmidt, F. L. (2004). *Methods of meta-analysis. Correcting error and bias in research findings.* Thousand Oaks, CA: Sage.

Hurley, S. F., & Kaldor, J. M. (1992). The benefits and risks of mammographic screening for breast cancer. [Review]. *Epidemiologic Reviews, 14,* 101–130.

Huss, K., Rand, C. S., Butz, A. M., Eggleston, P. A., Murigande, C., Thompson, L., et al. (1994). Home environmental risk factors in urban minority asthmatic children. *Annals of Allergy; 72,* 173–177.

Ingram, J. M., Sporik, R., Rose, G., Honsinger, R., Chapman, M. D., & Platts-Mills, T. A. (1995). Quantitative assessment of exposure to dog (Can f I) and cat (Fel d I) allergens: Relation to sensitization and asthma among children living in Los Alamos, New Mexico. *Journal of Allergy and Clinical Immunology, 96,* 449–456.

Institute of Medicine. (2002a). *Shaping the future for health: The future of the public's health in the 21st century.* Washington, DC: National Academy of Science.

Institute of Medicine (2002b). *Speaking of health: Assessing health communication strategies for diverse populations.* Washington, DC: National Academies Press.

Institute of Medicine (2004). *Health literacy: A prescription to end confusion.* Washington, DC: National Academies Press.

Institute of Medicine, Board on Health Promotion and Disease Prevention, Committee on Assuring the Health of the Public in the 21st Century. (1990). *Nutrition during pregnancy (Part I): Weight gain.* Washington, DC: National Academy Press.

Institute of Medicine, Committee on Understanding and Eliminating Racial and Ethnic Disparities in Health Care. (2003). *Unequal treatment: Confronting racial and ethnic disparities in health care.* Washington, DC: Institute of Medicine.

Instructions for authors. (2005). *JAMA: Journal of the American Medical Association, 293,* 108–115. Retrieved March 9, 2005, from http://jama.ama-assn.org

International Union for Health Promotion and Education & European Commission. (1999). *The evidence of health promotion effectiveness: Shaping public health in a new Europe* (Vols. ECSC EC EAEC). Brussels, Belgium: Author.

Irwin, J. C., & Davis, C. A. (1980). Measuring the readability of selected patient education materials: The CLOSE procedure. *Journal of Reading, 24,* 124–130.

Iscoe, I. (1974). Community psychology and the competent community. *American Psychologist, 29,* 607–613.

Isenberg, D. J. (1986). Group polarization: A critical review and meta analysis. *Journal of Personality and Social Psychology, 50,* 1141–1151.

Israel, A. C., Guile, C. A., Baker, J. E., & Silverman, W. K. (1994). An evaluation of enhanced self-regulation training in the treatment of childhood obesity. *Journal of Pediatric Psychology, 19,* 737–749.

Israel, B. A. (1982). Social networks and health status: Linking theory, research, and practice. *Patient Counseling and Health Education, 4*(2), 65–79.

Israel, B. A., Checkoway, B., Schulz, A., & Zimmerman, M. A. (1994). Health education and community empowerment: Conceptualizing and measuring perceptions of individual, organizational, and community control. *Health Education Quarterly, 21,* 149–170.

Israel, B. A., & Rounds, K. A. (1987). Social networks and social support: A synthesis of health educators. *Advances in Health Education and Promotion, 2,* 311–351.

Israel, B. A., Schulz, A. J., Parker, E. A., Becker, A. B., Allen, A. J., & Guzman, R. (2003). Critical issues in developing and following community-based participatory research principles. In M. Minkler & N. Wallerstein (Eds.), *Community-based participatory research for health* (pp. 53–76). San Francisco: Jossey-Bass.

Issel, L. M., & Searing, L. (2000). Community landscape asset mapping (CLAM) report to Chicago Department of Public Health and Lawndale Health Promotion Planning Council. Unpublished manuscript.

Jaccard, J., Blanton, H., & Dodge, T. (2005). Peer influences on risk behavior: an analysis of the effects of a close friend. *Developmental Psychology, 41,* 135–147.

Jackson, C., Fortmann, S. P., Flora, J. A., Melton, R. J., Snider, J. P., & Littlefield, D. (1994). The capacity-building approach to intervention maintenance implemented by the Stanford Five-City Project. *Health Education Research, 9,* 385–396.

Jacobs, I. J., Oram, D. H., & Bast, R. C., Jr. (1992). Strategies for improving the specificity of screening for ovarian cancer with tumor-associated antigens CA 125, CA 15-3, and TAG 72.3. *Obstetrics and Gynecology, 80*(3 Pt 1), 396–399.

Janis, I. L., & Mann, L. (1977). *Decision making: A psychological analysis of conflict, choice, and commitment.* New York: Free Press.

Janssen, R. S., Holtgrave, D. R., Valdisserri, R. O., Shepherd, M., Gayle, H. D., & De Cock, K. M. (2001). The serostatus approach to fighting the HIV epidemic: Prevention strategies for infected individuals. *American Journal of Public Health, 91,* 1019–1024.

Janz, N. K., & Becker, M. H. (1984). The Health Belief Model: A decade later. *Health Education Quarterly, 11,* 1–47.

Janz, N. K., Champion, V. L., & Strecher, V. J. (2002). The Health Belief Model. In K. Glanz, F. M. Lewis, & B. K. Rimer (Eds.), *Health behavior and health education: Theory, research and practice* (3rd ed., pp. 45–66). San Francisco: Jossey-Bass.

Jarvis, K. L., Friedman, R. H., Heeren, T., & Cullinane, P. M. (1997). Older women and physical activity: using the telephone to walk. *Women's Health Issues, 7,* 24–29.

Jemmott, J. B., Jemmott, L. S., & Fong, G. T. (1992). Reduction in HIV risk-associated sexual behaviors among black male adolescents: Effects of an AIDS prevention intervention. *American Journal of Public Health, 82,* 372–377.

Jemmott, J. B., III, Jemmott, L. S., Fong, G. T. (1998). Abstinence and safer sex HIV risk-reduction interventions for African American adolescents. *JAMA: Journal of the American Medical Association, 279,* 1529–1536.

Jencks, C., & Mayer, S. E. (1990). Residential segregation, job proximity, and black job opportunities. In L. E. Lynn & M. McGeary (Eds.), *Inner-city poverty in the United States* (pp. 243–267). Washington, DC: National Academy Press.

Joffe, H. (1989). Emotional factors in pregnancy. *Australian Family Physician, 18,* 493–497.

John, P. (2003). Is there life after policy streams, advocacy coalitions, and punctuations? Using evolutionary theory to explain policy change. *Policy Studies Journal, 31,* 481–498.

Johnson, A., & Baum, F. (2001). Health promoting hospitals: A typology of different organizational approaches to health promotion. *Health Promotion International, 16,* 281–287.

Johnson, D. W., & Johnson, F. P. (1994). *Joining together: Group theory and group skills* (5th ed.). Boston: Allyn and Bacon.

Johnson, K., Grossman, W., & Cassidy, A. (1996). *Collaborating to improve community health: Workbook and guide to best practices in creating healthier communities and populations.* San Francisco: Jossey-Bass.

Johnson, R. E., Newhall, W. J., Papp, J. R., Knapp, J. S., Black, C. M., Gift, T. L., et al. (2002). Screening tests to detect Chlamydia trachomatis and Neisseria gonorrhaeae infections. *Morbidity and Mortality Weekly Report, 51,* 1–38.

Johnson, S., McCarter, R., & Ferencz, C. (1987). Changes in alcohol, cigarette, and recreational drug use during pregnancy: Implications for intervention. *American Journal of Epidemiology, 126*(4), 695–702.

Johnson, S. B., Pollak, R. T., Silverstein, J. H., Rosenbloom, A. L., Spillar, R., McCallum, M., & Harkavy, J. (1982). Cognitive and behavioral knowledge about insulin-dependent diabetes among children and parents. *Pediatrics, 69*(6), 708–713.

Johnston, D. W., Johnston, M., Pollard, B., Kinmonth, A. L., & Mant, D. (2004). Motivation is not enough: prediction of risk behavior following diagnosis of coronary heart disease from the theory of planned behavior. *Health Psychology, 23,* 533–538.

Johnston, J. J., Hendricks, S. A., & Fike, J. M. (1994). Effectiveness of behavioral safety belt interventions. *Accident Analysis and Prevention, 26,* 315–323.

Jones, B. D. (2003). Bounded rationality and political science: Lessons from public administration and public policy. *Journal of Public Administration Research and Theory 13,* 395–412.

Jones, C. P. (2000). Levels of racism: theoretic framework and a gardener's tale. *American Journal of Public Health, 90,* 1212–1215.

Jones, E. F. (1986). *Teenage pregnancy in industrialized countries.* New Haven, CT: Yale University Press.

Jones, E. F., Forrest, J. D., Henshaw, S. K., Silverman, J., & Torres, A. (1988). Unintended pregnancy, contraceptive practice, and fmaily planning service in developed countries. *Family Planning Perspectives, 20,* 53–67.

Jones, S. C., & Donovan, R. J. (2004). Does theory inform practice in health promotion in Australia? *Health Education Research, 19,* 1–14.

Jones, S. E., Brener, N. D., & McManus, T. (2003). Prevalence of school policies, programs, and facilities that promote a healthy physical school environment. *American Journal of Public Health, 93,* 1570–1575.

Joseph, C. L., Foxman, B., Leickly, F. E., Peterson, E., & Ownby, D. (1996). Prevalence of possible undiagnosed asthma and associated morbidity among urban schoolchildren. *Journal of Pediatrics, 129,* 735–742.

Joseph, K. E., Adams, C. D., Cottrell, L., Hogan, M. B., & Wilson, N. W. (2003). Providing dust mite-proof covers improves adherence to dust mite control measures in children with mite allergy and asthma. *Annals of Allergy, Asthma, and Immunology, 90,* 550–553.

Julian, D. A. (1997). The utilization of the logic model as a system level planning and evaluation device. *Evaluation and Program Planning, 20,* 251–257.

Julian, D. A., Jones, A., & Deyo, D. (1995). Open systems evaluation and the logic model: Program planning and evaluation tools. *Evaluation and Program Planning, 18,* 333–341.

Juniper, E. F., Kline, P. A., Vanzieleghem, M. A., Ramsdale, E. FL, O'Byrne, P. M., & Hargreave, F. E. (1990). Effect of long-term treatment with an inhaled corticosteroid (budesonide) on airway hyperresponsiveness and clinical asthma in nonsteroid-dependent asthmatics. *American Review of Respiratory Disease, 142,* 832–836.

Kaaya, S. F., Flisher, A. J., Mbwambo, J. K., Schaalma, H., Aaro, L. E., & Klepp, K. I. (2002). A review of studies of sexual behaviour of school students in sub-Saharan Africa. *Scandinavian Journal of Public Health, 30,* 148–160.

Kahan, B., & Goodstadt, M. (1998). An exploration of best practices in health promotion. *Health Promotion in Canada, 34,* 9–11.

Kahan, B., & Goodstadt, M. (2001). The Interactive Domain Model of best practices in health promotion: Developing and implementing a best practices approach to health promotion. *Health Promotion Practice, 2,* 43–67.

Kahn, R. S., Certain, L., & Whitaker, R. C. (2002). A reexamination of smoking before, during, and after pregnancy. *American Journal of Public Health, 92,* 1801–1808.

Kalichman, S. C., & Rompa, D. (2000). Functional health literacy is associated with health status and health-related knowledge in people living with HIV-AIDS. *Journal of Acquired Immune Deficiency Syndrome, 25,* 337–344.

Kang, B. C., Johnson, J., & Veres-Thorner, C. (1993). Atopic profile of inner-city asthma with a comparative analysis on the cockroach-sensitive and ragweed-sensitive subgroups. *Journal of Allergy and Clinical Immunology, 92,* 802–811.

Kannel, W. B., D'Agostino, R. B., Sullivan, L., & Wilson, P. W. (2004). Concept and usefulness of cardiovascular risk profiles. *American Heart Journal, 148,* 16–26.

Kaplan, B. H., & Cowley, R. A. (1991). Seatbelt effectiveness and cost of noncompliance among drivers admitted to a trauma center. *American Journal of Emergency Medicine, 9,* 4–10.

Kattan, M., Mitchell, H., Eggleston, P., Gergen, P., Crain, E. Redline, S., et al. (1997). Characteristics of inner-city children with asthma: The National Cooperative Inner-City Asthma Study. *Pediatric Pulmonology 24,* 253–262.

Kauffold, A., Zuroweste, E., Garcia, D., & Drewes, C. T. (2004). *Breast, cervical and colon cancer in mobile underserved populations.* Austin, TX: Migrant Clinicians Network.

Kawachi, I., & Berkman, L. S. (2000). Social cohesion, social capital, and health. In I. Kawachi & L. S. Berkman (Eds.), *Social epidemiology* (pp. 174–190). New York: Oxford University Press.

Kawachi, I., Kennedy, B. P., Lochner, K., & Prothrow-Stith, D. (1997). Social capital, income inequality, and mortality. *American Journal of Public Health, 87,* 1491–1498.

Kawachi, I., Kim, D., Coutts, A., & Subramanian, S. V. (2004). Commentary: Reconciling the three accounts of social capital. *International Journal of Epidemiology, 33,* 682–690.

Kegeles, S. M., Hays, R. B., & Coates, T. J. (1996). The Mpowerment Project: A community-level HIV prevention intervention for young gay men. *American Journal of Public Health, 86,* 1129–1136.

Kegler, M. C., & McLeroy, K. R. (2003). Commentary on "Conceptualizing dissemination research and activity: The case of the Canadian Heart Health Initiative." *Health Education and Behavior, 30,* 283–286.

Kelly, D. L., Zito, M. A., & Weber, D. (2003). Using a stage model of behavior change to prompt action in an immunization project. *Joint Commission Journal on Quality and Safety, 29,* 321–323.

Kelly, J. A., St. Lawrence, J. S., Stevenson, L. Y., Hauth, A. C., Kalichman, S. C., Diaz, Y. E., et al. (1992). Community AIDS/HIV risk reduction: The effects of endorsements by popular people in three cities. *American Journal of Public Health, 82,* 1483–1489.

Kelly, J. A., Sogolow, E. D., & Neumann, M. S. (2000). Future directions and emerging issues in technology transfer between HIV prevention researchers and community-based service providers. *AIDS Education and Prevention, 12,* 126–141.

Kelsey, J. L., Whittemore, A. S., Evans, A. S., & Thompson, W. D. (1996). *Methods in observational epidemiology.* New York: Oxford University Press.

Kennelly, B., O'Shea, E., & Garvey, E. (2003). Social capital, life expectancy and mortality: A cross-national examination. *Social Science and Medicine, 56,* 2367–2377.

Kiecolt-Glaser, J. K., McGuire, L., Robles, T. F., & Glaser, R. (2002). Psychoneuroimmunology and psychosomatic medicine: Back to the future. *Psychosomatic Medicine, 64,* 15–28.

Kilburn, K. H. (1998). Pulmonary responses to gases and particles. In R. B. Wallace (Ed.), *Maxcy-Rosenau-Last public health and preventive medicine* (14th ed., pp. 577–591). Stamford, CT: Appleton & Lange.

King, A. C., Friedman, R., Marcus, B., Castro, C., Forsyth, L., Napolitano, M., et al. (2002). Harnessing motivational forces in the promotion of physical activity: the Community Health Advice by Telephone Project (CHAT). *Health Education Research, 17,* 627–636.

Kingdon, J. W. (2003). *Agendas, alternatives, and public policies* (2nd ed.). New York: Longman.

Kinney, P. L., Aggarwal, M., Northridge, M. E., Janssen, N. A., & Shepard, P. (2000). Airborne concentrations of PM (2.5) and diesel exhaust particles on Harlem sidewalks: A community-based pilot study. *Environmental Health Perspectives, 108,* 213–218.

Kirby, D. (2004). *BDI Logic models: A useful tool for designing, strengthening and evaluating programs to reduce adolescent sexual risk-taking, pregnancy, HIV and other STDs.* Retrieved November 23, 2004, from http://www.etr.org/recapp/BDILOGICMODEL20030924.pdf

Kirby, D. B., Baumler, E., Coyle, K. K., Basen-Engquist, K., Parcel, G. S., Harrist, R., et al. (2004). The "Safer Choices" intervention: Its impact on the sexual behaviors of different subgroups of high school students. *Journal of Adolescent Health, 35,* 442–452.

Kirby, D., Coyle, K., & Gould, J. B. (2001). Manifestations of poverty and birthrates among young teenagers in California zip code areas. *Family Planning Perspectives, 33,* 63–69.

Kirby, D., Korpi, M., Barth, R. P., & Cagampang, H. H. (1997). The impact of the Postponing Sexual Involvement curriculum among youths in California. *Family Planning Perspectives, 29,* 100–108.

Kirby, D., Short, L., Collins, J., Rugg, D., Kolbe, L., Howard, M., et al. (1994). School-based programs to reduce sexual risk behaviors: A review of effectiveness. *Public Health Reports, 109,* 339–360.

Kirk, J., & Miller, M. L. (1986). *Reliability and validity in qualitative research.* Thousand Oaks, CA: Sage.

Kirsch, I. S., Jungeblut, A., Jenkins, L., & Kolstad, A. (1993). *Adult literacy in America.* Washington, DC: U. S. Department of Education.

Kirtland, K. A., Porter, D. E., Addy, C. L., Neet, M. J., Williams, J. E., Sharpe, P. A., et al. (2003). Environmental measures of physical activity supports: Perception versus reality. *American Journal of Preventive Medicine, 24,* 323–331.

Kocken, P. (2001). Intermediates' satisfaction with a loneliness intervention program aimed at older adults: Linkage of program plans and users' needs. *Patient Education and Counseling, 43,* 189–197.

Koelen, M. A., Vaandrager, L., & Colomer, C. (2001). Health promotion research: Dilemmas and challenges. *Journal of Epidemiology and Community Health, 55,* 257–262.

Koffka, K. (1935). *Principles of Gestalt psychology* (1st ed.). New York: Harcourt Brace.

Kok, G., Den Boer, D. J., De Vries, H., Gerards, F., Hospers, H. J., & Mudde, A. N. (1992). Self-efficacy and attribution theory in health education. In R. Schwarzer (Ed.), *Self-efficacy: Thought control of action* (pp. 245–262). Washington: Hemisphere.

Kok, G., Schaalma, H., De Vries, H., Parcel, G., & Paulussen, T. (1996). Social psychology and health education. In W. Stroebe & M. Hewstone (Eds.), *European Review of Social Psychology* (pp. 241–282). New York: Wiley.

Kok, G., Schaalma, H., Ruiter, R. A., van Empelen, P., & Brug, J. (2004). Intervention mapping: Protocol for applying health psychology theory to prevention programmes. *Journal of Health Psychology, 9,* 85–98.

Kok, G. J., & Green, L. W. (1990). Research to support health promotion in practice: A plea for increased cooperation. *Health Promotion International, 5,* 303–308.

Kools, M., Ruiter, R. A., van de Wiel, M. W., & Kok, G. (2004). Increasing readers' comprehension of health education brochures: A qualitative study into how professional writers make texts coherent. *Health Education and Behavior, 31,* 720–740.

Kools, M., Van de Wiel, M., Ruiter, R., Crûts, A., & Kok, G. (2005). The effect of graphic organizers on subjective and objective comprehension of a health education text: Maastricht University. Unpublished manuscript.

Kolbe, L. J., & Iverson, D. C. (1981). Implementing comprehensive health education: Educational innovations and social change. *Health Education Quarterly, 8,* 57–80.

Kostelnick, C. (1996). Supra-textual design: The visual rhetoric of whole documents. *Technical Communication Quarterly, 5,* 9–33.

Kotses, H., Lewis, P., & Creer, T. L. (1990). Environmental control of asthma self-management. *Journal of Asthma, 27,* 375–384.

Kotses, H., Stout, C., McConnaughy, K., Winder, J. A., & Creer, T. L. (1996). Evaluation of individualized asthma self-management programs. *Journal of-Asthma, 33,* 113–118.

Kraft, J. M., Beeker, C., Stokes, J. P., & Peterson, J. L. (2000). Finding the "community" in community-level HIV/AIDS interventions: Formative research with young African American men who have sex with men. *Health Education and Behavior, 27,* 430–441.

Kremers, S. P., De Vries, H., Mudde, A. N., & Candel, M. (2004). Motivational stages of adolescent smoking initiation: Predictive validity and predictors of transitions. *Addictive Behaviors, 29,* 781–789.

Kremers, S. P., Mudde, A. N., & De Vries, H. (2004). Model of unplanned smoking initiation of children and adolescents: An integrated stage model of smoking behavior. *Preventive Medicine, 38,* 642–650.

Kretzmann, J. P., & McKnight, J. L. (1993). *Building communities from the inside out: A path toward finding and mobilizing a community's assets.* Chicago: ACTA.

Kreuger, R. A. (1988). *Focus groups: A practical guide for applied research.* Thousand Oaks, CA: Sage.

Kreuger, R. A. (1994). *Focus groups: A practical guide for applied research* (2nd ed.). Thousand Oaks, CA: Sage.

Kreuger, R. A., & Casey, M. A. (2000). *Focus groups: A practical guide for applied research* (3rd ed.). Thousand Oaks, CA: Sage.

Kreuter, M., Farrell, D., Olevitch, L., & Brennan, L. (2000). *Tailoring health messages: Customizing communication with computer technology.* Mahwah, NJ: Erlbaum.

Kreuter, M. W., Caburnay, C. A., Chen, J. J., & Donlin, M. J. (2004). Effectiveness of individually tailored calendars in promoting childhood immunization in urban public health centers. *American Journal of Public Health, 94,* 122–127.

Kreuter, M. W., De Rosa, C., Howze, E. H., & Baldwin, G. T. (2004). Understanding wicked problems: A key to advancing environmental health promotion. *Health Education and Behavior, 31,* 441–454.

Kreuter, M. W., & Lezin, N. (2002). Social capital theory: Implications for community-based health promotion. In R .J. DiClemente, R. A. Crosby, & M. C. Kegler (Eds.), *Emerging theories in health promotion practice and research: Strategies for improving public health* (pp. 228–254). San Francisco: Jossey-Bass.

Kreuter, M. W., Lezin, N. A., Kreuter, M. W., & Green, L. W. (1997). *Community health promotion ideas that work: A field-book for practitioners.* Sudbury, MA: Jones and Bartlett.

Kreuter, M. W., Lukwago, S. N., Bucholtz, R. D., Clark, E. M., & Sanders-Thompson, V. (2002). Achieving cultural appropriateness in health promotion programs: targeted and tailored approaches. *Health Education and Behavior, 30,* 133–146.

Kreuter, M. W., & Strecher, V. J. (1996). Do tailored behavior change messages enhance the effectiveness of health risk appraisal? Results from a randomized trial. *Health Education Research, 11,* 97–105.

Kreuter, M. W., & Wray, R. J. (2003). Tailored and targeted health communication: Strategies for enhancing information relevance. *American Journal of Health Behavior, 27*(Suppl. 3), S227–S232.

Krieger, J., Allen, C., Cheadle, A., Ciske, S., Schier, J. K., Senturia, K., et al. (2002). Using community-based participatory research to address social determinants of health: Lessons learned from Seattle Partners for Healthy Communities. *Health Education and Behavior, 29,* 361–382.

Krishnan, J. A., Diette, G. B., Skinner, E. A., Clark, B. D., Steinwachs, D., & Wu, A. W. (2001). Race and sex differences in consistency of care with national asthma guidelines in managed care organizations. *Archives of Internal Medicine, 161,* 1660–1668.

Kruse, J., LeFevre, M., & Zweig, S. (1986). Changes in smoking and alcohol consumption during pregnancy: A population-based study in a rural area. *Obstetrics and Gynecology, 67*(5), 627–632.

Kubler, D. (2001). Understanding policy change with the advocacy coalition framework: An application to Swiss drug policy. *Journal of European Public Policy, 8,* 623–642.

Kurtz, M. E., Given, B., Given, C. W., & Kurtz, J. C. (1993). Relationships of barriers and facilitators to breast self-examination, mammography, and clinical breast examination in a worksite population. *Cancer Nursing, 16,* 251–259.

Kuttner, M. J., Delamater, A. M., & Santiago, J. V. (1990). Learned helplessness in diabetic youths. *Journal of Pediatric Psychology, 15,* 595–604.

Kuzel, A. (1999). Sampling in qualitative inquiry. In B. Crabtree & W. Miller (Eds.), *Doing qualitative research: Research methods for primary care* (pp. 31–44). Thousand Oaks, CA: Sage.

Labarthe, D. R. (1998). *Epidemiology and prevention of cardiovascular diseases: A global challenge.* Gaithersburg, MD: Aspen.

Labarthe, D. R. (1999). Prevention of cardiovascular risk factors in the first place. *Preventive Medicine, 29,* S72-S78.

Labonte, R. (1997). Community, community development, and the forming of authentic partnerships: Some critical reflections. In M. Minkler (Ed.), *Community organizing and community building for health* (pp. 88–102). New Brunswick, NJ: Rutgers University Press.

Labonte, R., & Laverack, G. (2001). Capacity building in health promotion, part 2: Whose use? And with what measurement? *Critical Public Health, 11,* 129–138.

Ladson-Billings, G. (1992). Culturally relevant teaching: The key to making multicultural education work. In C.A.Grant (Ed.), *Research and multicultural education: From the margins to the mainstream* (pp. 106–121). Washington, DC: The Fulmer Press.

Ladson-Billings, G. (1995). Toward a theory of culturally relevant pedagogy. *American Educational Research Journal, 35,* 465–491.

Lam, T. K., McPhee, S. J., Mock, J., Wong, C., Doan, H. T., Nguyen, T., et al. (2003). Encouraging Vietnamese-American women to obtain pap tests through lay health worker outreach and media education. *Journal of General Internal Medicine, 18,* 516.

Lantz, P. M., Dupuis, L., Reding, D., Krauska, M., & Lappe, K. (1994). Peer discussions of cancer among Hispanic migrant farm workers. *Public Health Reports, 109,* 512–520.

Lantz, P. M., & Reding, D. (1994). Cancer: Beliefs and attitudes of migrant Latinos. *JAMA: Journal of the American Medical Association, 272,* 31–32.

Laraque, D., McLean, D. E., Brown-Peterside, P., Ashton, D., & Diamond, B. (1997). Predictors of reported condom use in central Harlem youth as conceptualized by the health belief model. *Journal of Adolescent Health, 21,* 318–327.

Larson, A. (2002). *Migrant and seasonal farmworkers enumeration profiles study: TEXAS final.* Rockville, MD: Health Resources and Services Administration.

Laumann, E. O., & Knoke, D. (1987). *The organizational state: Social choice in national policy domains.* Madison, WI: University of Wisconsin Press.

Laver, S. M., van den Borne, B., Kok, G., & Woelk, G. (1997). A pre-intervention survey to determine understanding of HIV and AIDS in farm worker communities in Zimbabwe. *AIDS Education and Prevention, 9,* 94–110.

Lazarus, R. S. (1993). Coping theory and research: Past, present, and future. *Psychosomatic Medicine, 55,* 234–247.

Lazarus, R. S., & Folkman, S. (1991). The concept of coping. In A. Monat & R. S. Lazarus (Eds.), *Stress and coping: An anthology* (3rd ed., pp. 189–206). New York: Columbia University Press.

Lechner, L., Brug, J., de Vries, H., Van Assema, P., & Mudde, A. (1998). Stages of change for fruit, vegetable and fat intake: Consequence of misconception. *Health Education Research, 13,* 1–13.

Lefebvre, R. C., & Flora, J. A. (1988). Social marketing and public health intervention. *Health Education Quarterly, 15,* 299–315.

Lefebvre, R. C., & Flora, J. A. (1992). The social marketing imbroglio in health promotion. *Health Promotion International, 7,* 61–64.

Lefebvre, R. C., Lurie, D., Goodman, L. S., Weinberg, L., & Loughrey, K. (1995). Social marketing and nutrition education: Inappropriate or misunderstood? *Journal of Nutrition Education, 27,* 146–150.

Lefebvre, R. C., & Rochlin, L. (1997). Social marketing. In K. Glanz, F. M. Lewis, & B. K. Rimer (Eds.), *Health behavior and health education: Theory, research, and practice* (2nd ed., pp. 384–402). San Francisco: Jossey-Bass.

Legler, J., Meissner, H. I., Coyne, C., Breen, N., Chollette, V., & Rimer, B. K. (2002). The effectiveness of interventions to promote mammography among women with historically lower rates of screening. *Cancer Epidemiology, Biomarkers and Prevention, 11*, 59–71.

Legorreta, A. P., Christian-Herman, J., O'Connor, R. D., Hasan, M. M., Evans, R., & Leung, K. M. (1998). Compliance with national asthma management guidelines and specialty care: A health maintenance organization experience. *Archives of Internal Medicine, 158*, 457–464.

Levinson, R. A. (1995). Reproductive and contraceptive knowledge, contraceptive self-efficacy, and contraceptive behavior among teenage women. *Adolescence, 30*, 65–85.

Leviton, L., Mrazek, P., & Stoto, M. (1996). Social marketing to adolescents and minority populations. *Social Marketing Quarterly, 3*, 6–23.

Levy, J. (1991). A conceptual meta-paradigm for the study of health behavior and health promotion. *Health Education Research, 6*, 195–202.

Levy, S. R., Anderson, E. E., Issel, L. M., Willis, M. A., Dancy, B. L., Jacobson, K. M., et al. (2004). Using multilevel, multisource needs assessment data for planning community interventions. *Health Promotion Practice, 5*, 59–68.

Levy, S. R., Perhats, C., Weeks, K., Handler, A. S., Zhu, C., & Flay, B. R. (1995). Impact of a school-based AIDS prevention program on risk and protective behavior for newly sexually active students. *Journal of School Health, 65*, 145–151.

Lewin, K. (1947). Quasi-stationary social equilibria and the problem of social change. In E. L. Newcomb & E. L. Hartley (Eds.), *Readings in social psychology*. New York: Holt, Rinehart & Winston.

Lewin, S. A., Dick, J., Pond, P., Zwarenstein, M., Aja, G., van Wyk, B., et al. (2003). Lay health workers in primary and community health care: Cochrane Review Retreived March 3, 2005, from http://www.chchrane.org/cochrane/revabstr/ab004015.htm.

Lewis, C. E., Rachelefsky, G., Lewis, M. A., de la Sota, A., & Kaplan, M. (1984). A randomized trial of A.C.T. (Asthma Care Training) for kids. *Pediatrics, 74*, 478–486.

Lewis, M. J., Yulis, S. G., Delnevo, C., & Hrywna, M. (2004). Tobacco industry direct marketing after the Master Settlement Agreement. *Health Promotion Practice, 5*, 75S–83S.

Lichtenstein, E., Thompson, B., Nettekoven, L., Corbett, K., & for the COMMIT Research Group (1996). Durability of tobacco control activities in 11 North American communities: Life after the community intervention trial for smoking cessation (COMMIT). *Health Education Research, 11*, 527–534.

Lieberman, D. A. (1997). Interactive video games for health promotion: Effects on knowledge, self-efficacy, social support and health. In R. Street, W. Gold, & T. Manning (Eds.), *Health promotion and interactive technology: Theoretical applications and future directions* (pp. 103–120). Mahwah, NJ: Erlbaum.

Lieberman, D. A. (2001). Management of chronic pediatric diseases with interactive health games: Theory and research findings. *Journal of Ambulatory Care Management, 24*, 26–38.

Lieberman, D. A., & Linn, M. (1991). Learning to learn revisited: Computers and the development of self-directed learning skills. *Journal of Research on Computing in Education, 23*, 373–394.

Lieberman, E., Gremy I., Lang, S. M., & Cohen, A. P. (1994). Low birthweight at term and the timing of fetal exposure to maternal smoking. *American Journal of Public Health, 84*(7), 1127–1131.

Lieu, T. A., Lozano, P., Finkelstein, J. A., Chi, F. W., Jensvold, N. G., Capra, A. M., et al. (2002). Racial/ethnic variation in asthma status and management practices among children in managed medicaid. *Pediatrics, 109*, 857–865.

Lieu, T. A., Quesenberry, C. P., Capra, M. A., Sorel, M. E., Martin, K. E., & Mendoza, G. R. (1997). Outpatient management practices associated with reduced risk of pediatric asthma hospitalization and emergency department visits. *Pediatrics, 100,* 334–341.

Lincoln, Y. S., & Guba, E. G. (1985). *Naturalistic inquiry.* Thousand Oaks, CA: Sage.

Ling, J. C., Franklin, B.A.K., Lindsteadt, J. F., & Gearon, S.A.N. (1992). Social marketing: Its place in public health. *Annual Review of Public Health, 13,* 341–362.

Linnan, L., & Steckler, A. (2002). Process evaluation for public health interventions and research: An overview. In A. Steckler & L. Linnan (Eds.), *Process evaluation for public health interventions and research* (pp. 1–23). San Francisco: Jossey-Bass.

Lipkus, I. M., Lyna, P. R., & Rimer, B. K. (2000). Colorectal cancer risk perceptions and screening intentions in a minority population. *Journal of the National Medical Association, 92,* 492–500.

Lipsey, M. W., & Wilson, D. B. (2001). *Practical meta-analysis.* Thousand Oaks, CA: Sage.

Livingstone, J., Axton, R. A., Mennie, M., Gilfillan, A., & Brock, D. J. (1993). A preliminary trial of couple screening for cystic fibrosis: Designing an appropriate information leaflet. *Clinical Genetics, 43*(2), 57–62.

Lochner, K. A., Kawachi, I., Brennan, R. T., & Buka, S. L. (2003). Social capital and neighborhood mortality rates in Chicago. *Social Science and Medicine, 56,* 1797–1805.

Locke, D. C. (1986). Cross-cultural counseling issues. In W. J. Weikel & A. J. Palmo (Eds.), *Foundation of mental health counseling.* Springfield, IL: Charles C. Thomas.

Locke, D. C. (1992). *Increasing multicultural understanding: A comprehensive model.* Thousand Oaks, CA: Sage.

Locke, E. A., & Latham, G. P. (1990). *A theory of goal setting and task performance.* Englewood Cliffs, NJ: Prentice Hall.

Locke, E. A., & Latham, G. P. (2002). Building a practically useful theory of goal setting and task motivation: A 35-year odyssey. *American Psychologist, 5,* 705–717.

Loeber, R., & Dishion, T. (1983). Early predictors of male delinquency: A review. *Psychological Bulletin, 94,* 68–99.

Loeber, R., Stouthamer-Loeber, M., van Kammen, W., & Farrington, D. P. (1991). Initiation, escalation, and desistence in juvenile offending and their correlates. *Journal of Criminal Law and Criminology, 94,* 68–99.

Longest, B. B., Jr. (2002). *Health policymaking in the United States* (3rd ed.). Chicago: Health Administration Press.

Loomes, G., & Sugden, R. (1982). Regret theory: An alternative theory of rational choice under uncertainty. *Economic Journal, 92,* 805–825.

Lopez, A. (2004). *Hispanic mothers describing asthma: A qualitative study.* Unpublished Master's Thesis, University of Texas Health Science Center School of Public Health, Houston.

Lorig, K., & Holman, H. (1993). Arthritis self-management studies: A twelve-year review. *Health Education Quarterly, 20,* 17–28.

Luepker, R. V. (1998). Heart disease. In R. B. Wallace (Ed.), *Maxcy-Rosenau-Last public health and preventive medicine* (14th ed.). Stamford, CT: Appleton & Lange.

Lusk, S. L., Ronis, D. L., Kazanis, A. S., Eakin, B. L., Hong, O., & Raymond, D. M. (2003). Effectiveness of a tailored intervention to increase factory workers' use of hearing protection. *Nursing Research, 52,* 289–295.

Lux, K. M., & Petosa, R. (1994). Using the health belief model to predict safer sex intentions of incarcerated youth. *Health Education Quarterly, 21,* 487–497.

Lynch, B. S., & Bonnie, R. J. (Eds.) and Committee on Preventing Nicotine Addiction in Children and Youths, Institute of Medicine (1994). *Growing up tobacco free: Preventing nicotine addiction in children and youths.* Washington, DC: National Academy Press.

Lytle, L. A., & Perry, C. L. (2001). Applying research and theory in program planning: An example from a nutrition education intervention. *Health Promotion Practice, 2,* 68–80.

Lytle, L. A., Ward, J., Nader, P. R., Pedersen, S., & Williston, B. J. (2003). Maintenance of a health promotion program in elementary schools: Results from the CATCH-ON study key informant interviews. *Health Education and Behavior, 30,* 503–518.

Macaulay, A. C., Commanda, L. E., Freeman, W. L., Gibson, N., McCabe, M. L., Robbins, C. M., et al. (1999). Participatory research maximises community and lay involvement. North American Primary Care Research Group. *British Medical Journal, 319,* 774–778.

MacKinnon, D. P. (1994). Analysis of mediating variables in prevention and intervention research. *NIDA Research Monograph, 139,* 127–153.

MacKinnon, D. P., Lockwood, C. M., Hoffman, J. M., West, S. G., & Sheets, V. (2002). A comparison of methods to test mediation and other intervening variable effects. *Psychological Methods, 7,* 83–104.

MacQueen, K. M., McLellan, E., Metzger, D. S., Kegeles, S., Strauss, R. P., Scotti, R., et al. (2001). What is community? An evidence-based definition for participatory public health. *American Journal of Public Health, 91,* 1929–1938.

Mager, R. F. (1984). *Preparing instructional objectives* (rev. 2nd ed.). Belmont, CA: Lake Publishing Company.

Mahoney, C. A., Thombs, D. L., & Howe, C. Z. (1995). The art and science of scale development in health education research. *Health Education Research, 10,* 1–10.

Maibach, E. W., & Cotton, D. (1995). Moving people to behavior change: A staged social cognitive approach to message design. In E. W. Maibach & R. L. Parrott (Eds.), *Designing health messages: Approaches from communication theory and public health practice* (pp. 41–64). Thousand Oaks, CA: Sage.

Maibach, E. W., Ladin, K., Maxfield, A., & Slater, M. (1996). Translating healthy psychology into effective health communication: The American health styles audience segmentation project. *Journal of Health Psychology, 1,* 261–278.

Maibach, E., & Murphy, D. A. (1995). Self-efficacy in health promotion research and practice: Conceptualization and measurement. *Health Education Research, 10,* 37–50.

Maibach, E. W., & Parrott, R. L. (1995). *Designing health messages: Approaches from communication theory and public health practice.* Thousand Oaks, CA: Sage.

Maibach, E. W., Rothchild, M. L., & Novelli, W. D. (2002). Social marketing. In K. Glanz, F. M. Lewis, & B. K. Rimer (Eds.), *Health behavior and health education: Theory, research, and practice* (3rd ed., pp. 437–461). San Francisco: Jossey-Bass.

Maiburg, H. J., Hiddink, G. J., van't Hof, M. A., Rethans, J. J., & van Ree, J. W. (1999). The NECTAR study: Development of nutrition modules for general practice vocational training; determinants of nutrition guidance practices of GP trainees. Nutrition education by computerized training and research. *European Journal of Clinical Nutrition, 53*(Suppl. 2), S83–S88.

Majumdar, B., & Roberts, J. (1998). AIDS awareness among women: The benefit of culturally sensitive educational programs. *Health Care Women International, 19,* 141–153.

Mak, H., Johnston, P., Abbey, H., & Talamo, R. C. (1982). Prevalence of asthma and health utilization of asthmatic children in an inner city. *Journal of Allergy and Clinical Immunology 70,* 367–372.

Mallett, S., Hopewell, S., & Clarke, M. (2002, July). Grey literature in systematic reviews: The first 1000 Cochrane systematic reviews. Paper presented at the 4th Symposium on Systematic Reviews: Pushing the Boundaries, Oxford, England.

Malloy, M. H., Hoffman, H. J., & Peterson, D. R. (1992). Sudden Infant Death Syndrome and maternal smoking. *American Journal of Public Health, 82,* 1380–1382.

Malloy, M. H., Kleinman, J. C., Land, G. H., & Schramm, W. F. (1988). The association of maternal smoking with age and cause of infant deaths. *American Journal of Epidemiology, 128*(1), 46–55.

Manders, A. J., Banerjee, A., van den Borne, H. W., Harries, A. D., Kok, G. J., & Salaniponi, F. M. (2001). Can guardians supervise TB treatment as well as health workers? A study on adherence during the intensive phase. *International Journal of Tuberculosis and Lung Disease, 5,* 838–842.

Manfredi, C., Lacey, L., Warnecke, R., & Balch, G. (1997). Method effects in survey and focus group findings: Understanding smoking cessation in low-SES African American women. *Health Education and Behavior, 24,* 786–800.

Manlove, J., Ryan, S., & Franzetta, K. (2004). Contraceptive use and consistency in U.S. teenagers' most recent sexual relationships. *Perspectives on Sexual and Reproductive Health, 36,* 265–275.

Mann, K. V. (1994). Educating medical students: Lessons from research in continuing education. *Academic Medicine, 69,* 41–47.

Mann, K. V., Linsday, E. A., Putnam, R. W., & Davis, D. A. (1996). Increasing physician involvement in cholesterol-lowering practices. *Journal of Continuing Education in the Health Professions, 16,* 225–240.

Mannino, D. M., Homa, D. M., Akinbami, L. J., Moorman, J. E., Gwynn, C., Redd, S. C., et al. (2002). Surveillance for asthma—United States—1980–1999. *Morbidity and Mortality Weekly Report, 51,* 1–13.

Mannino, D. M., Homa, D. M., Pertowski, M. D., Ashizawa, A., Nixon, L. L., Johnson, C. A., et al. (1998). Surveillance for asthma—United States, 1960–1995. *Morbidity and Mortality Surveillance Summaries, 47,* 1–27.

Manson, A. (1988). Language concordance as a determinant of patient compliance and emergency room use in patients with asthma. *Medical Care, 26,* 1119–1128.

Manstead, T., & Parker, D. (1995). Evaluating and extending the theory of planned behavior. In W. Stroebe & M. Hewstone (Eds.), *European review of social psychology* (pp. 69–95). Chichester, England: Wiley.

Marcus, A. C., & Crane, L. A. (1998). A review of cervical cancer screening intervention research: Implications for public health programs and future research. *Preventive Medicine, 27,* 13–31.

Margai, F., & Henry, N. (2003). A community-based assessment of learning disabilities using environmental and contextual risk factors. *Social Science and Medicine, 56,* 1073–1085.

Mark, M. M., & Shotland, R. L. (1985). Stakeholder-based evaluations and value judgements. *Evaluation Review, 9,* 605–626.

Marlatt, G. A., & Gordon, J. R. (1985). *Relapse prevention: Maintenance strategies in the treatment of addictive behaviors.* New York: Guilford Press.

Marmot, M. (2000). Social determinants of health: From observation to policy. *The Medical Journal of Austrailia, 172,* 379–382.

Martinez-Donate, A. P., Hovell, M. F., Blumberg, E. J., Zellner, J. A., Sipan, C. L., Shillington, A. M., et al. (2004). Gender differences in condom-related behaviors and attitudes among Mexican adolescents living on the U.S.-Mexico border. *AIDS Education and Prevention, 16,* 172–186.

Masse, L. C., Ainsworth, B. E., Tortolero, S., Levin, S., Fulton, J. E., Henderson, K. A., et al. (1998). Measuring physical activity in midlife, older, and minority women: Issues from an expert panel. *Journal of Women's Health, 7,* 57–67.

Mattessich, P., & Monsey, B. (1997). *Community building: What makes it work? A review of factors influencing successful community building.* St. Paul, MN: Amherst H. Wilder Foundation.

Maurer, T. J., & Pierce, H. R. (1998). A comparison of Likert scale and traditional measures of self-efficacy. *Journal of Applied Psychology, 83,* 324–329.

Mayer, R. E. (1984). Twenty-five years of research on advance organizers. *Instruction Science, 8,* 133–169.

Maziak, W., Rzehak, P., Keil, U., & Weiland, S. K. (2003). Smoking among adolescents in Muenster, Germany: Increase in prevalence (1995–2000) and relation to tobacco advertising. *Preventive Medicine, 36,* 172–176.

McAlister, A. (1995). Behavioral journalism: Beyond the marketing model for health communication. *American Journal of Health Promotion, 9,* 417–420.

McAlister, A., & Fernandez, M. (2001). "Behavioral journalism" accelertes diffusion of health innovations. In R. C. Hornik (Ed.), *Public health communication: Evidence for behavior change* (pp. 315–326). Mahwah, NJ: Erlbaum.

McAlister, A. L. (1991). Population behavior change: a theory-based approach. *Journal of Public Health Policy, 12,* 345–361.

McAlister, A. L., Fernandez-Esquer, M. E., Ramirez, A. G., Trevino, F., Gallion, K. J., Villarreal, R., et al. (1995). Community level cancer control in a Texas barrio, part II: Base-line and preliminary outcome findings (Monograph Nos. 123–126). *Journal of the National Cancer Institute.*

McBride, C. M., Pirie, P. L., & Curry, S. J. (1992). Postpartum relapse to smoking: A prospective study. *Health Education Research, 7,* 381–390.

McCallister, L., & Fischer, C. S. (1978). A procedure for surveying personal networks. *Sociological Methods and Research, 7,* 131–148.

McCullum, C., Pelletier, D., Barr, D., Wilkins, J., & Habich, J. P. (2004). Mechanisms of power within a community-based food security planning process. *Health Education and Behavior, 31,* 206–222.

McDonald, M. A., Thomas, J. C., & Eng, E. (2001). When is sex safe? Insiders' views on sexually transmitted disease prevention and treatment. *Health Education and Behavior, 28,* 624–642.

McFarlane, J., & Fehir, J. (1994). De Madres a Madres: A community, primary health care program based on empowerment. *Health Education Quarterly, 21,* 381–394.

McGrath, J. (1995). The gatekeeping process: The right combinations to unlock the gates. In E. W. Maibach & R. L. Parrott (Eds.), *Designing health messages: Approaches from communication theory and public health practice* (pp. 199–216). Thousand Oaks, CA: Sage.

McGuire, W. J. (1964). Inducing resistance to persuasion: Some contemporary approaches. In L. Berkowitz (Ed.), *Advances in experimental social psychology, 1* (pp. 191–229). New York: Academic Press.

McGuire, W. J. (1985). Attitudes and attitude change. In G. Lindzey & E. Aronson (Eds.), *The handbook of social psychology: Vol. 2. Special fields and applications* (3rd ed., pp. 233–346). New York: Knopf.

McGuire, W. J. (1986). The myth of massive media impact: Savagings and salvagings. In G. Comstock (Ed.), *Public communication and behavior* (pp. 175–234). Orlando, FL: Academic Press.

McKinlay, J. B., & Marceau, L. D. (2000). To boldly go . . . *American Journal of Public Health, 90,* 25-33.

McKnight, J. (1995). *The careless society: A community and its counterfeits.* New York: Basic Books.

McKnight, J. L., & Kretzmann, J. P. (1997). Mapping community capacity. In M. Minkler (Ed.), *Community organizing and community building for health* (pp. 157–172). New Brunswick, NJ: Rutgers University Press.

McLaughlin, G. (1969). The SMOG readability formula. *Journal of Reading, 12,* 639–646.

McLeroy, K. (1996, February). Community capacity: What is it? How do we measure it? What is the role of the Prevention Centers and CDC? Paper presented at the Sixth Annual Prevention Centers Conference, Centers for Disease Control and Prevention, Atlanta, GA.

McLeroy, K. R., Bibeau, D., Steckler, A., & Glanz, K. (1988). An ecological perspective on health promotion programs. *Health Education Quarterly, 15,* 351–377.

McLeroy, K. R., Gottlieb, N. H., & Heaney, C. A. (2001). Social health in the workplace. In M. P. O'Donnell (Ed.), *Health promotion in the workplace* (3rd ed., pp. 459–486). Albany, NY: Delmar.

McLeroy, K. R., Norton, B. L., Kegler, M. C., Burdine, J. N., & Sumaya, C. V. (2003). Community-based interventions. *American Journal of Public Health, 93,* 529–533.

McLeroy, K. R., Steckler, A. B., Simonsmorton, B., Goodman, R. M., Gottlieb, N., & Burdine, J. N. (1993). Social-science theory in health education: Time for a new model? *Health Education Research, 8,* 305–312.

McMillan, D. W., & Chavis, D. M. (1986). Sense of community: A definition and theory. *Journal of Community Psychology, 14,* 6–23.

McNabb, W. L., Wilson-Pessano, S. R., & Jacobs, A. M. (1986). Critical self-management competencies for children with asthma. *Journal of Pediatric Psychology 11,* 103–117.

McPherson, R. S., Hoelscher, D. M., Alexander, M., Scanlon, K. S., & Serdula, M. K. (2000). Dietary assessment methods among school-aged children: Validity and reliability. *Preventive Medicine, 31,* S11-S33.

Meister, J. S., Warrick, L. H., de Zapien, J. G., & Wood, A. H. (1992). Using lay health workers: Case study of a community-based prenatal intervention. *Journal of Community Health, 17,* 37–51.

Menashe, C. L., & Siegel, M. (1998). The power of a frame: An analysis of newspaper coverage of tobacco issues—United States, 1985–1996. *Journal of Health Communication, 3,* 307–325.

Menon, S. C., Pandey, D. K., & Morgenstern, L. B. (1998). Critical factors determining access to acute stroke care. *Neurology, 51,* 427–432.

Mercer, S. L., Green, L. W., Rosenthal, A. C., Husten, C. G., Khan, L. K., & Dietz, W. H. (2003). Possible lessons from the tobacco experience for obesity control. *American Journal of Clinical Nutrition, 77,* 1073S–1082S.

Mermelstein, R., Cohen, S., Lichtenstein, E., Baer, J. S., & Kamarck, T. (1986). Social support and smoking cessation and maintenance. *Journal of Consulting and Clinical Psychology, 54,* 447–453.

Merriam, S. B. (1988). *Case study research in education: A qualitative approach.* San Francisco: Jossey-Bass.

Merriam, S. B. (1998). *Case study research in education: A qualitative approach* (2nd ed.). San Francisco: Jossey-Bass.

Mesters, I., Meertens, R., Crebolder, H., & Parcel, G. (1993). Development of a health education program for parents of preschool children with asthma. *Health Education Research, 8,* 53–68.

Mesters, I., van Nunen, M., Crebolder, H., & Meertens, R. (1995). Education of parents about pediatric asthma: effects of a protocol on medical consumption. *Patient Education and Counseling, 25,* 131–136.

Metzler, C. W., Noell, J., Biglan, A., Ary, D., & Smolkowski, K. (1994). The social context for risky sexual behavior among adolescents. *Journal of Behavioral Medicine, 17,* 419–438.

Meyer-Weitz, A., Reddy, P., van den Borne, B., Kok, G., & Pietersen, J. (2003). Determinants of multi-partner behavior of male patients with sexually transmitted diseases in South Africa: Implications for interventions. *International Journal of Men's Health, 2,* 149–162.

Michielutte, R., Bahnson, J., Dignan, M. B., & Schroeder, E. M. (1992). The use of illustrations and narrative text style to improve readability of a health education brochure. *Journal of Cancer Education, 7,* 251–260.

Miles, M. B., & Huberman, A. M. (1984). *Qualitative data analysis: An expanded sourcebook* (2nd ed.). Thousand Oaks, CA: Sage.

Milio, N. (1981). *Promoting health through public policy.* Philadelphia: Davis.

Milio, N. (1988). Strategies for health promoting policy: A study of four national case studies. *Health Promotion, 3*(3), 307–311.

Milio, N. (2001). Glossary: Health public policy. *Journal of Epidemiology and Community Health, 55,* 622–623.

Miller, D., Shewchuk, R., Elliot, T. R., & Richards, S. (2000). Nominal group technique: A process for identifying diabetes self-care issues among patients and caregivers. *Diabetes Educator, 26,* 305–310, 312, 314.

Milne, S., Orbell, S., & Sheeran, P. (2002). Combining motivational and volitional interventions to promote exercise participation: Protection motivation theory and implementation intentions. *British Journal of Health Psychology, 7,* 163–184.

Mink, B. P., Downes, E. A., Owen, K. Q., & Mink, O. G. (1994). *Open organizations: A model for effectiveness, renewal, and intelligent change.* San Francisco: Jossey-Bass.

Minkler, M. (1997a). Community organizing among the elderly poor in San Francisco's Tenderloin District. In M. Minkler (Ed.), *Community organizing and community building* (pp. 244–258). New Brunswick, NJ: Rutgers University Press.

Minkler, M. (1997b). *Community organizing and community building for health* (1st ed.). New Brunswick, NJ: Rutgers University Press.

Minkler, M., Thompson, M., Bell, J., Rose, K., & Redman, D. (2002). Using community involvement strategies in the fight against infant mortality: Lessons from a multisite study of the national healthy start experience. *Health Promotion Practice, 3,* 176–187.

Minkler, M., & Wallerstein, N. (1997a). Improving health through community organization and community building: A health education perspective. In M. Minkler & N. Wallerstein (Eds.), *Community organizing and community building for health* (pp. 30–52). New Brunswick, NJ: Rutgers University Press.

Minkler, M. & Wallerstein, N. (1997b). Improving health through community organization and community building. In K. Glanz, F. M. Lewis, & B. K. Rimer (Eds.), *Health behavior and health education: Theory, research, and practice* (2nd ed., pp. 241–269). San Francisco: Jossey-Bass.

Misovich, S. J., Fisher, J. D., & Fisher, W. A. (1997). Close relationships and elevated HIV risk behavior: Evidence and possible underlying psychological processes. *Review of General Psychology, 1,* 72–107.

Mogilner, A. (1992). *Children's writer's word book.* Cincinnati, OH: Writer's Digest Books.

Monahan, J. (1995). Thinking positively: Using positive affect when designing health messages. In E. Maibach & R. L. Parrott (Eds.), *Designing health messages: Approaches from communication theory and public health practice.* Thousand Oaks, CA: Sage.

Monahan, J. L., & Scheirer, M. A. (1988). The role of linking agents in the diffusion of health promotion programs. *Health Education Quarterly, 15,* 417–433.

Mongoven, M., Dolan-Mullen, P., Groff, J. Y., Nicol, L., & Burau, K. (1996). Weight gain associated with prenatal smoking cessation in white, non-Hispanic women. *American Journal of Obstetrics and Gynecology, 174,* 72–77.

Montaño, D. E., & Kasprzyk, D. (2002). The theory of reasoned action and the theory of planned behavior. In K. Glanz, F. M. Lewis, & B. K. Rimer (Eds.), *Health behavior and health education: Theory, research, and practice.* (3rd ed., pp. 67–98). San Francisco: Jossey-Bass.

Montaño, D. E., Kasprzyk, D., & Taplin, S. H. (1997). The theory of reasoned action and the theory of planned behavior. In K. Glanz, F. M. Lewis, & B. K. Rimer (Eds.), *Health behavior and health education: Theory, research, and practice* (2nd ed.). San Francisco: Jossey-Bass.

Montaño, D. E., Thompson, B., Taylor, V. M., & Mahloch, J. (1997). Understanding mammography intention and utilization among women in an inner-city public hospital clinic. *Preventive Medicine, 26,* 817–824.

Moore, C. M. (1994). *Group techniques for idea building* (2nd ed.). Thousand Oaks, CA: Sage.

Morgan, C., Park, E., & Cortes, D. E. (1995). Beliefs, knowledge, and behavior about cancer among urban Hispanic women. *Journal of the National Cancer Institute, 18,* 57–63.

Morgan, D. L. (1988). *Focus groups as qualitative research.* Thousand Oaks, CA: Sage.

Morgan, D. L. (1997). *Focus groups as qualitative research* (2nd ed.). Thousand Oaks, CA: Sage.

Morgenstern, L. B., Bartholomew, L. K., Grotta, J. C., Staub, L., King, M., & Chan, W. (2003). Sustained benefit of a community and professional intervention to increase acute stroke therapy. *Archives of Internal Medicine, 163,* 2198–2202.

Morgenstern, L. B., Staub, L., Chan, W., Wein, T. H., Bartholomew, L. K., King, M., et al. (2002). Improving delivery of acute stroke therapy: The TLL Temple Foundation Stroke Project. *Stroke, 33,* 160–166.

Morgenstern, L., Wein, T. H., Staub, L., Hickenbottom, S. L., & Bartholomew, L. K. (2000, February). *Who are the appropriate targets to increase FDA-approved acute stroke therapy?* Paper presented at the 25th American Heart Association International Stroke Conference New Orleans, LA.

Moriarty, S. (1995). Visual communication as primary system. *Journal of Visual Literacy, 14,* 11–21.

Morisky, D. E., DeMuth, N. M., Field-Fass, M., Green, L. W., & Levine, D. M. (1985) Evaluation of family health education to build social support for long-term control of high blood pressure. *Health Education Quarterly, 12*(1), 35–50.

Morris, D. L., Felkner, M., & McLean, C. H. (1994). Pap screening in the Rio Grande Valley: A case study. *Family and Community Health, 17,* 1–14.

Morris, D. L., Rosamond, W., Madden, K., Schultz, C., & Hamilton, S. (2000). Prehospital and emergency department delays after acute stroke: The Genentech Stroke Presentation Survey. *Stroke, 31,* 2585–2590.

Mosenthal, P. B., & Kirsch, I. S. (1998). A new measure for assessing document complexity: The PMOSE/KIRSCH document readability formula. *Journal of Adolescent and Adult Literacy, 41,* 638–658.

Mukoma, W., & Flisher, A. J. (2004). Evaluations of health promoting schools: A review of nine studies. *Health Promotion International, 19,* 357–368.

Mullen, P. D. (1993). Using the research base to improve program design. In B. E. Giloth (Ed.), *Managing hospital-based patient education* (pp. 313–326). Chicago: American Hospital Association.

Mullen, P. D. (1999). Smoking during pregnancy and intervention to promote cessation: A meta-analysis. In J. G. Spangler (Ed.), *Primary care: Clinics in office practice* (Vol. 6, pp. 577–589). Philadelphia: W. B. Saunders.

Mullen, P. D. (2000). *How can more smoking suspension during pregnancy become lifelong abstinence? Lessons learned about predictors, interventions, and gaps in our accumulated knowledge.* Paper presented at the World Conference on Tobacco on Health, Chicago.

Mullen, P. D. (2004). How can more smoking suspension during pregnancy become lifelong abstinence? Lessons learned about predictors, interventions and gaps in our accumulated knowledge. *Nicotine and Tobacco Research, 6,* S127-S238.

Mullen, P. D., & Bartholomew, L. K. (1991, Nov.). *Project PANDA: Development of a program to reduce return to smoking by new mothers.* Atlanta, GA: Society for Health Education.

Mullen, P. D., Carbonari, J. P., & Glenday, M. (1991). Identfying pregnant women who drink alcoholic beverages. *American Journal of Obstetrics & Gynecology, 165,* 1429–1430.

Mullen, P. D., Carbonari, J. P., Tabak, E. R., & Glenday, M. (1991). Improving disclosure of smoking by pregnant women. *American Journal of Obstetrics & Gynecology, 165,* 409–413.

Mullen, P. D., & DiClemente, C. (1992). *Sustaining women's non-smoking postpartum.* Paper presented at the 8th World Conference on Tobacco and Health, Buenos Aires, Argentina.

Mullen, P. D., DiClemente, C. C., Carbonari, J. P., Nicol, L., Richardson, M. A., Sockrider, M. M., et al. (1999). Project PANDA: Maintenance of prenatal smoking abstinence 12 months postpartum. Unpublished manuscript.

Mullen, P. D., DiClemente, C. C., Carbonari, J. P., Nicol, L., Sockrider, M. M., & Richardson, M., et al (1997). Project PANDA maintenance of prenatal smoking abstinence postpartum at 6 weeks, and 3, 6, and 12 months [Abstract]. *Annals of Behavioral Medicine, 19,* 130.

Mullen, P. D., Gottlieb, N. H., Biddle, A. K., McCuan, R. A., & McAlister, A. L. (1988). Predictors of safety belt initiative by primary care physicians. A social learning theory perspective. *Medical Care, 26,* 373–382.

Mullen, P. D., Green, L. W., & Persinger, G. S. (1985). Clinical trials of patient education for chronic conditions: A comparative meta-analysis of intervention types. *Preventive Medicine, 14,* 753–781.

Mullen, P. D., Mains, D. A., & Velez, R. (1992). A meta-analysis of controlled trials of cardiac patient education. *Patient Education and Counseling, 19,* 143–162.

Mullen, P. D., & Mullen, L. R. (1983). Implementing asthma self-management education in medical care settings: Issues and strategies. *Journal of Allergy and Clinical Immunology, 72,* 611–622.

Mullen, P. D., Pollak, K. I., Kok, G. (1999). Success attributions for stopping smoking during pregnancy, self-efficacy, and postpartum maintenance. *Psychology of Addictive Behaviors, 13*(3), 198–206.

Mullen, P. D., Quinn, V. P., & Ershoff, D. H. (1990). Maintenance of nonsmoking postpartum by women who stopped during pregnancy. *American Journal of Public Health, 80,* 992–994.

Mullen, P. D., & Ramirez, G. (1987). Information synthesis and meta-analysis. In W. Ward, M. H. Becker, P. D. Mullen, & S. Simonds (Eds.), *Advances in health education and promotion: Vol. 2* (pp. 201–239). Greenwich, CT: JAI Press.

Mullen, P. D., & Ramirez, G. (2001). Efforts to reduce tobacco use among women: Pregnant women and mothers. In U.S. Public Health Service, Office on Smoking and Health. *The health consequences of smoking for women. A report of the Surgeon General.* Rockville, MD: U.S. Department of Health and Human Services.

Mullen, P. D., Ramirez, G., Strouse, D., Hedges, L. V., & Sogolow, E. (2002). Meta-analysis of the effects of behavioral HIV prevention interventions on the sexual risk behavior of sexually experienced adolescents in controlled studies in the United States. *Journal of Acquired Immune Deficiency Syndromes, 30*(Suppl. 1), S94-S105.

Mullen, P. D., Richardson, M. A., Quinn, V. P., & Ershoff, D. H. (1997). Postpartum return to smoking: Who is at risk and when? *American Journal of Health Promotion, 11,* 323–330.

Mullen, P. D., Simons-Morton, D. G., Ramirez, G., Frankowski, R. F., Green, L. W., & Mains, D. A. (1997). A meta-analysis of trials evaluating patient education and counseling for three groups of preventive behaviors. *Patient Education and Counseling, 32,* 157–173.

Mulvihill, C. K. (1996). AIDS education for college students: Review and proposal for a research-based curriculum. *AIDS Education and Prevention, 8,* 11–25.

Murphy, S., & Bennett, P. (2004). Health psychology and public health: Theoretical possibilities. *Journal of Health Psychology, 9,* 13–27.

Murphy-Smith, M., Meyer, B., Hitt, J., Taylor-Seehafer, M. A., & Tyler, D. O. (2004). Put Prevention into Practice implementation model: Translating practice into theory. *Journal of Public Health Management Practice, 10,* 109–115.

Murray A. B. (1988). Dust mite avoidance in the treatment of asthma. *Annals of Allergy, 60,* 84.

Murray, A. B., & Morrison, B. J. (1989). Passive smoking by asthmatics: Its greater effect on boys than girls and older than younger children. *Pediatrics, 84,* 451–459.

Murray, N., Kelder, S., Parcel, G., & Orpinas, P. (1998). Development of an intervention map for a parent education intervention to prevent violence among Hispanic middle school students. *Journal of School Health, 68,* 46–52.

Musick, J. S. (1991). The high-stakes challenge of programs for adolescent mothers. In P. B. Edelman & J. Ladner (Eds.), *Adolescence and poverty: Challenge for the 1990s.* Washington, DC: Center for National Policy Press.

Myers, R. E., Chodak, G. W., Wolf, T. A., Burgh, D. Y., McGrory, G. T., Marcus, S. M., et al. (1999). Adherence by African American men to prostate cancer education and early detection. *Cancer, 86,* 88–104.

Nader, P. R., Sellers, D. E., Johnson, C. C., Perry, C. L., Stone, E. J., Cook, K. C., et al. (1996). The effect of adult participation in a school-based family intervention to improve children's diet and physical activity: The child and adolescent trial for cardiovascular health. *Preventive Medicine, 25*(4), 455–464.

Nakkash, R., Afifi Soweid, R. A., Nehlawi, M. T., Shediac-Rizkallah, M. C., Hajjar, T. A., & Khogali, M. (2003). The development of a feasible community-specific cardiovascular disease prevention program: Triangulation of methods and sources. *Health Education and Behavior, 30,* 723–739.

National Asthma Education and Prevention Program school asthma education subcommittee (1998). How asthma friendly is your school? *Journal of School Health, 68,* 167–168.

National Cancer Institute, Office of Cancer Communications. (2002). *Making health communication programs work: A planner's guide.* Bethesda, MD: National Institutes of Health.

National Cancer Institute. (2005). Cancer control planet: Links to comprehensive cancer control resources for public health professionals. Retrieved from http://cancercontrol planet.cancer.gov/

National Center for Bicycling and Walking. (2002). Community assessment tool. Retrieved February 21, 2003.

National Center for Farmworker Health. (2002). Fact sheet about farmworkers. Retrieved January 23, 2005, from http://www.ncfh.org/factsheets.php.

National Heart, Lung, and Blood Institute (NHLBI). (1991). *Expert panel report: Executive summary. Guidelines for the diagnosis and management of asthma* (Publication No. 91–3042A). Bethesda, MD: National Institutes of Health.

National Heart, Lung, and Blood Institute (NHLBI). (1997). *National asthma education and prevention program expert panel 2 report: Guidelines for the diagnosis and management of asthma* (Report No. 97–4051). Bethesda, MD: National Institutes of Health.

National Institute of Neurological Disorders and Stroke. (1997). *Proceedings of a national symposium of rapid identification and treatment of acute stroke, December 12–13, 1996* (Publication No. 97–4239). Bethesda, MD: National Institutes of Health.

National Institute of Neurological Disorders and Stroke rtPA Stroke Study Group. (1995). Tissue plasminogen activator for acute ischemic stroke. *New England Journal of Medicine, 333,* 1581–1588.

National Institutes of Health. (1994). *Clear and simple: Developing effective print materials for low-literate readers* [Pamphlet]. Bethesda, MD: Author.

National Institutes of Health (2003). *Clear and to the point: Guidelines for using plain language at NIH.* Retrieved October 21, 2003, from http://execsec.od.nih.gov/plainlang/guidelines/index.html

Nationale Commissie AIDS Bestrijding. (1995). Epidemiology: The Netherlands. *AIDS Bestrijding, 20,* 12–13.

Natowicz, M. R., & Prence, E. M. (1996). Heterozygote screening for Tay-Sachs disease: Past successes and future challenges. *Current Opinion in Pediatrics, 8,* 625–629.

Navarro, A. M., Senn, K. L., Kaplan, R. M., McNicholas, L., Campo, M. C., & Roppe, B. (1995). Por La Vida intervention model for cancer prevention in Latinas. *Journal of the National Cancer Institute, 18* 137–145.

Needleman, H. L., Riess, J. A., Tobin, M. J., Biesecker, G. E., & Greenhouse, J. B. (1996). Bone lead levels and delinquent behavior. JAMA: *JAMA: Journal of the American Medical Association, 275,* 363–369.

Neuberger, J. S., Newkirk, D. D., Cotter, J., Thorpe, A., Wood, C., & Irwin, J. C. (1991). Diminished air quality and health problems in a Kansas City, Kansas, elementary school. *Journal of School Health, 61,* 439–442.

Neumann, M. S., & Sogolow, E. D. (2000). Replicating effective programs: HIV/AIDS prevention technology transfer. *AIDS Education and Prevention, 12,* 35–48.

Newacheck, P. W., & Halfon, N. (2000). Prevalence, impact, and trends in childhood disability due to asthma. *Archives of Pediatrics and Adolescent Medicine, 154,* 287–293.

Newes-Adeyi, G., Helitzer, D. L., Caulfield, L. E., & Bronner, Y. (2000). Theory and practice: Applying the ecological model to formative research for a WIC training program in New York State. *Health Education Research, 15,* 283–291.

Nigg, C. R., Allegrante, J. P., & Ory, M. (2002). Theory-comparison and multiple-behavior research: Common themes advancing health behavior research. *Health Education Research, 17,* 670–679.

Nodora, J. (1995). *Ethnic comparisons of adolescent sexual risk-taking and preventive behavior.* Unpublished doctoral dissertation, University of Texas, Houston.

Norback, D., Torgen, M., & Edling, C. (1990). Volatile organic compounds, respirable dust, and personal factors related to prevalence and incidence of sick building syndrome in primary schools. *British Journal of Industrial Medicine, 47,* 733–741.

Northridge, M. E., & Sclar, E. (2003). A joint urban planning and public health framework: Contributions to health impact assessment. *American Journal of Public Health, 93,* 118–121.

Northridge, M. E., Yankura, J., Kinney, P. L., Santella, R. M., Shepard, P., Riojas, Y., et al. (1999). Diesel exhaust exposure among adolescents in Harlem: A community-driven study. *American Journal of Public Health, 89,* 998–1002.

Norton, B. L., McLeroy, K. R., Burdine, J. N., Felix, M.R.J., & Dorsey, A. M. (2002). Community capacity: Concept, theory and methods. In R. J. DiClemente, R. A. Crosby, & M. C. Kegler (Eds.), *Emerging theories in health promotion practice and research: Strategies for improving public health* (pp. 194–227). San Francisco: Jossey-Bass.

Nutbeam, D. (1998). Health promotion glossary. *Health Promotion International, 13,* 349–364.

Nutbeam, D., & Harris, E. (1995). Creating supportive environments for health—A case study from Australia in developing national goals and targets for healthy environments. *Health Promotion International, 10,* 51–59.

O'Brien, K. (1993). Using focus groups to develop health surveys: An example from research on social relationships and AIDS-preventive behavior. *Health Education Quarterly, 20,* 361–372.

O'Campo, P., Faden, R. R., Brown, H., & Gielen, A. C. (1992). The impact of pregnancy on women's prenatal and postpartum smoking behavior. *American Journal of Preventive Medicine, 8,* 8–13.

Ohkubo, T., Imai, Y., Tsuji, I., Nagai, K., Watanabe, N., Minami, N., et al. (1997). Prediction of mortality by ambulatory blood pressure monitoring versus screening blood pressure measurements: A pilot study in Ohasma. *Journal of Hypertension, 15*(4), 357–364.

O'Keefe, D. J. (1990). *Persuasion.* Thousand Oaks, CA: Sage.

Oldenburg, B., Hardcastle, D. M., & Kok, G. (1997). Diffusion of innovations. In K. Glanz, B. K. Rimer, & F. M. Lewis (Eds.), *Health behavior and health education* (2nd ed., pp. 270–286). San Francisco: Jossey-Bass.

Oldenburg, B., & Parcel, G. S. (2002). Diffusion of innovations. In K. Glanz, F. M. Lewis, & B. K. Rimer (Eds.), *Health behavior and health education: Theory, research, and practice* (3rd ed., pp. 312–334). San Francisco: Jossey Bass.

Oldenburg, B. F., Sallis, J. F., French, M. L., & Owen, N. (1999). Health promotion research and the diffusion and institutionalization of interventions. *Health Education Research, 14,* 121–130.

Oldenburg, B., Sallis, J. F., Harris, D., & Owen, N. (2002). Checklist of Health Promotion Environments at Worksites (CHEW): Development and measurement characteristics. *American Journal of Health Promotion, 16,* 288–299.

O'Malley, A. S., Kerner, J., Johnson, A. E., & Mandelblatt, J. (1999). Acculturation and breast cancer screening among Hispanic women in New York City. *American Journal of Public Health, 89,* 219–227.

O'Malley, M. S., Earp, J. A., & Harris, R. P. (1997). Race and mammography use in two North Carolina counties. *American Journal of Public Health, 87,* 782–786.

Orbell, S., Hodgkins, S., & Sheeran, P. (1997). Implementation intentions and the theory of planned behavior. *Personality and Social Psychology Bulletin, 23,* 945–954.

Orlandi, M. A. (1986). The diffusion and adoption of worksite health promotion innovations: An analysis of barriers. *Preventive Medicine, 15,* 522–536.

Orlandi, M. A. (1987). Promoting health and preventing disease in health care settings: An analysis of barriers. *Preventive Medicine, 16,* 119–130.

Orlandi, M. A., Landers, C., Weston, R., & Haley, N. (1990). Diffusion of health promotion innovations. In K. Glanz, F. M. Lewis, & B. K. Rimer (Eds.), *Health behavior health education—theory, research, and practice* (1st ed., pp. 288–313). San Francisco: Jossey-Bass.

Orum, A. M. (1988). Political sociology. In N. J. Smelser (Ed.), *Handbook of sociology* (pp. 393–423). Thousand Oaks, CA: Sage.

Ory, M. G., Jordan, P. J., & Bazzarre, T. (2002). The Behavior Change Consortium: setting the stage for a new century of health behavior-change research. *Health Education Research, 17,* 500–511.

Osterlind, S. J. (1989). *Test item bias.* Thousand Oaks, CA: Sage.

Otero-Sabogal, R., Stewart, S., Sabogal, F., Brown, B. A., & Perez-Stable, E. (2003). Access and attitudinal factors related to breast and cervical cancer rescreening: Why are Latinas still under screened? *Health Education and Behavior, 30,* 337–359.

Ottoson, J. M., & Green, L. W. (1987). Reconciling concept and context: Theory of implementation. In W. B. Ward & M. H. Becker (Eds.), *Advances in health education and promotion* (pp. 358–382). Greenwich, CT: JAI Press.

Overpeck, M. D., & Moss, J. A. (1991). *Children's exposure to environmental cigarette smoke before and after birth: Advance data from Vital and Health Statistics #202* (Publication No. 91–1250). Hyattsville, MD: Department of Health and Human Services, National Center for Health Statistics.

Ovrebo, B., Ryan, M., Jackson, K., & Hutchinson, K. (1994). The Homeless Prenatal Program: A model for empowering homeless pregnant women. *Health Education Quarterly, 21,* 187–198.

Palmer, R., Fernandez, M. E., Tortolero-Luna, G., Mullen, P., & Gonzales, A. (in press). Correlates of Mammography screening among Hispanic women living in farmworker communities in the Lower Rio Grande Valley. *Health Education and Behavior.*

Palmer, R. C., Mayer, J. A., Eckhardt, L., & Sallis, J. F. (1998). Promoting sunscreen in a community drugstore [Research letter]. *American Journal of Public Health, 88,* 681.

Paluck, E. C., Green, L. W., Frankish, C. J., Fielding, D. W., & Haverkamp, B. (2003). Assessment of communication barriers in community pharmacies. *Evaluation and the Health Professions, 26,* 380–403.

Pamuk, E., Makuc, D., Heck, K., Reuben, C., (1998). *Socioeconomic status and health chartbook.* Hyattsville, MD: National Center for Health Statistics.

Papineau, D., & Kiely, M. C. (1996). Peer evaluation of an organization involved in community economic development. *Canadian Journal of Community Mental Health, 15,* 83–96.

Parcel, G. S. (1995). Diffusion research: The Smart Choices Project. *Health Education Research, 10,* 279–281.

Parcel, G. S., Eriksen, M. P., Lovato, C. Y., Gottlieb, N. H., Brink, S. G., & Green, L. W. (1989). The diffusion of a school-based tobacco-use prevention program: Project description and baseline data. *Journal of Health Education, 4,* 111–124.

Parcel, G. S., & Nader, P. R. (1977). Evaluation of a pilot school health education program for asthmatic children. *Journal of School Health, 47,* 433–456.

Parcel, G. S., Nader, P. R., & Tiernan, K. (1980). A health education program for children with asthma. *Journal of Developmental and Behavioral Pediatrics 1*, 128–132.

Parcel, G. S., O'Hara-Tompkins, N. M., Harrist, R. B., Basen-Engquist, K. M., McCormick, L. K., Gottlieb, N. H., et al. (1995). Diffusion of an effective tobacco prevention program. Part II: Evaluation of the adoption phase. *Health Education Research, 10*, 297–307.

Parcel, G. S., Perry, C. L., & Taylor, W. C. (1990). Beyond demonstration: Diffusion of health promotion interventions. In N. Bracht (Ed.), *Health promotion at the community level.* Thousand Oaks, CA: Sage.

Parcel, G. S., Simons-Morton, B. G., O'Hara, N. M., Baranowski, T., Kolbe, L. J., & Bee, D. E. (1987). School promotion of healthful diet and exercise behavior: An integration of organizational change and social learning theory interventions. *Journal of School Health, 57,* 150–156.

Parcel, G. S., Taylor, W. C., Brink, S. G., Gottlieb, N. H., Engquist, K. E., O'Hara, N. M., et al. (1989). Translating theory into practice: Intervention strategies for the diffusion of a health promotion innovation. *Family and Community Health, 12,* 1–13.

Parikh, N. S., Parker, R. M., Nurss, J. R., Baker, D. W., & Williams, M. V. (1996). Shame and health literacy: The unspoken connection 5. *Patient Education and Counseling, 27,* 33–39.

Parker, E. A., Baldwin, G. T., Israel, B., & Salinas, M. A. (2004). Application of health promotion theories and models for environmental health. *Health Education and Behavior, 31,* 491–509.

Parker, E. A., Schulz, A. J., Israel, B. A., & Hollis, R. (1998). Detroit's east side village health worker partnership: Community-based lay health advisor intervention in an urban area. *Health Education and Behavior, 25,* 24–45.

Parker, L. E., & Lepper, M. R. (1992). Effects of fantasy contexts on children's learning and motivation: Making learning more fun. *Journal of Personality and Social Psychology 62,* 625–633.

Parker, R., & Ehrhardt, A. A. (2001). Through an ethnographic lens: Ethnographic methods, comparative analysis, and HIV/AIDS research. *AIDS and Behavior, 5,* 105–114.

Parker, R. C. (1988). *Looking good in print: A guide to basic design for desktop publishing.* Chapel Hill, NC: Ventana Press.

Parker, R. M., Baker, D. W., Williams, M. V., & Nurss, J. R. (1995). The test of functional health literacy in adults: A new instrument for measuring patients' literacy skills. *Journal of General Internal Medicine, 10,* 537–541.

Partin, M. R., & Slater, J. S. (2003). Promoting repeat mammography use: Insights from a systematic needs assessment. *Health Education Health Behavior, 30,* 97–112.

Pasick, R. J. (1997). Socioeconomic and cultural factors in the development and use of theory. In K. Glanz, F. M. Lewis, & B. K. Rimer (Eds.), *Health behavior and health education: Theory, research, and practice* (2nd ed., pp. 425–440). San Francisco: Jossey-Bass.

Pasick, R. J., D'Onofrio, C. N., & Hiatt, R. A. (1996). Promoting cancer screening in ethnically diverse and underserved communities: The Pathways Project. *Health Education Quarterly, 23S,* 7-16.

Pate, R. R., Saunders, R. P., Ward, D. S., Felton, G., Trost, S. G., & Dowda, M. (2003). Evaluation of a community-based intervention to promote physical activity in youth: Lessons from Active Winners. *American Journal of Health Promotion, 17,* 171–182.

Patterson, G. R. (1986). Performance models for aggressive boys. *American Psychologist, 41,* 432–444.

Patterson, G. R., & Stouthamer-Loeber, M. (1984). The correlation of family management practices and delinquency. *Child Development, 55,* 1299–1307.

Patton, M. Q. (1990). *Qualitative research and evaluation methods* (2nd ed.). Thousand Oaks, CA: Sage.

Patton, M. Q. (1997). *Utilization focused evaluation: The new century text* (3rd ed.). Thousand Oaks, CA: Sage.

Patton, M. Q. (2001). *Qualitative research and evaluation methods* (3rd ed.). Thousand Oaks, CA: Sage.

Paulussen, T., Kok, G., & Schaalma, H. (1994). Antecedents to adoption of classroom-based AIDS education in secondary schools. *Health Education Research, 9,* 485–496.

Paulussen, T., Kok, G., Schaalma, H., & Parcel, G. S. (1995). Diffusion of AIDS curricula among Dutch secondary school teachers. *Health Education Quarterly, 22,* 227–243.

Payne, S. (2004). Designing and conducting qualitative studies. In S. Michie & C. Abraham (Eds.), *Health psychology in practice* (pp. 126–149). Malden, MA: Blackwell.

Pereira, M. A., FitzGerald, S. J., Gregg, E. W., Joswiak, M. L., Ryan, W. J., Suminski, R. R., et al. (1997). A collection of physical activity questionnaires for health-related research. *Medicine and Science in Sports and Exercise, 29,* S1–S205.

Perez-Stable, E. J., Sabogal, F., & Otero-Sabogal, R. (1995). Use of cancer-screening tests in the San Francisco Bay Area: Comparison of Latinos and Anglos *Journal of the National Cancer Institute, 18,* 147–153.

Peroni, D. G., Boner, A. L., Vallone, G., Antolini, I., & Warner, J. O. (1994). Effective allergen avoidance at high altitude reduces allergen-induced bronchial hyperresponsiveness. *American Journal of Respiratory and Critical Care Medicine, 149,* 1442–1446.

Perry, C. L., & Jessor, R. (1985). The concept of health promotion and the prevention of adolescent drug abuse. *Health Education Quarterly, 12,* 169–184.

Perry, C. L., Parcel, G. S., Stone, E., Nader, P., McKinley, S. M., Luepker, R. V., et al. (1992). The Child and Adolescent Trial for Cardiovascular Health (CATCH): Overview of the intervention program and evaluation methods. *Cardiovascular Risk Factors, 2,* 36–44.

Perry, C. L., Sellers, D. E., Johnson, C., Pedersen, S., Bachman, K. J., Parcel, G. S., et al. (1997). The Child and Adolescent Trial for Cardiovascular Health (CATCH): Intervention, implementation, and feasibility for elementary schools in the United States. *Health Education and Behavior, 24,* 716–735.

Perry, C. L., Stone, E. J., Parcel, G. S., Ellison, R. C., Nader, P., Webber, L. S., et al. (1990). School-based cardiovascular health promotion: The Child and Adolescent Trial for Cardiovascular Health (CATCH). *Journal of School Health, 60,* 406–413.

Perry, D. G., Perry, C. L., & Boldizar, J. P. (1990). Learning of aggression. In M. Lewis & S. M. Miller (Eds.), *Handbook of developmental psychopathology: Perspectives in developmental psychology* (pp. 135–146). New York: Plenum.

Petersen, D. J., & Alexander, G. R. (2001). *Needs assessment in public health: A practical guide for students and professionals.* New York: Kluwer Academic/Plenum.

Petticrew, M., & Gilbody, S. (2004). Planning and conducting systematic reviews. In S. Michie & C. Abraham (Eds.), *Health psychology in practice* (pp. 150–179). Malden, MA: Blackwell.

Petty, R. E., Barden, J., & Wheeler, S. C. (2002). The elaboration likelihood model of persuasion: Health promotions that yield sustained behavioral change. In R. J. DiClemente, R. A. Crosby, & M. C. Kegler (Eds.), *Emerging theories in health promotion practice and research* (pp. 71–99). San Francisco: Jossey-Bass.

Petty, R. E., & Cacioppo, J. T. (1986a). *Communication and persuasion: Central and peripheral routes to attitude change.* New York: Springer-Verag.

Petty, R. E., & Cacioppo, J. T. (1986b). The elaboration likelihood model of persuasion. In L. Berkowitz (Ed.), *Advances in experimental social psychology* (pp. 123–205). New York: Academic Press.

Petty, R. E., & Wegener, D. T. (1998). Attitude change: Multiple roles for persuasion variables. In D. T. Gilbert, S. T. Fiske, & G. Lindzey (Eds.), *The handbook of social psychology* (4th ed., pp. 323–390). Boston, MA: McGraw-Hill.

Pierce, J. P., Choi, W. S., & Gilpin, E. A. (1999). Sharing the blame: Smoking experimentation and future smoking-attributable mortality due to Joe Camel and Marlboro advertising and promotions. *Tobacco Control, 8,* 37–44.

Pierce, J. P., Choi, W. S., Gilpin, E. A., Farkas, A. J., & Berry, C. C. (1998). Tobacco industry promotion of cigarettes and adolescent smoking. *JAMA: Journal of the American Medical Association, 279,* 511–515.

Pieterse, M., Kok, G., & Verbeek, J. (1992). Determinants of the acquisition and utilization of automobile child restraint devices: A survey among Dutch parents. *Health Education Research, 7,* 349–358.

Pignone, M., Rich, M., Teutsch, S. M., Berg, A. O., & Lohr, K. N. (2002). Screening for colorectal cancer in adults at average risk: A summary of the evidence for the U.S. Preventive Services Task Force. *Annals of Internal Medicine, 137,* 132–141.

Pirie, P. L., McBride, C. M., Hellerstedt, W., Jeffery, R. W., Hatsukami, D., Allen, S., & Lando, H. (1992). Smoking cessation in women concerned about weight. *American Journal of Public Health, 82*(9), 1238–1243.

Platts-Mills, T. A. (1994). How environment affects patients with allergic disease: Indoor allergens and asthma. *Annals of Allergy, 72,* 381–384.

Platts-Mills, T. A., & Pollart Squillace, S. (1997). Allergen sensitization and perennial asthma. *International Archives of Allergy and lmmunology, 113,* 83–86.

Pollak, K. I., & Mullen, P. D. (1997). An exploration of the effects of partner smoking, type of social support, and stress on postpartum smoking in married women who stopped smoking during pregnancy. *Psychology of Addictive Behaviors, 11*(3), 182–189.

Pollart, S. M., Chapman, M. D., Fiocoo, G. P., Rose, G., & Platts-Mills, T. A. (1989). Epidemiology of acute asthma: IgE antibodies to common inhalant allergens as a risk factor for emergency room visits. *Journal of Allergy and Clinical Immunology, 83,* 875–882.

Pollay, R. W., Siddarth, S., Siegel, M., Haddix, A., Merrit, R. K., Giovino, G. A., et al. (1996). The last straw? Cigarette advertising and realized market shares among youth and adults, 1979–1993. *Journal of Marketing, 60,* 1–16.

Pope, A., Patterson, R., & Burge, H. (Eds.), (with the Committee on the Health Effects of Indoor Allergens, Division of Health Promotion and Disease Prevention, Institute of Medicine). (1993). *Indoor allergens: Assessing and controlling adverse health effects.* Washington, DC: National Academy Press.

Pope, C., & Mays, N. (1995). Reaching the parts other methods cannot reach: An introduction to qualitative methods in health and health services research. *British Medical Journal, 311,* 42–45.

Porras, J. I., & Robertson, P. J. (1987). Organizational development theory: A typology and evaluation. In R. W. Woodman & W. A. Pasmore (Eds.), *Research in organizational change and development.* Greenwich, CT: JAI Press.

Portes, A. (1998). Social capital: Its origins and applications in modern sociology. *Annual Review of Sociology, 24,* 1–24.

Preskill, H. (1994). Evaluation's roles in facilitating organizational learning: A model for practice. *Evaluation and Program Planning, 17,* 291–298.

Prochaska, J. O., & DiClemente, C. C. (1984). *The transtheoretical approach: Crossing traditional boundaries of therapy.* Homewood, IL: Dow Jones-Irwin.

Prochaska, J. O., DiClemente, C. C., & Norcross, J. C. (1997). In search of how people change: Applications to addictive behaviors. In G. A. Marlatt & G. R. VandenBos (Eds.), *Addictive behaviors: Readings on etiology, prevention, and treatment* (pp. 671–696). Washington, DC: American Psychological Association.

Prochaska, J. O., DiClemente, C. C., Velicer, W. F., & Rossi, J. S. (1993). Standardized, individualized, interactive, and personalized self-help programs for smoking cessation. *Health Psychology, 12,* 399–405.

Prochaska, J. O., Redding, C. A., & Evers, K. E. (2002). The Transtheoretical Model and Stages of Change. In K. Glanz, C. E. Lewis, & B. K. Rimer (Eds.), *Health behavior and health education: Theory, research, and practice* (3rd ed., pp. 99–120). San Francisco: Jossey-Bass.

Prochaska, J. O., Velicer, W. F., DiClemente, C. C., & Fava, J. (1988). Measuring processes of change: Applications to the cessation of smoking. *Journal of Consulting and Clinical Psychology, 56,* 520–528.

Prochaska,, J. O., Velicer, W. F., Guadagnoli, E., Rossi, J. S., et al. (1991). Patterns of change: Dynamic typology applied to smoking cessation. *Multivariate Behavioral Research, 26*(1), 83–107.

Prokhorov, A. V., Murray, D. M., & Whitbeck, J. (1993). Three approaches to adolescent smoking detection: A comparison of "expert" assessment, anonymous self-report, and comeasurement. *Addictive Behaviors, 18,* 407–414.

Provan, K. G., Veazie, M. A., Teufel-Shone, N. I., & Huddleston, C. (2004). Network analysis as a tool for assessing and building community capacity for provision of chronic disease services. *Health Promotion Practice, 5,* 174–181.

Pryor, J. B., Reeder, G. D., & Landau, S. (1999). A social-psychological analysis of HIV-related stigma: A two-factor theory. *American Behavioral Scientist, 42,* 1212–1228.

Pulley, L. V., McAlister, A. L., Kay, L. S., & O'Reilly, K. (1996). Prevention campaigns for hard-to-reach populations at risk for HIV infection: Theory and implementation. *Health Education Quarterly, 23,* 488–496.

Putnam, R. D. (1993). The prosperous community: Social capital and public life. *American Prospect, 13,* 35–42.

Putnam, R. D. (1995). Bowling alone: America's declining social capital. *Journal of Democracy, 6,* 65–78.

Putnam, R. D. (2000). *Bowling alone: The collapse and revival of American community.* New York: Simon & Schuster.

Quinn, V. P., Mullen, P. D., & Ershoff, D. H. (1991). Women who stop smoking spontaneously prior to prenatal care and predictors of relapse before delivery. *Addictive Behaviors, 6,* 153–160.

Rafaelcli, S. (1988). Interactivity: From new media to communication. In R. P. Hawkins, J. M. Wiemann, & S. Pingree (Eds.), *Advancing communication science: Merging mass and interpersonal processes.* Thousand Oaks, CA: Sage.

Rakowski, W., & Breslau, E. S. (2004). Perspectives on behavioral and social science research on cancer screening. *Cancer, 101,* 1118–1130.

Rakowski, W., Dube, C. E., Marcus, B. H., Prochaska, J. O., Velicer, W. F., & Abrams, D. B. (1992). Assessing elements of women's decisions about mammography. *Health Psychology, 11,* 111–118.

Rakowski, W., Fulton, J. P., & Feldman, J. P. (1993). Women's decision making about mammography: A replication of the relationship between stages of adoption and decisional balance. *Health Psychology, 12,* 209–214.

Ramelson, H. Z., Friedman, R. H., & Ockene, J. K. (1999). An automated telephone-based smoking cessation education and counseling system. *Patient Education and Counseling, 36,* 131–144.

Ramirez, A. G., McAlister, A., Gallion, K. J., Ramirez, V., Garza, I. R., Stamm, K., et al. (1995). Community-level cancer control in a Texas barrio, Part 1: Theoretical basis, implementation, and process evaluation *Journal of the National Cancer Institute,* pp. 117–122.

Ramirez, A. G., Villarreal, R., McAlister, A., Gallion, K. J., Suarez, L., & Gomez, P. (1999). Advancing the role of participatory communication in the diffusion of cancer screening among Hispanics. *Journal of Health Communication, 4,* 31–36.

Ramirez, R. R., & Cruz, G. P. (2003). *The Hispanic population in the United States* (Report No. P20–545). Washington, DC: U.S. Census Bureau.

Rapoff, M. A. (1999). *Adherence to pediatric medical regimens.* New York: Kluwer Academic/Plenum.

Reddy, P., Meyer-Weitz, A., van den Borne, B., & Kok, G. (2000). Determinants of condom-use behaviour among STD clinic attenders in South Africa. *International Journal of STD & AIDS, 11,* 521–530.

Reineke, R. A. (1991). Stakeholder involvement in evaluation: Suggestions for practice. *Evaluation Practice, 12,* 39–44.

Reis, J. (2001). Consumers' self-care algorithms for the common cold: Implications for health education interventions. *Journal of American College Health, 50,* 27–32.

Reiss, A., Miczek, K., & Roth, J. (1993). *Understanding and preventing violence.* Washington, D.C.: National Academy Press.

Renaud, L., & Paradis, G. (2001). Au coeur de la vie: the Quebec Heart Health Dissemination Project. *Promotion and Education*(Suppl. 1), 22–26.

Rennison, C. M., Rand, M. R., & U.S. Department of Justice (2003). *Criminal victimization, 2002: A National Crime Victimization Survey* (Report No. NCJ 199994). Washington, DC: United States Department of Justice.

Reno, R. (1981). Sex differences in attribution for occupational success. *Journal of Research in Personality, 15*(1), 81–92.

Resnicow, K., Baranowski, T., Ahluwalia, J. S., & Braithwaite, R. L. (1999). Cultural sensitivity in public health: Defined and demystified. *Ethnicity and Disease, 9,* 10–21.

Resnicow, K., Braithwaite, R. L., Dilorio, C., & Glanz, K. (2002). Applying theory to culturally diverse and unique populations. In K. Glanz, F. M. Lewis, & B. K. Rimer (Eds.), *Health behavior and health education: Theory, research, and practice* (3rd ed., pp. 485–509). San Francisco: Jossey-Bass.

Resnicow, K., Dilorio, C., Soet, J. E., Ernst, D., Borrelli, B., & Hecht, J. (2002). Motivational interviewing in health promotion: It sounds like something is changing. *Health Psychology, 21,* 444–451.

Resnicow, K., Vaughan, R., Futterman, R., Weston, R. E., Royce, J., Parms, C., et al. (1997). A self-help smoking cessation program for inner-city African Americans: Results from the Harlem Health Connection Project. *Health Education and Behavior, 24,* 201–217.

Revere, D., & Dunbar, P. J. (2001). Review of computer-generated outpatient health behavior interventions: Clinical encounters "in absentia." *JAMA: Journal of the American Medical Informatics Association, 8,* 62–79.

Rhodes, F., Fishbein, M., & Reis, J. (1997). Using behavioral theory in computer-based health promotion and appraisal. *Health Education and Behavior, 24,* 20–34.

Rhodes, J. E., Contreras, J. M., & Mangelsdorf, S. C. (1994). Natural mentor relationships among Latina adolescent mothers: psychological adjustment, moderating processes, and the role of early parental acceptance. *American Journal of Community Psychology, 22,* 211–227.

Richard, L., Gauvin, L., Potvin, L., Denis, J. L., & Kishchuk, N. (2002). Making youth tobacco control programs more ecological: Organizational and professional profiles. *American Journal of Health Promotion, 16,* 267–279.

Richard, L., Potvin, L., Kishchuk, N., Prlic, H., & Green, L. W. (1996). Assessment of the integration of the ecological approach in health promotion programs. *American Journal of Health Promotion, 10,* 318–328.

Richard, R., Van der Pligt, J., & de Vries, N. (1995). Anticipated affective reactions and prevention of AIDS. *British Journal of Social Psychology, 34,* 9–21.

Richardson, M. A., Mullen, P. D., & DiClemente, C. C. (1993, March). *Smoking during pregnancy: A man's perspective.* Poster presented at the Society of Behavioral Medicine annual meeting, San Francisco, CA.

Richardson, W. S., Wilson, M. C., Nishikawa, J., & Hayward, R. S. (1995). The well-built clinical question: A key to evidence-based decisions. *ACP Journal Club, 123,* A12–A13.

Riekert, K. A., & Drotar, D. (2000). Adherence to medical treatment in pediatric chronic illness: Critical issues and answered questions. In D. Drotar (Ed.), *Promoting adherence to medical treatment in chronic childhood illness* (pp. 3–32). Mahwah, NJ: Erlbaum.

Ries, L.A.G., Eisner, M. P., Kosary, C. L., Hankey, B. F., Miller, B. A., CLegg, L., et al. (2002). SEER cancer statistics review, 1973–1999. Surveillance, epidemiology and end results. Retrieved December 24, 2004, from http://seer.cancer.gov/csr/1973_1999/sections.html

Riley, B. L. (2003). Dissemination of heart health promotion in the Ontario Public Health System: 1989–1999. *Health Education Research, 18,* 15–31.

Riley, B. L., Taylor, S. M., & Elliott, S. J. (2003). Organizational capacity and implementation change: A comparative case study of heart health promotion in Ontario public health agencies. *Health Education Research, 18,* 754–769.

Rimal, R. N., & Flora, J. A. (1997). Interactive technology attributes in health promotion: Practical and theoretical issues. In R. Street, W. Gold, & T. Manning (Eds.), *Health promotion and interactive technology: Theoretical applications and future directions* (pp. 19–38). Mahwah, NJ: Erlbaum.

Rimer, B. K. (2002). Perspectives on intrapersonal theories of health behavior. In K. Glanz, B. K. Rimer, & F. M. Lewis (Eds.), *Health behavior and health education: Theory, research and Practice* (3rd ed., pp. 144–159). San Francisco: Jossey-Bass.

Rimer, B. K., Briss, P. A., Zeller, P. K., Chan, E. C., & Woolf, S. H. (2004). Informed decision making: What is its role in cancer screening? *Cancer, 101,* 1214–1228.

Rimer, B. K., Conaway, M. R., Lyna, P. R., Rakowski, W., Woods-Powell, C. T., Tessaro, I., et al. (1996). Cancer screening practices among women in a community health center population. *American Journal of Preventive Medicine, 12,* 351–357.

Rimer, B. K., Orleans, C. T., Fleisher, L., Cristinzio, S., Resch, N., Telepchak, J., et al. (1994). Does tailoring matter? The impact of a tailored guide on ratings and short-term smoking-related outcomes for older smokers. *Health Education Research, 9,* 69–84.

Ringwalt, C., Ennett, S., Johnson, R., Rohrback, L. A., Simons-Rudolph, A., Vincus, A., et al. (2004). Factors associated with fidelity to substance use prevention curriculum guides in the nation's middle schools. *Health Education and Behavior, 30,* 375–391.

Rios, R. A., McDaniel, J. E., & Stowell, L. P. (1998). Pursuing the possibilities of passion: The affective domain of multicultural education. In M. Dillworth (Ed.), *Being responsive to cultural differences: How teachers learn* (pp. 160–181). Thousand Oaks, CA: Corwin Press.

Roberts-Gray, C., Solomon, T., Gottlieb, N., & Kelsey, E. (1985). Managing the implementation of innovations. *Education and Program Planning, 8,* 261–269.

Roberts-Gray, C., Solomon, T., Gottlieb, N., & Kelsey, E. (1998). Heart Partners: A strategy for promoting effective diffusion of school health promotion programs. *Journal of School Health, 68,* 106–110.

Robertson, A., & Minkler, M. (1994). New health promotion movement: A critical examination [Review]. *Health Education Quarterly, 21,* 295-312.

Roese & Jamieson. (1993). Twenty years of bogus pipeline research: A critical review and meta-analysis. *Psychology Bulletin, 114,* 363–375.

Rogers, E. M. (1983). *Diffusion of innovations.* (3rd ed.). New York: The Free Press.

Rogers, E. M. (1995). *Diffusion of innovations.* (4th ed.). New York: The Free Press.

Rogers, E. M. (2002). Diffusion of preventive innovations. *Addictive Behaviors, 27,* 989–993.

Rogers, E. M. (2003). *Diffusion of innovations.* (5th ed.). New York: The Free Press.

Rogers, E. M., & Antola, L. (1985). Telenovelas in Latin America: A success story. *Journal of Communication, 35,* 24–35.

Rogers, R. (1983). Cognitive and physiological processes in fear-based attitude change: A revised theory of protection motivation. In J. T. Cacioppo & R. E. Petty (Eds.), *Social psychophysiology: A sourcebook* (pp. 153–176). New York: Guilford Press.

Rogers, R. W. (1975). A protection motivation theory of fear appeals and attitude change. *Journal of Psychology, 91,* 93–114.

Ronda, G., Van Assema, P., & Brug, J. (2001). Stages of change, psychological factors and awareness of physical activity levels in The Netherlands. *Health Promotion International, 16,* 305–314.

Rosamond, W. D., Gorton, R. A., Hinn, A. R., Hohenhaus, S. M., & Morris, D. L. (1998). Rapid response to stroke symptoms: The Delay in Accessing Stroke Healthcare (DASH) study. *Academic Emergency Medicine, 5,* 45–51.

Rosen, R. H. (1992). *Healthy company: Eight strategies to develop people, productivity, and profits.* New York: Jeremy P. Tarcher/Putnam.

Rosenstock, I. M., Strecher, V. J., & Becker, M. H. (1988). Social learning theory and the health belief model. *Health Education Quarterly, 15,* 175–183.

Rosenstreich, D. L., Eggleston, P., Kattan, M., Baker, D., Slavin, R G., Gergen, P., et al. (1997). The role of cockroach allergy and exposure to cockroach allergen in causing morbidity among inner-city children with asthma. *New England Journal of Medicine, 336,* 1356–1363.

Rosenthal, R., Rosnow, R. L., & Rubin, D. B. (2000). *Contrasts and effect sizes in behavioral research: A correlational approach.* Cambridge, England: Cambridge University Press.

Rosnow, R. L. (2003). Effect sizes for experimenting psychologists. *Candian Journal of Experimental Psychology, 57,* 221–237.

Rosnow, R. L., & Rosenthal, R. (1996). Computing contrasts, effect sizes and counternulls on other people's published data: General procedures for research consumers. *Psychological Methods, 1,* 331–340.

Ross, M. W., Tikkanen, R., & Mansson, S. A. (2000). Differences between Internet samples and conventional samples of men who have sex with men: Implications for research and HIV interventions. *Social Science and Medicine, 51,* 749–758.

Rossi, P. H., & Freeman, H. E. (1993). *Evaluation: A systematic approach* (5th ed.). Thousand Oaks, CA: Sage.

Rossi, P. H., Freeman, H. E., & Lipsey, M. W. (1999). *Evaluation: A systematic approach* (6th ed.). Thousand Oaks, CA: Sage.

Rossi, P. H., Lipsey, M. W., & Freeman, H. E. (2004). *Evaluation: A systematic approach* (7th ed.). Thousand Oaks, CA: Sage.

Rothman, A. J., Baldwin, A. S., & Hertel, A. W. (2004). Self-regulation and behavior change. In R. F. Baumeister & K. D. Vohs (Eds.), *Handbook of self-regulation: Research, theory and applications* (pp. 130–148). New York: Guilford Press.

Rothman, J. (2004). Three models of community organization practice, their mixing and phasing. In F. M. Cox, J. L. Erlich, J. Rothman, & J. E. Tropman (Eds.), *Strategies of community organization: A book of readings* (3rd ed.). Itasca, IL: F. E. Peacock.

Rothman, K. J. (2002). *Epidemiology: An introduction.* Oxford, England: Oxford University Press.

Rothman, K. J., & Greenland, S. (1998). *Modern epidemiology* (2nd ed.). Philadelphia: Lippincott-Raven.

Rowling, L. (1996). The adaptability of the health promoting schools concept: A case study from Australia. *Health Education Research, 11,* 519–526.

Rudd, R. E. (2002). How to create and assess print materials. Harvard School of Public Health, Health Literacy Series. Retrieved February 14, 2005, from http://www.hsph. harvard.edu/healthliteracy/materials.html

Rudd, R. E., & Comings, J. P. (1994). Learner developed materials: An empowering product. *Health Education Quarterly, 21,* 313–327.

Rudd, R. E., Comings, J. P., & Hyde, J. N. (2003). Leave no one behind: Improving health and risk communication through attention to literacy. *Journal of Health Communication, 8*(Suppl. 1), 104–115.

Rudd, R. E., Moeykens, B. A., & Colton, T. C. (1999). Health and literacy: A review of medical and public health literature. In B. Comings, C. Garners, & C. Smith (Eds.), *Annual review of adult learning and literacy* (pp. 158–199). San Francisco: Jossey-Bass.

Ruhl, R, Chang, C., Halpern, G., & Gershwin, M. E. (1993). The sick building syndrome: II. Assessment and regulation of indoor air quality. *Journal of Asthma, 30,* 297–308.

Ruiter, R. A., Abraham, C., & Kok, G. (2001). Scary warnings and reactional precautions: A review of the psychology of fear appeals. *Psychology and Health, 16,* 613–630.

Rumelhart, D. E. (1980). Schemata: The building blocks of cognition. In R. J. Spiro, B. C. Bruce, & W. F. Brewer (Eds.), *Theoretical issues in reading comprehension: Perspectives from cognitive psychology, linguistics, artificial intelligence and education* (pp. 33–58). Mahwah, NJ: Erlbaum.

Russell, D. (1982). The causal dimension scale: A measure of how individuals perceive causes. *Journal of Personality and Social Psychology, 42*(6), 1137–1145.

Russell, J., Kresnow, M. J., & Brackbill, R. (1994). The effect of adult belt laws and other factors on restraint use for children under age 11. *Accident Analysis and Prevention, 26,* 287–295.

Ryan, G. W., & Bernard, H. R. (2000). Data management and analysis methods. In N. K. Denzin & Y. S. Lincoln (Eds.), *Handbook of qualitative research*. Thousand Oaks, CA: Sage.

Sabatier, P. A. (2003). Policy change over a decade or more. In P. R. Lee, C. L. Estes, & F. M. Rodriguez (Eds.), *The nation's health* (pp. 143–174). Sudbury, MA: Jones and Bartlett.

Sabido, M. (1989, March). *Soap operas in Mexico*. Paper presented at the Entertainment for Social Change Conference, Los Angeles, CA.

Sabogal, F., Otero-Sabogal, R. A., Pasick, R., Jenkins, C., & Perez-Stable, E. (1996). Printed health education materials for diverse communities: Suggestions learned from the field. *Health Education Quarterly, 23*, S123–S141.

Sackett, D. L. (1980). Evaluation of health services. In J. Last (Ed.), *Maxcy-Rosenau public health and preventive medicine*. Norwalk, CT: Appleton-Century-Crofts.

Sackett, D. L., & Snow, J. C. (1979). The magnitude of compliance and noncompliance. In R. B. Haynes, D. W. Taylor, & D. L. Sackett (Eds.), *Compliance in health care* (pp. 11–22). Baltimore, MD: Johns Hopkins University Press.

Saint-Germain, M. A., Bassford, T. L., & Montaño, G. (1993). Surveys and focus groups in health research with older Hispanic women. *Qualitative Health Research, 3*, 341–367.

Salmeron, S., Guerin, J. C., Godard, P., Renon, D., Henry-Amar, M., Duroux, P., et al. (1989). High doses of inhaled corticosteroids in unstable chronic asthma: A multi-center, double-blind, placebo-controlled study. *American Review of Respiratory Disease, 140*, 167–171.

Salovey, P., Rothman, A. J., & Rodin, J. (1998). Health behavior. In D. T. Gilbert, S. T. Fiske, & G. Lindzey (Eds.), *The handbook of social psychology* (4th ed., pp. 633–683). Boston: McGraw-Hill.

Samet, J., Cain, W., & Leaderer, B. (1991). Environmental tobacco smoke. In J. Samet & J. Spengler (Eds.), *Indoor air pollution: A health perspective* (pp. 131–169). Baltimore: Johns Hopkins University Press.

Sampson, E. E., & Marthas, M. (1990). *Group process for the health professions* (3rd ed.). Albany, NY: Delmar Thomson Learning.

Sandelowski, M. (1986). The problem of rigor in qualitative research. *Advances in Nursing Science, 3*, 27–37.

Saraiya, M., Hall, H. I., Thompson, T., Hartman, A., Glanz, K., Rimer, B., et al. (2004). Skin cancer screening among U.S. adults from 1992, 1998, and 2000 National Health Interview Surveys. *Preventive Medicine, 39*, 308–314.

Sarsfield, J. K., Gowland, G., Toy, R, & Normal, A. L. (1974). Mite-sensitive asthma of childhood: Trial of avoidance measures. *Archives of Disease in Childhood, 49*, 716–721.

Sartourius, R. (1991). The logical framework approach to project design and management. *Evaluation Practice, 12*, 139–147.

Saunders, R. B., & Robins, E. (1987). Changes in the marital relationship during the first pregnancy. *Health Care for Women International, 8*, 361–377.

Sawicki, P. T. (1999). A structured teaching and self-management program for patients receiving oral anticoagulation: A randomized controlled trial. *JAMA: Journal of the American Medical Association, 281*, 145–150.

Schaalma, H. P., Kok, G., Bosker, R., Parcel, G., Peters, L., Poelman, & J. Reinders, J. (1996). Planned development and evaluation of AIDS/STD education for secondary school students in the Netherlands: Short-term effects. *Health Education Quarterly, 23*, 469–487.

Schaalma, H. P., Kok, G., Poelman, J., & Reinders, J. (1994). The development of AIDS education for Dutch secondary schools: A systematic approach based on research, theories, and co-operation. In D. R. Rutter & L. Quine (Eds.). *Social psychology and health: European perspectives* (pp. 175–194). Aldershot, UK: Avebury Publishers.

Schaalma, H. P., Abraham, C., Gillmore, M. R., & Kok, G. (2004). Sex education as health promotion: What does it take? *Archives of Sexual Behavior, 33,* 259–269.

Schaalma, H., & Kok, G. (1995). Promoting health through education: The surplus value of a systematic approach. *Odyssey, 1,* 44–51.

Schaalma, H. P., Kok, G., Bosker, R. J., Parcel, G. S., Peters, L., Poelman, J., et al. (1996). Planned development and evaluation of AIDS/STD education for secondary school students in the Netherlands: Short-term effects. *Health Education Quarterly, 23,* 469–487.

Schaalma, H. P., Kok, G., Braeken, D., Schopman, M., & Deven, F. (1991). Sex and AIDS education for adolescents. *Tijdschrift voor Seksuologie* [Journal of Sexology], *15,* 140–149.

Schaalma, H., Kok, G., & Paulussen, T. (1996). HIV behavioural interventions in young people in The Netherlands [Review]. *International Journal of STD and AIDS, 7,* 43–46.

Schaalma, H., Kok, G., & Peters, L. (1993). Determinants of consistent condom use by adolescents: The impact of experience of sexual intercourse. *Health Education Research, 8,* 255–269.

Schaalma, H., Kok, G., Poelman, J., & Reinders, J. (1994). The development of AIDS education for Dutch secondary schools: A systematic approach based on research, theories, and co-operation. In D. R. Rutter & L. Quine (Eds.), *Social psychology and health: European perspectives* (pp. 175–194). Aldershot, England: Avery.

Schaffer, L. C., & Hannafin, M. J. (1986). The effects of progressively enriched interactivity on learning from interactive video. *Educational Communication and Technology Journal, 34,* 89–96.

Schein, E. H. (2004). *Organizational culture and leadership* (3rd ed.). San Francisco: Jossey-Bass.

Scheier, M. F., & Carver, C. S. (2003). Goals and confidence as self-regulatory elements underlying health and illness behavior. In L. D. Cameron & H. Leventhal (Eds.), *The self-regulation of health and illness behavior* (pp. 17–41). New York: Routledge.

Scheirer, M. A. (1981). *Program implementation: The organizational context.* Thousand Oaks, CA: Sage.

Scheirer, M. A. (1990). The life cycle of an innovation: Adoption versus discontinuation of the Fluoride Mouth Rinse Program in schools. *Journal of Health and Social Behavior, 31,* 203–215.

Scheirer, M. A. (1994). Designing and using process evaluation. In J. S. Wholey, H. P. Hatry, & K. E. Newcomer (Eds.), *Handbook of practical program evaluation* (pp. 40–68). San Francisco: Jossey-Bass.

Scheirer, M. A., & Rezmovic, E. L. (1983). Measuring the degree of program implementation: A methodological review. *Evaluation Review, 7,* 599–633.

Scheirer, M. A., Shediac, M. C., & Cassady, C. E. (1995). Measuring the implementation of health promotion programs: The case of the Breast and Cervical Cancer Program in Maryland. *Health Education Research, 10,* 11–25.

Schiffman, C. (1995). Ethnovisual and sociovisual elements of design: Visual dialect as a basis for creativity in public service graphic design. *Journal of Visual Literacy, 14,* 23–39.

Schillinger, D., Bindman, A., Wang, F., Stewart, A., & Piette, J. (2004). Functional health literacy and the quality of physician-patient communication among diabetes patients. *Patient Education and Counseling, 52,* 315–323.

Schillinger, D., Grumbach, K., Piette, J., Wang, F., Osmond, D., Daher, C., et al. (2002). Association of health literacy with diabetes outcomes. *JAMA: Journal of the American Medical Association, 288*, 475–482.

Schmidt, F., & Taylor, T. K. (2002). Putting empirically supported treatments into practice: Lessons learned in a children's mental health center. *Professional Psychology-Research and Practice, 33*, 483–489.

Schooler, C., Feighery, E., & Flora, J. A. (1996). Seventh graders' self-reported exposure to cigarette marketing and its relationship to their smoking behavior. *American Journal of Public Health, 86*(9), 1216–1221.

Schroeder, E. B., Rosamond, W. D., Morris, D. L., Evenson, K. R., & Hinn, A. R. (2000). Determinants of use of emergency medical services in a population with stroke symptoms: The Second Delay in Accessing Stroke Healthcare (DASH II) Study. *Stroke, 31*, 2591–2596.

Schulz, A., & Northridge, M. E. (2004). Social determinants of health: Implications for environmental health promotion. *Health Education and Behavior, 31*, 455–471.

Schulz, A. J., Williams, D. R., Israel, B. A., & Lempert, L. B. (2002). Racial and spatial relations as fundamental determinants of health in Detroit. *The Milbank Quarterly, 80*, 677–707.

Schunk, D. H. (1998). Teaching elementary students to self-regulate practice of mathematical skills with modeling. In D. H. Schunk & B. J. Zimmerman (Eds.), *Self-regulated learning: From teaching to self-reflective practice* (pp. 137–159). New York: Gilford Press.

Schunk, D. H., & Ertmer, P. A. (2000). Self-regulation and academic learning: Self-efficacy enhancing interventions. In M.Boekaerts, P. R. Pintrich, & M. Zeider (Eds.), *Handbook of self-regulation* (pp. 631–650). San Diego: Academic Press.

Schunk, D. H., & Zimmerman, B. J. (1994). *Self-regulation of learning and performance: Issues and educational applications.* Mahwah, NJ: Erlbaum.

Schwartz, R., Smith, C., Speers, M. A., Dusenbury, L. J., Bright, F., Hedlund, S., et al. (1993). Capacity building and resource needs of state health agencies to implement community-based cardiovascular disease programs. *Journal of Public Health Policy, 14*, 480–494.

Schwartz, R., Wasserman, E. A., & Robbins, S. J. (2001). *Psychology of learning and behavior* (5th ed.). New York: Norton.

Schwartz, S. H., & Howard, J. A. (1982). Helping and cooperation: A self-based motivational model. In V. J. Derlaga & J. Grzelak (Eds.), *Cooperation and helping behavior: Theories and research* (pp. 327–353). San Diego, CA: Academic Press.

Scorpiglione, N., el Shazly, M., Abdel-Fattah, M., Belfiglio, M., Cavaliere, D., Carinci, F., et al. (1996). Epidemiology and determinants of blood glucose self-monitoring in clinical practice. *Diabetes Research and Clinical Practice, 34*, 115–125.

Scrimshaw, S.C.M., & Gleason, G. R. (Eds.). (1992). *Rapid assessment procedures: Qualitative methodologies for planning and evaluation of health-related programmes.* Boston: International Nutrition Foundation for Developing Countries.

Scrimshaw, S.C.M., & Hurtado, E. (1987). *Rapid assessment procedures for nutrition and primary health care.* Los Angeles, CA: UCLA Latin American Center Publications.

Scrimshaw, S.C.M., & Hurtado, E. (1992). *Rapid assessment procedures: Qualitative methodology for planning and evaluation of health related programmes.* Boston: International Nutrition Foundation for Developing Countries.

Secker-Walker, R. H., Solomon, L. J., Flynn, B. S., Skelly, J. M., Lepage, S. S., Goodwin, G. D., & Mead, P. B. (1995). Smoking relapse prevention counseling during prenatal and early postnatal care. *American Journal of Preventive Medicine, 11*(2), 86–93. Published erratum appears in *American Journal of Preventive Medicine, 12*(2), 71–72.

Seeman, T. E. (2000). Health promoting effects of friends and family on health outcomes in older adults. *American Journal of Health Promotion, 14*, 362–370.

Senge, P., Kleiner, A., Roberts, C., Ross, R. B., & Smith, B. J. (1994). *The fifth discipline fieldbook: Strategies and tools for building a learning organization.* New York: Doubleday.

Severson, H. H., Andrews, J. A., Lichtenstein, E., Wall, M., & Zoref, L. (1995). Predictors of smoking during and after pregnancy: A survey of mothers of newborns. *Preventive Medicine, 24*(1), 23–28.

Shadish, W. R., Cook, T. D., & Campbell, D. T. (2002). *Experimental and quasi-experimental designs for generalized causal inference.* Boston: Houghton-Mifflin.

Shaffer, R. (1993). *Beyond the dispensary.* Neirobi, Kenya: African Medical and Research Foundation.

Shavelson, R. J., & Stern, P. (1981). Research on teachers' pedagogical thoughts, judgements, decisions, and behavior. *Review of Educational Research, 51*, 455–498.

Shea, J. A., Beers, B. B., McDonald, V. J., Quistberg, D. A., Ravenell, K. L., & Asch, D. A. (2004). Assessing health literacy in African American and Caucasian adults: Disparities in rapid estimate of adult literacy in medicine (REALM) scores. *Family Medicine, 36*, 575–581.

Shediac-Rizkallah, M. C., & Bone, L. R. (1998). Planning for the sustainability of community-based health programs: Conceptual frameworks and future directions for research, practice and policy. *Health Education Research, 13*, 87–108.

Sheeran, P. (2002). Intention-behaviour relations: A conceptual and emperical review. In W. Stroebe & M. Hewstone (Eds.), *European review of social psychology* (Vol. 12, pp. 1–36). Chichester, England: Wiley.

Sheeran, P., Abraham, C., & Orbell, S. (1999). Psychosocial correlates of heterosexual condom use: A meta-analysis. *Psychological Bulletin, 125*, 90–132.

Sheeran, P., & Orbell, S. (2000). Using implementation intentions to increase attendance for cervical cancer screening. *Health Psychology, 19*, 283–289.

Sheeran, P., & Silverman, M. (2003). Evaluation of three interventions to promote workplace health and safety: Evidence for the utility of implementation intentions. *Social Science & Medicine, 56*, 2153–2163.

Shegog, R., Bartholomew, L. K., Gold, R. S., Parcel, G. S., Czyzewski, D. I., Sockrider, M. M., et al. (1999). Demonstration of an effective computer-based pediatric asthma self-management training program [Abstract]. *American Journal of Respiratory and Critical Care Medicine, 159*, A268.

Shegog, R., Bartholomew, L. K., Gold, R. S., Pierrel, E., Parcel, G. S., Sockrider, M. M., et al. (1999). Self-management education for pediatric chronic disease: A description of the Watch, Discover, Think, and Act asthma computer program. Unpublished manuscript.

Shegog, R., Bartholomew, L. K., Parcel, G. S., Sockrider, M. M., Masse, L., & Abramson, S. L. (2001). Impact of a computer-assisted education program on factors related to asthma self-management behavior. *JAMA: Journal of the American Medical Informatics Association, 8*, 49–61.

Shekelle, R. B., Shryock, A. M., Paul, O., Lepper, M., Stamler, J., Liu, S., & Raynor, W. J., Jr. (1981). Diet, serum cholesterol, and death from coronary health disease: The Western Electric study. *New England Journal of Medicine, 304*(2), 65–70.

Sherman, C. B., Tosteson, T. D., Tager, I. B., Speizer, F. E., & Weiss, S. T (1990). Early childhood predictors of asthma. *American Journal of Epidemiology 132,* 83–95.

Sherman, S. J., Cialdini, R. B., Schwartzman, D. F., & Reynolds, K. D. (1985). Imagining can heighten or lower the perceived likelihood of contracting a disease: The mediating effect of ease of imagery. *Personality and Social Psychology Bulletin, 11,* 118–127.

Shiffman, S. (1984). Cognitive antecedents and sequela of smoking relapse crises. *Journal of Applied Social Psychology, 14,* 296–309.

Sidney, S., Jacobs, D. R., Jr., Haskell, W. L., Armstrong, M. A., Dimicco, A., Oberman, A., et al. (1991). Comparison of two methods of assessing physical actvity in the Coronary Artery Risk Development in Young Adults (CARDIA) study. *American Journal of Epidemiology, 133,* 1231–1245.

Siegel, D., DiClemente, R., Durbin, M., Krasnovsky, F., & Saliba, P. (1995). Change in junior high school students' AIDS-related knowledge, misconceptions, attitudes, and HIV-preventive behaviors: Effects of a school-based intervention. *AIDS Education and Prevention, 7,* 534–543.

Siero, S., Boon, M., Kok, G., & Siero, F. (1989). Modification of driving behavior in a large transport organization: A field experiment. *Journal of Applied Psychology, 74,* 417–423.

Simons-Morton, B. G. (2004). The protective effect of parental expectations against early adolescent smoking initiation. *Health Education Research, 19,* 561–569.

Simons-Morton, B. G., Brink, S. G., Simons-Morton, D. G., McIntyre, R., Chapman, M., Longoria, J., et al. (1989). An ecological approach to the prevention of injuries due to drinking and driving. *Health Education Quarterly, 16,* 397–411.

Simons-Morton, B. G., Greene, W. H., & Gottlieb, N. H. (1995). *Introduction to health education and health promotion* (2nd ed.). Prospect Heights, IL: Waveland Press.

Simons-Morton, B. G., Parcel, G. S., & O'Hara, N. M. (1988). Implementing organizational changes to promote healthful diet and physical activity at school. *Health Education Quarterly, 15,* 115–130.

Simons-Morton, D. G., Simons-Morton, B. G., Parcel, G. S., & Bunker, J. F. (1988). Influencing personal and environmental conditions for community health: A multilevel intervention model. *Family and Community Health, 11,* 25–35.

Singer, H. H., & Kegler, M. C. (2004). Assessing interoranizational networks as a dimension of community capacity: Illustrations from a community intervention to prevent lead poisoning. *Health Education and Behavior, 31,* 808–821.

Singer, J. L., & Singer, D. G. (1979). Come back, Mr. Rogers, come back. *Psychology Today, 12,* 56–60.

Singh, G. K., & Yu, S. M. (1996). Trends and differentials in adolescent and young adult mortality in the United States, 1950 through 1993. *American Journal of Public Health, 86,* 560–564.

Singhal, A. (1990). *Entertainment-educational communication strategies for development.* Los Angeles: University of Southern California.

Singhal, A., & Rogers, E. M. (1999). *Entertainment-education: A community strategy for social change.* Mahwah, NJ: Erlbaum.

Skinner, B. F. (1963). Operant behavior. *American Psychologist, 18,* 25–35.

Skinner, C. S., Strecher, V. J., & Hospers, H. (1994). Physicians' recommendations for mammography: Do tailored messages make a difference? *American Journal of Public Health, 84,* 43–49.

Skinner, C. S., Sykes, R. K., Monsees, B. S., Andriole, D. A., Arfken, C. L., & Fisher, E. B. (1988). Learn, Share, and Live: Breast cancer education for older, urban minority women. *Health Education and Behavior, 25,* 60–78.

Slaby, R. G., & Guerra, N. G. (1988). Cognitive mediators of aggression in adolescent offenders: 1. Assessment. *Developmental Psychology, 24,* 580–588.

Slater, M. D. (1995). *Choosing audience segmentation strategies and methods for health communications.* Thousand Oaks, CA: Sage.

Smalley, S. E., Wittler, R. R., & Oliverson, R. H. (2004). Adolescent assessment of cardiovascular heart disease risk factor attitudes and habits. *Journal of Adolescent Health, 35,* 374–379.

Smart, C. R., Hendrick, R. E., Rutledge, J. H., & Smith, R. A. (1995). Benefit of mammography screening in women ages 40 to 49 years: Current evidence from randomized controlled trials. *Cancer, 75*(11), 1619–1626.

Smelser, N. J. (1998). Social structure. In N. J. Smelser (Ed.), *Handbook of sociology* (pp. 103–130). Thousand Oaks, CA: Sage.

Smith, D. W., Steckler, A. B., McCormick, L. K., & McLeroy, K. R. (1995). Lessons learned about disseminating health curricula to schools. *Journal of Health Education, 26,* 37–43.

Smith, R. A., Cokkinides, V., & Eyre, H. J. (2003). American Cancer Society guidelines for the early detection of cancer, 2003. *CA: A Cancer Journal for Clinicians, 53,* 27–43.

Sockrider, M. M., Bartholomew, L. K., Tortolero, S. R., Abramson, S., Jones, J., Tyrrell, S., et al. (2005). Prevalence of possible asthma among inner-city elementary school children: Results of a school-based asthma screening. Unpublished manuscript.

Sockrider, M. M., Craver, J., Pilney, S., et al. (2004). Development of an expert system knowledge base: A novel approach to promote guideline-congruent asthma care. *Journal of Asthma, 41,* 385–402.

Soet, J. E., & Basch, C. E. (1997). The telephone as a communication medium for health education. *Health Education and Behavior, 24,* 759–772.

Sogolow, E., Peersman, G., Semaan, S., Strouse, D., & Lyles, C. M. (2002). The HIV/AIDS Prevention Research Synthesis Project: Scope, methods, and study classification results. *Journal of Acquired Immune Deficiency Syndromes, 30*(Suppl. 1), S15-S29.

Sorensen, G., Fagan, P., Hunt, M. K., Stoddard, A. M., Girod, K., Eisenberg, M., et al. (2004). Changing channels for tobacco control with youth: Developing an intervention for working teens. *Health Education Research, 19,* 250–260.

Soriano, F. I. (1995). *Conducting needs assessments: A multidisciplinary approach.* Thousand Oaks, CA: Sage.

Sormanti, M., Pereira, L., El Basel, N., Witte, S., & Gilbert, L. (2001). The role of community consultants in designing an HIV prevention intervention. *AIDS Education and Prevention, 13,* 311–328.

Snell-Johns, J., Imm, P., Wandersman, A., & Claypoole, J. (2003). Roles assumed by a community coalition when creating environmental and policy-level changes. *Journal of Community Psychology, 31,* 661–670.

Snow, D. A. (2004). Framing processes, ideology, and discursive fields. In D. A. Snow, S. A. Soule, & H. Kriesi (Eds.), *The Blackwell companion to social movements* (pp. 380–412). Oxford, England: Blackwell.

Snow, D. A., Soule, S. A., & Kriesi, H. (2004a). *The Blackwell companion to social movements.* Oxford, England: Blackwell.

Snow, D. A., Soule, S. A., & Kriesi, H. (2004b). Mapping the terrain. In D. A. Snow, S. A. Soule, & H. Kriesi (Eds.), *The Blackwell companion to social movements* (pp. 3–16). Oxford, England: Blackwell.

Stake, R. E. (1995). *The art of case study research.* Thousand Oaks, CA: Sage.

Steadman, L., & Quine, L. (2004). Encouraging young males to perform testicular self-examination: A simple, but effective, implementation intentions intervention. *British Journal of Health Psychology, 9,* 479–487.

Steckler, A., Allegrante, J. P., Altman, D., Brown, R., Burdine, J. N., Goodman, R. M., et al. (1995). Health education intervention strategies: Recommendations for future research. *Health Education Quarterly, 22,* 307–328.

Steckler, A., Goodman, R. M., & Kegler, M. C. (2002). Mobilizing organizations for health enhancement: Theories of organizational change. In K. Glanz, C. E. Lewis, & B. K. Rimer (Eds.), *Health behavior and health education: Theory, research, and practice* (3rd ed., pp. 335–360). San Francisco: Jossey-Bass.

Steckler, A., Goodman, R. M., McLeroy, K. R., Davis, S., & Koch, G. (1992). Measuring the diffusion of innovative health promotion programs. *American Journal of Health Promotion, 6,* 214–224.

Steckler, A., & Linnan, L. (2002). *Process evaluation for public health interventions and research.* San Francisco: Jossey-Bass.

Steckler, A., McLeroy, K. R., Goodman, R. M., Bird, S. T., & McCormick, L. (1992). Toward integrating qualitative and quantitative methods: An introduction. *Health Education Quarterly, 19,* 1–8.

Steenhuis, I. H., Van Assema, P., & Glanz, K. (2001). Strengthening environmental and educational nutrition programmes in worksite cafeterias and supermarkets in The Netherlands. *Health Promotion International, 16,* 21–33.

Steuart, G. W. (1993). Social and behavioral change strategies. *Health Education Quarterly,* S113-S136.

Stevens, V., De Bourdeaudhuij, I, & Van Oost, P. (2001). Anti-bullying interventions at school: Aspects of programme adaptation and critical issues for further programme development. *Health Promotion International, 16,* 155–167.

Stokking, K. M., & Leenders, F. J. (1992). *Heeft de verspreiding van informatie zin?* [Does the spread of information make sense?] Utrecht, The Netherlands: ISOR.

Stockbauer, J. W., & Land, G. H. (1991). Changes in characteristics of women who smoke during pregnancy: Missouri, 1978–1988. *Public Health Reports, 106,* 52–58.

Stokols, D. (1996). Translating social ecological theory into guidelines for community health promotion. *American Journal of Health Promotion, 10,* 282–298.

Stone, E. G., Morton, S. C., Hulscher, M. E., Maglione, M. A., Roth, E. A., Grimshaw, J. M., et al. (2002). Interventions that increase use of adult immunization and cancer screening services: A meta-analysis. *Annals of Internal Medicine, 136,* 641–651.

Stotts, A. L., DiClemente, C. C., Carbonari, J. P., & Mullen (1996). Pregnancy smoking cessation: A case of mistaken identity. *Addictive Behaviors, 21,* 459-471.

Stotts, A. L., DiClemente, C. C., Carbonari, J. P. & Mullen, P. D. (2000). Postpartum return to smoking: Staging a "suspended" behavior. *Health Psychology, 19,* 324–332.

Strategies for reducing exposure to environmental tobacco smoke, increasing tobacco-use cessation, and reducing initiation in communities and health-care systems: A report on recommendations of the Task Force on Community Preventive Services (2005). *Morbidity and Mortality Weekly Report, 49 (No. RR12)*.

Strauss, A., & Corbin, J. (1990). *Basics of qualitative research: Grounded theory procedure and techniques*. Thousand Oaks, CA: Sage.

Strauss, A. L. (1988). *Qualitative analysis for social scientists*. Cambridge, England: Cambridge University Press.

Strecher, V. J. (1999). Computer-tailored smoking cessation materials: Review and discussion. *Patient Education and Counseling, 36*, 107–117.

Strecher, V. J., Bishop, K. R., Bernhardt, J., Thorp, J. M., Cheuvront, B., & Potts, P. (2000). Quit for keeps: Tailored smoking cessation guides for pregnancy and beyond. *Tobacco Control, 9*(Suppl. 3), III78-III79.

Strecher, V. J., DeVellis, B. M., Becker, M. H., & Rosenstock, I. M. (1986). The role of self-efficacy in achieving health behavior change. *Health Education Quarterly, 13*(1), 73–92.

Strecher, V. J., Greenwood, T., Wang, C., & Dumont, D. (1999). Interactive multimedia and risk communication. *Journal of the National Cancer Institute Monographs, XX*, 134–139.

Strecher, V. J., Kreuter, M., Den Boer, D. J., Kobrin, S., Hospers, H. J., & Skinner, C. S. (1994). The effects of computer-tailored smoking cessation messages in family practice settings. *The Journal of Family Practice, 39*, 262–270.

Strecher, V. J., Seijts, G. H., Kok, G. J., Latham, G. P., Glasgow, R., DeVellis, B., et al. (1995). Goal setting as a strategy for health behavior change. *Health Education Quarterly, 22*, 190–200.

Strecher, V., Wang, C., Derry, H., Wildenhaus, K., & Johnson, C. (2002). Tailored interventions for multiple risk behaviors. *Health Education Research, 17*, 619–626.

Street, R. L., Jr., & Rimal, R. N. (1997). Health promotion and interactive technology: A conceptual foundation. In R. Street, W. Gold, & T. Manning (Eds.), *Health promotion and interactive technology: Theoretic applications and future directions* (pp. 1–18). Mahwah, NJ: Erlbaum.

Strong, L. V. (1990). *The how-to book of advertising: Creating it; preparing it; presenting it* (3rd ed.). New York: Fairchild.

Suarez, L., Nichols, D. C., Pulley, L., Brady, C. A., & McAlister, A. (1993). Local health departments implement a theory-based model to increase breast and cervical cancer screening. *Public Health Reports, 108*, 477–482.

Suarez, L., Roche, R. A., Pulley, L. V., Weiss, N. S., Goldman, D., & Simpson, D. M. (1997). Why a peer intervention program for Mexican-American women failed to modify the secular trend in cancer screening. *American Journal of Preventive Medicine, 13*, 411–417.

Suarez-Balcazar, Y. (1992). Problem identification in social intervention research. In F. B. Bryant, J. Edwards, R. C. Tindale, E. Posavac, L. Heath, L. Henderson, & Y. Suarez-Balcazar (Eds.), *Methodological issues in applied social psychology: Volume 2* (pp. 25–42). New York: Plenum.

Sullivan, M., Chao, S. S., Allen, C. A., Kone, A., Pierre-Louise, M., & Krieger, J. (2003). Community-research partnerships: Perspectives from the field. In M. Minkler & N. Wallerstein (Eds.), *Community-based participatory research for health*. San Francisco: Jossey-Bass.

Suls, J. M., Wheeler, L., & Suls, J. (2000). *Handbook of social comparisons: Theory and research*. London: Kluwer Academic.

Suls, J., & Wills, T. A. (1991). *Social comparison: Contemporary theory and research*. Mahwah, NJ: Erlbaum.

Susser, E., Valencia, E., & Torres, J. (1994). Sex, games, and videotapes: An HIV-prevention intervention for men who are homeless and mentally ill. *Psychosocial Rehabilitation Journal, 17*, 31–40.

Sussman, S. (1991). Curriculum development in school-based prevention research. *Health Education Research, 6,* 339–351.

Svenson, G. R., Ostergren, P. O., Merlo, J., & Rastam, L. (2002). Action control and situational risks in the prevention of HIV and STIs: individual, dyadic, and social influences on consistent condom use in a university population. *AIDS Education and Prevention, 14,* 515–531.

Swanson, M., & Thompson, P. (1994). Managing asthma triggers in school. *Pediatric Nursing, 20,* 181–184.

Syme, S. L. (1988). Social epidemiology and the work environment. *International Journal of Health Services, 18,* 635–645.

Tabak, E. R., Simons-Morton, D. G., Green, L. W., Mains, D. A., Eilat-Greenberg, S., Frankowski, R. F., et al. (1991). The definition and yield of inclusion criteria for a meta-analysis of patient education studies in clinical preventive services. *Evaluation and the Health Professions, 14,* 388–411.

Tanner, W. M., & Pollack, R. H. (1988). The effect of condom use and erotic instructions on attitudes toward condoms. *Journal of Sex Research, 25,* 537–541.

Tapert, S. F., Aarons, G. A., Sedlar, G. R., & Brown, S. A. (2001). Adolescent substance use and sexual risk-taking behavior. *Journal of Adolescent Health, 28,* 181–189.

Task Force on Community Preventive Services (2000). Recommendations regarding interventions to improve vaccination coverage in children, adolescents, and adults. *American Journal of Preventive Medicine, 18,* 92–96.

Task Force on Community Preventive Services (2001). Recommendations regarding interventions to reduce tobacco use and exposure to environmental tobacco smoke. *American Journal of Preventive Medicine, 20,* 10–15.

Taylor, S. M., Elliott, S., & Riley, B. (1998). Heart health promotion: Predisposition, capacity and implementation in Ontario Public Health Units, 1994–1996. *Canadian Journal of Public Health, 89,* 410–414.

Taylor, S. M., Elliott, S., Robinson, K., & Taylor, S. (1998). Community-based heart health promotion: Perceptions of facilitators and barriers. *Canadian Journal of Public Health, 89,* 406–409.

Taylor, V., & Van Dyke, N. (2004). "Get up, stand up": Tactical repertoires of social movements. In D. A. Snow, S. A. Soule, & H. Kriesi (Eds.), *The Blackwell companion to social movements* (pp. 263–293). Oxford, England: Blackwell.

Taylor, V. M., Taplin, S. H., Urban, N., White, E., & Peacock, S. (1995). Repeat mammography use among women ages 50–75. *Cancer Epidemiology, Biomarkers and Prevention, 4,* 409–413.

Taylor, W. L. (1953). Cloze procedure: A new tool for measuring readability. *Journalism Quarterly, 30,* 415–433.

Taylor, W. R., & Newacheck, P. W. (1992). Impact of asthma on health. *Pediatrics, 90,* 657–662.

Taylor, W. C., Richardson, M. A., & Mullen, P. D. (1993, March). *Intrinsic and extrinsic motivation: Implications for smoking cessation during pregnancy.* Poster presented at the Society of Behavioral Medicine annual meeting, San Francisco, CA.

Tempkin, K., & Robe, W. (with the Fannie Mae Foundation). (1998). *Social capital and neighborhood stability: An empirical investigation. Housing Policy Debate, 9,* 61–88.

Texas Department of State Health Services. (2003a). *Texas population (estimates) by county, 1998.* Retrieved May 25, 2003, from http://www.tdh.state.tx.us/dpa/popdata/ST1998.htm

Texas Department of State Health Services. (2003b). *Texas population (estimates) by county, 1999.* Retrieved February 8, 2003, from http://www.tdh.stat.tx.us/dpa/popdata/ST1999.htm

Texas Department of State Health Services. (2004). *Worksite wellness index.* Retrieved April 6, 2005, from http://www.tdh.state.tx.us/wellness/agency/default.htm

Texas Department of State Health Services. (2005a). *Cardiovascular health and wellness program.* Retrieved March 4, 2005, from http://www.dshs.state.tx.us/wellness/healthed.shtm

Texas Department of State Health Services. (2005b). *Texas cancer registry.* Retrieved July 7, 2005, from http://www.dshs.state.tx.us/tcr

Texas Diabetes Program/Council & Texas Department of State Health Services. (1998). *Walk Texas!* Retrieved from http://www.tdh.texas.gov/diabetes/walktx/index.html

Themba, M. N., & Minkler, M. (2003). Influencing policy through community-bsed participatory research. In M. Minkler & N. Wallerstein (Eds.), *Community-based participatory research for health* (pp. 349–370). San Francisco: Jossey-Bass.

Third Workshop of National/Regional Health Promoting Hospitals Network Coordinators. (2005). *The Vienna recommendations on health promoting hospitals.* Retrieved July 7, 2005, from http://www.euro.who.int/document/IHB/hphviennarecom.pdf

Thomas, S. B. (2001). The color line: Race matters in the elimination of health disparities. *American Journal of Public Health, 91,* 1046–1048.

Thompson, E. J., & Russell, M. L. (1994). Risk factors for non-use of seatbelts in rural and urban Alberta. *Revue Canadienne de Sante Publique* [Canadian Journal of Public Health], *85,* 304–306.

Thompson, F. E., & Byers, T. (1994). Dietary assessment resource manual. *Journal of Nutrition, 124,* 2245S–2317S.

Thompson, S. G., Pyke, S. D., & Hardy, R. J. (1997). The design and analysis of paired cluster randomized trials: An application of meta-analysis techniques. *Statistics in Medicine, 16,* 2063–2079.

Thompson, S. G., Pyke, S. D., & Wood, D. A. (1996). Using a coronary risk score for screening and intervention in general practice. British Family Heart Study. *Journal of Cardiovascular Risk, 3*(3), 301–306.

Thompson, S. J., Gifford, S. M., & Thorpe, L. (2000). The social and cultural context of risk and prevention: Food and physical activity in an urban Aboriginal community. *Health Education and Behavior, 27,* 725–743.

Thorensen, C. E., & Kirmil-Gray, K. (1983). Self-management psychology and the treatment of childhood asthma. *Journal of Allergy and Clinical Immunology, 72,* 596–610.

Thurmond, V. A. (2001). The point of triangulation. *Journal of Nursing Scholarship: An official publication of Sigma Theta Tau International Honor Society of Nursing / Sigma Theta Tau, 33,* 253–258.

Tilley, B. C., Vernon, S. W., Myers, R., Glanz, K., Lu, M., Hirst, K., et al. (1999). The Next Step Trial: Impact of a worksite colorectal cancer screening promotion program. *Preventive Medicine, 28,* 276–283.

The Tobacco Use and Dependence Clinical Practice Guideline Panel, Staff, and Consortium Representatives. (2000). A clinical practice guideline for treating tobacco use and dependence. *JAMA: Journal of the American Medical Association, 283,* 3244–3254.

Tolan, P. H., & Guerra, N. G. (1994). *What works in reducing adolescent violence: An empirical review of the field.* Boulder, CO: University of Colorado, Institute for Behavioral Sciences, Center for the Study and Prevention of Violence.

Tolan, P. H., & Guerra, N. G. (1996). Progress and prospects in youth violence-prevention evaluation. *American Journal of Preventive Medicine, 12,* 129–131.

Torrence, D. R., & Torrence, J. A. (1987). Training in the face of illiteracy. *Training and Development Journal, 41,* 44–48.

Torrens, P. R., Lynch, B. S., & Bonnie, R. J. (1995). Growing up tobacco free. *JAMA: Journal of the American Medical Association, 273,* 1326.

Torres, R. T., Preskill, H. S., & Piontek, M. E. (1996). *Evaluation strategies for communicating and reporting: Enhancing learning in organizations.* Thousand Oaks, CA: Sage.

Tortolero, S. R., Bartholomew, L. K., Abramson, S. L., Sockrider, M. M., Jones, J., Tyrrell, S., et al. (2005). Prevalence of asthma symptoms in an urban school-age population. Unpublished manuscript.

Tortolero, S. R., Bartholomew, L. K., Tyrrell, S., Abramson, S. L., Sockrider, M. M., Markham, C. M., et al. (2002). Environmental allergens and irritants in schools: A focus on asthma. *Journal of School Health, 72,* 33–38.

Tortolero, S. R., Markham, C. M., Parcel, G. S., Peters, R. J., Escobar-Chaves, S. L., & Lewis, H. (2005) Using intervention mapping to adapt an effective HIV, STD, and pregnancy prevention program for high-risk minority youth. *Health Promotion Practice, 6,* 286–298.

Toseland, R. W., & Rivas, R. F. (2005). *An introduction to group work practice* (5th ed.). New York: MacMillan.

Trapini, F., & Walmsley, S. A. (1981). Five readability estimates: Differential effects of simplifying a document. *Journal of Reading, 24,* 398–403.

Treuth, M. S., Sherwood, N. E., Baranowski, T., Butte, N. F., Jacobs, D. R., Jr., McClanahan, B., et al. (2004). Physical activity self-report and accelerometry measures from the Girls Health Enrichment Multi-Site Studies. *Preventive Medicine, 38*(Suppl. 1), S43-S49.

Triandis, H. C. (1994). *Culture and social behavior.* New York: McGraw Hill.

Trice, H. M., Beyer, J. M., & Hunt, R. E. (1978). Evaluating implementation of a job-based alcoholism policy. *Journal of Studies on Alcohol, 39*(3), 448–465.

Tripp, M. K., Carvajal, S. C., McCormick, L. K., Mueller, N. H., Hu, S. H., Parcel, G. S., et al. (2003). Validity and reliability of the parental sun protection scales. *Health Education Research, 18,* 58–73.

Tripp, M. K., Herrmann, N. B., Parcel, G. S., Chamberlain, R. M., & Gritz, E. R. (2000). Sun protection is fun! A skin cancer prevention program for preschools. *Journal of School Health, 70,* 395–401.

Trochim, W. M., Cook, J. A., & Setze, R. J. (1994). Using concept mapping to develop a conceptual framework of staff's views of a supported employment program for individuals with severe mental illness. *Journal of Consulting and Clinical Psychology, 62,* 766–775.

Trochim, W. M., Milstein, B., Wood, B. J., Jackson, S., & Pressler, V. (2004). Setting objectives for community and systems change: An application of concept mapping for planning a statewide health improvement initiative. *Health Promotion Practice, 5,* 8–19.

Trochim, W.M.K. (1989). An introduction to concept mapping for planning and evaluation. *Evaluation and Program Planning, 12,* 1–16.

Tross, S. (2001). Women at heterosexual risk for HIV in inner-city New York: Reaching the hard to reach. *AIDS and Behavior, 5,* 131–139.

Truman, B. I., Smith-Akin, C. K., Hinman, A. R., Gebbie, K. M., Brownson, R., Novick, L. F., et al. (2000). Developing the Guide to Community Preventive Services: Overview and rationale. *American Journal of Preventive Medicine, 18,* 18–26.

Trusty, J., Thompson, B., & Petrocelli, J. V. (2004). Practical guide for reporting effect size in quantitative research in the Journal of Counseling and Development. *Journal of Counseling and Development, 82,* 107–110.

Tryon, W. W. (1985). *Activity measurement in psychology and medicine.* New York: Plenum Press.

Tufte, E. R. (1983). *The visual display of quantitative information.* Cheshire, CT: Graphics Press.

Tsoukasas, T., & Glantz, S. A. (2003). The Duluth Clean Indoor Air Ordinance: Problems and success in fighting the tobacco industry at the local level in the 21st Century. *American Journal of Public Health. 93,* 1214–1221.

Tufte, E. R. (1990). *Envisioning information.* Cheshire, CT: Graphics Press.

Tufte, E. R. (1997). *Visual explanations: Images and quantities, evidence and narrative.* Cheshire, CT: Graphics Press.

Tulving, E., & Thomson, D. M. (1973). Encoding specificity and retrieval processes in episodic memory. *Psychological Review, 80,* 359–380.

Turbin, M. S., Jessor, R., & Costa, F. M. (2000). Adolescent cigarette smoking: Health-related behavior or normative transgression? *Prevention Science, 1,* 115–124.

Turner, J. C. (1991). *Social influence.* Milton Keynes, England: Open University Press.

Turner, J. C. (2005). Explaining the nature of power: A three-process theory. *European Journal of Social Psychology, 35,* 1–22.

Turner, L., Mermelstein, R., & Flay, B. (2004). Individual and contextual influences on adolescent smoking. *Annals of the New York Academy of Sciences, 1021,* 175–197.

Tversky, A., & Kahneman, D. (1983). Extensional versus intuitive reasoning: The conjunction fallacy in probability judgment. *Psychological Review, 90,* 293–315.

Tyler, D. O., Taylor-Seehafer, M. A., & Murphy-Smith, M. (2004). Utilizing "PPIP Texas style!" in a medically underserved population. *Journal of Public Health Management Practice, 10,* 100–108.

Tyrrell, S. (2000). Program to improve the asthma-related environment of urban elementary schools: An application to the Intervention Mapping framework. Master's thesis, University of Texas Health Science Center at Houston, School of Public Health.

Uchino, B. N., Cacioppo, J. T., & Kiecolt-Glaser, J. K. (1996). The relationship between social support and physiological processes: A review with emphasis on underlying mechanisms and implications for health. *Psychological Bulletin, 119*(3), 488–531.

Uchino, B. N., Holt-Lunstad, J., Uno, D., Betancourt, R., & Garvey, T. S. (1999). Social support and age-related differences in cardiovascular function: An examination of potential mediators. *Annals of Behavioral Medicine, 21,* 135–142.

Unger, J. B., & Chen, X. (1999). The role of social networks and media receptivity in predicting age of smoking initiation: A proportional hazards model of risk and protective factors. *Addictive Behaviors, 24,* 371–381.

U.S. Census Bureau & Bernstein, R. (2004). Hispanic and Asian Americans increasing faster than overall population. Retrieved from http://www.census.gov/Press-Release/www/releases/archives/race/oo1839.html

U.S. Department of Health and Human Services. (1991). *Healthy People 2000: National health promotion and disease prevention objectives* (Full report with commentary; DHHS Publication No. PHS 91-502212). Washington, DC: Author.

U.S. Department of Health and Human Services. (1994). Preventing tobacco use among young people: A report of the Surgeon General. Washington, DC: Government Printing Office.

U.S. Department of Health and Human Services. (1998). *Healthy People 2010 objectives: Draft for public comment.* Washington, DC: Author.

U.S. Department of Health and Human Services. (2000). *Reducing tobacco use: A report of the Surgeon General.* Atlanta, GA: Author.

U.S. Department of Health and Human Services. (2005). *Healthy People 2010.* Retrieved from http://www.healthypeople.gov/

U.S. Department of Health and Human Services, Agency for Healthcare Research and Quality. (2000). *Clincal practice guidelines: Treating tobacco and dependence.* Washington, DC: Author.

U.S. Department of Health and Human Services, Centers for Disease Control, National Center for Health Statistics. (1998). *Health, United States 1998 with socioeconomic status and health chartbook.* Retrieved from http://www.cdc.gov/nchs/data/hus/hus98.pdf

U.S. Department of Health and Human Services, Health Resourses Services Administration (HRSA), Bureau of Primary Health Care. (2005). *U.S. Mexico border health.* Retrieved from http://bphc.hrsa.gov/bphc/borderhealth/default.htm

U.S. Department of Health and Human Services, National Cancer Institute. (1984). *Methods, examples and resources for improving health messages and materials.* Bethesda, MD: Author.

U.S. Department of Health and Human Services, National Institute on Alcohol Abuse and Alcoholism (NIAAA); J. P. Allen & M. Columbus (Eds.). (1995). *Assessing alcohol problems: A guide for clinicians and researchers.* Bethesda, MD: Author.

U.S. Department of Health and Human Services, National Institute on Drug Abuse (NIDA); L. Harrison & A. Hughes (Eds.). (1995). *The validity of self-reported drug use: Improving the accuracy of survey estimates.* Rockville, MD: Author.

U.S. Department of Health and Human Services, Office of Cancer Communications, National Cancer Institute. (2002). *Making health communication programs work: A planner's guide* (2nd ed.). Bethesda, MD: Author.

U.S. Department of Health and Human Services, Public Health Service: Office on Smoking and Health, (1980). *The health consequences of smoking for women: A report of the Surgeon General.* Rockville, MD: Author.

U.S. Department of Health and Human Services, Public Health Service: Office on Smoking and Health. (1984a). *The health consequences of smoking: Cardiovascular disease. A report of the Surgeon General.* Rockville, MD: Author.

U.S. Department of Health and Human Services, Public Health Service: Office on Smoking and Health. (1984b). *The health consequences of smoking: Chronic obstructive lung disease. A report of the Surgeon General.* Rockville, MD: Author.

U.S. Department of Health and Human Services, Public Health Service: Office on Smoking and Health. (1985). *The health consequences of smoking: Cancer and chronic lung disease in the workplace. A report of the Surgeon General.* Rockville, MD: Author.

U.S. Environmental Protection Agency (EPA). (1995). *Indoor air quality tools for schools: Action kit* (Publication No. 402-K-95–001). Cleveland, OH: National Service Center for Environmental Publications.

U.S. Environmental Protection Agency (EPA), Indoor Air Division. (1991). *Building air quality: A guide for building owners and facility managers.* Washington, DC: U.S. Government Printing Office.

U.S. Preventive Services Task Force. (2004). *Guide to clinical preventive services: Periodic updates.* (3rd ed.). Rockville, MD: Agency for Healthcare Research and Quality.

United Way of America. (1996). Measuring program outcomes: A practical approach. 1–170. Accessed November 2004 at http://national.unitedway.org/outcomes/resources/What/ndpaper.cfm

University of Texas Health Science Center. (1996). *Interventions to improve asthma management and prevention at school* (First Technical Progress Report, Contract No. NOl-HR-56079). Houston, TX: Author.

Urban, N., Anderson, G. L., & Peacock, S. (1994). Mammography screening: How important is cost as a barrier to use? *American Journal of Public Health, 84,* 50–55.

Uutela, A., Absetz, P., Nissinen, A., Valve, R., Talja, M., & Fogelholm, M. (2004). Health psychological theory in promoting population health in Paijat-Hame, Finland: First steps toward a type 2 diabetes prevention study. *Journal of Health Psychology, 9,* 73–84.

Vacha-Hasse, T., & Thompson, B. (2004). How to estimate and interpret various effect sizes. *Journal of Counseling Psychology, 51,* 473–481.

Van Assema, P., Martens, M., Ruiter, R. A., & Brug, J. (2001). Framing of nutrition education messages in persuading consumers of the advantages of a healthy diet. *Journal of Human Nutrition and Dietetics, 14,* 435–442.

van Bokhoven, M. A., Kok, G., & van der Weijden, T. (2003). Designing a quality improvement intervention: A systematic approach. *Quality and Safety in Health Care, 12,* 215–220.

van den Bree, M. B., Whitmer, M. D., & Pickworth, W. B. (2004). Predictors of smoking development in a population-based sample of adolescents: A prospective study. *Journal of Adolescent Health, 35,* 172–181.

Van der Pligt, J. (1994). Risk appraisal and health behavior. In D. R. Rutter & L. Quine (Eds.), *Social psychology and health: European perspectives* (pp. 131–152). Aldershot, England: Avebury.

Van der Pligt, J., Otten, W., Richard R., & Van der Velde, F. (1993). Perceived risk of AIDS: Unrealistic optimism and self-protective action. In B. J. Pryor & G. D. Reeder (Eds.), *The social psychology of HIV infection* (pp. 39–58). Mahwah, NJ: Erlbaum.

van Empelen, P., & Kok, G. (2005). Social cognitive prerequisites of preparatory actions in the context of condom use among young people. Unpublished manuscript.

van Empelen, P., & Kok, G. (in press). On planning, preparation and willingness to take risks in the context of safe sex. *Psychology & Health.*

van Empelen, P., Kok, G., Schaalma, H. P., & Bartholomew, L. K. (2003). An AIDS risk reduction program for Dutch drug users: An Intervention Mapping approach to planning. *Health Promotion Practice, 4,* 402–412.

van Empelen, P., Kok, G., van Kesteren, N. M., van den Borne, Bos, A. E., & Schaalma, H. P. (2003). Effective methods to change sex risk among drug users: A review of psychosocial interventions. *Social Science and Medicine, 57,* 1593–1608.

van Empelen, P., Schaalma, H. P., Kok, G., & Jansen, M. W. (2001). Predicting condom use with casual and steady sex partners among drug users. *Health Education Research, 16,* 293–305.

van Kesteren, N., Hospers, H., & Kok, G. (2005). HIV and sex: Using Intervention Mapping to develop an HIV preventive intervention for HIV positive MSM. Unpublished manuscript.

van Kesteren, N.M.C., Kospers, H. J., Kok, G., & van Empelen, P. (2005). Sex and sexual risk behavior in HIV positive men who have sex with men. *Qualitative Health Research, 15,* 145–168.

Vandelanotte, C., de Bourdeaubhuij, B., I, & Brug, J. (2004). Acceptability and feasibility of an interactive computer-tailored fat intake intervention in Belgium. *Health Promotion International, 19,* 463–470.

Veen, P. (1985). *Sociale psychologie toegepast: van probleem naar oplossing* [Applying social psychology: From problem to solution]. Alphen aan den Rijn: Samson.

Veenstra, G. (2002). Social capital and health (plus wealth, income inequality and regional health governance). *Social Science and Medicine, 54,* 849–868.

Velicer, W. F., DiClemente, C. C., Prochaska, J. O., & Brandenburg, N. (1985). Decisional balance measure for assessing and predicting smoking status. *Journal of Personality and Social Psychology, 48,* 1279–1289.

Velicer, W. F., & Prochaska, J. O. (1999). An expert system intervention for smoking cessation. *Patient Education and Counseling, 36,* 119–129.

Velicer, W. F., Prochaska, J. O., Bellis, J. M., DiClemente, C. C., Rossi, J. S., Fava, J. L., et al. (1993). An expert system intervention for smoking cessation. *Addictive Behaviors, 18,* 269–290.

Vernon, S. W. (2004). Tailored interactive intervention to increase CRC screening. Retrieved from http://crisp.cit.nih.gov/crisp/crisp_query.generate_screen

Verplanken, B., & Aarts, H. (1999). Habit, attitude, and planned behavior: Is habit an empty construct or an interesting case of goal-directed automaticity? In W. Stroebe & M. Hewstone (Eds.), *European review of social psychology: Volume 10* (pp. 101–134). Chichester, England: Wiley.

Villar-Cordova, C., Morgenstern, L. B., Barnholtz, J. S., Frankowski, R. F., & Grotta, J. C. (1998). Neurologists' attitudes regarding rt-PA for acute ischemic stroke. *Neurology, 50,* 1491–1494.

Vinicor, F., Burton, B., Foster, B., & Eastman, R. (2000). Healthy People 2010: Diabetes. *Diabetes Care, 23,* 853–855.

Virginia Department of Health, Division of HIV/AIDS, Regional Consortia. (2005). *Virginia HIV prevention evaluation system: follow-up referral form.* Retrieved July 7, 2005, from http://www.vdh.state.va.us/std/follow%20up%20referral.pdf

Vogels, T., & van der Vliet, R. (1990). *Jeugd en sex* [Youth and sex]. The Hague, Netherlands: SDU.

Wall, M. A., Severson, H. H., Andrews, J. A., Lichtenstein, E., & Zoref, L. (1995). Pediatric office-based smoking intervention: impact on maternal smoking and relapse. *Pediatrics, 96*(4 Pt 1), 622–628.

Wallace, H. M., McQueen, J. C., Biehl, R., & Blackman, J. A. (2005). *Mosby's resource guide to children with disabilities and chronic illness.* St. Louis, MO: C. V. Mosby.

Wallace, L. S., & Lennon, E. S. (2004). American Academy of Family Physicians patient education materials: Can patients read them? *Family Medicine, 36,* 571–574.

Wallack, L., Dorfman, L., Jernigan, D., & Themba, M. (1993). *Media advocacy and public health: Power for prevention.* Thousand Oaks, CA: Sage.

Wallerstein, N. (1992). Powerlessness, empowerment, and health: Implications for health promotion programs. *American Journal of Health Promotion, 6,* 197–205.

Wallerstein, N. B., & Sanchez-Merki, V. (1994). Freirian praxis in health education: Research results from an adolescent prevention program. *Health Education Research, 9,* 105–118.

Wallerstein, N. B., Sanchez-Merki, V., & Dow, L. (1997). Freirian praxis in health education and community organizing: A case study of an adolescent prevention program. In M. Minkler (Ed.), *Community organizing and community building for health* (pp. 195–215). New Brunswick, NJ: Rutgers University Press.

Walsh, J. M., & Terdiman, J. P. (2003). Colorectal cancer screening: Scientific review. *JAMA: Journal of the American Medical Association, 289,* 1288–1296.

Walter, H. J., & Vaughan, R. D. (1993). AIDS risk reduction among a multiethnic sample of urban high school students. *JAMA: Journal of the American Medical Association, 11,* 725–730.

Walter, R. S., & Kuo, A. R. (1993). Taxicabs and child restraint. *American Journal of Diseases of Children, 147,* 561–564.

Walters, J. L., Canady, R., & Stein, T. (1994). Evaluating multicultural approaches in HIV/ AIDS educational material. *AIDS Education and Prevention, 6,* 446–453.

Wang, C., & Burris, M. A. (1994). Empowerment through photo novella: Portraits of participation. *Health Education Quarterly, 21,* 171–186.

Wang, C. C. (2003). Using photovoice as a participatory assessment and issue select tool. In M. Minkler & N. Wallerstein (Eds.), *Community-based participatory research for health* (pp. 179–196). San Francisco: Jossey-Bass.

Wang, C. C., Cash, J. L., & Powers, L. S. (2000). Who knows the streets as well as the homeless? Promoting personal and community action through photovoice. *Health Promotion Practice, 1,* ??-81.

Wang, C. C., Yi, W. K., Tao, Z. W., & Carovano, K. (1998). Photovoice as a participatory health promotion strategy. *Health Promotion International, 13,* 75–86.

Warneke, C. L., Davis, M., De Moor, C., & Baranowski, T. (2001). A 7-item versus 31-item food frequency questionnaire for measuring fruit, juice, and vegetable intake among a predominantly African-American population. *Journal of the American Dietetic Association, 101,* 774–779.

Wasilewski, Y., Clark, N. M., Evans, D., Levison, M. J., Levin, B., & Mellins, R. B. (1996). Factors associated with emergency department visits by children with asthma: Implications for health education. *American Journal of Public Health, 86,* 1410–1415.

Webber, G. C. (1990). Patient education. A review of the issues. *Medical Care, 28,* 1089–1103.

Weber, M. (1947). *The theory of social and economic organization: Vol. 1.* New York: Oxford University Press.

Webster, D. W., Wilson, M. E., Duggan, A. K., & Pakula, L. C. (1992). Parents' beliefs about preventing gun injuries to children. *Pediatrics, 89,* 908–914.

Weick, K. E., & Quinn, R. E. (19999). Organizational change and development. *Annual Review of Psychology, 50,* 36–86.

Weiner, B. (1985). An attributional theory of achievement motivation and emotion. *Psychological Review, 92,* 548–573.

Weiner, B. (1986). *An attributional theory of motivation and emotion.* New York: Springer-Verlag.

Weiner, B., Perry, R. P., & Magnusson, J. (1988). An attributional analysis of reactions to stigmas. *Journal of Personality and Social Psychology, 55,* 738–748.

Weinstein, N. D. (1988). The precaution-adoption process. *Health Psychology, 7,* 355–386.

Weinstein, N. D. (1989). Effects of personal experience on self-protective behavior. *Psychological Bulletin, 105,* 31–50.

Weinstein, N. D., & Sandman, P. M. (2002). The Precaution Adoption Process Model. In K. Glanz, F. M. Lewis, & B. K. Rimer (Eds.), *Health behavior and health education: Theory, research, and practice* (3rd ed., pp. 121–143). San Francisco: Jossey-Bass.

Weiss, B. D., & Coyne, C. (1997). Communicating with patients who cannot read. *New England Journal of Medicine, 337,* 272–274.

Weiss, C. H. (1997). How can theory-based evaluation make greater headway? *Evaluation Review, 21,* 501–524.

Weiss, K. B., Gergen, P. J., & Hodgson, T. (1992). An economic evaluation of asthma in the United States. *New England Journal of Medicine, 326,* 862–866.

Weiss, K. B., Gergen, Y. J., & Wagener, D. K. (1993). Breathing better or wheezing worse? The changing epidemiology of asthma morbidity and mortality. *Annual Review of Public Health, 14,* 491–531.

Weitzman, E. R., & Kawachi, I. (2000). Giving means receiving: The protective effect of social capital on binge drinking on college campuses. *American Journal of Public Health, 90,* 1936–1939.

Weitzman, M., Gortmaker, S., & Sobol, A. (1990). Racial, social, and environmental risks for childhood asthma. *American Journal of Diseases of Children, 144,* 1189–1194.

Welk, T. A. (1999). Clinical and ethical considerations of fluid and electrolyte management in the terminally ill client. *Journal of Intravenous Nursing, 22,* 43–47.

Wells, W., Burnett, J., & Moriarty, S. (1998). *Advertising principles and practice* (4th ed.). Upper Saddle River, NJ: Prentice Hall.

Wen, S. W., Goldenberg, R. L., Cutter, G. R., & Hoffman, H. J. (1989). Intrauterine growth retardation and preterm delivery: Risk factors in an indigent population. *American Journal of Obstetrics and Gynecology, 162,* 213–218.

Wenzel, L., Glanz, K., & Lerman, C. (2002). Stress, coping and health behavior. In K. Glanz, F. M. Lewis, & B. K. Rimer (Eds.), *Health behavior and health education: Theory, research, and practice* (3rd ed., pp. 121–143). San Francisco: Jossey-Bass.

Werner, O., & Campbell, D. T. (1973). Translation, working through interpreters and the problem of decentering. In R. Naroll & R. Cohen (Eds.), *A handbook of method in cultural anthropology* (pp. 398–422). New York: Columbia University Press.

Westen, D. (1997). *Psychology: Mind, brain, and culture.* New York: Wiley.

Wester, P., Radberg, J., Lundgren, B., & Peltonen, M. (1999). Factors associated with delayed admission to hospital and in-hospital delays in acute stroke and TIA: A prospective, multicenter study. Seek-Medical-Attention-in-Time Study Group. *Stroke, 30,* 40–48.

White, J. V. (1988). *Graphic design for the electronic age: The manual for traditional and desktop publishing.* New York: Watson-Guptill.

Whitehead, D. (2004). The European Health Promoting Hospitals Project: How far on? *Health Promotion International, 19,* 259–267.

Wholey, J. S. (1994). Assessing the feasibility and likely usefulness of evaluation. In J. S. Wholey, H. P. Hatry, & K. E. Newcomer (Eds.), *Handbook of practical program evaluation* (pp. 15–39). San Francisco: Jossey-Bass.

Wholey, J. S., Hatry, H. P., & Newcomer, K. E. (1994). *Handbook of practical program evaluation.* San Francisco, Jossey-Bass.

Wigal, J. K., Stout, C., Brandon, M., Winder, J. A., McConnaughy, K., Creer, T. L., et al. (1993). The knowledge, attitude, and self-efficacy asthma questionnaire. *Chest, 104,* 1144–1148.

Wight, D., Raab, G. M., Henderson, M., Abraham, C., Buston, K., Hart, G., et al. (2002). Limits of teacher-delivered sex education: Interim behavioural outcomes from randomised trial. *British Medical Journal, 324,* 1430.

Wilcher, R. A., Gilbert, L. K., Siano, C. S., & Arredondo, E. M. (1999). From focus groups to workshops: Developing a culturally appropriate cervical cancer prevention intervention for rural Latinas. *International Quarterly of Community Health Education, 19,* 83–102.

Williams, D. M., Counselman, F. L., & Caggiano, C. D. (1996). Emergency department discharge instructions and patient literacy: A problem of disparity. *American Journal of Emergency Medicine, 14,* 19–22.

Williams, D. R., & Jackson, J. S. (2000). Race/ethnicity and the 2000 census: Recommendations for African American and other black populations in the United States. *American Journal of Public Health, 90,* 1728–1730.

Williams, L. S., Bruno, A., Rouch, D., Marriott, D. J., & Mas, D. J. (1997). Stroke patients' knowledge of stroke: Influence on time to presentation. *Stroke, 28,* 912–915.

Williams, M. V., Baker, D. W., Honig, E. G., Lee, T. M., & Nowlan, A. (1998). Inadequate literacy is a barrier to asthma knowledge and self-care. *Chest, 114,* 1008–1015.

Williams, M. V., Baker, D. W., Parker, R. M., & Nurss, J. R. (1998). Relationship of functional health literacy to patients' knowledge of their chronic disease. A study of patients with hypertension and diabetes. *Archives of Internal Medicine, 158,* 166–172.

Williams, M. V., Davis, T., Parker, R. M., & Weiss, B. D. (2002). The role of health literacy in patient-physician communication. *Family Medicine, 34,* 383–389.

Williams, P. L., Innis, S. M., Vogel, A. M., & Stephen, L. J. (1999). Factors influencing infant feeding practices of mothers in Vancouver. *Canadian Journal of Public Health, 90,* 114–119.

Williams, R. (1994). *The non-designer's design book: Design and typographic principles for the visual novice.* Berkeley, CA: Peachpit Press.

Williams, R. M., Jr. (1970). *American society: A sociological interpretation.* New York: Knopf.

Williams, W. (2004). The cultural contexts of collective action: Constraints, opportunities, and the symbolic life of social movements. In D. A. Snow, S. A. Soule, & H. Kriesi (Eds.), *The Blackwell companion to social movements* (pp. 91–115). Oxford, England: Blackwell.

Williamson, J. W. (1978). The estimation of achievable health care benefit. In *Assessing and improving health care outcomes* (pp. 51–69). Cambridge, MA: Ballinger Publishers.

Wilson-Pessano, S. R., Scamagas, P., Arsham, G. M., Chardon, L., Coss, S., German, D. F., et al. (1987). An evaluation of approaches to asthma self-management education for adults: The AIR Kaiser-Permanente study. *Health Education Quarterly, 14,* 333–343.

Windham, G. C., Swan, S. H., & Fenter, L. (1992). Parental smoking and the risk of spontaneous abortion. *American Journal of Epidemiology, 35*(12), 1394–1403.

Windsor, R., Baranowski, T., Clark, N., & Cutter, G. (1994). *Evaluation of health promotion, health education and disease prevention programs* (2nd ed.). Mountain View, CA: Mayfield.

Windsor, R., Clark, N., Boyd, N. R., & Goodman, R. M. (2004). *Evaluation of health promotion, health education and disease prevention programs* (3rd ed.). New York: McGraw-Hill.

Wingood, G. M., Hunter-Gamble, D., & DiClemente, R. J. (1993). A pilot study of sexual communication and negotiation among young African American women: Implications for HIV prevention. *Journal of Black Psychology, 19,* 190–203.

Winkleby, M. A., Robinson, T. N., Sundquist, J., & Kraemer, H. C. (1999). Ethnic variation in cardiovascular disease risk factors among children and young adults: Findings from the Third National Health and Nutrition Examination Survey, 1988–1994. *JAMA: Journal of the American Medical Association, 281,* 1006–1013.

Wissow, S., Gittelsohn, A. M., Szklo, M., Starfield, B., & Mussman, M. (1988). Poverty, race, and hospitalization for childhood asthma. *American Journal of Public Health, 78,* 777–782.

Witkin, R. B., & Altschuld, J. W. (1995). *Planning and conducting needs assessments: A practical guide.* Thousand Oaks, CA: Sage.

Witte, K. (1995). Fishing for success: Using the persuasive health message framework to generate effective campaign messages. In E. Maibach & R. L. Parrott (Eds.), *Designing health messages: Approaches from communication theory and public health practice* (pp. 145–166). Thousand Oaks, CA: Sage.

Witte, K., & Allen, M. (2000). A meta-analysis of fear appeals: Implications for effective public health campaigns. *Health Education and Behavior, 27,* 615.

Witte, K., Meyer, G., & Martell, D. (2001). *Effective health risk messages: A step-by-step guide.* Thousand Oaks, CA: Sage.

Witte, K., & Morrison, K. (1995). Intercultural and cross-cultural health communication: Understanding people and motivating healthy behaviors. In R. L. Wiseman (Ed.), *Intercultural communication theory.* Thousand Oaks, CA: Sage.

W. K. Kellogg Foundation. (1998). *W. K. Kellogg Foundation evaluation handbook.* Battle Creek, MI: Author.

Wohlfeiler, D. (1997). Community organizing and community building among gay and bisexual men: The STOP AIDS Project. In M. Minkler (Ed.), *Community organizing and community building for health* (pp. 230–243). New Brunswick, NJ: Rutgers University Press.

Wolcott, H. F. (1994). *Transforming qualitative data: Description, analysis, and interpretation.* Thousand Oaks, CA: Sage.

Wolff, T. (2001). Community coalition building—contemporary practice and research: Introduction. *American Journal of Community Psychology, 29,* 165–172.

Wood, P. R., Hidalgo, H. A., Prihoda, T. J., & Kromer, M. E. (1993). Hispanic children with asthma: Morbidity. *Pediatrics, 91,* 62–69.

Woodby, L. L., Windsor, R. A., Snyder, S. W., Kohler, C. L., & Diclemente, C. C. (1999). Predictors of smoking cessation during pregnancy. *Addiction, 94*(2), 283–292.

World Health Organization (1978, September). *Primary health care.* Report of the International Conference on Primary Health Care, Alma-Ata, USSR. Geneva, Switzerland: Author.

World Health Organization (1986). Ottawa charter for health promotion. *Health Promotion International, 1,* iii-iv. Retrieved from http://www.euro.who.int/aboutwho/policy/20010827_2

World Health Organization. (1997). *Vienna recommendations on health promoting hospitals.* Retrieved from http://www.euro.who.int/document/IHB/hphviennarecom.pdf

World Health Organization. (2002a). *Community participation in local health and sustainable development: Approaches and techniques.* (EUR/ICP/POLC 060305D ed.). Retrieved February 23, 2005, from http://www.euro.who.int/document/e78653.pdf

World Health Organization. (2002b). *World report on violence and health.* Geneva, Switzerland: Author.

Wraight, J. M., Cowan, J. O., Flannery, E. M., Town, G. I., & Taylor, D. R. (2002). Adherence to asthma self-management plans with inhaled corticosteroid and oral prednisone: A descriptive analysis. *Respirology, 7,* 133–139.

Yabroff, K. R., & Mandelblatt, J. S. (1999). Interventions targeted toward patients to increase mammography use. *Cancer Epidemiology, Biomarkers and Prevention, 8,* 749–757.

Yabroff, K. R., O'Malley, A., Mangan, P., & Mandelblatt, J. (2001). Inreach and outreach interventions to improve mammography use. *JAMA: Journal of the American Medical Women's Association, 56,* 166–73, 188.

Yates, B. T. (1996). *Analyzing costs, procedures, processes, and outcomes in human services.* Thousand Oaks, CA: Sage.

Yawn, B. P., Wollan, P., Kurland, M., & Scanlon, P. (2002). A longitudinal study of the prevalence of asthma in a community population of school-age children. *The Journal of Pediatrics, 140,* 576–581.

Yin, R. (1994). *Case study research: Design and methods* (2nd ed.). Thousand Oaks, CA: Sage.

Yin, R. (2002). *Case study research: Design and methods* (3rd ed.). Thousand Oaks, CA: Sage.

Yin, R. K. (1979). *Changing urban bureaucracies: How new practices become routinized.* Lexington, MA: D.C. Heath.

Yoo, S., Wood, N. E., Lampa, M. L., Mbondo, M., Shado, R. E., & Goodman, R. (2004). Collaborative community empowerment: An illustration of a six-step process. *Health Promotion Practice, 5,* 256–265.

Yoshikawa, H. (1994). Prevention as cumulative protection: Effects of early family support and education on chronic delinquency and its risks. *Psychological Bulletin, 115,* 28–54.

Young, D. R., Gittelsohn, J., Charleston, J., Felix-Aaron, K., & Appel, L. J. (2001). Motivations for exercise and weight loss among African-American women: Focus group results and their contribution towards program development. *Ethnicity and Health, 6,* 227–245.

Zajonc, R. B. (1980). Feeling and thinking: Preferences need no inferences. *American Psychologist, 35,* 151–175.

Zaltman, G., & Duncan, R. (1977). *Strategies for planned change.* New York: Wiley.

Zaza, S., Briss, P. A., & Harris, K. W. (2005). *The guide to community preventive services: What works to promote health?* New York: Oxford University Press.

Zaza, S., Lawrence, R. S., Mahan, C. S., Fullilove, M., Fleming, D., Isham, G. J., et al. (2000). Scope and organization of the Guide to Community Preventive Services. *American Journal of Preventive Medicine, 18,* 27–34.

Zhu, S. H., Stretch, V., Balabanis, M., Rosbrook, B., Sadler, G., & Pierce, J. P. (1996). Telephone counseling for smoking cessation: Effects of single-session and multiple-session interventions. *Journal of Consulting Clinical Psychology, 64,* 202–211.

Zimbardo, P. G., & Leippe, M. R. (1991). *The psychology of attitude change and social influence.* Philadelphia: McGraw-Hill.

Zimmerman, B. (2000). Attaining self-regulation: A social cognitive perspective. In M. Boekaerts, M. Pintrich, & M. Zeider (Eds.), *Handbook of self-regulation* (pp. 13–39). San Diego, CA: Academic Press.

Zimmerman, B. J., Bonner, S., Evans, D., & Mellins, R. B. (1999). Self-regulating childhood asthma: A developmental model of family change. *Health Education and Behavior, 26,* 55–71.

Zimmerman, M. A. (1990). Taking aim on empowerment research: On the distinction between individual and psychological conception. *American Journal of Community Psychology, 18,* 169–177.

Zimmerman, M. A. (1995). Psychological empowerment: Issues and illustrations. *American Journal of Community Psychology, 23,* 581–599.

NAME INDEX

A

Aarons, G. A., 45
Aarts, H., 109
Abbema, E. A., 304
Abbey, H., 551
Abbott, R. D., 485
Abel, E., 257
Abraham, C., 76, 90, 98, 101, 107, 111, 270, 275, 349, 527
Abrams, D., 527
Abramson, S. L., 30, 31, 549
Adams, C. D., 222
Adams, H. P., 243
Adams, J., 111
Adams, R. J., 222
Aday, L. A., 225, 498
Adler, N. E., 152
Affonso, D. D., 581, 582
Agars, J., 257
Aggarwal, M., 262
Ahluwalia, J. S., 237, 299, 369–370
Airhihenbuwa, C. O., 426
Ajzen, I., 35, 46, 47, 68, 69, 97, 100, 101, 338, 460, 513, 516, 538, 616
Akinbami, L. J., 217

Albers, G. W., 243, 249
Alberts, M. J., 246–247
Albuqureque, 262
Alcoe, S. Y., 256
Alderson, P., 41, 49, 60–61
Alewijnse, D, 257
Alexander, M., 498
Alinsky, S. D., 173
Allegrante, J. P., 118–119, 202
Allen, 285
Allen, A. J., 28
Allen, C. A., 28, 200
Allen, D. B., 67
Allen, J., 114, 157, 158
Allen, J. D., 616
Allen, M., 76
Allen, R., 157
Allensworth, D., 140
Altman, D. G., 175, 176–177, 178, 385
Altschuld, J. W., 195, 207, 215, 224, 225, 228, 231, 238
Altschuler, A., 152
Ammerman, A. S., 115, 292, 448
Anderson, C., 484
Anderson, E. E., 15
Anderson, G. L., 616

Anderson, J. R., 94
Anderson, P. S., 263
Andreasen, A. R., 384
Andrews, J. A., 580, 585
Andrews, J. S., 208
Antola, L., 627
Antolini, I., 550
Appel, L. J., 230
Argys, L. M., 46
Arita, I., 454
Arizmendi, T. G., 581, 582
Armitage, C. J., 107
Arredondo, E. M., 613
Ary, D., 47
Ashton, D., 46
Auslander, W., 201
Austin, S. B., 220
Averch, H. A., 272
Averett, S. L., 46
Awofeso, N., 139, 263
Axton, R. A., 257
Azzimondi, G., 247

B

Backbier, E., 100, 103, 111
Baddeley, A. D., 96

SUBJECT INDEX

A

A Su Salud, 384

Abstracts, 60. *See also* Behavioral journalism

Access to Air Pollution Data, 227

ACT UP, 175

Action control, methods to promote, 335, 336

Action planning, 155–156

Action research model, 155

Action stage of change, 110, 113; processes in, 113; in Project PANDA, 597

Active learning: modeling combined with, 347; parameters for use of, 334, 335, 347; theories related to, 334, 335

Active processing of information, 337, 528

ActKnowledge, 25

Adaptation, of existing program to new population, 300–303

Adherence, 257–258

Adolescent Social Action Program, 166, 167

Adopters: early, 132–133, 134; identification of, 446–447, 576–577, 638. *See also* Implementers; Linkage system; Program users; Service providers

Adoption, Implementation, and Sustainability Planning (Step 5), 443–471; in Cultivando la Salud, 609, 638–643; determinants for, 457–461; in Dutch school HIV-prevention program, 537–540; evaluation planning in, 467, 471; identification of users in, 446–447; importance of, 443–446; linkage system reevaluation in, 447–450; matrices in, 21, 461–465, 640–641; methods and strategies for, 465–467, 468–470, 642; overview of, 20–21; in Partners in School Asthma Program, 576–577; performance objectives for, 451–457; perspectives in, 444–446; in Project PANDA, 603; scope and sequence plan for, 467, 470; in

Stroke Project example, 471; tasks in, 16, 21. *See also* Adoption planning; Implementation planning; Sustainability

Adoption-of-innovation theories: for individual behavior, 78, 131–135; for organizations, 158–160. *See also* Diffusion of Innovations Theory (DIT)

Adoption planning: adoption determinants and, 457–459; importance of, 23–24, 443–446; methods and strategies for, 465–467, 468–470; performance objectives for, 451–452, 454–455; pretesting for, 430. *See also* Adoption, Implementation, and Sustainability Planning (Step 5)

Advance organizers: parameters for use of, 335; theory related to, 94, 335

Advocacy: concepts of, 175–179; counteradvocacy and, 177–178; design documents for, 406–408; guidelines for, 178;